HANDBOOK OF

Signs & Symptoms

Second Edition

HANDBOOK OF

Signs & Symptoms

Second Edition

Lippincott Williams & Wilkins
A **Wolters Kluwer** Company
Philadelphia • Baltimore • New York • London
Buenos Aires • Hong Kong • Sydney • Tokyo

STAFF

Publisher
Judith A. Schilling McCann, RN, MSN

Editorial Director
H. Nancy Holmes

Clinical Director
Joan M. Robinson, RN, MSN, CCRN

Senior Art Director
Arlene Putterman

Clinical Project Manager
Beverly Ann Tscheschlog, RN, BS

Editors
Jennifer P. Kowalak (senior associate editor), Audrey S. Hughes

Copy Editors
Peggy Williams (supervisor), Kimberly Bilotta, Dolores P. Matthews, Celia McCoy, Dorothy P. Terry, Pamela Wingrod

Designers
Lesley Weissman-Cook (book designer and design project manager), Donna S. Morris, Jeffrey Sklarow

Associate Editor (electronic)
Liz Schaeffer

Electronic Production Services
Diane Paluba (manager), Joyce Rossi Biletz

Manufacturing
Patricia K. Dorshaw (senior manager), Beth Janae Orr

Editorial Assistants
Danielle J. Barsky, Beverly Lane, Linda Ruhf

Indexer
Ellen S. Brennan

Cover
Risa Clow, Larry Didona/Didona Designs

The clinical treatments described and recommended in this publication are based on research and consultation with nursing, medical, and legal authorities. To the best of our knowledge, these procedures reflect currently accepted practice. Nevertheless, they can't be considered absolute and universal recommendations. For individual applications, all recommendations must be considered in light of the patient's clinical condition and, before administration of new or infrequently used drugs, in light of the latest package-insert information. The authors and the publisher disclaim any responsibility for any adverse effects resulting from the suggested procedures, from any undetected errors, or from the reader's misunderstanding of the text.

Printed in the United States of America.
HBSS2 – D N O S A J J M A M
04 03 02 10 9 8 7 6 5 4 3 2 1

Library of Congress Cataloging-in-Publication Data

Handbook of signs & symptoms.— 2nd ed. / editors, Jennifer P. Kowalak (senior associate editor), Audrey S. Hughes.
p. ; cm.
Includes bibliographical references and index.
1. Symptoms — Handbooks, manuals, etc.
[DNLM: 1. Signs and Symptoms — Handbooks. WB 39 H23633 2002]
I. Title: Handbook of signs and symptoms. II. Title: Signs & symptoms. III. Kowalak, Jennifer P. IV. Hughes, Audrey S. V. Lippincott Williams & Wilkins.
RC69 .H246 2002
616′.047 — dc21
ISBN 1-58255-159-6 (alk. paper) 2001054907

CONTENTS

CONTRIBUTORS AND CONSULTANTS

Cheryl L. Brady, RN, MSN
Nursing Instructor
Kent State University
Liverpool, Ohio

Janice T. Chussil, RN,C, MSN, ANP, DNC
Nurse Practitioner
Dermatology Associates, P.C.
Portland, Ore.

Diane Dixon, PA-C, MA, MMSC
Assistant Professor, Department of Physician Assistant Studies
University of South Alabama
Mobile

Lisa L. Dutton, PT, MS
Assistant Dean for Health Professions and Associate Professor of Physical Therapy
University of Findlay (Ohio)

Michael R. France, PA-C
Liver Disease Fellow; Research Coordinator
Digestive Diseases Center at South Texas
San Antonio

Nancy Hutton Haynes, RN, MN, CCRN
Assistant Professor
St. Luke's College
Kansas City, Mo.

Connie S. Heflin, RN, MSN
Professor of Nursing
Paducah (Ky.) Community College

Erin Jaynes, RN, MSN
Administrative Nurse Specialist
Medical College of Ohio
Toledo

Nancy L. Kranzley, RN, MS
Pulmonary Clinical Nurse Specialist
The Christ Hospital
Cincinnati

Pamela S. Messer, RN, MSN
Drug Safety Surveillance, Product Manager
AstraZeneca (USA Division)
Wilmington, Del.

E. Ann Myers, MD
Endocrine Consultant
San Francisco

Glenn H. Nordehn, DO
Assistant Professor
University of Minnesota Duluth School of Medicine

Wendy J. Smith, RN, MSN, ACNP, AOCN
Nurse Practitioner
North Mississippi Hematology and Oncology Associates, Ltd.
Tupelo

Kathleen M. Speer, RN, PhD, CPNP
Pediatric Nurse Practitioner
Children's Medical Center of Dallas

We extend special thanks to the following people, who contributed to the previous edition.

Sherry L. Altschuler, PhD

Charold L. Baer, RN, PhD, FCCM, CCRN

Laura P. Barnes, RN, MSN, CNAA

Roxanne Aubol Batterden, RN, MS, CCRN

Jack M. Becker, MD

John M. Bertoni, MD, PhD

Heather Boyd-Monk, RN, SRN, BSN

Barbara Gross Braverman, RN, MSN, CS

Sally A. Brozenec, RN, MS, PhD

Laura J. Burke, RN, MSN, PhD

Dorothea Caldwell-Brown, RN, NP, BSN, MPH, JD

Paul L. Carmichael, MD, MSc(Med), FAAO, FACS, FICS

Robert B. Cooper, MD

Jerome M. Cotler, MD, FAAOS, FACS

Mary Helen Davis, MD

Nancy B. Davis, RN, MSN, NP, CNOR, CRNFA

Gloria Donnelly, RN, PhD, FAAN

Brian Doyle, MD

Stephen C. Duck, MD

Kenneth H. Einhorn, MD

Mary Jo Sagaties Farmer, RN,C, MS, PhD

Susan Gauthier, RN, MSN, PhD

Jalal K. Ghali, MD

Roslyn M. Gleeson, RN,C, MSN, CS, APN, CRNP

Kelly J. Henrickson, MD

Barbara S. Henzel, RN, BSN, CGRN

Denise A. Hess, RN

Marcia J. Hill, RN, MSN

Esther Holzbauer, RN,C, BS, MSN

Sheila Scannell Jenkins, RN, MSN

Lee Ann Kelly, RN, MS, PNP

Robert L. Klaus, MD, FACS

Karen A. Landis, RN, MS, CRNP, CCRN

Gizell Rosetti Larson, MD

Herbert A. Luscombe, MD

Neil MacIntyre, MD

Steven Margulis, MD, FACP

Margaret E. Miller, RN, MSN

Chris Platt Moldovanyi, RN, MSN

Mary Lou Moore, RN,C, PhD, FAAN, FACCE

Roger M. Morrell, MD, PhD, FACP

Frances W. Quinless, RN, PhD

Patricia L. Radzewicz, RN, BSN

Amy Perrin Ross, RN, MSN, CNRN

Grannum R. Sant, MD

Kristine A. Scordo, RN, MS, PhD

Ellen Shapiro, MD

Harrison J. Shull, Jr., MD

Eric Silfen, MD, MSHA

Carol E. Smith, RN, PhD

June Stark, RN, BSN, MEd

Frances J. Storlie, RN, PhD, CANP

Richard W. Tureck, MD

Dharmapuri Vidyasagar, MD, MSc, FCCM

Naomi Walpert, RN, MS, CDE

Maryann Banko Wee, RN, BSN

John K. Wiley, MD, FACES

Sandi Wind, RN, ET

Janette R. Yanko, RN, MN, CNRN

Joseph A. Zeccardi, MD, FACEP

FOREWORD

Assuring quality patient care while containing costs is essential in today's pressured health care environment. Both goals rely on the quality and accuracy of the initial patient evaluation and ongoing assessments during patient care. Accurate evaluation of each patient's signs and symptoms means better choice of diagnostic studies to further evaluate findings and arrive at an accurate diagnosis, saving unnecessary test costs. Accurate diagnosis of signs and symptoms also helps the health care provider prescribe the most appropriate treatment. And monitoring signs and symptoms for changes during the course of care helps the provider alter treatment as appropriate for each patient.

Thus, a thorough knowledge of clinical signs and symptoms is paramount to the course and outcome of disease management. Such knowledge can enable the clinician to make effective use of reduced time for patient encounters while avoiding diagnostic and therapeutic errors. Quickly recognizing telltale indicators, knowing what signs and symptoms to look for next, and understanding their clinical significance can help ensure appropriate — even life-saving — patient care in a succinct timeframe.

Handbook of Signs and Symptoms, Second Edition, is an invaluable resource in this critical endeavor. This comprehensive resource on more than 525 signs and symptoms has been completely reviewed and expanded. Signs and symptoms are arranged alphabetically to increase efficiency for the time-pressured clinician. The discussion of a sign or symptom guides the clinician's history taking and physical examination, describes the sign or symptom's most probable causes, and relates each cause to its typical associated findings. This new edition includes diseases that are currently high in the public's awareness, such as the West Nile virus and increasingly alarming drug-resistant infections.

An attention-grabbing icon makes signs and symptoms of life-threatening disorders stand out and details emergency interventions for a rapid response.

New to this edition is latest information on herbal and other alternative medicines that can cause specific signs and symptoms — important knowledge now that more and more patients are using alternative and complementary remedies. An *Herb alert* icon makes these unexpected causes readily visible on the page. Also included are other nonclinical causes, such as specific drugs, diagnostic tests, surgeries, and clinical procedures.

Hundreds of helpful illustrations and tables clarify the appearance of certain signs, show how to correctly use examination equipment, and make it easy to compare findings and differentiate among possible causes. Another standout icon, *Examination tip,* shows how to elicit certain signs. In addition, the format and style of the book make it a practical reference for the busy clinician. It's small enough to carry to the clinic, and its valuable pointers alert the clinician to important information, such as tips on differences in a sign or symptom's presentation or significance in pediatric and geriatric populations.

The *Handbook of Signs and Symptoms* in its second edition remains the authoritative handbook for eliciting and recognizing patient signs and symptoms and for interpreting them in the context of today's evidence-based medicine.

Michael H. Crawford, MD
Professor of Medicine
Mayo Medical School
Consultant in Cardiovascular Diseases
Mayo Clinic Scottsdale (Ariz.)

A

Abdominal distention

Abdominal distention refers to increased abdominal girth; it occurs when increased intra-abdominal pressure forces the abdominal wall outward. Distention may be mild or severe, depending on the amount of pressure. It may be localized or diffuse and may occur gradually or suddenly. Acute abdominal distention may signal life-threatening peritonitis or acute bowel obstruction.

Causes of abdominal distention include fat, fluid, flatus, or a fetus (intrauterine or ectopic pregnancy). Fluid and gas are normally present in the GI tract, but not in the peritoneal cavity; however, if they can't pass freely through the GI tract, abdominal distention occurs. Distention originating in the peritoneal cavity may reflect acute bleeding, accumulation of ascitic fluid, or air from perforation of an abdominal organ.

Abdominal distention doesn't always signal pathology. For example, in anxious patients or those with digestive distress, localized distention in the left upper quadrant can result from aerophagia — the unconscious swallowing of air. Generalized distention can result from ingestion of fruits or vegetables with large quantities of unabsorbable carbohydrates, such as legumes, or from abnormal food fermentation by microbes. Don't forget to rule out pregnancy in all females with abdominal distention.

Emergency interventions

When a patient displays abdominal distention, quickly check for signs of hypovolemia, such as pallor, diaphoresis, hypotension, rapid thready pulse, rapid shallow breathing, decreased urine output, poor capillary refill, and altered mentation. Ask the patient if he's experiencing severe abdominal pain or difficulty breathing. Find out about any recent accidents, and observe the patient for signs of trauma and peritoneal bleeding, such as Cullen's sign (a bluish tinge around the umbilicus) or Turner's sign (ecchymosis of the abdomen or flank area). Then auscultate all abdominal quadrants, noting rapid and high-pitched, diminished, or absent bowel sounds. (If you don't hear bowel sounds immediately, listen for at least 5 minutes.) *Gently* palpate the abdomen for rigidity. Remember that deep or extensive palpation may increase pain.

If you detect abdominal distention and rigidity along with abnormal bowel sounds in a patient who complains of pain, begin emergency interventions. Place the patient in the supine position, administer oxygen, and insert an I.V. line for fluid replacement. Prepare to insert a nasogastric tube to relieve acute intraluminal distention. Reassure the patient and prepare him for surgery.

Abdominal distention: Common causes and associated findings

CAUSES	MAJOR ASSOCIATED SIGNS AND SYMPTOMS							
	Abdominal mass	Abdominal pain	Abdominal rigidity	Anorexia	Bowel sounds, absent	Bowel sounds, hyperactive	Constipation	Diarrhea
Abdominal trauma		◆	◆		◆			
Cirrhosis		◆		◆			◆	◆
Heart failure								
Irritable bowel syndrome		◆					◆	◆
Large-bowel obstruction		◆				◆	◆	
Nephrotic syndrome				◆				
Ovarian cysts	◆	◆						
Paralytic ileus		◆			◆		◆	
Peritonitis		◆	◆		◆			
Small-bowel obstruction		◆				◆	◆	

History and physical examination

If the patient's abdominal distention isn't acute, ask about its onset and duration and associated signs. A patient with localized distention may report a sensation of pressure, fullness, or tenderness in the affected area. A patient with generalized distention may report a bloated feeling, a pounding heart, and difficulty breathing deeply, especially when lying flat.

The patient may also feel unable to bend at his waist. Be sure to ask about abdominal pain, fever, nausea, vomiting, anorexia, altered bowel habits, and weight gain or loss. (See *Abdominal distention: Common causes and associated findings*.)

Obtain a medical history, noting GI or biliary disorders that may cause peritonitis or ascites, such as cirrhosis, hepatitis, or inflammatory bowel disease. (See *Detecting ascites*, page 4.) Also, ask about chronic constipation. Has the patient recently had abdominal surgery? Ask about recent accidents, even ones like falling off a stepladder.

Perform a complete physical examination. Don't restrict the examination to the abdomen or you could miss important clues to the cause of abdominal

	Edema	Fever	Hepatomegaly	Hypotension	Jaundice	Jugular vein distention	Nausea	Oliguria	Rebound tenderness	Tachycardia	Vomiting	Weight change
				◆							◆	
	◆	◆	◆		◆		◆				◆	◆
	◆		◆			◆	◆			◆	◆	
							◆					
											◆	
	◆							◆				
											◆	
		◆		◆			◆		◆	◆	◆	
							◆		◆		◆	

symptoms. Next, stand at the foot of the bed and observe the recumbent patient for abdominal asymmetry to determine if distention is localized or generalized. Also observe for any visible peristalsis, which may indicate obstruction. Then assess abdominal contour by stooping at his side. Inspect for tense, glistening skin and bulging flanks, which may indicate ascites. Note the umbilicus. Eversion suggests ascites or umbilical hernia; inversion may reflect distention from gas, but it's also common in obesity. Inspect the abdomen for signs of inguinal or femoral hernia and for incisions, which may suggest adhesions. Both may lead to intestinal obstruction.

Then auscultate for bowel sounds, abdominal friction rubs (indicating peritoneal inflammation), and bruits (indicating an aneurysm). Listen for succussion splash—a splashing sound normally heard in the stomach when the patient moves or when palpation disturbs the viscera. However, an abnormally loud splash indicates fluid accumulation, suggesting gastric dilation or obstruction.

Next, percuss and palpate the abdomen to determine if distention results from air, fluid, or both. A tympanic note

EXAMINATION TIP

Detecting ascites

To differentiate ascites from other causes of distention, check for shifting dullness, fluid wave, and puddle sign.

SHIFTING DULLNESS
With the patient supine, percuss from the umbilicus outward to the flank, as shown. Draw a line on the patient's skin to mark the change from tympany to dullness.

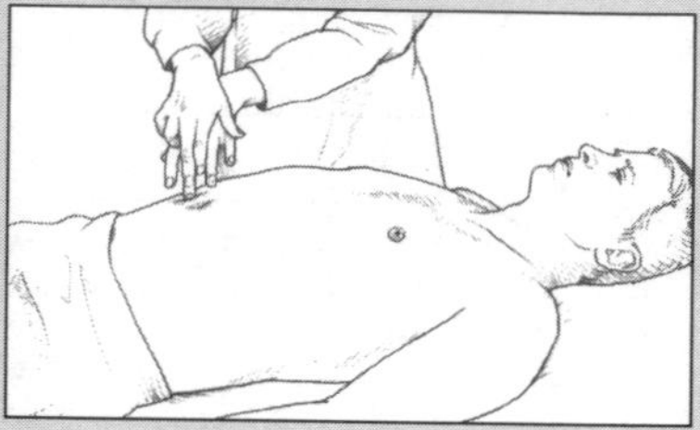

Turn the patient onto his side, which causes ascitic fluid to shift. Percuss again and mark the change from tympany to dullness. Any difference between these lines suggests the presence of ascites.

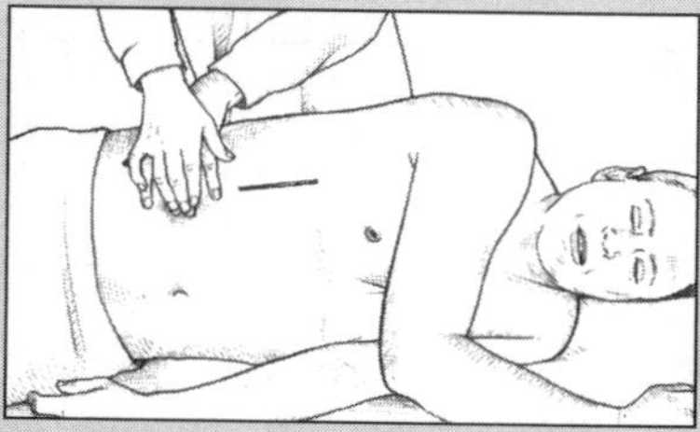

FLUID WAVE
Have another person press deeply into the patient's midline to prevent vibration from traveling along the abdominal wall. Place one of your palms on one of the patient's flanks. Strike the opposite flank with your other hand. If you feel the blow in the opposite palm, ascitic fluid is present.

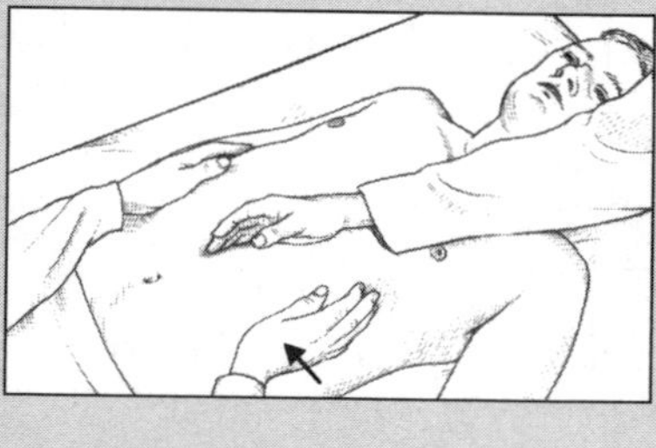

PUDDLE SIGN
Position the patient on his elbows and knees, which causes ascitic fluid to pool in the most dependent part of the abdomen, forming a puddle. Percuss the abdomen from the flank to the midline. The percussion note becomes louder at the edge of the puddle.

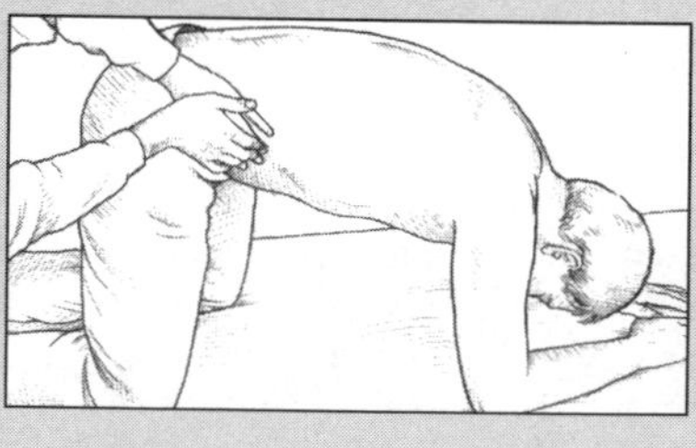

in the left lower quadrant suggests an air-filled descending or sigmoid colon. A tympanic note throughout a generally distended abdomen suggests an air-filled peritoneal cavity. A dull percussion note throughout a generally distended abdomen suggests a fluid-filled peritoneal cavity. Shifting of dullness laterally with the patient in the decubitus position also indicates a fluid-filled abdominal cavity. A pelvic or intra-abdominal mass causes local dullness upon percussion and should be palpable. Obesity causes a large abdomen without shifting dullness, prominent tympany, or palpable bowel or other masses, and dullness is generalized rather then localized.

Palpate the abdomen for tenderness, noting whether it's localized or generalized. Watch for peritoneal signs, such as rebound tenderness, guarding, rigidity, McBurney's sign, obturator sign, and psoas sign. Female patients should undergo a pelvic examination, and males should undergo a genital examination. All patients who report abdominal pain should undergo a digital rectal examination with fecal occult blood testing. Finally, measure abdominal girth for a baseline value. Mark the flanks with a felt-tipped pen as a reference for subsequent measurements.

Common medical causes

◆ ***Abdominal trauma.*** When brisk internal bleeding accompanies trauma, abdominal distention may be acute and dramatic. Associated signs of this life-threatening disorder include abdominal rigidity with guarding, decreased or absent bowel sounds, vomiting, tenderness, and abdominal bruising. Pain may occur over the trauma site or over the scapula if abdominal bleeding irritates the phrenic nerve. Signs of hypovolemic shock, such as hypotension and rapid, thready pulse, reflect significant blood loss.

◆ ***Cirrhosis.*** In this disorder, ascites causes generalized distention and is confirmed by a fluid wave, shifting dullness, and a puddle sign. Umbilical eversion and caput medusae (dilated veins around the umbilicus) are common. The patient may report a feeling of fullness or weight gain. Associated findings include vague abdominal pain, fever, anorexia, nausea, vomiting, constipation or diarrhea, bleeding tendencies, severe pruritus, palmar erythema, spider angiomas, leg edema and, possibly, splenomegaly. Hematemesis, encephalopathy, gynecomastia, or testicular atrophy may also be present. Jaundice is usually a late sign. Hepatomegaly occurs initially, but the liver may not be palpable in advanced disease.

◆ ***Heart failure.*** Generalized abdominal distention due to ascites typically accompanies severe cardiovascular impairment and is confirmed by shifting dullness and a fluid wave. Signs and symptoms of heart failure are numerous and depend on the disease stage and degree of cardiovascular impairment. The hallmarks include peripheral edema, jugular vein distention, dyspnea, and tachycardia. Common associated signs include hepatomegaly (which may cause right-upper-quadrant pain), nausea, vomiting, productive cough, crackles, cool extremities, cyanotic nail beds, nocturia, exercise intolerance, nocturnal wheezing, diastolic hypertension, and cardiomegaly.

◆ ***Irritable bowel syndrome.*** In this disorder, periodic intestinal spasms may produce intermittent, localized distention, typically with lower abdominal pain or cramping. The pain is usually relieved by defecation or by passage of intestinal gas and is aggravated by stress. Other possible signs and symptoms include diarrhea that may alternate with constipation or normal bowel function; nausea; dyspepsia; straining and urgency at defecation; feeling of incomplete evacuation; and small, mucus-streaked stools.

◆ ***Large-bowel obstruction.*** Dramatic abdominal distention is characteristic in this life-threatening disorder; in fact, loops of the large bowel may become visible on the abdomen. Constipation precedes the distention and, in fact, may be the only symptom for days. Associated findings may include tympany, high-pitched bowel sounds, and sudden onset of colicky lower abdominal pain that becomes persistent. Fecal vomiting and diminished peristaltic waves and bowel sounds are late signs.

♦ ***Paralytic ileus.*** This disorder, which produces generalized distention with a tympanic percussion note, is accompanied by absent or hypoactive bowel sounds and, occasionally, mild abdominal pain and vomiting. The patient may be severely constipated or may pass flatus and small, liquid stools.

♦ ***Peritonitis.*** In this life-threatening disorder, abdominal distention may be localized or generalized, depending on the extent of peritonitis. Fluid accumulates first within the peritoneal cavity and then within the bowel lumen, causing a fluid wave and shifting dullness. Typically, distention is accompanied by sudden and severe abdominal pain that worsens with movement, rebound tenderness, and abdominal rigidity.

The skin over the patient's abdomen may appear taut. Associated signs and symptoms usually include hypoactive or absent bowel sounds, fever, chills, hyperalgesia, nausea, and vomiting. Signs of shock, such as tachycardia and hypotension, reflect significant fluid loss into the abdomen.

♦ ***Small-bowel obstruction.*** Abdominal distention, which is characteristic in this life-threatening disorder, is most pronounced during late obstruction, especially in the distal small bowel. Auscultation reveals hypoactive or hyperactive bowel sounds; percussion produces a tympanic note. Accompanying symptoms include colicky periumbilical pain, constipation, nausea, and vomiting; the higher the obstruction, the earlier and more severe the vomiting. Rebound tenderness reflects intestinal strangulation with ischemia. Associated signs and symptoms may include drowsiness, malaise, and signs of dehydration. Signs of hypovolemic shock appear with progressive dehydration and plasma loss.

♦ ***Toxic megacolon (acute).*** This life-threatening complication of infectious or ulcerative colitis produces dramatic abdominal distention that usually develops gradually and is accompanied by a tympanic percussion note, diminished or absent bowel sounds, and mild rebound tenderness. The patient presents with abdominal pain and tenderness, fever, tachycardia, and dehydration.

Special considerations

Position the patient comfortably, using pillows for support. Place him on his left side to help flatus escape. Or, if he has ascites, elevate the head of the bed to ease his breathing. Administer drugs to relieve pain, and offer emotional support.

Prepare the patient for diagnostic tests, such as abdominal X-rays, endoscopy, laparoscopy, ultrasonography, computed tomography scan or, possibly, paracentesis.

Pediatric pointers

Because a young child's abdomen is normally rounded, distention may be difficult to observe. Fortunately, however, a child's abdominal wall is less well developed than an adult's, so that palpation is easier. When percussing the abdomen, remember that children normally swallow air when eating and crying, resulting in louder-than-normal tympany. In a child, air swallowing and incomplete abdominal muscle development also make the fluid wave difficult to interpret. To check for abdominal fluid, test for shifting dullness instead of for a fluid wave. Minimal tympany with abdominal distention suggests fluid accumulation or solid masses.

Some children won't cooperate with a physical examination. Try to gain the child's confidence, and consider allowing him to remain in the parent's or caregiver's lap. You can gather clues by observing the child while he's coughing, walking, or even climbing on office furniture. Remove all the child's clothing to avoid missing any diagnostic clues. Also, perform a gentle rectal examination.

In neonates, ascites usually results from GI or urinary perforation; in older children, from heart failure, cirrhosis, or nephrosis. Besides ascites, congenital malformations of the GI tract (such as intussusception and volvulus) may cause abdominal distention. A hernia may cause distention if it obstructs the intestine. Overeating and constipation also can cause distention.

Geriatric pointers

As people age, fat tends to accumulate in the lower abdomen and near the hips, even when body weight is stable. This accumulation, together with weakening abdominal muscles, commonly produces a potbelly, which some elderly patients may interpret as fluid collection or evidence of disease.

Abdominal mass

Commonly detected on routine physical examination, localized swelling in one of the abdominal quadrants indicates an abdominal mass, such as an enlarged organ, a neoplasm, an abscess, a vascular defect, or a fecal mass. (See *Abdominal mass: Locations and common causes*, page 8.) Typically, this sign develops insidiously. Distinguishing an abdominal mass from normal structures requires skillful palpation. At times, palpation must be repeated with the patient in a different position or performed by a second examiner to verify initial findings. A palpable abdominal mass is an important clinical sign and usually represents a serious — and perhaps life-threatening — disorder.

Emergency interventions

If the patient has a pulsating midabdominal mass and severe abdominal or back pain, suspect an aortic aneurysm. Quickly take his vital signs. Because the patient may require emergency surgery, withhold food or fluids until the patient is examined. Prepare to administer oxygen and to start an I.V. infusion for fluid and blood replacement. Obtain routine preoperative tests, and prepare the patient for angiography. Frequently monitor blood pressure, pulse, respirations, and urine output. Be alert for signs of shock, such as tachycardia, hypotension, and cool, clammy skin, which may indicate significant blood loss.

History and physical examination

If the patient's abdominal mass doesn't suggest an aortic aneurysm, continue with a detailed history. Ask the patient if the mass is painful. If so, ask if the pain is constant or occurs only on palpation. Is it localized or generalized? Determine if the patient was already aware of the mass. If he was, ask if he has noticed any change in its size or location.

Next, review the patient's medical history, paying special attention to GI disorders. Ask the patient about GI signs and symptoms, such as constipation, diarrhea, rectal bleeding, abnormally colored stools, and vomiting. Has the patient noticed a change in appetite? Ask a female patient if her menstrual cycles are regular and when her last menstrual period began.

A complete physical examination should be performed. Auscultate for bowel sounds in each quadrant. Listen for bruits or friction rubs, and check for enlarged veins. Lightly palpate and then deeply palpate the abdomen, assessing any painful or suspicious areas last. Be sure to note the patient's position when

Abdominal mass: Locations and common causes

The location of an abdominal mass provides an important clue to the causative disorder. Here are the disorders most commonly responsible for abdominal masses in each of the four abdominal quadrants.

RIGHT UPPER QUADRANT
- Aortic aneurysm (epigastric area)
- Cholecystitis or cholelithiasis
- Gallbladder, gastric, or hepatic carcinoma
- Hepatomegaly
- Hydronephrosis
- Pancreatic abscess or pseudocysts
- Renal cell carcinoma

LEFT UPPER QUADRANT
- Aortic aneurysm (epigastric area)
- Gastric carcinoma (epigastric area)
- Hydronephrosis
- Pancreatic abscess (epigastric area)
- Pancreatic pseudocysts (epigastric area)
- Renal cell carcinoma
- Splenomegaly

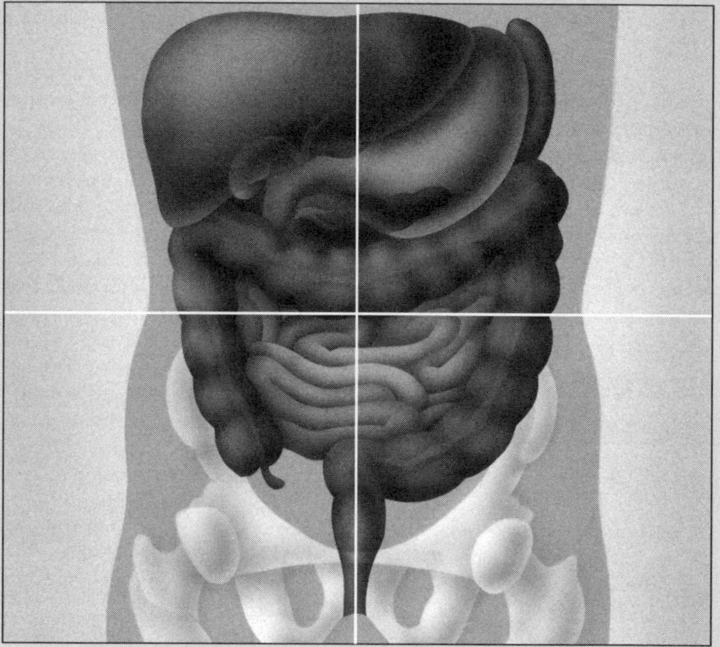

RIGHT LOWER QUADRANT
- Bladder distention (suprapubic area)
- Colon cancer
- Crohn's disease
- Inguinal hernia
- Ovarian cyst (suprapubic area)
- Uterine leiomyomas (suprapubic area)

LEFT LOWER QUADRANT
- Bladder distention (suprapubic area)
- Colon cancer
- Diverticulitis
- Inguinal hernia
- Ovarian cyst (suprapubic area)
- Uterine leiomyomas (suprapubic area)
- Volvulus

you locate the mass. Some masses can be detected only with the patient supine; others only when the patient lies on his side.

Estimate the size of the mass in centimeters. Determine its shape. Is it round or sausage shaped? Describe its contour as smooth, rough, sharply defined, nodular, or irregular. Determine the consistency of the mass. Is it doughy, soft, solid, or hard? Also, percuss the mass; a dull sound indicates a fluid-filled or solid mass; a tympanic sound, an air-filled mass.

Next, determine if the mass moves with your hand or in response to respiration. Is it free floating or attached to intra-abdominal structures? To determine whether the mass is located in the abdominal wall or in the abdominal cavity, ask the patient to lift his head and shoulders off the examination table, thereby contracting his abdominal muscles. While these muscles are contracted, try to palpate the mass. If you can, the mass is in the abdominal wall; if you can't, the mass is within the abdominal cavity. After the abdominal examination is complete, perform pelvic, genital, and rectal examinations.

Common medical causes

♦ ***Abdominal aortic aneurysm.*** This disorder may persist for years, producing only a pulsating periumbilical mass, noticeable in a supine position, with a systolic bruit over the aorta. However, it may become life-threatening if the aneurysm expands and its walls weaken. In such cases, the patient initially reports constant upper abdominal pain or, less commonly, lower back or dull abdominal pain. If the aneurysm ruptures, he'll report severe abdominal and back pain. And, after rupture, the aneurysm no longer pulsates.

Associated signs and symptoms may include mottled skin below the waist, absent femoral and pedal pulses, lower blood pressure in the legs than in the arms, mild to moderate tenderness with guarding, and abdominal rigidity. Signs of shock — such as tachycardia and cool, clammy skin — appear with significant blood loss.

♦ ***Cholecystitis.*** Deep palpation below the liver border may reveal a smooth, firm, sausage-shaped mass. However, in acute inflammation, the gallbladder is usually too tender to be palpated. Cholecystitis can cause severe right-upper-quadrant pain that may radiate to the right shoulder, chest, or back; abdominal rigidity and tenderness; fever; pallor; diaphoresis; anorexia; nausea; and vomiting. Recurrent attacks usually occur 1 to 6 hours after meals. Murphy's sign (inspiratory arrest elicited when the examiner palpates the right upper quadrant as the patient takes a deep breath) is common.

♦ ***Colon cancer.*** A right-lower-quadrant mass may reflect cancer of the right colon, which may also cause occult bleeding with anemia and abdominal aching, pressure, or dull cramps. Associated findings include weakness, fatigue, exertional dyspnea, vertigo, and signs of intestinal obstruction, such as obstipation and vomiting.

Occasionally, cancer of the left colon causes a palpable mass. Most commonly, however, it produces rectal bleeding, intermittent abdominal fullness or cramping, and rectal pressure. The patient may also report fremitus and pelvic discomfort. Later, he develops obstipation, diarrhea, or pencil-shaped, grossly bloody, or mucus-streaked stools. Typically, defecation relieves pain.

♦ ***Crohn's disease.*** In this disorder, tender, sausage-shaped masses are usually palpable in the right lower quadrant and, at times, in the left lower quadrant. Attacks of colicky right-lower-quadrant pain and diarrhea are common. Associated signs and symptoms include fever, anorexia, weight loss, hyperactive bowel sounds, nausea, abdominal tenderness with guarding, and perirectal, skin, or vaginal fistulas.

◆ ***Hepatomegaly.*** This produces a firm, blunt, irregular mass in the epigastric region or below the right costal margin. Associated signs and symptoms vary with the causative disorder but commonly include ascites, right-upper-quadrant pain and tenderness, anorexia, nausea, vomiting, leg edema, jaundice, palmar erythema, spider angiomas, gynecomastia, testicular atrophy or, possibly, splenomegaly.

◆ ***Hernia.*** The soft and typically tender bulge is usually an effect of prolonged increased intra-abdominal pressure on weakened areas of the abdominal wall. The bulge may be the only sign until strangulation occurs.

◆ ***Hydronephrosis.*** Enlarging one or both kidneys, this disorder produces a smooth, boggy mass in one or both flanks. Other findings vary with the degree of hydronephrosis. The patient may have severe colicky renal pain or dull flank pain that radiates to the groin, vulva, or testes. Hematuria, pyuria, dysuria, alternating oliguria and polyuria, nocturia, accelerated hypertension, nausea, and vomiting may also occur.

◆ ***Ovarian cyst.*** A large ovarian cyst may produce a smooth, rounded, fluctuant mass, similar to a distended bladder, in the suprapubic region. Large or multiple cysts may cause mild pelvic discomfort, lower back pain, menstrual irregularities, and hirsutism. A twisted or ruptured cyst may cause abdominal tenderness, distention, and rigidity.

◆ ***Renal abscess.*** These infections cause a palpable mass in the flank. The abscess may be localized to the renal cortex or extend into the fatty tissue around the kidney. Findings include chills, fever, leukocytosis, and abdominal pain with guarding.

◆ ***Splenomegaly.*** Lymphomas, leukemias, hemolytic anemias, and inflammatory diseases are among the many disorders that may cause splenomegaly. Typically, the smooth edge of the enlarged spleen is palpable in the left upper quadrant. Associated signs and symptoms vary with the causative disorder but commonly include a feeling of abdominal fullness, left-upper-quadrant abdominal pain and tenderness, splenic friction rub, splenic bruits, and low-grade fever.

◆ ***Uterine leiomyomas (fibroids).*** If large enough, these common, benign uterine tumors produce a round, multinodular mass in the suprapubic region. The patient's chief complaint is usually menorrhagia; she may also experience a feeling of heaviness in the abdomen, and pressure on surrounding organs may cause back pain, constipation, and urinary frequency or urgency. Edema and varicosities of the lower extremities may develop. Rapid fibroid growth in perimenopausal or postmenopausal women needs further evaluation.

Special considerations

Discovery of an abdominal mass often causes anxiety. Offer emotional support to the patient and his family as they await the diagnosis. Position the patient comfortably, and administer drugs for pain or anxiety, as needed.

If an abdominal mass causes bowel obstruction, watch for signs of peritonitis — abdominal pain and rebound tenderness — and for signs of shock, such as tachycardia and hypotension.

Pediatric pointers

Detecting an abdominal mass in an infant can be quite a challenge. However, these tips will make palpation easier for you: Allow the infant to suck on his bottle or pacifier to prevent crying, which causes abdominal rigidity and interferes with palpation. Avoid tickling him because laughter also causes abdominal rigidity. Also, reduce his apprehension by distracting him with cheerful conversation. Rest your hand on his abdomen for a few moments before palpation. If he remains sensitive, place his hand under yours as you palpate. Consider allowing the child to remain on the parent's or caregiver's lap. A gentle rectal examination should also be performed.

In neonates, most abdominal masses result from renal disorders, such as polycystic kidney disease or congenital hydronephrosis. In older infants and children, most abdominal masses are caused by enlarged organs, such as the liver and spleen.

Other common causes include Wilms' tumor, neuroblastoma, intussusception, volvulus, Hirschsprung's disease (congenital megacolon), pyloric stenosis, and abdominal abscess.

Geriatric pointers

Ultrasonography should be used to evaluate a prominent midepigastric mass in a thin, elderly patient.

ABDOMINAL PAIN

Abdominal pain usually results from GI disorders, but it can be caused by reproductive, genitourinary, musculoskeletal, and vascular disorders or injury as well as drug use and ingestion of toxins. At times, such pain signals life-threatening complications.

Abdominal pain arises from the abdominopelvic viscera, the parietal peritoneum, or the capsules of the liver, kidney, or spleen. It may be acute or chronic, diffuse or localized. Visceral pain develops slowly into a deep, dull, aching pain that's poorly localized in the epigastric, periumbilical, or lower midabdominal (hypogastric) region. In contrast, somatic (parietal, peritoneal) pain produces a sharp, more intense, and well-localized discomfort that rapidly follows the insult. Movement or coughing aggravates this pain. (See *Abdominal pain: Types and locations,* page 12.)

Pain may also be referred to the abdomen from another site with the same or similar nerve supply. This sharp, well-localized, referred pain is felt in skin or deeper tissues and may coexist with skin hyperesthesia and muscle hyperalgesia.

Mechanisms that produce abdominal pain include stretching or tension of the gut wall, traction on the peritoneum or mesentery, vigorous intestinal contraction, inflammation, ischemia, and sensory nerve irritation.

Emergency interventions

If the patient is experiencing sudden and severe abdominal pain, quickly take his vital signs and palpate pulses below the waist. Be alert for signs of hypovolemic shock, such as tachycardia and hypotension. Obtain I.V. access and keep the patient on nothing-by-mouth status.

Emergency surgery may be required if the patient also has mottled skin below the waist and a pulsating epigastric mass or rebound tenderness and rigidity.

History and physical examination

If the patient has no life-threatening signs or symptoms, take his history. Ask the patient if the pain is constant or intermittent and when the pain began. Constant, steady abdominal pain suggests organ perforation, ischemia, or inflammation or blood in the peritoneal cavity. Intermittent, cramping abdominal pain suggests the patient may have obstruction of a hollow organ.

If pain is intermittent, find out the duration of a typical episode. In addition, ask the patient where the pain is located, if it radiates to other areas, and if there are any precipitating factors.

Find out if movement, coughing, exertion, vomiting, eating, elimination, or walking worsens or relieves the pain. The patient may report abdominal pain as indigestion or gas pain, so have him describe it in detail.

Ask the patient about all drug (over-the-counter and street) and alcohol use and any history of vascular, GI, geni-

Abdominal pain: Types and locations

AFFECTED ORGAN	VISCERAL PAIN	PARIETAL PAIN	REFERRED PAIN
Appendix	Periumbilical area	Right lower quadrant	Right lower quadrant
Distal colon	Hypogastrium and left flank for descending colon	Over affected area	Left lower quadrant and back (rare)
Gallbladder	Middle epigastrium	Right upper quadrant	Right subscapular area
Ovaries, fallopian tubes, and uterus	Hypogastrium and groin	Over affected area	Inner thighs
Pancreas	Middle epigastrium and left upper quadrant	Middle epigastrium and left upper quadrant	Back and left shoulder
Proximal colon	Periumbilical area and right flank for ascending colon	Over affected site	Right lower quadrant and back (rare)
Small intestine	Periumbilical area	Over affected site	Midback (rare)
Stomach	Middle epigastrium	Middle epigastrium and left upper quadrant	Shoulders
Ureters	Costovertebral angle	Over affected site	Groin: scrotum, labia in women (rare)

tourinary, or reproductive disorders. When appropriate, ask the female patient about the date of her last menses, changes in her menstrual pattern, or dyspareunia.

Ask the patient about appetite changes. In addition, ask about the onset and frequency of nausea or vomiting. Find out about any changes in bowel habits, such as constipation, diarrhea, and changes in stool consistency. When was the last bowel movement? Ask about urinary frequency, urgency, or pain. Is the urine cloudy or pink?

Perform a physical examination. Take the patient's vital signs, and assess skin turgor and mucous membranes. Inspect his abdomen for distention or visible peristaltic waves and, if indicated, measure his abdominal girth.

Auscultate for bowel sounds and characterize their motility. Percuss all quadrants, carefully noting the percussion sounds. Palpate the entire abdomen for masses, rigidity, and tenderness. Check specifically for costovertebral angle (CVA) tenderness, abdominal tenderness with guarding, and rebound tenderness.

(See *Abdominal pain: Common causes and associated findings*, pages 14 to 17.)

Common medical causes

◆ ***Abdominal aortic aneurysm (dissecting).*** Initially, this life-threatening disorder may produce dull lower abdominal, lower back, or severe chest pain. More commonly, it produces constant upper abdominal pain, which may worsen when the patient lies down and abate when he leans forward or sits up. Palpation may reveal an epigastric mass that pulsates before rupture but not after it.

Other findings may include mottled skin below the waist, absent femoral and pedal pulses, lower blood pressure in the legs than in the arms, mild to moderate abdominal tenderness with guarding, and abdominal rigidity. Signs of shock, such as tachycardia and tachypnea, may appear.

◆ ***Abdominal trauma.*** Generalized or localized abdominal pain occurs with possible ecchymoses on the abdomen, abdominal tenderness, vomiting, and, with hemorrhage into the peritoneal cavity, abdominal rigidity. Bowel sounds are decreased or absent. The patient may have signs of hypovolemic shock, such as hypotension and a rapid, thready pulse.

◆ ***Adrenal crisis.*** Severe abdominal pain appears early, along with nausea, vomiting, profound weakness, anorexia, and fever. Later signs are progressive loss of consciousness; hypotension; tachycardia; oliguria; cool, clammy skin; and increased motor activity, which may progress to delirium or seizures.

◆ ***Appendicitis.*** In this life-threatening disorder, dull discomfort in the epigastric or umbilical region typically follows anorexia. The pain is followed by nausea and vomiting. Pain localizes at McBurney's point in the right lower quadrant and is accompanied by abdominal rigidity, increasing tenderness (especially over McBurney's point), rebound tenderness, and retractive respirations. Later signs include constipation (or diarrhea), slight fever, and tachycardia.

◆ ***Cholelithiasis.*** Patients may suffer sudden, severe, and paroxysmal pain in the right upper quadrant lasting several minutes to several hours. The pain may radiate to the epigastrium, back, or shoulder blades. The pain is accompanied by anorexia, nausea, vomiting (sometimes bilious), diaphoresis, restlessness, and abdominal tenderness with guarding over the gallbladder or biliary duct. The patient may also experience fatty food intolerance and frequent indigestion.

◆ ***Cirrhosis.*** Dull abdominal aching occurs early and is usually accompanied by anorexia, indigestion, nausea, vomiting, constipation, or diarrhea. Subsequent right-upper-quadrant pain worsens when the patient sits up or leans forward. Associated signs include fever, ascites, leg edema, weight gain, hepatomegaly, jaundice, severe pruritus, bleeding tendencies, palmar erythema, and spider angiomas. Gynecomastia and testicular atrophy may also be present.

◆ ***Crohn's disease.*** An acute attack causes severe cramping pain in the lower abdomen, typically preceded by weeks or months of milder cramping pain. Crohn's disease may also cause diarrhea or constipation, bloody stools, hyperactive bowel sounds, high fever, abdominal tenderness with guarding and, possibly, a palpable mass in a lower quadrant. Abdominal pain is commonly relieved by defecation. Milder chronic symptoms include right-lower-quadrant pain with diarrhea, steatorrhea, weight loss, and perirectal or vaginal fistulas.

◆ ***Duodenal ulcer.*** Localized abdominal pain — described as steady, gnawing, burning, aching, or hungerlike — may occur high in the midepigastrium, slightly off center, usually on the right. The pain usually doesn't radiate unless pancreatic penetration occurs. It typically begins 2 to 4 hours after a meal and may cause nocturnal awakening. Ingestion of

(Text continues on page 16.)

Abdominal pain: Common causes and associated findings

S&S

CAUSES	Abdominal distention	Abdominal mass	Abdominal rigidity	Abdominal tenderness	Amenorrhea	Anorexia	Bowel sounds, absent	Bowel sounds, hyperactive	Bowel sounds, hypoactive
	MAJOR ASSOCIATED SIGNS AND SYMPTOMS								
Abdominal aortic aneurysm		◆	◆	◆					
Abdominal cancer	◆	◆				◆			
Adrenal crisis						◆			
Appendicitis			◆	◆		◆			
Cholelithiasis		◆		◆		◆			
Cirrhosis	◆					◆			
Crohn's disease		◆		◆				◆	
Diverticulitis		◆	◆						
Duodenal ulcer									
Ectopic pregnancy		◆			◆				
Endometriosis				◆					
Gastric ulcer						◆			
Gastroenteritis								◆	
Heart failure	◆								
Hepatitis				◆		◆			
Herpes zoster				◆					
Intestinal obstruction	◆			◆			◆	◆	◆
Ovarian cyst	◆	◆		◆	◆				
Pancreatitis			◆	◆					◆
Pelvic inflammatory disease		◆		◆					

	Chest pain	Constipation	Cough	Costovertebral angle tenderness	Diarrhea	Dyspnea	Fever	Nausea	Oliguria or anuria	Skin lesions	Skin mottling	Tachycardia	Tachypnea	Urinary frequency	Vomiting	Weakness	Weight change
	◆										◆	◆	◆				
																◆	◆
							◆	◆	◆			◆			◆	◆	
		◆			◆		◆	◆				◆			◆		
							◆	◆							◆		
		◆			◆		◆	◆							◆		
		◆			◆		◆										◆
		◆					◆	◆									
	◆	◆			◆												◆
								◆					◆		◆		
		◆															
								◆									◆
					◆			◆							◆		
			◆			◆		◆				◆			◆		
								◆							◆		
	◆						◆			◆							
		◆						◆				◆	◆		◆		
							◆	◆							◆		
							◆	◆				◆			◆		
							◆	◆							◆		

(continued)

Abdominal pain: Common causes and associated findings *(continued)*

S&S

CAUSES	MAJOR ASSOCIATED SIGNS AND SYMPTOMS								
	Abdominal distention	Abdominal mass	Abdominal rigidity	Abdominal tenderness	Amenorrhea	Anorexia	Bowel sounds, absent	Bowel sounds, hyperactive	Bowel sounds, hypoactive
Perforated ulcer			◆	◆			◆		
Peritonitis	◆		◆	◆			◆		◆
Pneumothorax									
Prostatitis									
Pyelonephritis				◆					
Renal calculi									
Sickle cell crisis									
Ulcerative colitis				◆		◆			◆

food or antacids brings relief until the cycle starts again, but it also may produce weight gain. Other symptoms include changes in bowel habits and heartburn or retrosternal burning.

◆ ***Ectopic pregnancy.*** Lower abdominal pain may be sharp, dull, or cramping and constant or intermittent in this potentially life-threatening disorder. Vaginal bleeding, nausea, and vomiting may occur, along with urinary frequency, a tender adnexal mass, and a 1- to 2-month history of amenorrhea. Rupture of the fallopian tube produces sharp lower abdominal pain, which may radiate to the shoulders and neck and become extreme with cervical or adnexal palpation. Signs of shock, such as pallor, tachycardia, and hypotension, may also appear.

◆ ***Endometriosis.*** Constant, severe pain in the lower abdomen usually begins 5 to 7 days before the start of menstruation and may be aggravated by defecation. Depending on the location of the ectopic tissue, the pain may be accompanied by constipation, abdominal tenderness, dysmenorrhea, dyspareunia, and deep sacral pain.

◆ ***Gastric ulcer.*** Diffuse, gnawing, burning pain in the left upper quadrant or epigastric area commonly occurs 1 to 2 hours after meals and may be relieved by food or antacids. Vague bloating and nausea after eating are common. Indigestion, weight change, anorexia, and episodes of GI bleeding also occur.

◆ ***Heart failure.*** Right-upper-quadrant pain commonly accompanies this disorder's hallmarks: neck vein distention, dyspnea, tachycardia, and peripheral edema. Other findings may include nausea, vomiting, ascites, productive cough,

Chest pain	Constipation	Cough	Costovertebral angle tenderness	Diarrhea	Dyspnea	Fever	Nausea	Oliguria or anuria	Skin lesions	Skin mottling	Tachycardia	Tachypnea	Urinary frequency	Vomiting	Weakness	Weight change
						♦					♦		♦	♦	♦	♦
						♦	♦				♦	♦		♦		
♦					♦						♦	♦				
						♦										
			♦			♦	♦							♦	♦	
			♦			♦	♦							♦		
♦					♦										♦	
				♦		♦	♦							♦		♦

crackles, cool extremities, and cyanotic nail beds. Clinical signs are numerous and vary according to the stage of the disease and amount of cardiovascular impairment.

♦ ***Hepatitis.*** Liver enlargement from any type of hepatitis causes discomfort or dull pain and tenderness in the right upper quadrant. Associated signs and symptoms may include dark urine, clay-colored stools, nausea, vomiting, anorexia, jaundice, malaise, and pruritus.

♦ ***Intestinal obstruction.*** Short episodes of intense, colicky, cramping pain alternate with pain-free intervals in this life-threatening disorder. Accompanying signs and symptoms may include abdominal distention, tenderness, and guarding; visible peristaltic waves; anorexia; high-pitched, tinkling, or hyperactive sounds proximal to obstruction and hypoactive or absent sounds distally; obstipation; and pain-induced agitation. In jejunal and duodenal obstruction, nausea and bilious vomiting occur early. In distal small-bowel or large-bowel obstruction, nausea and vomiting are commonly feculent. Complete obstruction produces absent bowel sounds. Late-stage obstruction produces signs of hypovolemic shock, such as hypotension and tachycardia.

♦ ***Ovarian cyst.*** Torsion or hemorrhage causes pain and tenderness in the right or left lower abdominal quadrant. Sharp and severe if the patient suddenly stands or stoops, the pain becomes brief and intermittent if the torsion self-corrects, or dull and diffuse after several hours if it doesn't. Pain is accompanied by slight fever, mild nausea and vomiting, abdominal tenderness, a palpable abdominal mass and, possibly, amenorrhea. Abdominal distention may occur with large cysts. Peritoneal irritation, or rupture and ensuing peritonitis, causes high fever and severe nausea and vomiting.

♦ ***Pancreatitis.*** Life-threatening acute pancreatitis produces fulminating, continuous upper abdominal pain that may radiate to both flanks and to the back. To relieve this pain, the patient may bend forward, draw his knees to his chest, or move restlessly about. Early findings include abdominal tenderness, nausea, vomiting, fever, anorexia, pallor, tachycardia and, in some patients, abdominal rigidity, rebound tenderness, and hypoactive bowel sounds. Turner's sign (ecchymosis of the abdomen or flank) or Cullen's sign (a bluish tinge around the umbilicus) signals hemorrhagic pancreatitis. Jaundice may occur as inflammation subsides.

Chronic pancreatitis produces severe left-upper-quadrant or epigastric pain that radiates to the back. Abdominal tenderness, a midepigastric mass, jaundice, fever, and splenomegaly may occur. Steatorrhea, weight loss, maldigestion, and diabetes mellitus are common.

♦ ***Pelvic inflammatory disease.*** Pain in the right or left lower quadrant ranges from vague discomfort worsened by movement to deep, severe, and progressive pain. Sometimes, metrorrhagia precedes or accompanies the onset of pain. Extreme pain accompanies cervical or adnexal palpation. Associated findings may include abdominal tenderness, a palpable abdominal or pelvic mass, fever, occasional chills, nausea, vomiting, urinary discomfort, and abnormal vaginal bleeding.

♦ ***Perforated ulcer.*** In this life-threatening disorder, sudden, severe, and prostrating epigastric pain may radiate through the abdomen to the back or right shoulder. Other signs and symptoms include boardlike abdominal rigidity, tenderness with guarding, generalized rebound tenderness, absent bowel sounds, grunting and shallow respirations and, commonly, fever, tachycardia, hypotension, and syncope.

♦ ***Peritonitis.*** In this life-threatening disorder, sudden and severe pain can be diffuse or localized in the area of the underlying disorder; movement worsens the pain. The degree of abdominal tenderness usually varies according to the extent of disease. Typical findings include fever; chills; nausea; vomiting; hypoactive or absent bowel sounds; abdominal tenderness, distention, and rigidity; rebound tenderness and guarding; hyperalgesia; tachycardia; hypotension; tachypnea; and positive psoas and obturator signs.

♦ ***Prostatitis.*** Vague abdominal pain or discomfort in the lower abdomen, groin, perineum, or rectum may develop. Other findings may include dysuria, urinary frequency and urgency, fever, chills, lower back pain, myalgia, arthralgia, and nocturia. Scrotal pain, penile pain, and pain on ejaculation may occur in chronic cases.

♦ ***Pyelonephritis (acute).*** Progressive lower quadrant pain in one or both sides, flank pain, and CVA tenderness characterize this disorder. Pain may radiate to the lower midabdomen or to the groin. Additional signs and symptoms may include abdominal and back tenderness, high fever, shaking chills, nausea, vomiting, and urinary frequency and urgency.

♦ ***Renal calculi.*** Depending on the location of calculi, severe abdominal or back pain may occur. However, the classic symptom is severe, colicky pain that travels from the CVA to the flank, suprapubic region, and external genitalia. The pain may be excruciating or dull and constant. Pain-induced agitation, nausea, vomiting, abdominal distention, fever, chills, hypertension, and urinary urgency with hematuria and dysuria may occur.

♦ ***Splenic infarction.*** Fulminating pain in the left upper quadrant occurs along with chest pain that may worsen on inspiration. Pain commonly radiates to the left shoulder with splinting of the left diaphragm, abdominal guarding and, occasionally, a splenic friction rub.

♦ ***Ulcerative colitis.*** This disorder may begin with vague abdominal discomfort that leads to cramping lower abdominal pain. As the disorder progresses, pain can become steady and diffuse, increasing with movement and coughing. The most common symptom — recurrent and possibly severe diarrhea with blood, pus, and mucus — may relieve the pain. The abdomen may feel soft, squashy, and extremely tender. High-pitched, infrequent bowel sounds may accompany nausea, vomiting, anorexia, weight loss, and mild, intermittent fever.

Other causes

♦ ***Drugs.*** Salicylates and nonsteroidal anti-inflammatory drugs commonly cause burning, gnawing pain in the left upper quadrant or epigastric area, along with nausea and vomiting.

Special considerations

Help the patient find a comfortable position to ease his distress. The patient should lie supine, with his head flat on the table, arms at his sides, and knees slightly flexed to relax the abdominal muscles. Monitor him closely because abdominal pain can signal a life-threatening disorder. Especially important indications include tachycardia, hypotension, clammy skin, abdominal rigidity, rebound tenderness, a change in the pain's location or intensity, or sudden relief from the pain.

Withhold analgesics from the patient because they may mask symptoms. Also withhold food and fluids because surgery may be needed. Prepare for I.V. infusion and insertion of a nasogastric or other intestinal tube. Peritoneal lavage or abdominal paracentesis may be required.

You may have to prepare patients for diagnostic procedures, which may include pelvic or rectal examination; blood, urine, and stool tests; X-rays; barium studies; ultrasonography; endoscopy; or biopsy.

Pediatric pointers

Because a child commonly has difficulty describing abdominal pain, you should pay close attention to nonverbal cues, such as wincing, lethargy, or unusual positioning (such as a side-lying position with knees flexed to the abdomen). Observing the child while he coughs, walks, or climbs may offer some diagnostic clues. Also, remember that a parent's description of the child's complaints is a subjective interpretation of what the parent believes is wrong.

In children, abdominal pain can signal a disorder with greater severity or different associated signs than in adults. Appendicitis, for example, has a higher rupture rate and mortality in children, and vomiting may be the only other sign. Acute pyelonephritis may cause abdominal pain, vomiting, and diarrhea but not the classic urologic signs found in adults. Peptic ulcer, which is becoming increasingly common in teenagers, causes nocturnal pain and colic that, unlike peptic ulcer in adults, may not be relieved by food.

Abdominal pain in children can also result from lactose intolerance, allergic-tension-fatigue syndrome, volvulus, Meckel's diverticulum, intussusception, mesenteric adenitis, diabetes mellitus, juvenile rheumatoid arthritis, and many uncommon disorders, such as heavy metal poisoning. Remember, too, that a child's complaint of abdominal pain may reflect an emotional need, such as a wish to avoid school or to gain adult attention.

Geriatric pointers

Advanced age may decrease the manifestations of acute abdominal disease. Pain may be less severe, fever is commonly less pronounced, and signs of peritoneal inflammation may be diminished or absent.

Abdominal Rigidity

[Abdominal muscle spasm, involuntary guarding]

Detected by palpation, abdominal rigidity refers to abnormal muscle tension or inflexibility of the abdomen. Rigidity may be voluntary or involuntary. Voluntary rigidity reflects the patient's fear or nervousness upon palpation; involuntary rigidity reflects potentially life-threatening peritoneal irritation or inflammation. (See *Recognizing voluntary rigidity.*)

Involuntary rigidity most commonly results from GI disorders but may also result from pulmonary and vascular disorders and from the effects of insect toxins. Usually, it's accompanied by fever, nausea, vomiting, and abdominal tenderness, distention, and pain.

Emergency interventions

After palpating abdominal rigidity, quickly take the patient's vital signs. Even though the patient may not appear gravely ill or have markedly abnormal vital signs, abdominal rigidity calls for emergency interventions.

Prepare to administer oxygen and to insert an I.V. line for fluid and blood replacement. The patient may require drugs to support blood pressure. Also, prepare him for catheterization, and monitor intake and output.

A nasogastric tube may have to be inserted to relieve abdominal distention. Because emergency surgery may be necessary, the patient should be prepared for laboratory tests and X-rays and kept on nothing-by-mouth status.

History and physical examination

If the patient's condition allows further assessment, take a brief history. Find out when the abdominal rigidity began. Is it associated with abdominal pain? If so, did the pain begin at the same time? Determine whether abdominal rigidity is localized or generalized. Is it always present? Has its site changed or remained constant? Next, ask about aggravating or alleviating factors, such as position changes, coughing, vomiting, elimination, and walking.

Then explore other signs and symptoms. Inspect the abdomen for peristaltic waves, which may be visible in very thin patients. Also, check for a visible distended bowel loop. Next, auscultate bowel sounds. Perform light palpation to locate the rigidity and determine its severity. Avoid deep palpation, which may exacerbate abdominal pain. Finally, check for poor skin turgor and dry mucous membranes, indicating dehydration.

Common medical causes

♦ ***Abdominal aortic aneurysm (dissecting).*** Mild to moderate abdominal rigidity occurs in this life-threatening disorder. Typically, it's accompanied by constant upper abdominal pain that may radiate to the lower back. The pain may worsen when the patient lies down and may be relieved when he leans forward or sits up. Before rupture, the aneurysm may produce a pulsating mass in the epigastrium, accompanied by a systolic bruit over the aorta. However, the mass stops pulsating after rupture. Associated signs and symptoms may include mottled skin below the waist, absent femoral and pedal pulses, lower blood pressure in the legs than in the arms, and mild to moderate tenderness with guarding. Significant blood loss causes signs of shock, such as tachycardia, tachypnea, and cool, clammy skin.

♦ ***Insect toxins.*** Insect stings and bites, especially black widow spider bites, release toxins that can produce generalized, cramping abdominal pain, usually accompanied by rigidity. These toxins may also cause low-grade fever, nausea, vomiting, tremors, and burning sensations in the hands and feet. Some patients develop increased salivation, hypertension, paresis, and hyperactive reflexes. Children commonly are restless, have an expiratory grunt, and keep their legs flexed.

◆ ***Mesenteric artery ischemia.*** Two to three days of persistent, low-grade abdominal pain and diarrhea leading to sudden, severe abdominal pain and rigidity characterize this life-threatening disorder. Rigidity occurs in the central or periumbilical region and is accompanied by severe abdominal tenderness, fever, and signs of shock such as tachycardia and hypotension. Other findings may include vomiting, anorexia, diarrhea, or constipation. Always suspect mesenteric artery ischemia in patients over age 50 who have a history of heart failure, arrhythmia, cardiovascular infarct, or hypotension.

◆ ***Peritonitis.*** Depending on the cause of peritonitis, abdominal rigidity may be localized or generalized. For example, if an inflamed appendix causes local peritonitis, rigidity may be localized in the right lower quadrant. If a perforated ulcer causes widespread peritonitis, rigidity may be generalized and, in severe cases, boardlike.

Peritonitis also causes sudden and severe abdominal pain that can be localized or generalized. It can, in addition, produce abdominal tenderness and distention, rebound tenderness, guarding, hyperalgesia, hypoactive or absent bowel sounds, nausea, and vomiting. Usually, the patient also displays fever, chills, tachycardia, tachypnea, and hypotension.

Special considerations

Continue to monitor the patient closely for signs of shock. Position him as comfortably as possible. The patient should lie supine, with his head flat on the table, arms at his sides, and knees slightly flexed to relax the abdominal muscles. Because analgesics may mask symptoms, withhold them until a tentative diagnosis has been made. Because emergency surgery may be required, withhold food and fluids and administer I.V. antibiotics. Prepare the patient for diagnostic tests, which may include blood, urine, and stool studies; chest and abdominal X-rays; peritoneal lavage; and gastroscopy or colonoscopy. A pelvic or rectal examination may also be done.

EXAMINATION TIP

Recognizing voluntary rigidity

Distinguishing voluntary from involuntary abdominal rigidity is a must for accurate assessment. Review this comparison so that you can quickly tell the two apart.

VOLUNTARY RIGIDITY

- Usually symmetrical
- More rigid on inspiration (expiration causes muscle relaxation)
- Eased by relaxation techniques, such as positioning the patient comfortably and talking to him in a calm, soothing manner
- Painless when the patient sits up using his abdominal muscles alone

INVOLUNTARY RIGIDITY

- Usually asymmetrical
- Equally rigid on inspiration and expiration
- Unaffected by relaxation techniques
- Painful when the patient sits up using his abdominal muscles alone

Pediatric pointers

Voluntary rigidity may be difficult to distinguish from involuntary rigidity if associated pain makes the child restless, tense, or apprehensive. However, in any child with suspected involuntary rigidity, your priority is early detection of dehydration and shock, which can rapidly become life-threatening.

Abdominal rigidity in the child can stem from gastric perforation, hypertrophic pyloric stenosis, duodenal obstruction, meconium ileus, intussusception, cystic fibrosis, celiac disease, and appendicitis.

Geriatric pointers

Advanced age and impaired cognition decrease pain perception and intensity. Weakening of abdominal muscles may decrease muscle spasms and rigidity.

ACCESSORY MUSCLE USE

When breathing requires extra effort, the accessory muscles — the sternocleidomastoid, scalene, pectoralis major, trapezius, internal intercostals, and abdominal muscles — stabilize the thorax during ventilation. Some accessory muscle use normally takes place during such activities as singing, talking, coughing, defecating, and exercising. (See *Role of accessory muscles in respiration.*) However, more pronounced use of these muscles may signal acute respiratory distress, diaphragmatic weakness, or fatigue. It may also result from chronic respiratory disease. Typically, the extent of accessory muscle use reflects the severity of the underlying cause.

Emergency interventions

If the patient displays increased accessory muscle use, immediately look for signs of acute respiratory distress. These include decreased level of consciousness, shortness of breath when speaking, tachypnea, intercostal and sternal retractions, cyanosis, audible breath sounds (such as wheezing or stridor), diaphoresis, nasal flaring, and extreme apprehension or agitation. Quickly auscultate for abnormal, diminished, or absent breath sounds. Check for airway obstruction and, if detected, attempt to restore airway patency. Insert an airway or intubate the patient. Then begin suctioning and manual or mechanical ventilation. Assess oxygen saturation using pulse oximetry, if available. Administer oxygen; if the patient has chronic obstructive pulmonary disease (COPD), use a low flow rate. An I.V. line may be required.

History and physical examination

If the patient's condition allows, examine him more closely. Ask him about the onset, duration, and severity of associated symptoms, such as dyspnea, chest pain, cough, or fever.

Explore his medical history, focusing on respiratory disorders, such as infection or COPD. Ask about cardiac disorders, such as heart failure, which may lead to pulmonary edema; also inquire about neuromuscular disorders, such as amyotrophic lateral sclerosis, which may affect respiratory muscle function. Note a history of allergies or asthma. Because collagen vascular diseases can cause diffuse infiltrative lung disease, ask about such conditions as rheumatoid arthritis and lupus erythematosus.

Ask about recent trauma, especially to the spine or chest. Find out if the patient has recently undergone pulmonary function tests or received respiratory therapy. Ask about smoking, which can aggravate respiratory disorders, and about occupational exposure to chemical fumes or mineral dusts such as asbestos, which can cause diffuse infiltrative lung disease. Explore the family history for such disorders as cystic fibrosis and neurofibromatosis, which can cause diffuse infiltrative lung disease.

Perform a detailed chest examination, noting abnormal respiratory rate, pattern, or depth. Assess the color, temperature, and turgor of the patient's skin, and check for clubbing. (See *Accessory*

Role of accessory muscles in respiration

Physical exertion and pulmonary disease often increase the work of breathing, taxing the diaphragm and external intercostal muscles. When this happens, accessory muscles provide the extra effort needed to maintain ventilation.

In inspiration, the scalene muscles elevate, fix, and expand the upper chest. The sternocleidomastoid muscles raise the sternum, expanding the chest's anteroposterior and longitudinal dimensions. The pectoralis major muscles elevate the chest, increasing its antoroposterior size, and the trapezius muscles raise the thoracic cage.

In expiration, the internal intercostals depress the ribs, decreasing the chest size. The abdominal muscles pull the lower chest down, depress the lower ribs, and compress the abdominal contents, which exert pressure on the diaphragm.

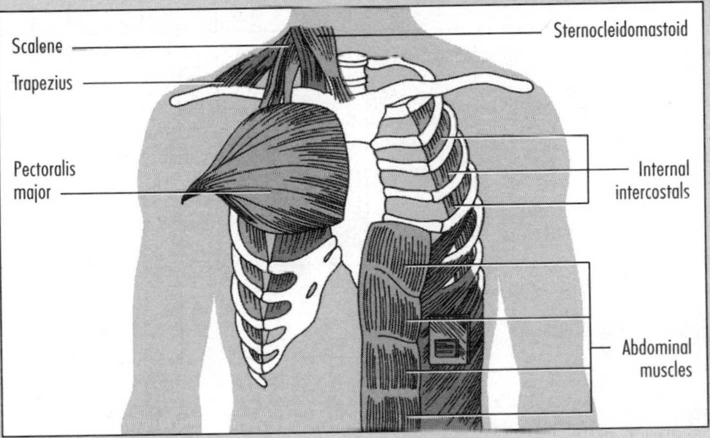

muscle use: Common causes and associated findings, page 24.)

Common medical causes

◆ ***Adult respiratory distress syndrome.*** In this life-threatening disorder, accessory muscle use increases in response to hypoxia. It's accompanied by intercostal, supracostal, and sternal retractions on inspiration and by grunting on expiration. Other characteristics include tachypnea, dyspnea, diaphoresis, and diffuse crackles. Worsening hypoxia produces anxiety, tachycardia, and mental sluggishness.

◆ ***Amyotrophic lateral sclerosis.*** Typically, this progressive motor neuron disorder affects the diaphragm more than the accessory muscles. As a result, increased accessory muscle use is characteristic. Other symptoms include fasciculations, muscle atrophy and weakness, spasticity, bilateral Babinski's reflex, and hyperactive deep tendon reflexes. Incoordination makes carrying out routine activities difficult for the patient. Associated signs and symptoms include impaired speech, difficulty chewing or swallowing and breathing; urinary frequency and urgency; and, occasionally, choking and excessive drooling. (*Note:* Other neuromuscular disorders may produce similar symptoms.) Although the

Accessory muscle use: Common causes and associated findings

S&S

CAUSES	Barrel chest	Chest pain	Cough	Crackles	Cyanosis	Diaphoresis	Dyspnea	Fever	Muscle weakness	Paralysis	Stridor	Tachycardia	Tachypnea	Wheezing
	MAJOR ASSOCIATED SIGNS AND SYMPTOMS													
Adult respiratory distress syndrome			◆	◆		◆	◆					◆	◆	
Airway obstruction			◆		◆		◆				◆	◆	◆	◆
Asthma	◆		◆	◆	◆	◆	◆					◆	◆	◆
Emphysema	◆		◆		◆		◆						◆	
Pneumonia		◆	◆	◆	◆	◆	◆	◆				◆	◆	
Pneumothorax		◆					◆					◆	◆	
Pulmonary edema			◆	◆	◆		◆					◆	◆	◆
Pulmonary embolism		◆	◆	◆	◆		◆	◆				◆	◆	◆
Spinal cord injury									◆	◆				

patient's mental status remains intact, his poor prognosis may cause depression.

♦ ***Asthma.*** During acute asthmatic attacks, the patient usually displays increased accessory muscle use. Accompanying it may be severe dyspnea, tachypnea, wheezing, productive cough, nasal flaring, and cyanosis. Auscultation reveals faint or possibly absent breath sounds, musical crackles, and rhonchi. Other signs and symptoms include tachycardia, diaphoresis, and apprehension caused by air hunger. Chronic asthma may also cause barrel chest.

♦ ***Emphysema.*** This form of COPD is the most common cause of chronic increased accessory muscle use. Dyspnea on exertion is always present as well as dyspnea at rest in severe cases. Sometimes called a "pink puffer," the patient will display pursed-lip breathing and tachypnea. Associated signs and symptoms include anorexia, weight loss, malaise, and barrel chest. Auscultation reveals diminished breath sounds and distant heart sounds; percussion detects hyperresonance.

♦ ***Pneumonia.*** Bacterial pneumonia may produce increased accessory muscle use. Initially, this infection produces sudden high fever with chills. Its associated signs and symptoms include chest pain, productive cough, dyspnea, tachypnea, tachycardia, expiratory grunting, cyanosis, diaphoresis, and fine crackles.

♦ ***Pneumothorax.*** Increased accessory muscle use may occur, especially in the presence of chronic respiratory disease or tension pneumothorax. Associated signs and symptoms are dyspnea, unilateral decreased chest wall movement, unilateral decreased breath sounds, tracheal deviation, and chest pain. Tension pneumothorax may also cause elevated neck veins and decreased blood pressure progressing to cardiopulmonary arrest.

♦ ***Pulmonary edema.*** In acute pulmonary edema, increased accessory muscle use is accompanied by dyspnea, tachypnea, orthopnea, crepitant crackles, wheezing, and a cough with pink, frothy sputum. Other findings include restlessness, tachycardia, ventricular gallop, and cool, clammy, cyanotic skin.

♦ ***Pulmonary embolism.*** Although signs and symptoms vary with the size, number, and location of the emboli, this life-threatening disorder may cause increased accessory muscle use. Commonly, it produces dyspnea and tachypnea that may be accompanied by pleuritic or substernal chest pain. Other signs include restlessness, tachycardia, productive cough, low-grade fever and, with a large embolus, hemoptysis, cyanosis, syncope, neck vein distention, scattered crackles, and focal wheezing.

♦ ***Spinal cord injury.*** Increased accessory muscle use may occur, depending on the location and severity of the injury. An injury below Ll typically doesn't affect the diaphragm or accessory muscles, whereas an injury between C3 and C5 affects the upper respiratory muscles and diaphragm, causing increased accessory muscle use.

Associated signs and symptoms of spinal cord injury may include unilateral or bilateral Babinski's reflex, hyperactive deep tendon reflexes, spasticity, and variable or total loss of pain and temperature sensation, proprioception, and motor function. Horner's syndrome (unilateral ptosis, pupillary constriction, facial anhidrosis) may occur with lower cervical cord injury.

♦ ***Thoracic injury.*** Increased accessory muscle use may occur, depending on the type and extent of injury. Associated signs and symptoms of this potentially life-threatening injury may include an obvious chest wound or bruising, chest pain, dyspnea, asymmetrical chest wall movement, cyanosis, and agitation. Signs of shock, such as tachycardia and hypotension, occur with significant blood loss.

Other causes

♦ ***Diagnostic tests and treatments.*** Pulmonary function tests, incentive spirometry, and intermittent positive-pressure breathing can increase accessory muscle use by increasing respiratory effort.

Special considerations

If the patient is alert, elevate the head of the bed to make his breathing as easy as possible. Allow him to get plenty of rest, and encourage fluid intake to liquefy secretions. Administer oxygen. Prepare him for such tests as pulmonary function studies, chest X-rays, lung scans, arterial blood gas analysis, complete blood count, and sputum culture.

If appropriate, stress how smoking endangers the patient's health, and refer him to an organized program to stop smoking. Also, teach him how to prevent infection. Explain the purpose of prescribed drugs, such as bronchodilators and mucolytics, and make sure he knows their dosage and schedule.

Pediatric pointers

Because an infant or child tires sooner than an adult, respiratory distress can more rapidly precipitate respiratory failure. Upper airway obstruction — caused by edema, bronchospasm, or a foreign object — usually produces respiratory distress and increased accessory muscle use. Disorders associated with airway obstruction include acute epiglottitis, croup, pertussis, cystic fibrosis, and asthma. Supraventricular, intercostal, or abdominal retractions indicate accessory muscle use.

Geriatric pointers

Because of age-related loss of elasticity in the rib cage, accessory muscle use may be part of the older person's normal breathing pattern.

AGITATION

Agitation refers to a state of hyperarousal, increased tension, and irritability that can lead to confusion, hyperactivity, and overt hostility. This common sign can result from various disorders, pain, fever, anxiety, drug use and withdrawal, and hypersensitivity reactions. It can arise gradually or suddenly and last for minutes or months. Whether it's mild or severe, agitation worsens with increased fever, pain, stress, or external stimuli.

Agitation alone merely signals a change in the patient's condition; however, it's a useful indicator of a developing disorder when considered with his history, current status, and other findings.

History and physical examination

Determine the severity of the patient's agitation by examining the number and quality of agitation-induced behaviors, such as emotional lability, confusion, memory loss, hyperactivity, and hostility. Obtain a history from the patient or a family member, including diet and known allergies.

Ask if the patient is being treated for any illnesses. Has the patient had any recent infections, trauma, stress, or changes in sleep patterns? Ask the patient about prescribed or over-the-counter drug use. Check for signs of drug abuse, such as needle tracks and dilated pupils. Ask about alcohol intake. Obtain baseline vital signs and neurologic status for future comparison.

Common medical causes

- ***Alcohol withdrawal syndrome.*** Mild to severe agitation occurs with hyperactivity, tremors, and anxiety. In delirium tremens, the potentially life-threatening stage of alcohol withdrawal, severe agitation accompanies visual hallucinations, insomnia, diaphoresis, and depression. Pulse rate and temperature rise as withdrawal progresses; status epilepticus, cardiac exhaustion, and shock can occur.
- ***Bipolar disorder.*** Agitation may occur in both depressed and manic phases of this disorder. In its depressive form, chronic anxiety occurs with varying severity. The hallmark is depression upon awakening, which eases during the day. Psychomotor agitation may be characterized by an inability to sit still, handwringing, pacing, and irritability. Other findings in manic states may include decreased sleep, pressured speech, and grandiosity.
- ***Drug withdrawal syndrome.*** Mild to severe agitation occurs. Related findings vary with the drug but may include anxiety, abdominal cramps, diaphoresis, and anorexia. In narcotic or barbiturate withdrawal, a decreased level of consciousness, seizures, and elevated blood pressure, heart rate, and respiratory rate can occur.
- ***Hypersensitivity reaction.*** Moderate to severe agitation appears, possibly as the first sign of a reaction. Depending on the severity of the reaction, agitation may be accompanied by urticaria, pruritus, and facial and dependent edema.

  In *anaphylactic shock,* a potentially life-threatening reaction, agitation occurs rapidly along with apprehension, urticaria or diffuse erythema, skin that's warm and moist, paresthesia, pruritus, edema, dyspnea, wheezing, stridor, hypotension, and tachycardia. Abdominal cramps, vomiting, and diarrhea can also occur.

♦ ***Hyperthyroidism.*** This is also called thyrotoxicosis; an imbalance in the body's metabolism may occur from overproduction of thyroid hormone. Mild agitation in the form of nervousness or restlessness may result. Other symptoms include weight loss, increased appetite, heat intolerance, increased sweating, and fatigue.

♦ ***Hypoxemia.*** Beginning as restlessness, agitation rapidly worsens. The patient may be confused and have impaired judgment and motor coordination. He may also have tachycardia, tachypnea, dyspnea, and cyanosis.

♦ ***Increased intracranial pressure (ICP).*** Agitation usually precedes other early symptoms, such as headache, nausea, and vomiting. Increased ICP produces respiratory changes, such as Cheyne-Stokes, cluster, ataxic, or apneustic breathing; sluggish, nonreactive, or unequal pupils; widening pulse pressure; tachycardia; decreased level of consciousness; seizures; and motor changes, such as decerebrate or decorticate posture.

♦ ***Post-head-trauma syndrome.*** Shortly after injury, or even years later, mild to severe agitation develops, characterized by disorientation, loss of concentration, angry outbursts, and emotional lability. Other findings include fatigue, wandering behavior, and poor judgment.

♦ ***Vitamin B deficiency.*** Agitation can range from mild to severe. Other effects include seizures, peripheral paresthesia, and dermatitis. Oculogyric crisis may also occur.

Other causes

♦ ***Drugs.*** Mild to moderate agitation, frequently dose related, develops as an adverse effect of central nervous system stimulants — especially appetite suppressants, such as amphetamines and amphetamine-like drugs; sympathomimetic drugs such as ephedrine; caffeine; and theophylline. Agitation is especially common in patients with cocaine or phencyclidine intoxication.

♦ ***Herbal medicines.*** Ephedra (ma huang) stimulates the central nervous system by increasing the heart rate and strength of cardiac contractions. Agitation is an adverse effect, especially if the drug is taken in large amounts.

♦ ***Radiographic contrast media.*** Reaction to the contrast medium injected during various diagnostic tests produces moderate to severe agitation along with other signs of hypersensitivity.

Special considerations

Because agitation can be an early sign of diverse disorders, you must continue to monitor the patient's vital signs and neurologic status while the cause is being determined. Eliminate stressors, which can increase agitation. Provide adequate lighting, maintain a calm environment, and allow the patient ample time to sleep. Ensure a balanced diet, and provide vitamin supplements.

Remain calm, nonjudgmental, and nonargumentative. Use restraints sparingly because they tend to increase agitation. If appropriate, prepare the patient for diagnostic tests, such as computed tomography scanning, skull X-rays, magnetic resonance imaging, and blood studies.

Pediatric pointers

A common sign in children, agitation accompanies the expected childhood diseases as well as more severe disorders that can lead to brain damage: hyperbilirubinemia, phenylketonuria, vitamin A deficiency, hepatitis, frontal lobe syndrome, increased ICP, and lead poisoning. In neonates, agitation can stem from alcohol or drug withdrawal if the mother abused these substances.

When evaluating an agitated child, remember to use words that he can understand and to look for nonverbal clues. For instance, if you suspect that pain is causing agitation, ask him to tell you where it hurts, but be sure to watch for other indicators, such as wincing, crying, or moving away.

Geriatric pointers

Any deviation from an older person's usual activities or rituals may provoke anxiety or agitation. Any environmental change, such as a transfer to a nursing home or a visit from a stranger in the patient's home, may trigger a need for treatment.

AMENORRHEA

The absence of menstrual flow, amenorrhea can be classified as primary or secondary. In *primary amenorrhea,* menstruation fails to begin by age 16. *Secondary amenorrhea* is absence of menses for 3 or more months without a nonpathologic cause, such as pregnancy, lactation, or menopause.

Pathologic amenorrhea can be episodic or chronic and can result from anovulation or physical obstruction, imperforate hymen, cervical stenosis, or intrauterine adhesions. Anovulation can be the result of hormonal imbalance, ovarian failure, disease, stress, emotional disturbances, prolonged pattern of strenuous exercise, malnutrition, obesity, or anatomic abnormalities, such as congenital absence of the ovaries. Amenorrhea may also be an adverse effect of drug therapy or hormonal treatments. (See *How amenorrhea develops,* pages 30 and 31.)

History and physical examination

Determine whether amenorrhea is primary or secondary. Assess the patient's physical, mental, and emotional development because these factors, as well as heredity and climate, may delay menarche until after the age of 16. Age at menarche is generally consistent in females. Ask the patient about her own, her mother's and her sisters' menstrual histories, including age at menarche, length and pattern of cycles, and episodes of amenorrhea.

When secondary amenorrhea is suspected, determine the date of her last menses. Ask her about the onset and nature of any changes in her normal menstrual pattern. Ask if she has experienced any signs of pregnancy, such as breast swelling or weight changes. Ask about reproductive history and birth control use.

Review her health history, noting any long-term illnesses, such as anemia. Ask about exercise and nutritional patterns and excessive or recent weight changes (gain or loss). Does she experience excessive stress? What's her sleep pattern, and is she experiencing depression or any change in emotional status?

Regardless of the patient's age, rule out pregnancy before considering other causes of amenorrhea. Determine if she is experiencing other symptoms, such as hirsutism, acne, blood pressure changes, libido changes, galactorrhea, or vitilization. If performing a pelvic examination, check for anatomic aberrations of the outflow tract, such as cervical adhesions, fibroids, vaginal agenesis, vaginal septum, fusion of labia, or imperforate hymen.

Common medical causes

- ***Adrenal tumor.*** Amenorrhea may be accompanied by acne, thinning scalp hair, hirsutism, increased blood pressure, truncal obesity, and psychotic changes. Asymmetrical ovarian enlargement in conjunction with rapid onset of virilizing signs is usually indicative.
- ***Adrenocortical hyperplasia.*** Amenorrhea precedes characteristic cushingoid signs, such as truncal obesity, moon face, buffalo hump, bruises, purple striae, hypertension, renal calculi, psychiatric disturbances, and widened pulse pressure. Acne, thinning scalp hair, and hirsutism typically appear.

♦ ***Adrenocortical hypofunction.*** Besides amenorrhea, this disorder may cause fatigue, irritability, weight loss, increased pigmentation (including bluish black discoloration of the areolas and mucous membranes of the lips, mouth, rectum, and vagina), nausea, vomiting, and orthostatic hypotension.

♦ ***Amenorrhea-lactation disorders.*** These disorders, such as Forbes-Albright and Chiari-Frommel syndromes, produce secondary amenorrhea accompanied by lactation in the absence of breastfeeding. Associated features may include hot flashes, dyspareunia, vaginal atrophy, and large, engorged breasts.

♦ ***Anorexia nervosa.*** This psychological disorder can cause either primary or secondary amenorrhea. Related findings commonly include significant weight loss, a thin or emaciated appearance, compulsive behavior patterns, blotchy or sallow complexion, constipation, reduced libido, decreased pleasure in once-enjoyable activities, dry skin, loss of scalp hair, lanugo on the face and arms, skeletal muscle atrophy, and sleep disturbances.

♦ ***Congenital absence of the ovaries.*** This anomaly results in primary amenorrhea and absence of secondary sex characteristics.

♦ ***Congenital absence of the uterus.*** Primary amenorrhea occurs in this disorder. The patient may or may not develop breasts.

♦ ***Corpus luteum cysts.*** Commonly causing sudden amenorrhea, these cysts may also produce acute abdominal pain and breast swelling. Examination may reveal a tender adnexal mass as well as vaginal and cervical hyperemia.

♦ ***Hypothalamic tumor.*** In addition to amenorrhea, a hypothalamic tumor can cause endocrine and visual field defects, gonadal underdevelopment or dysfunction, and short stature.

♦ ***Hypothyroidism.*** Deficient thyroid hormone levels can cause primary or secondary amenorrhea. Typically vague, early findings include fatigue, forgetfulness, cold intolerance, unexplained weight gain, and constipation. Subsequent signs include bradycardia; decreased mental acuity; dry, flaky, inelastic skin; puffy face, hands, and feet; hoarseness; periorbital edema; ptosis; dry, sparse hair; and thick, brittle nails. Other common findings include anorexia, abdominal distention, decreased libido, ataxia, intention tremor, nystagmus, and delayed reflex relaxation time, especially in the Achilles tendon.

♦ ***Ovarian insensitivity to gonadotropins.*** This hormonal disturbance leads to amenorrhea and an absence of secondary sex characteristics.

♦ ***Pituitary tumor.*** Amenorrhea may be the first sign of a pituitary tumor. Associated findings may include headache; vision disturbances, such as bitemporal hemianopsia; and acromegaly. Cushingoid signs include moon face, buffalo hump, hirsutism, hypertension, truncal obesity, bruises, purple striae, widened pulse pressure, and psychiatric disturbances.

♦ ***Polycystic ovary syndrome.*** Typically, menarche occurs at a normal age, followed by irregular menstrual cycles, oligomenorrhea, and secondary amenorrhea. Or, periods of profuse bleeding may alternate with periods of amenorrhea. Obesity, hirsutism, slight deepening of the voice, and enlarged, "oyster-like" ovaries may also accompany this disorder.

♦ ***Pseudoamenorrhea.*** An anatomic anomaly such as imperforate hymen obstructs menstrual flow, causing primary amenorrhea and, possibly, cyclic episodes of abdominal pain. Examination may reveal a pink or blue bulging hymen.

♦ ***Pseudocyesis.*** Amenorrhea may be accompanied by lordosis, abdominal distention, nausea, and breast enlargement in this disorder.

♦ ***Testicular feminization.*** Primary amenorrhea may signal this form of male pseudohermaphroditism. The patient,

How amenorrhea develops

A disruption at any point in the menstrual cycle can produce amenorrhea, as illustrated in the flowchart below.

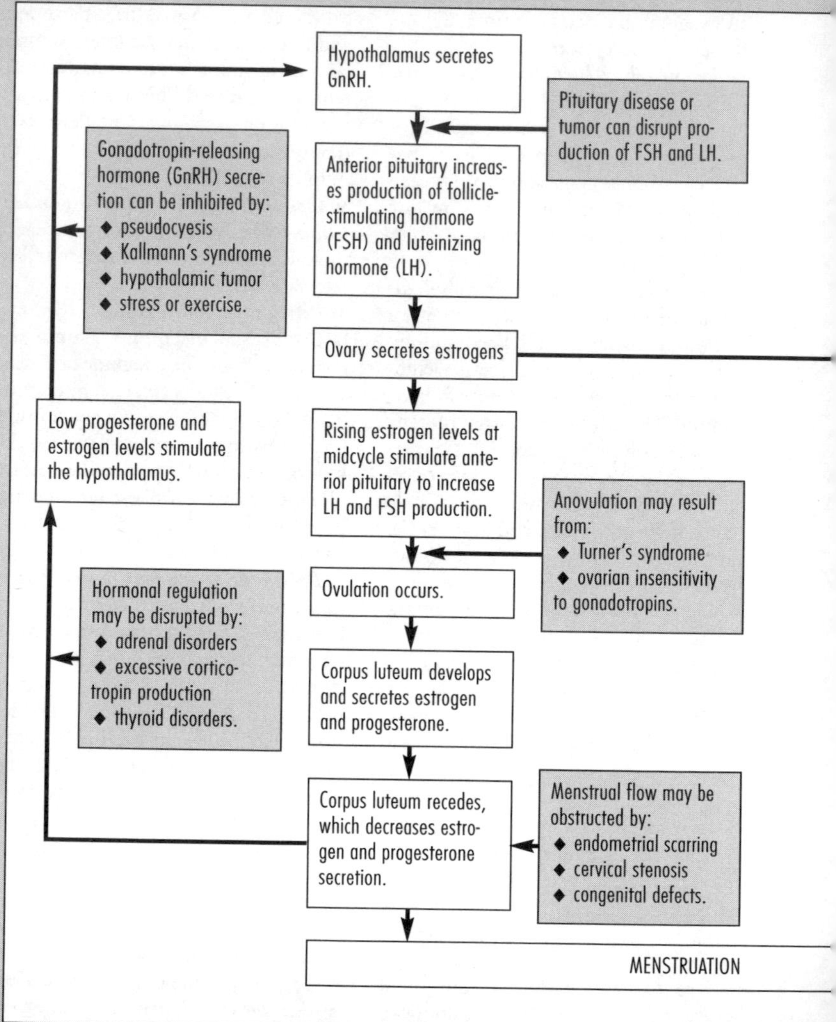

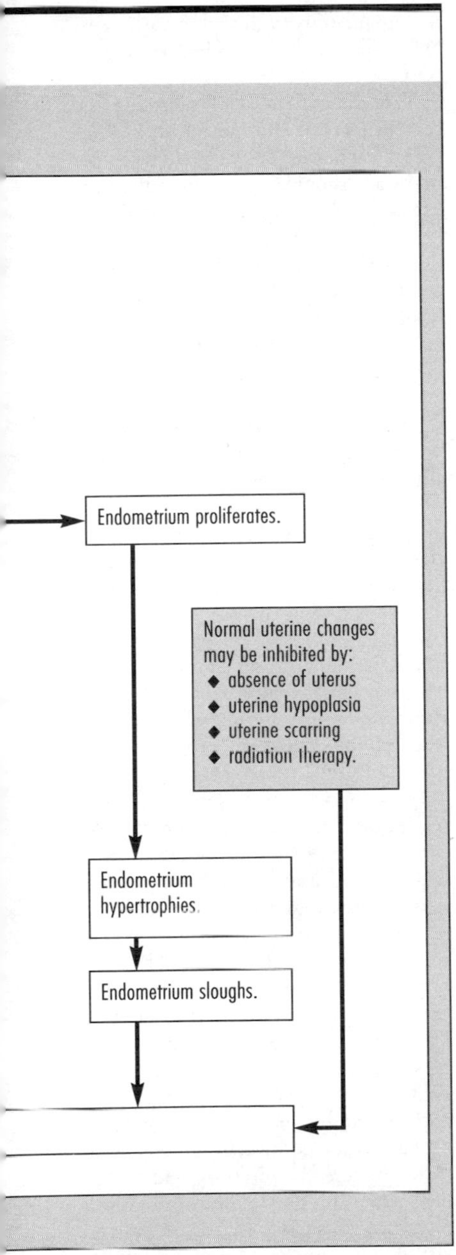
Endometrium proliferates.
Normal uterine changes may be inhibited by:
♦ absence of uterus
♦ uterine hypoplasia
♦ uterine scarring
♦ radiation therapy.
Endometrium hypertrophies.
Endometrium sloughs.

outwardly female but genetically male, shows breast and external genital development but scant or absent pubic hair.

♦ ***Turner's syndrome.*** Primary amenorrhea and failure to develop secondary sex characteristics may signal this syndrome of genetic ovarian dysgenesis. Typical features include short stature, webbing of the neck, low nuchal hairline, a broad chest with widely spaced nipples and poor breast development, underdeveloped genitalia, and edema of the legs and feet.

♦ ***Uterine hypoplasia.*** Primary amenorrhea results from underdevelopment of the uterus, which is detectable on physical examination.

Other causes

♦ ***Drugs.*** Cyclophosphamide, busulfan, chlorambucil, phenothiazines, and injectable or implanted contraceptives may cause amenorrhea. Anovulation and amenorrhea initially caused by oral contraceptives can continue after the drug is discontinued.

♦ ***Radiation therapy.*** Irradiation of the abdomen may destroy the endometrium or ovaries, causing amenorrhea.

♦ ***Surgery.*** Surgical removal of both ovaries or of the uterus produces amenorrhea.

Special considerations

In patients with secondary amenorrhea, physical and pelvic examinations must rule out pregnancy before diagnostic testing begins. Typical tests include progestin withdrawal, serum hormone and thyroid function studies, and endometrial biopsy.

Pediatric pointers

Adolescent girls are especially prone to amenorrhea caused by emotional upsets, typically stemming from school, social, or family problems.

Geriatric pointers

In women over age 50, amenorrhea commonly represents the onset of menopause;

however, pregnancy should be ruled out before any hormone therapy is considered.

Amnesia

Amnesia—a disturbance in, or loss of, memory—may be classified as partial or complete and as anterograde or retrograde. *Anterograde amnesia* denotes memory loss for events that occurred *after* the onset of the causative trauma or disease; *retrograde amnesia* denotes memory loss for events that occurred *before* the onset. Depending on the cause, amnesia may arise suddenly or slowly and may be temporary or permanent.

Organic (or true) amnesia results from temporal lobe dysfunction, and it characteristically spares patches of memory. A common symptom in patients with seizures or head trauma, organic amnesia can also be an early indicator of Alzheimer's disease. *Hysterical amnesia* has a psychogenic origin and characteristically causes complete memory loss. *Treatment-induced amnesia* is usually transient.

History and physical examination

Because the patient commonly isn't aware of his amnesia, you'll usually need help in gathering information from his family or friends. Throughout your assessment, notice the patient's general appearance, behavior, mood, and train of thought. Ask when the amnesia first appeared and what types of things the patient is unable to remember. Can he learn new information? How long does he remember it? Does the amnesia encompass a recent or a remote time period?

Test the patient's recent memory by asking him to identify and repeat three items. Retest after 3 minutes. Test his intermediate memory by asking, "Who was the president before this one?" "What was the last type of car you bought?" Test remote memory with such questions as "How old are you?" "Where were you born?"

Take the patient's vital signs and assess his level of consciousness (LOC). Check his pupils: They should be equal in size and should constrict quickly when exposed to direct light. Also assess his extraocular movements. Test motor function by having the patient move his arms and legs through their range of motion. Evaluate sensory function with pinpricks on the patient's skin. (See *Amnesia: Common causes and associated findings.*)

Common medical causes

♦ ***Alzheimer's disease.*** This disease usually begins with retrograde amnesia, which progresses slowly over many months or years to include anterograde amnesia, producing severe and permanent memory loss. Associated findings include agitation, inability to concentrate, disregard for personal hygiene, confusion, irritability, and emotional lability. Later signs include aphasia, dementia, incontinence, and muscle rigidity.

♦ ***Cerebral hypoxia.*** After recovery from hypoxia (brought on by such conditions as carbon monoxide poisoning or acute respiratory failure), the patient may experience total amnesia for the event, along with sensor disturbances, such as numbness and tingling.

♦ ***Head trauma.*** Depending on the trauma's severity, amnesia may last for minutes, hours, or longer. Usually, the patient experiences brief retrograde and longer anterograde amnesia as well as persistent amnesia about the traumatic event. Severe head trauma can cause permanent amnesia or difficulty retaining recent memories. Related findings may include altered respirations and LOC; headache; dizziness; confusion; vision disturbances, such as blurred or double vision; and motor and sensory disturbances, such as hemiparesis and paresthesia, on the side of the body opposite the injury.

Amnesia: Common causes and associated findings

CAUSES	Agitation	Ataxia	Confusion	Decreased level of consciousness	Diplopia	Dizziness	Emotional lability	Headache	Nausea	Paresthesia	Vertigo	Visual blurring	Vomiting
Alzheimer's disease	♦		♦				♦						
Cerebral hypoxia	♦		♦	♦	♦		♦	♦		♦			
Head trauma	♦		♦	♦	♦	♦	♦	♦	♦	♦	♦	♦	♦
Hysteria			♦				♦						
Seizures			♦	♦									
Wernicke-Korsakoff syndrome		♦	♦	♦	♦			♦		♦			

♦ ***Hysteria.*** Hysterical amnesia, a complete and long-lasting memory loss, begins and ends abruptly and is typically accompanied by confusion.

♦ ***Seizures.*** In temporal lobe seizures, amnesia occurs suddenly and lasts for several seconds to minutes. The patient may recall an aura or nothing at all. An irritable focus on the left side of the brain primarily causes amnesia for verbal memories, whereas an irritable focus on the right side of the brain causes graphic and nonverbal amnesia. Associated signs may include decreased LOC during the seizure, confusion, abnormal mouth movements, and visual, olfactory, and auditory hallucinations.

♦ ***Wernicke-Korsakaff syndrome.*** Retrograde and anterograde amnesia can become permanent without treatment in this syndrome. Accompanying clinical findings include apathy, an inability to concentrate or to put events into sequence, and confabulation to fill memory gaps. The syndrome may also cause diplopia, decreased LOC, headache, ataxia, and symptoms of peripheral neuropathy, such as numbness and tingling.

Other causes

♦ ***Drugs.*** Anterograde amnesia can be precipitated by general anesthetics, especially fentanyl, halothane, and isoflurane; barbiturates, most commonly thiopental and pentobarbital; and certain benzodiazepines, especially triazolam.

♦ ***Electroconvulsive therapy.*** Sudden onset of retrograde or anterograde amnesia occurs with electroconvulsive therapy. Typically, the amnesia lasts for several minutes to several hours, but severe, prolonged amnesia occurs with treatments given frequently over a prolonged period.

◆ ***Temporal lobe surgery.*** Usually performed on only one lobe, this surgery causes brief, slight amnesia. However, removal of both lobes leaves permanent amnesia.

Special considerations

Prepare the patient for diagnostic tests, such as computed tomography scan, magnetic resonance imaging, electroencephalography, or cerebral angiography.

Provide reality orientation for the patient with retrograde amnesia, and encourage his family to help by supplying familiar photos, objects, and music.

Adjust your patient-teaching techniques for the patient with anterograde amnesia because he can't acquire new information. Include his family in teaching sessions. In addition, write down all instructions — particularly medication dosages and schedules — so the patient won't have to rely on his memory.

Consider basic needs, such as safety, elimination, and nutrition, for the patient with severe amnesia. If necessary, arrange for placement in an extended-care facility.

Pediatric pointers

A child who suffers amnesia during seizures may be mistakenly labeled as "learning disabled." To prevent this mislabeling, stress the importance of adhering to the prescribed medication schedule, and discuss ways that the child, his parents, and his teachers can cope with amnesia.

Analgesia

Analgesia, the absence of sensitivity to pain, is an important sign of central nervous system disease, commonly indicating a specific type and location of spinal cord lesion. It always occurs with loss of temperature sensation (thermanesthesia) because these sensory nerve impulses travel together in the spinal cord. It can also occur with other sensory deficits, such as paresthesia, loss of proprioception and vibratory sense, and tactile anesthesia, in various disorders involving the peripheral nerves, spinal cord, and brain. However, when accompanied only by thermanesthesia, analgesia points to an incomplete lesion of the spinal cord.

Analgesia can be classified as partial or total below the level of the lesion and as unilateral or bilateral, depending on the cause and level of the lesion. Its onset may be slow and progressive with a tumor or abrupt with trauma. Commonly transient, analgesia may resolve spontaneously.

Emergency interventions

Suspect spinal cord injury if the patient complains of unilateral or bilateral analgesia over a large body area, accompanied by paralysis. Immobilize his spine in proper alignment, using a cervical collar and a long backboard, if possible. If a collar or backboard isn't available, position the patient supine on a flat surface, and place sandbags around his head, neck, and torso. Use correct technique and extreme caution when moving him to prevent exacerbating spinal injury. Continuously monitor respiratory rate and rhythm, and observe for accessory muscle use because a complete lesion above the T6 level may cause diaphragmatic and intercostal muscle paralysis. Have an artificial airway and a handheld resuscitation bag on hand, and be prepared to initiate emergency resuscitation measures in case of respiratory failure.

History and physical examination

Once you're satisfied that the patient's spine and respiratory status are stabilized — or if the analgesia isn't severe and isn't accompanied by signs of spinal cord injury — perform a physical examination and baseline neurologic evaluation. First, take the patient's vital signs and assess his level of consciousness. Then test pupillary, corneal, cough, and gag reflexes to rule out brain stem and cranial nerve involvement. If the patient is conscious, evaluate his speech and ability to swallow.

If possible, observe the patient's gait and posture, and assess his balance and coordination. Evaluate muscle tone and strength in all extremities. Test for other sensory deficits over all dermatomes (individual skin segments innervated by a specific spinal nerve) by applying light tactile stimulation with a tongue blade or cotton swab. Perform a more thorough check of pain sensitivity, if necessary, using a pin. Also test temperature sensation over all dermatomes, using two test tubes — one filled with hot water, the other with cold water. In each arm and leg, test vibration sense (using a tuning fork), proprioception, and both superficial and deep tendon reflexes. Check for increased muscle tone by extending and flexing the patient's elbows and knees as he tries to relax.

Focus your history taking on the onset of analgesia (sudden or gradual) and on any recent trauma — a fall, sports injury, or automobile accident. Obtain a complete medical history, noting especially any incidence of cancer in the patient or his family.

Common medical causes

♦ ***Anterior cord syndrome.*** In this syndrome, analgesia and thermanesthesia occur bilaterally below the level of the lesion, along with flaccid paralysis and hypoactive deep tendon reflexes.

♦ ***Central cord syndrome.*** Typically, analgesia and thermanesthesia occur bilaterally in several dermatomes, frequently extending in a capelike fashion over the arms, back, and shoulders. Early weakness in the hands progresses to weakness and muscle spasms in the arms and shoulder girdle. Hyperactive deep tendon reflexes and spastic weakness of the legs may develop. However, if the lesion affects the lumbar spine, hypoactive deep tendon reflexes and flaccid weakness may persist in the legs.

With brain stem involvement, additional findings may include facial analgesia and thermanesthesia, vertigo, nystagmus, atrophy of the tongue, and dysarthria. The patient may also have dysphagia, urine retention, anhidrosis, decreased intestinal motility, and hyperkeratosis.

♦ ***Spinal cord hemisection.*** Contralateral analgesia and thermanesthesia occur below the level of the lesion. In addition, loss of proprioception, spastic paralysis, and hyperactive deep tendon reflexes develop ipsilaterally. The patient may also experience urine retention with overflow incontinence.

Other causes

♦ ***Drugs.*** Analgesia may occur with use of topical and local anesthetics, although numbness and tingling are more common.

Special considerations

Prepare the patient for spinal X-rays, and maintain spinal alignment and stability during transport to the laboratory.

Focus your care on preventing further injury to the patient because analgesia can mask injury or developing complications. Prevent formation of decubiti through meticulous skin care, massage, use of lamb's wool pads, and frequent repositioning, especially when significant motor deficits hamper the patient's movement. Guard against scalding by testing the patient's bathwater temperature before he bathes; advise him to test it at home using a thermometer or a body part with intact sensation.

Pediatric pointers

Because a child may have difficulty describing analgesia, observe him carefully during the assessment for nonverbal clues to pain, such as facial expressions, crying, and retraction from stimuli. Remember that pain thresholds are high in infants, so your assessment findings may not be reliable. Also, remember to test bathwater carefully for a child who's too young to test it himself.

Anorexia

Anorexia, a lack of appetite in the presence of a physiologic need for food, is a common symptom of GI and endocrine disorders and is characteristic of certain severe psychological disturbances, such as anorexia nervosa. It can also result from such factors as anxiety, chronic pain, poor oral hygiene, increased blood temperature due to hot weather or fever, and changes in taste or smell that normally accompany aging. Anorexia also can result from drug therapy or abuse. Short-term anorexia rarely jeopardizes health, but chronic anorexia can lead to life-threatening malnutrition.

History and physical examination

Take the patient's vital signs and weight. Find out previous minimum and maximum weights. Explore dietary habits, such as when and what the patient eats. Ask what foods he likes and dislikes and why. The patient may identify tastes and smells that nauseate him and cause loss of appetite. Ask about dental problems that interfere with chewing, including poor-fitting dentures. Ask if he has difficulty or pain when swallowing or if he vomits or has diarrhea after meals. Ask the patient how frequently and intensely he exercises.

Check for a history of esophagus, stomach, or bowel disorders, which can interfere with the ability to mobilize, digest, absorb, or metabolize nutrients. Find out about changes in bowel habits. Ask about alcohol use and drug use and dosage.

If the medical history doesn't reveal an organic basis for anorexia, consider psychological factors. Ask the patient if he knows what's causing his decreased appetite. Situational factors — such as a death in the family or problems at school or at work — can lead to depression and subsequent loss of appetite. Be alert for signs of malnutrition, consistent refusal of food, and a 7% to 10% loss of body weight in the preceding month. (See *Is your patient malnourished?*)

Common medical causes

◆ ***Acquired immunodeficiency syndrome.*** An infection or Kaposi's sarcoma affecting the GI or respiratory tract may lead to anorexia. Other findings may include fatigue, afternoon fevers, night sweats, diarrhea, cough, bleeding, lymphadenopathy, oral thrush, gingivitis, and skin disorders, including persistent herpes zoster and recurrent herpes simplex, herpes labialis, or herpes genitalis.

◆ ***Adrenocortical hypofunction.*** In this disorder, anorexia may begin slowly and subtly, causing gradual weight loss. Other common signs and symptoms include nausea and vomiting, abdominal pain, diarrhea, weakness, fatigue, malaise, vitiligo, bronze-colored skin, and purple striae on the breasts, abdomen, shoulders, and hips.

◆ ***Alcoholism.*** Chronic anorexia commonly accompanies alcoholism, eventually leading to malnutrition. Other findings include signs of liver damage (jaundice, spider angiomas, ascites, edema), paresthesia, tremors, increased blood pressure, bruising, GI bleeding, and abdominal pain.

◆ ***Anorexia nervosa.*** Chronic anorexia begins insidiously and eventually leads to life-threatening malnutrition, as evidenced by skeletal muscle atrophy, loss of fatty tissue, constipation, amenorrhea, dry and blotchy or sallow skin, alopecia, sleep disturbances, distorted self-image, anhedonia, and decreased libido. Paradoxically, the patient commonly exhibits extreme restlessness and vigor and may exercise avidly. Many patients also have

EXAMINATION TIP

Is your patient malnourished?

When assessing a patient with anorexia, be sure to check for these common signs of malnutrition.

Hair. Dull, dry, thin, fine, straight; easily plucked; areas of lighter or darker spots; hair loss

Face. Generalized swelling, dark areas on cheeks and under eyes, lumpy or flaky skin around nose and mouth, enlarged parotid glands

Eyes. Dull appearance; dry and pale or red membranes; triangular, shiny gray spots on conjunctiva; red and fissured eyelid corners; bloodshot ring around cornea

Lips. Red and swollen, especially at corners

Tongue. Swollen, purple, raw-looking; sores or abnormal papillae

Teeth. Missing or emerging abnormally; visible cavities or dark spots; spongy, bleeding gums

Neck. Swollen thyroid gland

Skin. Dry, flaky, swollen; dark with lighter or darker spots, some resembling bruises; tight and drawn, with poor turgor

Nails. Spoon-shaped, brittle and ridged

Musculoskeletal system. Muscle wasting, knock-knee or bowlegs, bumps on ribs, swollen joints, musculoskeletal hemorrhages

Cardiovascular system. Heart rate above 100 beats/minute, arrhythmias, elevated blood pressure

Abdomen. Enlarged liver and spleen

Reproductive system. Decreased libido, amenorrhea

Nervous system. Irritability, confusion, paresthesia in hands and feet, loss of proprioception, decreased ankle and knee reflexes

complicated food preparation and eating rituals.

♦ ***Appendicitis.*** Anorexia closely follows the abrupt onset of generalized or localized epigastric pain, nausea, and vomiting. It can continue as pain localizes in the right lower quadrant (McBurney's point) and other signs appear: abdominal rigidity, rebound tenderness, constipation (or diarrhea), slight fever, and tachycardia.

♦ ***Cancer.*** Chronic anorexia occurs along with possible weight loss, weakness, apathy, and cachexia.

♦ ***Chronic renal failure.*** Chronic anorexia is common and insidious. It's accompanied by changes in all body systems, such as nausea, vomiting, mouth ulcers, ammonia breath odor, metallic taste in mouth, GI bleeding, constipation or diarrhea, drowsiness, confusion, tremors, pallor, dry and scaly skin, pruritus, alopecia, purpuric lesions, and edema.

♦ ***Cirrhosis.*** Anorexia occurs early and may be accompanied by weakness, nausea, vomiting, constipation or diarrhea, and dull abdominal pain. It continues after these early signs subside and is accompanied by lethargy, slurred speech, bleeding tendencies, ascites, severe pruritus, dry skin, poor skin turgor, hepatomegaly, fetor hepaticus, jaundice, edema of the legs, gynecomastia, and right-upper-quadrant pain.

♦ ***Crohn's disease.*** Chronic anorexia causes marked weight loss. Associated signs vary according to the site and extent of the lesion but may include diarrhea, abdominal pain, fever, abdominal mass, weakness, perianal or vaginal fistulas and, rarely, clubbing of the fingers. Acute inflammatory symptoms — right-lower-quadrant pain, cramping, tenderness, flatulence, fever, nausea, diarrhea (including nocturnal), and bloody stools — mimic those of appendicitis.

♦ ***Gastritis.*** In acute gastritis, the onset of anorexia may be sudden. The patient may experience epigastric distress after a meal, accompanied by nausea, vomiting (commonly with hematemesis), fever, belching, hiccups, and malaise.

♦ ***Hepatitis.*** In *viral hepatitis (hepatitis A, B, C, or D),* anorexia begins in the preicteric phase and is accompanied by fatigue, malaise, headache, arthralgia, myalgia, photophobia, nausea and vomiting, mild fever, hepatomegaly, and lymphadenopathy. It may continue throughout the icteric phase, along with mild weight loss, dark urine, clay-colored stools, jaundice, right-upper-quadrant pain and, possibly, irritability and severe pruritus.

Signs and symptoms of *nonviral hepatitis* usually resemble those of viral hepatitis but may vary, depending on the causative agent and the extent of liver damage.

♦ ***Hypothyroidism.*** Anorexia is common and usually insidious in thyroid hormone deficiency. Typically, vague early findings include fatigue, forgetfulness, cold intolerance, unexplained weight gain, and constipation. Subsequent findings include decreased mental stability; dry, flaky, and inelastic skin; edema of the face, hands, and feet; ptosis; hoarseness; thick, brittle nails; coarse, broken hair; and signs of decreased cardiac output, such as bradycardia. Other common findings include abdominal distention, menstrual irregularities, decreased libido, ataxia, intention tremor, nystagmus, dull facial expression, and slow reflex relaxation time.

♦ ***Ketoacidosis.*** Anorexia usually arises gradually and is accompanied by dry, flushed skin; fruity breath odor; polydipsia; polyuria and nocturia; hypotension; weak, rapid pulse; dry mouth; abdominal pain; and vomiting.

Other causes

♦ ***Drugs.*** Anorexia results from use of amphetamines, chemotherapeutic agents, sympathomimetics such as ephedrine, and some antibiotics. It also signals digoxin toxicity.

♦ ***Radiation therapy.*** Radiation treatments can cause anorexia, possibly as the result of metabolic disturbances.

♦ ***Total parenteral nutrition.*** Maintenance of blood glucose levels by I.V. therapy may cause anorexia.

Special considerations

Because the causes of anorexia are diverse, diagnostic procedures may include thyroid function studies, endoscopy, upper GI series, gallbladder series, barium enema, liver and kidney function tests, hormone assays, computed tomography scans, ultrasonography, and blood studies to assess nutritional status.

Promote protein and caloric intake by providing high-calorie snacks or frequent, small meals. You should encourage the patient's family to supply his favorite foods to help stimulate his appetite. Take a 24-hour diet history daily. The patient may consistently exaggerate his food intake (a common occurrence in anorexia nervosa), so you'll need to maintain strict calorie and nutrient counts for the patient's meals. In severe malnutrition, provide supplemental nutritional support, such as total parenteral nutrition or oral nutritional supplements.

Because anorexia and poor nutrition increase susceptibility to infection, monitor the patient's vital signs and white blood cell count and closely observe any wounds.

Pediatric pointers

In children, anorexia commonly accompanies many illnesses but usually resolves promptly. However, in preadolescent and adolescent girls, be alert for the subtle signs of anorexia nervosa.

ANURIA

Clinically defined as urine output of less than 75 ml daily, anuria indicates either urinary tract obstruction or acute renal failure due to various mechanisms. Fortunately, anuria is a rare occurrence; even in renal failure, the kidneys usually produce at least 75 ml of urine daily.

Because urine output is easily measured, anuria rarely goes undetected. However, without immediate treatment, it can rapidly cause uremia and other complications.

Emergency interventions

After detecting anuria, your priorities are to determine if urine formation is occurring and to intervene appropriately. Prepare to catheterize the patient to relieve any lower urinary tract obstruction and to check for residual urine. You may find that an obstruction hinders catheter insertion and that urine return is cloudy and foul smelling. If you collect more than 75 ml of urine, suspect lower urinary tract obstruction; less than 75 ml, renal dysfunction or obstruction higher in the urinary tract.

History and physical examination

Take the patient's vital signs and obtain a complete history. First ask about any changes in voiding pattern. Determine the amount of fluid normally ingested each day, the amount of fluid ingested in the last 24 to 48 hours, and the time and amount of his last urination. Review his medical history, noting especially previous kidney disease, urinary tract obstruction or infection, prostate enlargement, renal calculi, neurogenic bladder, or congenital abnormalities. Ask about drug use and about any abdominal, renal, or urinary tract surgery.

Inspect and palpate the abdomen for asymmetry, distention, or bulging. Inspect the flank area for edema or erythema, and percuss and palpate the bladder. Palpate the kidneys both anteriorly and posteriorly, and percuss them at the costovertebral angle. Auscultate over the renal arteries, listening for bruits.

Common medical causes

◆ ***Acute tubular necrosis.*** Prolonged (up to 2 weeks) anuria or, more commonly, oliguria (less than 400 ml/24 hours) is a common finding in this disorder. It precedes the onset of diuresis, which is heralded by polyuria. Associated findings reflect the underlying cause and may include signs of hyperkalemia (muscle weakness, cardiac arrhythmias), uremia (anorexia, nausea, vomiting, confusion, lethargy, twitching, seizures, pruritus, uremic frost, and Kussmaul's respirations), and heart failure (edema, jugular vein distention, crackles, and dyspnea).

◆ ***Cortical necrosis (bilateral).*** This disorder is characterized by a sudden change from oliguria to anuria, along with gross hematuria, flank pain, and fever.

◆ ***Glomerulonephritis (acute).*** This disorder produces anuria or oliguria. Related effects include mild fever, malaise, flank pain, gross hematuria, facial and generalized edema, elevated blood pressure, headache, nausea, vomiting, abdominal pain, and signs of pulmonary congestion (crackles, dyspnea).

◆ ***Hemolytic-uremic syndrome.*** Anuria commonly occurs in the initial stages of this disorder and may last from 1 to 10 days. The patient may experience vomiting, diarrhea, abdominal pain, hematemesis, melena, purpura, fever, elevated blood pressure, hepatomegaly, ecchymoses, edema, hematuria, and pallor. He may also show signs of upper respiratory tract infection.

◆ ***Renal artery occlusion (bilateral).*** This disorder produces anuria or severe oliguria, commonly accompanied by severe, continuous upper abdominal and flank pain; nausea and vomiting; decreased bowel sounds; fever up to 102° F (39° C); and diastolic hypertension.

◆ ***Urinary tract obstruction.*** Severe obstruction can produce acute and sometimes total anuria, alternating with or preceded by burning and pain on urination, overflow incontinence or dribbling, increased urinary frequency and nocturia, voiding of small amounts, or altered urine stream. Associated findings may include bladder distention, pain and a sensation of fullness in the lower abdomen and groin, upper abdominal and flank pain, nausea and vomiting, and signs of secondary infection, such as fever, chills, malaise, and cloudy, foul-smelling urine.

◆ ***Vasculitis.*** This disorder occasionally produces anuria. More typical findings include malaise, myalgia, polyarthralgia, fever, elevated blood pressure, hematuria, proteinuria, arrhythmia, pallor, and possibly skin lesions, urticaria, and purpura.

Other causes

◆ ***Diagnostic tests.*** Contrast media used in radiographic studies can cause nephrotoxicity, producing oliguria and, rarely, anuria.

◆ ***Drugs.*** Many classes of drugs can cause anuria or, more commonly, oliguria through their nephrotoxic effects. Antibiotics, especially the aminoglycosides, are the most commonly seen nephrotoxins. Anesthetic agents, heavy metals, ethyl alcohol, and organic solvents can also be nephrotoxic. Adrenergic and anticholinergic drugs can cause anuria by affecting the nerves and muscles of micturition to produce urinary retention.

Special considerations

If catheterization fails to initiate urine flow, prepare the patient for diagnostic studies, such as ultrasonography, cystoscopy, retrograde pyelography, and renal scan, to detect a possible obstruction higher in the urinary tract. If these tests reveal an obstruction, prepare him for immediate surgery to remove the obstruction, and insert a nephrostomy or ureterostomy tube to drain the urine. If these tests fail to reveal an obstruction, prepare the patient for further kidney function studies.

Carefully monitor the patient's vital signs and intake and output, initially saving any urine for analysis. Restrict daily fluid allowance to 600 ml more than the previous day's total urine output. Restrict foods and juices high in potassium and sodium, and make sure the patient maintains a balanced diet with moderate protein levels. Provide low-sodium hard candy to help decrease thirst. Record fluid intake and output, and weigh the patient daily.

Pediatric pointers

Anuria in neonates is clinically defined as the absence of urine output for 24 hours. It can be classified as primary or secondary. *Primary anuria* results from bilateral renal agenesis, aplasia, or multicystic dysplasia. *Secondary anuria,* associated with edema or dehydration, results from renal ischemia, renal vein thrombosis, or congenital anomalies of the genitourinary tract. Anuria in children commonly results from loss of renal function.

Geriatric pointers

In elderly patients, anuria is generally a gradual manifestation of underlying pathology. Hospitalized or bedridden elderly patients may be unable to generate the necessary pressure to void if they remain supine.

ANXIETY

A subjective reaction to a real or imagined threat, anxiety is a nonspecific feeling of uneasiness or dread. It may be mild, moderate, or severe. Mild anxiety may cause slight physical or psychological discomfort. Severe anxiety may be incapacitating or even life-threatening.

Everyone experiences anxiety from time to time — it's a normal response to actual danger, prompting the body (through stimulation of the sympathetic and parasympathetic nervous systems) to purposeful action. It's also a normal response to physical and emotional stress, which can be produced by virtually any illness. In addition, anxiety can be precipitated or exacerbated by many nonpathologic factors, including lack of sleep, poor diet, and excessive intake of caffeine or other stimulants. However, excessive, unwarranted anxiety may indicate an underlying psychological problem.

History and physical examination

If the patient displays acute, severe anxiety, quickly take his vital signs and determine his chief complaint; this will serve as a guide for how to proceed. For example, if the patient's anxiety occurs with chest pain and shortness of breath, you might suspect myocardial infarction and act accordingly. While examining the patient, try to keep him as calm as possible. Suggest relaxation techniques, and talk to the patient in a reassuring, soothing voice. Uncontrolled anxiety can alter vital signs and exacerbate the causative disorder.

ALTERNATIVE THERAPY

Relieving anxiety with yoga

Yoga is a form of mind-body exercise that uses certain postures, coordinated breathing techniques, and meditation to achieve physical and mental self-discipline. The postures help the person develop strength and flexibility by using all the muscles in the body, increasing circulation, and stretching and aligning the spinal column. Breathing exercises and meditation help reduce stress and anxiety.

If the patient displays mild or moderate anxiety, ask about its duration. Is the anxiety constant or sporadic? Did he notice any precipitating factors? Find out if the anxiety is exacerbated by stress, lack of sleep, or excessive caffeine intake and alleviated by rest, tranquilizers, or exercise.

Obtain a complete medical history, especially noting drug use. Then perform a physical examination, focusing on any complaints that may trigger or be aggravated by anxiety.

If significant physical signs don't accompany the patient's anxiety, suspect a psychological basis. Determine the patient's level of consciousness and observe his behavior. If appropriate, refer the patient for psychiatric evaluation. (See *Relieving anxiety with yoga*.)

Common medical causes

◆ ***Anaphylactic shock.*** Acute anxiety usually signals the onset of this shock state. It's accompanied by urticaria, angioedema, pruritus, and shortness of breath. Soon, other signs and symptoms develop: light-headedness, hypotension, tachycardia, nasal congestion, sneezing, wheezing, dyspnea, barking cough, abdominal cramps, vomiting, diarrhea, and urinary urgency and incontinence.

♦ ***Angina pectoris.*** Acute anxiety may either precede or follow an attack of angina pectoris. An attack produces sharp and crushing substernal or anterior chest pain that may radiate to the back, neck, arms, or jaw. The pain is commonly relieved by nitroglycerin or rest, which eases anxiety.

♦ ***Asthma.*** In allergic asthma attacks, acute anxiety occurs with dyspnea, wheezing, productive cough, accessory muscle use, hyperresonant lung fields, diminished breath sounds, coarse crackles, cyanosis, tachycardia, and diaphoresis.

♦ ***Cardiogenic shock.*** Acute anxiety is accompanied by cool, pale, clammy skin; tachycardia; weak and thready pulse; tachypnea; ventricular gallop; crackles; neck vein distention; decreased urine output; hypotension; narrowing pulse pressure; and peripheral edema.

♦ ***Chronic obstructive pulmonary disease.*** Acute anxiety, dyspnea on exertion, cough, wheezing, crackles, hyperresonant lung fields, tachypnea, and accessory muscle use characterize this disorder.

♦ ***Heart failure.*** In this disorder, acute anxiety is frequently the first symptom of inadequate oxygenation. Associated findings include restlessness, shortness of breath, tachypnea, decreased level of consciousness, edema, crackles, ventricular gallop, hypotension, diaphoresis, and cyanosis.

♦ ***Mitral valve prolapse.*** Panic may occur in patients with this valvular disorder, referred to as the click-murmur syndrome. The disorder also may cause paroxysmal palpitations accompanied by sharp, stabbing, or aching precordial pain. Its hallmark is a midsystolic click followed by an apical systolic murmur.

♦ ***Mood disorder.*** In the depressive form of this disorder, chronic anxiety occurs with varying severity. The hallmark is depression upon awakening, which abates during the day. Associated findings may include dysphoria; anger; insomnia or hypersomnia; decreased libido, interest, energy, and concentration; appetite disturbance; multiple somatic complaints; and suicidal thoughts.

♦ ***Myocardial infarction.*** In this life-threatening disorder, acute anxiety commonly occurs with persistent, crushing substernal pain that may radiate to the left arm, jaw, neck, or shoulder blades. It can be accompanied by shortness of breath, nausea, vomiting, diaphoresis, and cool, pale skin.

♦ ***Neurochemical imbalance.*** Gamma-aminobutyric acid (GABA) is the amino acid neurotransmitter believed to cause anxiety disorders. GABA is an inhibitory neurotransmitter reducing cell excitability and lowering the rate of neuronal firing. Because GABA reduces anxiety and the neurotransmitter norepinephrine increases anxiety, it's thought that there's a problem with the regulation of these neurotransmitters in the brain. The benzodiazepines enhance GABA's effect, thereby reducing anxiety.

♦ ***Obsessive-compulsive disorder.*** Chronic anxiety occurs in this disorder, along with recurrent, unshakable thoughts or impulses to perform ritualistic acts. The patient recognizes these acts as irrational but can't control them. Anxiety builds if he can't perform these acts and diminishes after he does.

♦ ***Pheochromocytoma.*** Acute, severe anxiety accompanies this disorder's cardinal sign: persistent or paroxysmal hypertension. Common associated signs and symptoms include tachycardia, diaphoresis, orthostatic hypotension, tachypnea, flushing, severe headache, palpitations, nausea, vomiting, epigastric pain, and paresthesia.

♦ ***Phobic disorders.*** In these disorders, chronic anxiety occurs along with persistent fear of an object, activity, or situation that results in a compelling desire to avoid it. The patient recognizes the fear as irrational but can't suppress it.

♦ ***Pneumothorax.*** Acute anxiety occurs in moderate to severe pneumothorax associated with profound respiratory distress. It's accompanied by sharp pleuritic pain, coughing, and shortness of breath, cyanosis, asymmetrical chest expansion, weak and rapid pulse, pallor, and neck vein distention.

♦ ***Posttraumatic stress disorder.*** This disorder produces chronic anxiety of varying severity and is accompanied by intrusive, vivid memories and thoughts of the traumatic event. The patient also relives the event in dreams and nightmares. Insomnia, depression, and feelings of numbness and detachment are common.

♦ ***Pulmonary edema.*** In this disorder, acute anxiety occurs with dyspnea, orthopnea, cough with frothy sputum, tachycardia, tachypnea, crackles, ventricular gallop, hypotension, and thready pulse. The patient's skin may be cool, clammy, and cyanotic.

♦ ***Pulmonary embolism.*** Acute anxiety is usually accompanied by dyspnea, tachypnea, chest pain, tachycardia, blood-tinged sputum, and low-grade fever.

♦ ***Rabies.*** Anxiety signals the beginning of the acute phase of this rare disorder, which is commonly accompanied by painful laryngeal spasms associated with difficulty swallowing and, as a result, hydrophobia.

♦ ***Somatoform disorder.*** Most common in adolescents and young adults, this disorder is characterized by chronic anxiety and various somatic complaints that have no physiologic basis. Anxiety and depression may be prominent or hidden by dramatic, flamboyant, or seductive behavior.

Other causes

♦ ***Drugs.*** Many drugs cause anxiety, especially sympathomimetics and central nervous system stimulants. In addition, many antidepressants may cause paradoxical anxiety.

Special considerations

Supportive care commonly can help relieve anxiety. Provide a calm, quiet atmosphere and make the patient comfortable. Encourage him to express his feelings and concerns freely. If it helps, take a short walk with him while you're talking. Or, try anxiety-reducing measures, such as distraction, relaxation techniques, or biofeedback.

Pediatric pointers

Anxiety in children usually results from painful physical illness or inadequate oxygenation. Its autonomic signs tend to be more common and dramatic than in adults.

Geriatric pointers

In elderly patients, distractions from the patient's ritual activity may provoke anxiety or agitation.

Aphasia
[Dysphasia]

Aphasia, impaired expression or comprehension of written or spoken language, reflects disease or injury of the brain's language centers. (See *Where language originates,* page 44.) Depending on its severity, aphasia may slightly impede communication or may make it impossible. It can be classified as Broca's, Wernicke's, anomic, or global aphasia. Anomic aphasia eventually resolves in more than 50% of patients, but global aphasia is commonly irreversible. (See *Identifying types of aphasia,* page 45.)

Emergency interventions

Quickly look for signs of increased intracranial pressure (ICP), such as pupillary changes, decreased level of consciousness (LOC), vomiting, seizures, bradycardia, widening pulse pressure, and irregular respirations. If you detect signs of increased ICP, administer mannitol I.V. to decrease cerebral edema. In addition, make sure that emergency resuscitation equipment is readily available to support respiratory and cardiac function, if necessary. You

Where language originates

Aphasia reflects damage to one or more of the brain's primary language centers, which in most persons is in the left hemisphere. *Broca's area* lies next to the region of the motor cortex that controls the muscles necessary for speech. *Wernicke's area* is the center of auditory, visual, and language comprehension. It lies between *Heschl's gyrus*, the primary receiver of auditory stimuli, and the *angular gyrus*, a "way station" between the brain's auditory and visual regions. Connecting Wernicke's and Broca's areas is a large nerve bundle, the *arcuate fasciculus*, which enables reception of speech.

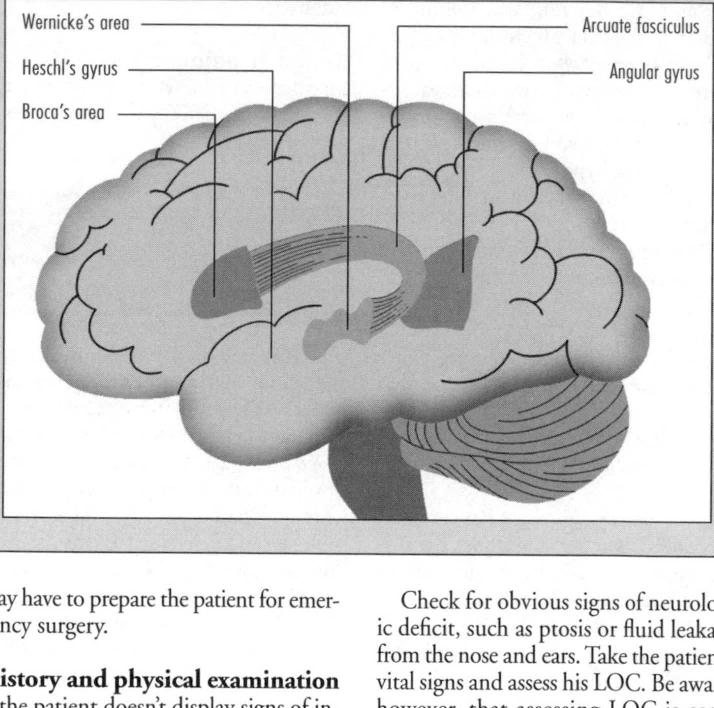

may have to prepare the patient for emergency surgery.

History and physical examination

If the patient doesn't display signs of increased ICP, or if his aphasia has developed gradually, perform a thorough neurologic examination, starting with the patient history. You'll probably need to obtain this history from the patient's family or companion because of the patient's impairment. Ask about a history of headaches, hypertension, or seizure disorders and about drug use. Also ask about the patient's ability to communicate and to perform routine activities before aphasia began.

Check for obvious signs of neurologic deficit, such as ptosis or fluid leakage from the nose and ears. Take the patient's vital signs and assess his LOC. Be aware, however, that assessing LOC is commonly difficult because the patient's verbal responses may be unreliable. Also recognize that dysarthria (impaired articulation due to weakness or paralysis of the muscles necessary for speech) or speech apraxia (inability to voluntarily control the muscles of speech) may accompany aphasia; so speak slowly and distinctly, and allow the patient ample time to respond. Keep questions simple and allow the patient time to comprehend basic components of the question. Assess the

Identifying types of aphasia

TYPE	LOCATION OF LESION	CLINICAL FINDINGS
Broca's (expressive) aphasia	Broca's area; usually in third frontal convolution of the left hemisphere	◆ Understanding of written and spoken language relatively spared ◆ Nonfluent speech — word-finding difficulty, jargon, paraphasias, limited vocabulary, simple sentence construction ◆ Can't repeat words and phrases ◆ If Wernicke's area is intact: recognizes speech errors and shows frustration; often hemiparetic
Wernicke's aphasia (receptive aphasia)	Wernicke's area; usually in posterior-superior temporal lobe	◆ Difficulty understanding written and spoken language ◆ Can't repeat words or phrases or follow directions ◆ Speech fluent but may be rapid and rambling, with paraphasias ◆ Difficulty naming objects (anomia) and no awareness of speech errors
Anomic aphasia	Temporal-parietal area; may extend to angular gyrus, but sometimes poorly localized	◆ Understanding of written and spoken language relatively unimpaired ◆ Speech fluent, but lacks meaningful content ◆ Word-finding difficulty and circumlocution characteristic ◆ Paraphasias rare
Global aphasia	Broca's and Wernicke's areas	◆ Profoundly impaired receptive and expressive ability ◆ Can't repeat words or phrases and can't follow directions ◆ Occasional paraphasias or jargon

patient's pupillary response, eye movements, and motor function, especially his mouth and tongue movement, swallowing ability, and spontaneous movements and gestures. To best assess motor function, first demonstrate the motions and then have the patient imitate them.

Common medical causes

◆ ***Alzheimer's disease.*** In this degenerative disease, anomic aphasia may begin insidiously and then progress to severe global aphasia. Associated signs and symptoms typically include behavioral changes, loss of memory, poor judgment, restlessness, myoclonus, and muscle rigidity. Incontinence is usually a late sign.

♦ ***Brain abscess.*** Any type of aphasia may occur in brain abscess. Usually, aphasia develops insidiously and may be accompanied by hemiparesis, ataxia, facial weakness, or signs of increased ICP.

♦ ***Brain tumor.*** This may cause any type of aphasia. As the tumor enlarges, other aphasias may occur along with behavioral changes, memory loss, motor weakness, seizures, auditory hallucinations, visual field deficits, and increased ICP.

♦ ***Cerebrovascular accident.*** The most common cause of aphasia, this disorder may produce Wernicke's, Broca's, or global aphasia. Associated findings usually include decreased LOC, right-sided hemiparesis, homonymous hemianopsia, and paresthesia and loss of sensation. (These symptoms may appear on the left side if the right hemisphere contains the language centers.)

♦ ***Head trauma.*** Any type of aphasia may accompany severe head trauma; typically, it occurs suddenly and may be transient or permanent, depending on the extent of brain damage. Associated signs and symptoms may include blurred or double vision, headache, pallor, diaphoresis, numbness and paresis, cerebrospinal otorrhea or rhinorrhea, altered respirations, tachycardia, disorientation, behavioral changes, and signs of increased ICP.

♦ ***Seizures.*** Seizures and the postictal state may cause a transient aphasia if the seizures involve the language centers.

♦ ***Transient ischemic attack.*** This disorder can produce any type of aphasia, which occurs suddenly and resolves within 24 hours of the attack. Associated symptoms include transient hemiparesis, hemianopsia, and paresthesia (all usually right sided), dizziness, and confusion.

Special considerations

Immediately after aphasia develops, the patient may become confused or disoriented. Help to restore a sense of reality by frequently telling him what has happened, where he is and why, and the date. Carefully explain diagnostic tests, such as skull X-rays, computed tomography scan or magnetic resonance imaging, angiography, and electroencephalography. Later, expect periods of depression as the patient recognizes his impairment. Be prepared for sudden outbursts of profanity, which usually reflects the patient's intense frustration with his impairment. Deal with such outbursts as gently as possible to ease embarrassment. Help him to communicate by providing a relaxed, accepting environment with a minimum of distracting stimuli.

When you speak to the patient, don't assume that he understands you. He may simply be interpreting subtle clues to meaning, such as social context, facial expressions, and gestures. To help avoid misunderstanding, use nonverbal techniques, speak to him in simple phrases, and use demonstration to clarify your verbal directions.

Remember that aphasia is a *language* disorder, not an emotional or auditory one, so speak to the patient in a normal tone of voice. Make sure he has necessary aids, such as eyeglasses or dentures, to facilitate communication. Refer the patient to a speech pathologist early to help him cope with his aphasia.

Pediatric pointers

Recognize that the term *childhood aphasia* is sometimes mistakenly applied to children who fail to develop normal language skills but who aren't considered mentally retarded or developmentally delayed. *Aphasia* refers solely to loss of previously developed communication skills. Brain damage associated with aphasia in children most commonly follows anoxia — the result of near-drowning or airway obstruction.

Common causes of apnea

AIRWAY OBSTRUCTION
- Asthma
- Bronchospasm
- Chronic bronchitis
- Foreign body aspiration
- Hemothorax or pneumothorax
- Mucus plug
- Obstruction by tongue or tumor
- Obstructive sleep apnea
- Secretion retention
- Tracheal or bronchial rupture

BRAIN STEM DYSFUNCTION
- Brain abscess
- Brain stem injury
- Brain tumor
- Central nervous system depressants
- Central sleep apnea
- Cerebral hemorrhage
- Cerebral infarction
- Encephalitis
- Head trauma
- Increased intracranial pressure
- Meningitis
- Pontine or medullary hemorrhage or infarction
- Transtentorial herniation

NEUROMUSCULAR FAILURE
- Amyotrophic lateral sclerosis
- Botulism
- Diphtheria
- Guillain-Barré syndrome
- Myasthenia gravis
- Phrenic nerve paralysis
- Rupture of the diaphragm
- Spinal cord injury

PARENCHYMAL DISEASE
- Adult respiratory distress syndrome
- Diffuse pneumonia
- Emphysema
- Near-drowning
- Pulmonary edema
- Pulmonary fibrosis
- Secretion retention

PLEURAL PRESSURE GRADIENT DISRUPTION
- Flail chest
- Open chest wounds

PULMONARY CAPILLARY PERFUSION DECREASE
- Arrhythmias
- Cardiac arrest
- Myocardial infarction
- Pulmonary embolism
- Pulmonary hypertension
- Shock

APNEA

Apnea, the cessation of spontaneous respiration, is occasionally temporary and self-limiting, as occurs during Cheyne-Stokes or Biot's respirations. More commonly, however, it's a life-threatening emergency that requires immediate intervention to prevent death.

Apnea usually results from one or more of six pathophysiologic mechanisms, each of which has numerous causes. Its most common causes include trauma, cardiac arrest, neurologic disease, aspiration of foreign objects, bronchospasm, and drug overdose. (See *Common causes of apnea*.)

Emergency interventions

If you detect apnea, first establish and maintain a patent airway. Position the patient supine and open his airway using the head-tilt or chin-lift technique. *Caution:* Use the jaw-thrust technique on a patient with an obvious or suspected head or neck injury to prevent hyperextending the neck. Next, quickly look, listen, and feel for spontaneous respiration; if it's absent, begin artificial ventilation until it occurs or until mechanical ventilation can be initiated.

Because apnea may result from cardiac arrest (or may cause it), be sure to assess the patient's carotid pulse immediately after you've established a patent airway. Or, if the patient is an infant or small child, assess the brachial pulse instead. If you can't palpate a pulse, begin cardiac compression.

History and physical examination

When the patient's respiratory and cardiac status is stable, investigate the underlying cause of apnea. Ask him (or, if he's unable to answer, anyone who witnessed the episode) about the onset of apnea and events immediately preceding it. The cause may become readily apparent, as in trauma.

Take a patient history, noting especially any reports of headache, chest pain, muscle weakness, sore throat, or dyspnea. Ask about any history of respiratory, cardiac, or neurologic disease and about allergies and drug use.

Inspect the head, face, neck, and trunk for soft-tissue injury, hemorrhage, or skeletal deformity. Don't overlook obvious clues, such as oral and nasal secretions reflecting fluid-filled airways and alveoli or facial soot and singed nasal hair suggesting thermal injury to the tracheobronchial tree.

Auscultate over all lung lobes for adventitious breath sounds, particularly crackles and rhonchi, and percuss the lung fields for increased dullness or hyperresonance. Move on to the heart, auscultating for murmurs, pericardial friction rub, and arrhythmia. Check for cyanosis, pallor, jugular vein distention, and edema. If appropriate, perform a neurologic assessment. Evaluate level of consciousness, orientation, and mental status; test cranial nerve function and motor function, sensation, and reflexes in all extremities.

Common medical causes

- ***Airway obstruction.*** Occlusion or compression of the trachea, central airways, or smaller airways can cause sudden apnea by blocking the patient's airflow and producing acute respiratory failure.
- ***Brain stem dysfunction.*** Primary or secondary brain stem dysfunction can cause apnea by destroying the brain stem's ability to initiate respirations. Apnea may arise suddenly (as in trauma, hemorrhage, or infarction) or gradually (as in degenerative disease or tumor). Apnea may be preceded by a decreased level of consciousness or by various motor and sensory deficits.
- ***Neuromuscular failure.*** Trauma or disease can disrupt the mechanics of respiration, causing sudden or gradual apnea. Associated findings may include diaphragmatic or intercostal muscle paralysis from injury or respiratory weakness or paralysis from acute or degenerative disease.
- ***Parenchymal lung disease.*** An accumulation of fluid within the alveoli causes apnea by interfering with pulmonary gas exchange and producing acute respiratory failure. Apnea may arise suddenly, as in near-drowning or acute pulmonary edema, or gradually, as in emphysema. Apnea also may be preceded by crackles and labored respirations with accessory muscle use.
- ***Pleural pressure gradient disruption.*** Conversion of normal negative pleural air pressure to positive pressure by chest wall injuries (such as flail chest) causes lung collapse, producing respiratory distress and, if untreated, apnea. Associated signs include an asymmetrical chest wall and asymmetrical or paradoxical respirations.
- ***Pulmonary capillary perfusion decrease.*** Apnea can stem from obstructed pulmonary circulation, most commonly due to heart failure or lack of cir-

culatory patency. It occurs suddenly in cardiac arrest, massive pulmonary embolism, and most cases of severe shock. In contrast, it occurs progressively in septic shock and pulmonary hypertension. Related findings include hypotension, tachycardia, and edema.

Other causes

◆ ***Drugs.*** Hypoventilation and apnea may be caused by central nervous system (CNS) depressants. Benzodiazepines may cause respiratory depression and apnea when given I.V. with other CNS depressants to elderly or acutely ill patients.

Neuromuscular blocking agents — such as curariform drugs and anticholinesterase inhibitors — may cause sudden apnea by causing respiratory muscle paralysis.

◆ ***Sleep-related apneas.*** These repetitive apneas that occur during sleep result from airflow obstruction or brain stem dysfunction.

Special considerations

Closely monitor the apneic patient's cardiac and respiratory status to prevent further apneic episodes.

Pediatric pointers

The immature CNS of premature infants makes them especially susceptible to periodic apneic episodes. Other common causes of apnea in infants include sepsis, intraventricular and subarachnoid hemorrhage, seizures, bronchiolitis, and sudden infant death syndrome.

In toddlers and older children, the most common cause of apnea is acute airway obstruction by aspirated foreign objects. Other causes include acute epiglottitis, croup, asthma, and systemic disorders such as muscular dystrophy or cystic fibrosis.

Geriatric pointers

In elderly patients, increased sensitivity to analgesics, sedative-hypnotics, or any combination of these drugs, even within normal dosage ranges, may cause apnea.

APNEUSTIC RESPIRATIONS

This irregular breathing pattern is characterized by prolonged, gasping inspiration, with a pause at each full inspiration. It's an important localizing sign of severe brain stem damage.

Involuntary breathing is primarily regulated by groups of neurons in respiratory centers in the medulla oblongata and the pons. In the medulla, neurons react to impulses from the pons and other areas to regulate respiratory rate and depth. In the pons, two respiratory centers regulate respiratory rhythm by interacting with the medullary respiratory center to smooth the transition from inspiration to expiration and back. The apneustic center in the pons stimulates inspiratory neurons in the medulla to initiate inspiration. These inspiratory neurons, in turn, stimulate the pneumotaxic center in the pons to initiate expiration. Destruction of neural pathways by pontine lesions disrupts normal regulation of respiratory rhythm, causing apneustic respirations.

Apneustic respirations must be differentiated from bradypnea and hyperpnea (disturbances of rate and depth, but not of rhythm), Cheyne-Stokes respirations (rhythmic alterations in rate and depth, followed by periods of apnea), and Biot's respirations (irregularly alternating periods of hyperpnea and apnea).

Emergency interventions

Your first priority for a patient with apneustic respirations is to provide adequate ventilation. The patient may need an artificial airway, oxygen, and mechanical ventilation. Arterial blood gas analysis will determine if the patient is able to maintain adequate oxygen and carbon dioxide levels. Next, use a standardized tool such as the Glasgow Coma Scale to thoroughly evaluate the patient's neurologic status. In addition, be sure to obtain a brief patient history from a family member or companion, if possible.

Common medical causes

◆ ***Pontine lesions.*** Apneustic breathing usually results from extensive damage to the upper or lower pons caused by infarction, hemorrhage, herniation, severe infection, tumor, or trauma. Typically, this breathing pattern is accompanied by profound stupor or coma; pinpoint midline pupils; ocular bobbing (a spontaneous downward jerk, followed by a slow drift up to midline); quadriplegia or, less commonly, hemiplegia with the eyes pointing toward the weak side; a positive Babinski's reflex; negative oculocephalic and oculovestibular reflexes; and, possibly, decorticate posture.

Special considerations

Constantly monitor the patient's neurologic and respiratory status. Watch for prolonged apneic periods or signs of neurologic deterioration. Monitor the patient's arterial blood gas levels or use a pulse oximetry device. If appropriate, prepare him for neurologic tests, such as electroencephalography and computed tomography scan or magnetic resonance imaging.

Pediatric pointers

The Glasgow Coma Scale isn't appropriate for use in young children because it requires verbal responses and assumes a certain level of language development.

ARM PAIN

Arm pain usually results from musculoskeletal disorders, but it can also stem from neurovascular or cardiovascular disorders. (See *Common causes of local pain.*) In some cases, it may be referred from another area, such as the chest, neck, or abdomen. Its location, onset, and character provide clues to its cause. The pain may affect the entire arm or only the upper arm or forearm. It may arise suddenly or gradually and be constant or intermittent. Arm pain can be described as sharp or dull, burning or numbing, shooting or penetrating. Diffuse arm pain, however, may be difficult to describe, especially if it isn't associated with injury.

History and physical examination

If the patient reports arm pain after an injury, take a detailed history of the injury from the patient or his companion. Then quickly assess for severe injuries requiring immediate treatment. If you've ruled out severe injuries, check pulses, capillary refill time, sensation, and movement distal to the affected area because circulatory impairment or nerve injury may require immediate surgery. Inspect the arm for deformities, assess the level of pain, and immobilize the arm to prevent further injury.

If the patient reports continuous or intermittent arm pain, ask him to describe it and relate when it began. Is the pain associated with repetitive or specific movements or positions? Ask him to point out other painful areas because arm pain may be referred. For example, arm pain commonly accompanies the characteristic chest pain of myocardial infarction, and right shoulder pain may be referred from the right-upper-quadrant abdominal pain of cholecystitis. Ask the patient if the pain worsens in the morning or in the evening, if it prevents him from performing his job, and if it restricts any movements. Also ask if heat, rest, or drugs relieve it. Finally, ask about any preexisting illnesses, a family history of gout or arthritis, and current drug therapy.

Next, perform a focused examination. Observe the way the patient walks, sits, and holds his arm. Inspect the entire arm, comparing it with the opposite arm for symmetry, movement, and muscle atrophy. (It's important to know if the patient is right- or left-handed.) Palpate the entire arm for swelling, nodules, and ten-

Common causes of local pain

Various disorders cause hand, wrist, elbow, or shoulder pain. In some disorders, pain may radiate from the injury site to other areas.

HAND PAIN
- Arthritis
- Buerger's disease
- Carpal tunnel syndrome
- Dupuytren's contracture
- Elbow tunnel syndrome
- Fracture
- Ganglion cyst
- Infection
- Occlusive vascular disease
- Radiculopathy
- Raynaud's disease
- Shoulder-hand syndrome (reflex sympathetic dystrophy)
- Sprain or strain
- Thoracic outlet syndrome
- Trigger finger

WRIST PAIN
- Arthritis
- Carpal tunnel syndrome
- Fracture
- Ganglion
- Sprain or strain
- Tenosynovitis (de Quervain's disease)

ELBOW PAIN
- Arthritis
- Bursitis
- Dislocation
- Fracture
- Lateral epicondylitis (tennis elbow)
- Tendinitis

SHOULDER PAIN
- Acromioclavicular separation
- Acute pancreatitis
- Adhesive capsulitis (frozen shoulder)
- Angina pectoris (usually left)
- Arthritis
- Bursitis
- Cholecystitis or cholelithiasis (right)
- Clavicle fracture
- Diaphragmatic inflammation or irritation
- Diaphragmatic pleurisy
- Dislocation
- Dissecting aortic aneurysm
- Gastritis
- Gastric ulcer
- Humeral neck fracture
- Infection
- Pancoast's syndrome
- Perforated ulcer
- Pneumothorax
- Ruptured spleen (left shoulder)
- Shoulder-hand syndrome
- Subluxation
- Subphrenic abscess
- Tendinitis

der areas. Compare bilateral active range of motion, muscle strength, and reflexes.

If the patient reports numbness or tingling, check his sensation to temperature or pain and vibration or proprioception and pinprick. Compare bilateral hand grasps and shoulder strength to detect weakness.

If a patient has a cast, splint, or restrictive dressing, check for circulation, sensation, and mobility distal to the dressing. Ask the patient about edema and if the pain has worsened during the past 24 hours. Also ask what activities he has been performing.

Examine the neck for pain on motion, point tenderness, muscle spasms, or arm pain when the neck is extended with the head toward the involved side. (See *Arm pain: Common causes and associated findings,* page 52.)

Common medical causes

◆ ***Angina.*** This disorder may cause inner arm pain as well as chest and jaw pain. The pain usually but not always af-

Arm pain: Common causes and associated findings

CAUSES	Chest pain	Crepitus	Decreased motion	Decreased reflex response	Deformity	Ecchymosis	Edema	Impaired circulation	Muscle weakness	Nausea	Parasthesia	Vomiting
	MAJOR ASSOCIATED SIGNS AND SYMPTOMS											
Angina	◆											
Biceps rupture					◆		◆		◆			
Cellulitis							◆					
Cervical nerve root compression				◆					◆		◆	
Compartment syndrome			◆				◆	◆	◆		◆	
Fractures		◆	◆		◆	◆	◆	◆			◆	
Muscle contusion						◆	◆					
Muscle strain			◆						◆			
Myocardial infarction	◆									◆		◆
Neoplasm of the arm							◆	◆			◆	
Osteomyelitis			◆				◆					

fects the left arm. Typically, the pain follows exertion and persists for a few minutes. Accompanied by dyspnea, diaphoresis, and apprehension, the pain is relieved by rest, nitroglycerin, or oxygen therapy.

◆ ***Biceps rupture.*** Rupture of the biceps after excessive weight lifting or osteoarthritic degeneration of bicipital tendon insertion at the shoulder can cause pain in the upper arm. Forearm flexion and supination aggravate the pain. Other signs include muscle weakness, deformity, and edema. The biceps bulges at rest; this is sometimes referred to as a pop-eyed look.

◆ ***Cellulitis.*** Typically, this disorder affects the legs, but it can also affect the arms. It produces pain as well as redness, tenderness, edema and, at times, fever, chills, tachycardia, headache, or hypotension. Cellulitis follows interruption of the skin's natural barrier to bacteria, usually by an abrasion, laceration, bite, or other injury.

◆ ***Cervical nerve root compression.*** Compression of the cervical nerves supplying the upper arm produces chronic arm and neck pain, which may worsen with movement or prolonged sitting. The patient may also experience muscle weakness, paresthesia, and decreased deep tendon response.

♦ ***Compartment syndrome.*** Severe pain on passive muscle stretching is the cardinal sign of this syndrome. It may also impair distal circulation and cause muscle weakness, decreased reflex response, paresthesia, and edema. Ominous signs include paralysis, reduced sensation, and absent pulse.

♦ ***Fractures.*** Fractures of the cervical vertebrae, humerus, scapula, clavicle, radius, or ulna can cause pain that begins at the injury site and radiates through the entire arm. Pain at a fresh fracture site is intense and worsens with movement. Associated signs and symptoms include swelling; crepitus, felt and heard when bone ends rub together (don't attempt to elicit this sign); deformity, if bones are misaligned; local ecchymosis and edema; paresthesia; and impaired circulation and sensation distal to the injury. Fractures of the small wrist bones can manifest with pain and swelling several days after the trauma.

♦ ***Muscle contusion.*** This injury may cause generalized pain in the area of injury. It may also cause local swelling and ecchymosis.

♦ ***Muscle strain.*** Acute or chronic muscle strain causes mild to severe pain with movement. The resultant reduction in arm movement may cause muscle weakness and atrophy.

♦ ***Myocardial infarction.*** In this life-threatening disorder, the patient may complain of arm pain, usually on the left, as well as the characteristic deep and crushing chest pain. He may display weakness, pallor, nausea, vomiting, diaphoresis, altered blood pressure, tachycardia, dyspnea, and feelings of apprehension, anxiety, or impending doom.

♦ ***Neoplasm of the arm.*** This disorder produces continuous, deep, and penetrating arm pain that worsens at night. Occasionally, redness and swelling accompany arm pain; later, skin breakdown, impaired circulation, and paresthesia may occur.

♦ ***Osteomyelitis.*** This disorder typically begins with fever and vague localized arm pain that comes and goes; it's accompanied by local tenderness, painful and restricted movement and, later, swelling. Associated findings include malaise and tachycardia.

Special considerations

If you suspect a fracture, apply a sling or a splint to immobilize the arm, and monitor for worsening pain, numbness, or decreased circulation distal to the injury. Also monitor vital signs, and be alert for tachycardia, hypotension, and diaphoresis. Withhold food, fluids, and analgesics until potential fractures are evaluated. Promote the patient's comfort by elevating his arm and applying ice. Clean abrasions and lacerations and apply dry, sterile dressings, if necessary. Also, prepare the patient for X-rays or other diagnostic tests.

Pediatric pointers

In children, arm pain commonly results from fractures, muscle sprain, muscular dystrophy, or rheumatoid arthritis. In young children especially, the exact location of the pain may be difficult to establish. Watch for nonverbal clues, such as wincing or guarding.

If the child has a fracture or sprain, obtain a complete account of the injury. Closely observe interactions between the child and his family, and don't rule out the possibility of child abuse.

Geriatric pointers

Elderly patients with osteoporosis may experience fractures from simple trauma or even from heavy lifting or unexpected movements. They're also prone to degenerative joint disease, which can involve several joints in the arm or neck.

Asterixis

[Liver flap, flapping tremor]

A bilateral, coarse movement, asterixis is characterized by sudden relaxation of muscle groups holding a sustained position. This elicited sign is most commonly observed in the wrists and fingers but may also appear during any sustained voluntary action. Typically, it signals hepatic, renal, or pulmonary disease, and it's considered a hallmark of hepatic encephalopathy.

To elicit asterixis, have the patient extend his arms, dorsiflex his wrists, and spread his fingers (or do this for him, if necessary). Briefly observe for asterixis. Alternately, if the patient has a decreased level of consciousness but can follow verbal commands, ask him to squeeze two of your fingers. Consider rapid clutching and unclutching positive for asterixis. Or, elevate the patient's leg off the bed and dorsiflex the foot, and observe for asterixis in the ankle. If the patient can tightly close his eyes and mouth, observe for irregular tremulous movements of the eyelids and corners of the mouth. If he can stick out his tongue, observe for continuous quivering.

Emergency interventions

Because asterixis may signal serious metabolic deterioration, quickly evaluate the patient's neurologic status and vital signs. Compare these data to his baseline, and watch carefully for acute changes. Continue to closely monitor neurologic status, vital signs, and urine output.

Watch for signs of respiratory insufficiency and be prepared to provide endotracheal intubation and ventilatory support. Also, be alert for complications of end-stage hepatic, renal, or pulmonary disease.

If the patient has hepatic disease, assess for early signs of hemorrhage, including restlessness, tachypnea, and cool, moist, pale skin. If the patient is jaundiced, check for pallor in the conjunctiva and mucous membranes of the mouth.

It's important to recognize that hypotension, oliguria, hematemesis, and melena are late signs of hemorrhage. Prepare to insert a large-bore I.V. line for fluid and blood replacement. Position the patient flat in bed with his legs elevated 20 degrees. Begin or continue to administer oxygen.

If the patient has renal disease, briefly review what type of therapy he has received. If he's on dialysis, ask about the frequency of treatments to help gauge the severity of disease. Question a family member if the patient's level of consciousness is significantly decreased.

Then assess for hyperkalemia and metabolic acidosis. Look for tachycardia, nausea, diarrhea, abdominal cramps, muscle weakness, hyperreflexia, and Kussmaul's respirations. Prepare to administer sodium bicarbonate, calcium gluconate, dextrose, insulin, or Kayexalate.

If the patient has pulmonary disease, assess for labored respirations, tachypnea, accessory muscle use, and cyanosis, which are critical signs. Prepare to provide ventilatory support via nasal cannula, mask, or intubation and mechanical ventilation.

Common medical causes

◆ ***Hepatic encephalopathy.*** A life-threatening disorder, hepatic encephalopathy initially causes mild personality changes and a slight tremor. The tremor progresses into asterixis and is accompanied by lethargy, aberrant behavior, and apraxia. Eventually, the patient becomes stuporous and displays hyperventilation. When he slips into a coma, hyperactive reflexes, a positive Babinski's sign, and fetor hepaticus are characteristic signs. The patient also may experience bradycardia, decreased respirations, and seizures.

◆ ***Portal systemic encephalopathy.*** Asterixis is a classic symptom of this complex neuropsychiatric syndrome. Other symptoms cover the wide range from lethargy and confusion to coma.

◆ ***Uremic syndrome.*** This life-threatening disorder initially causes lethargy, somnolence, confusion, disorientation, behavior changes, and irritability. Eventually, signs and symptoms appear in diverse body systems. Asterixis is accompanied by stupor, paresthesia, muscle twitching, fasciculations, and footdrop. Other signs and symptoms include polyuria and nocturia followed by oliguria and, then, anuria; elevated blood pressure; signs of heart failure and pericarditis; Kussmaul's respirations; anorexia; nausea; vomiting; diarrhea; GI bleeding; weight loss; ammonia breath odor; and metallic taste.

Other causes

◆ ***Drugs.*** Certain drugs, such as the anticonvulsant phenytoin and bronchodilators, may cause asterixis.

Special considerations

Provide simple comfort measures, such as frequent rest periods to minimize fatigue and elevating the head of the bed to relieve dyspnea and orthopnea. Administer oil baths and avoid soap to relieve itching caused by jaundice and uremia. Provide emotional support to the patient and his family.

Provide enteral or parenteral nutrition if the patient is intubated or has a decreased level of consciousness. Closely monitor serum and urine glucose levels to evaluate hyperalimentation. Because the patient will probably be on bed rest, reposition him at least once every 2 hours to prevent skin breakdown. Also, recognize that his debilitated state makes him prone to infection. Observe strict handwashing and aseptic technique when changing dressings and caring for invasive lines.

Pediatric pointers

End-stage hepatic, renal, and pulmonary disease may also cause asterixis in children.

Ataxia

Classified as cerebellar or sensory, ataxia refers to incoordination and irregularity of voluntary, purposeful movements. *Cerebellar ataxia* results from disease of the cerebellum and its pathways to and from the cerebral cortex, brain stem, and spinal cord. It causes gait, trunk, limb and, possibly, speech disorders. Sensory ataxia results from impaired position sense (proprioception) due to interruption of afferent nerve fibers in the peripheral nerves, posterior roots, posterior columns of the spinal cord, or medial lemnisci or is occasionally caused by a lesion in both parietal lobes. It causes gait disorders. (*See Identifying ataxia*, page 56.)

Ataxia occurs in acute and chronic forms. *Acute ataxia* may result from cerebrovascular accident (CVA), hemorrhage, or a large tumor in the posterior fossa. In this life-threatening condition, the cerebellum may herniate downward through the foramen magnum behind the cervical spinal cord or upward through the tentorium on the cerebral hemispheres. Herniation may also compress the brain stem. Acute ataxia may also result from drug toxicity or poisoning. *Chronic ataxia* can be progressive and, at times, can result from acute disease. It can also occur in metabolic and chronic degenerative neurologic disease.

Emergency interventions

If ataxic movements suddenly develop, examine the patient for signs of increased intracranial pressure and impending herniation. Determine his level of consciousness (LOC) and be alert for pupillary changes, motor weakness or paralysis, neck stiffness or pain, and vomiting. Check vital signs, especially respirations; abnormal respiratory patterns may quickly lead to respiratory arrest. Elevate the head of the bed to promote venous drainage. Have

Identifying ataxia

Ataxia may be observed in the patient's speech, in the movements of his trunk and limbs, or in his gait.

SPEECH ATAXIA

- A form of dysarthria
- Patient typically speaks slowly and stresses usually unstressed words and syllables
- Speech content not affected

TRUNCAL ATAXIA

- A disturbance in equilibrium
- Patient can't sit or stand without falling
- Head and trunk may bob and sway (titubation)
- Reeling gait if walking is possible

LIMB ATAXIA

- Loss of ability to gauge distance, speed, and power of movement, resulting in poorly controlled, variable, and inaccurate voluntary movements
- Movement may be too quick or too slow; movements may break down into component parts, giving appearance of a puppet or a robot
- Coarse, irregular tremor in purposeful movement (but not at rest) and reduced muscle tone

GAIT ATAXIA

- Wide-based, unsteady, irregular gait
- *Cerebellar ataxia:* patient may stagger or lurch in zigzag fashion, turn with extreme difficulty, and lose his balance when his feet are together
- *Sensory ataxia:* patient moves abruptly and stomps or taps his feet because he throws his feet forward and outward, then brings them down first on the heels, then on the toes; patient fixes his eyes on the ground, watching his steps or, if unable to watch them, staggering worsens; sways or loses balance when standing with feet together

emergency resuscitation equipment readily available. Prepare the patient for computed tomography scanning or surgery. Immediate interventions may include intubation followed by hyperventilation, osmotic diuretics, steroids, and elevation of the head of the bed.

History and physical examination

If the patient isn't in distress, review his history. Ask about multiple sclerosis, diabetes, central nervous system infection, neoplastic disease, previous CVA, and a family history of ataxia. Also, ask about chronic alcohol abuse or prolonged exposure to industrial toxins such as mercury. Find out if the patient's ataxia developed suddenly or gradually.

If necessary, perform the Romberg test to help distinguish between cerebellar and sensory ataxia. Instruct the patient to stand with his feet together and his arms at his side. Note his posture and balance, first with his eyes open, then closed. Test results may indicate normal posture and balance (minimal swaying), cerebellar ataxia (swaying and inability to maintain balance with eyes open or closed), or sensory ataxia (increased swaying and inability to maintain balance with eyes closed). Stand close to the patient during this test to prevent his falling.

If you test for gait and limb ataxia, be aware that motor weakness may mimic ataxic movements, so check motor strength, too. Gait ataxia may be severe, even when there is minimal limb ataxia. In gait ataxia, ask the patient if he tends to fall to one side or if falling occurs more commonly at night. In truncal ataxia, remember that the patient's inability to walk or stand, combined with the absence of other signs while he's lying down, may give the impression of hysteria or drug or alcohol intoxication.

Common medical causes

◆ ***Cerebellar abscess.*** This disorder commonly causes limb ataxia on the same side as the lesion as well as gait and truncal ataxia. Typically, the initial symptom is headache localized behind the ear or in the occipital region, followed by oculomotor palsy, fever, vomiting, altered LOC, and coma.

◆ ***CVA.*** In this disorder, occlusions in the vertebrobasilar arteries halt blood flow to cause infarction in the medulla, pons, or cerebellum that may lead to ataxia. Ataxia may occur at the onset of CVA and remain as a residual deficit. Worsening ataxia during the acute phase may indicate extension of the CVA or severe swelling. Ataxia may be accompanied by unilateral or bilateral motor weakness, possible altered LOC, sensory loss, vertigo, nausea, vomiting, oculomotor palsy, and dysphagia.

◆ ***Diabetic neuropathy.*** Peripheral nerve damage due to diabetes mellitus may cause sensory ataxia as well as extremity pain, slight leg weakness, skin changes, and bowel and bladder dysfunction.

◆ ***Diphtheria.*** Within 4 to 8 weeks of the onset of symptoms, a life-threatening neuropathy can produce sensory ataxia. Diphtheria can be accompanied by fever, paresthesia, and paralysis of the limbs and, sometimes, the respiratory muscles.

◆ ***Friedreich's ataxia.*** This progressive familial disorder affects the spinal cord and cerebellum. It causes gait ataxia, followed by truncal, limb, and speech ataxia. Other features include pes cavus, kyphoscoliosis, cranial nerve palsy, and motor and sensory deficits. A positive Babinski's reflex may appear.

◆ ***Hepatocerebral degeneration.*** Patients who survive hepatic coma are occasionally left with residual neurologic defects, including mild cerebellar ataxia with a wide-based, unsteady gait. Ataxia may be accompanied by altered LOC, dysarthria, rhythmic arm tremors, and choreoathetosis of the face, neck, and shoulders.

◆ ***Multiple sclerosis (MS).*** Nystagmus and cerebellar ataxia commonly occur in this disorder, but they aren't always accompanied by limb weakness and spasticity. Speech ataxia (especially scanning) may occur as well as sensory ataxia from spinal cord involvement. During remissions, ataxia may subside or even disappear. During exacerbations, it may reappear, worsen, or even become permanent. Multiple sclerosis also causes optic neuritis, optic atrophy, numbness and weakness, diplopia, dizziness, and bladder dysfunction.

◆ ***Olivopontocerebellar atrophy.*** This disease produces gait ataxia and, later, limb and speech ataxia. Rarely, it produces an intention tremor. It's accompanied by choreiform movements, dysphagia, and loss of sphincter tone.

◆ ***Poisoning.*** Chronic *arsenic poisoning* may cause sensory ataxia, along with headache, seizures, altered LOC, motor deficits, and muscle aching. Chronic *mercury poisoning* causes gait ataxia and limb ataxia, principally of the arms. It also causes tremors of the extremities, tongue, and lips; mental confusion; mood changes; and dysarthria.

◆ ***Polyneuropathy.*** Carcinomatous and myelomatous polyneuropathy may occur before detection of the primary tumor in cancer, multiple myeloma, or Hodgkin's disease. Signs and symptoms include ataxia, severe motor weakness, muscle atrophy, and sensory loss in the limbs. Pain and skin changes may also occur.

◆ ***Posterior fossa tumor.*** Gait, truncal, or limb ataxia is an early sign and may worsen as the tumor enlarges. It's accompanied by vomiting, headache, papilledema, vertigo, oculomotor palsy, decreased LOC, and motor and sensory impairments on the same side as the lesion.

◆ ***Spinocerebellar ataxia.*** In this disorder, the patient may initially experience fatigue, followed by stiff-legged gait ataxia. Eventually, limb ataxia, dysarthria, static tremor, nystagmus, cramps, paresthesia, and sensory deficits occur.

◆ ***Wernicke's disease.*** The result of thiamine deficiency, this disease produces gait ataxia and, rarely, intention tremor or speech ataxia. In severe ataxia, the patient may be unable to stand or walk. Ataxia decreases with thiamine therapy.

Associated signs include nystagmus, diplopia, ocular palsies, confusion, tachycardia, exertional dyspnea, and orthostatic hypotension.

Other causes

♦ ***Drugs.*** Toxic levels of anticonvulsants, especially phenytoin, anticholinergics, or tricyclic antidepressants may cause gait ataxia. Aminoglutethimide causes ataxia in about 10% of patients; however, this effect usually disappears 4 to 6 weeks after drug therapy is discontinued.

Special considerations

Prepare the patient for laboratory studies, such as blood tests for toxic drug levels and radiologic tests. Then focus on helping the patient adapt to his condition. Promote rehabilitation goals and help ensure the patient's safety. For example, instruct the patient with sensory ataxia to move slowly, especially when turning or getting up from a chair. Provide a cane or walker for extra support. Ask the patient's family to check his home for hazards, such as uneven surfaces or the absence of handrails on stairs. If appropriate, refer the patient with progressive disease for counseling.

Pediatric pointers

In children, ataxia occurs in acute and chronic forms. Acute ataxia may result from febrile infection, brain tumors, mumps, and other disorders. Causes of chronic ataxia include Gaucher's disease, Refsum's disease, and other inborn errors of metabolism.

When assessing a child for ataxia, consider his level of motor skills and emotional state. Your examination may be limited to observing the child in spontaneous activity and carefully questioning his parents about changes in his motor activity, such as increased unsteadiness or falling. If you suspect ataxia, refer the child for a neurologic evaluation to rule out brain tumor.

AURA

An aura is a sensory or motor phenomenon, idea, or emotion that marks the initial stage of a seizure or the approach of a classic migraine headache. Auras may be classified as cognitive, affective, psychosensory, or psychomotor. (See *Types of auras.*)

An aura associated with a seizure stems from an irritable focus in the brain that spreads throughout the cortex. Although once considered a sign of impending seizure, an aura is now considered the first stage of a seizure. Typically, it occurs seconds to minutes before the ictal phase. Its intensity, duration, and type depend on the origin of the irritable focus. For example, an aura of bitter taste commonly accompanies a frontal lobe lesion, or a seizure arising from a focus in the motor trip area may produce twitching in the thumb or finger. Unfortunately, an aura is difficult to describe because the postictal phase of a seizure temporarily alters the patient's level of consciousness, impairing his memory of the event.

The aura associated with a classic migraine headache results from cranial vasoconstriction. Diagnostically important, it helps distinguish a classic migraine from other types of headaches. Typically, an aura develops over 10 to 30 minutes and varies in intensity and duration. If the patient recognizes the aura as a warning sign, he may be able to prevent the headache by taking appropriate drugs.

Emergency interventions

When an aura rapidly progresses to the ictal phase of a seizure, quickly evaluate the seizure and be alert for life-threatening complications such as apnea (see "Seizure"). When an aura heralds a classic migraine, make the patient as comfortable as possible. Place him in a dark, quiet room and administer drugs to prevent the headache, if necessary.

History and physical examination
Later, obtain a thorough history of the patient's headaches or seizure history, asking him to describe any preceding sensory or motor phenomena. Find out how long each headache or seizure typically lasts. Does anything make it worse, such as bright lights, noise, or caffeine? Does anything make it better? Ask the patient about drugs he takes for pain relief.

Common medical causes
♦ ***Classic migraine headache.*** A migraine is preceded by a vague premonition and then, usually, a visual aura of flashing light. The aura lasts 10 to 30 minutes and may intensify until it completely obscures the patient's vision. A classic migraine may cause numbness or tingling of lips, face, or hands; slight confusion; and dizziness before the characteristic unilateral, throbbing headache. It slowly intensifies and, at its peak, may cause photophobia, nausea, and vomiting.
♦ ***Seizure, generalized tonic-clonic.*** A generalized tonic-clonic seizure may begin with or without an aura. The patient loses consciousness and falls to the ground. His body stiffens (tonic phase); then he experiences rapid, synchronous muscle jerking and hyperventilation (clonic phase). The seizure usually lasts 2 to 5 minutes.

Special considerations
Advise the patient to keep a diary of factors that precipitate each headache, as well as associated symptoms, to enable you to evaluate the effectiveness of drug therapy and to recommend lifestyle changes. Stress-reduction measures frequently play a role here.

Pediatric pointers
Watch for nonverbal clues possibly associated with aura, such as rubbing the eyes, coughing, and spitting. When taking the seizure history, recognize that children — like adults — tend to forget the aura. Ask simple, direct questions, such as "Do you see anything funny before the seizure?" "Do you get a bad taste in your mouth?" Give the child ample time to respond because he may have difficulty describing the aura.

Types of auras

Determining whether an aura marks the patient's thought processes, emotions, or sensory or motor function frequently requires keen observation. An aura is typically difficult to describe and is only dimly remembered when associated with seizure activity. Here you'll find the types of auras the patient may experience.

COGNITIVE
♦ Déjà vu (familiarity with unfamiliar events or environments)
♦ Jamais vu (unfamiliarity with a known event)
♦ Time standing still
♦ Flashback of past events

AFFECTIVE
♦ Fear
♦ Paranoia
♦ Other emotions

PSYCHOSENSORY
♦ *Visual:* flashes of light (scintillations)
♦ *Olfactory:* foul odors
♦ *Gustatory:* acidic, metallic, or bitter tastes
♦ *Auditory:* buzzing or ringing in the ears
♦ *Tactile:* numbness or tingling
♦ Vertigo

PSYCHOMOTOR AURAS
♦ Automatisms (inappropriate, repetitive movements): lip smacking, chewing, swallowing, grimacing, picking at clothes, climbing stairs

B

BABINSKI'S REFLEX
[Extensor plantar reflex]

Babinski's reflex — dorsiflexion of the great toe with extension and fanning of the other toes — is elicited by firmly stroking the lateral aspect of the sole of the foot with a blunt object. (See *How to elicit Babinski's reflex.*) A positive Babinski's reflex is normal in neonates and in infants up to 24 months old. An indicator of corticospinal damage, Babinski's reflex may occur unilaterally or bilaterally. In some patients, it can be triggered by noxious stimuli, such as pain, noise, or even bumping of the bed. It may also be temporary or permanent. A temporary Babinski's reflex commonly occurs during the postictal phase of a seizure, whereas a permanent Babinski's reflex reflects corticospinal damage.

History and physical examination
After eliciting a positive Babinski's reflex, evaluate the patient for other neurologic signs. Evaluate muscle strength in each extremity by having the patient push or pull against your resistance. Passively flex and extend the extremity to assess muscle tone. Intermittent resistance to flexion and extension indicates spasticity, and a lack of resistance indicates flaccidity.

Next, check for evidence of incoordination by asking the patient to perform a repetitive activity. Test deep tendon reflexes (DTRs) in the patient's elbow, antecubital area, wrist, knee, and ankle by striking the tendon with a reflex hammer. An exaggerated muscle response indicates hyperactive DTRs; little or no muscle response indicates hypoactivity.

Then evaluate pain sensation and proprioception in the feet. As you move the patient's toes up and down, ask the patient to identify the direction in which the toes have been moved without looking at his feet.

Common medical causes
♦ ***Amyotrophic lateral sclerosis (ALS).*** In this progressive motor neuron disorder, bilateral Babinski's reflex may occur with hyperactive DTRs and spasticity. Typically, ALS causes fasciculations accompanied by muscle atrophy and weakness. Incoordination makes carrying out activities of daily living difficult for the patient. Associated signs and symptoms include impaired speech; difficulty chewing, swallowing, and breathing; urinary frequency and urgency; and, occasionally, choking and excessive drooling. Although his mental status remains intact, the patient's poor prognosis may cause periodic depression. Progressive bulbar palsy involves the brain stem and may cause episodes of crying or inappropriate laughter.

♦ ***Brain tumor.*** When it involves the corticospinal tract, a brain tumor may produce Babinski's reflex. The reflex may

EXAMINATION TIP

How to elicit Babinski's reflex

To elicit Babinski's reflex, stroke the lateral aspect of the sole of the patient's foot with your thumbnail or another moderately sharp object. Normally, this elicits flexion of all toes (a negative Babinski's reflex), as shown at left. In a positive Babinski's reflex, the great toe dorsiflexes and the other toes fan out, as shown at right.

NEGATIVE BABINSKI'S REFLEX

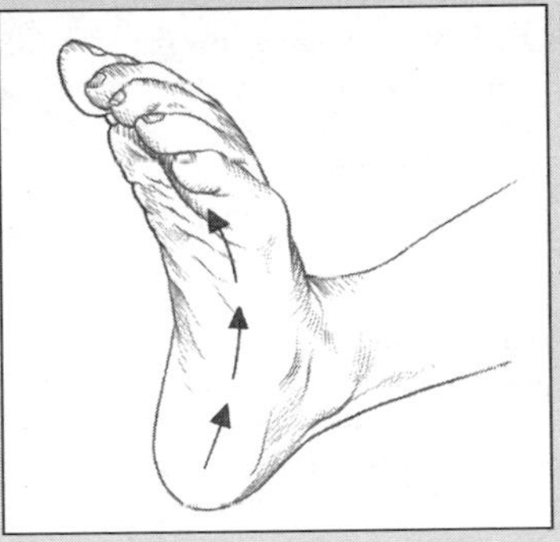

POSITIVE BABINSKI'S REFLEX

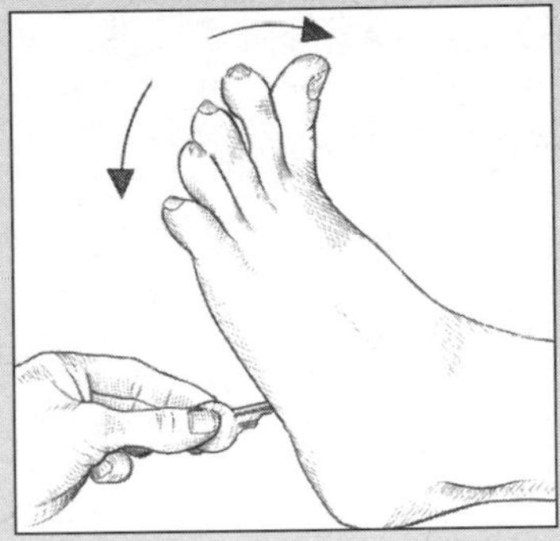

be accompanied by hyperactive DTRs (unilateral or bilateral), spasticity, seizures, cranial nerve dysfunction, hemiparesis or hemiplegia, decreased pain sensation, unsteady gait, incoordination, headache, emotional lability, and decreased level of consciousness (LOC).

♦ ***Cerebrovascular accident (CVA).*** Babinski's reflex varies with the site of the CVA. If the CVA involves the cerebrum, it produces unilateral Babinski's reflex accompanied by hemiplegia or hemiparesis, unilateral hyperactive DTRs, hemianopsia, and aphasia. If it involves the brain stem, it produces bilateral Babinski's reflex accompanied by bilateral weakness or paralysis, bilateral hyperactive DTRs, cranial nerve dysfunction, incoordination, and unsteady gait. Generalized signs and symptoms of CVA may include headache, vomiting, fever, disorientation, nuchal rigidity, seizures, and coma.

♦ ***Head trauma.*** Unilateral or bilateral Babinski's reflex may occur as the result of primary corticospinal damage or secondary injury associated with increased intracranial pressure. Hyperactive DTRs and spasticity commonly occur with Babinski's reflex. The patient may also exhibit weakness and incoordination. Other signs and symptoms vary with the type of head trauma and include headache, vomiting, behavior changes, altered vital signs, and decreased LOC with abnormal pupil size and response to light.

♦ ***Hepatic encephalopathy.*** Babinski's reflex occurs late in this disorder when the patient slips into a coma. It's accompanied by hyperactive DTRs and fetor hepaticus.

♦ ***Meningitis.*** In this infection, bilateral Babinski's reflex commonly follows fever, chills, and malaise and is accompanied by nausea and vomiting. As meningitis progresses, it also causes decreased LOC, nuchal rigidity, positive Brudzinski's and Kernig's signs, hyperactive DTRs, and opisthotonos. Associated signs and symptoms include irritability, photophobia, diplopia, delirium, and deep stupor that may progress to coma.

♦ ***Rabies.*** Bilateral Babinski's reflex — possibly elicited by nonspecific noxious stimuli alone — appears in the excitation phase of rabies. This phase occurs 2 to 10 days after the onset of prodromal symptoms, such as fever, malaise, and irritability (which occur 30 to 40 days after an animal bite). Rabies is characterized by marked restlessness and extremely painful pharyngeal muscle spasms. Difficulty swallowing causes excessive drooling and hydrophobia in about 50% of affected patients. Seizures and hyperactive DTRs may also occur.

♦ ***Spinal cord injury.*** In acute injury, spinal shock temporarily erases all reflexes. As shock resolves, Babinski's reflex occurs — unilaterally when injury affects only one side of the spinal cord (Brown-Séquard syndrome), bilaterally when injury affects both sides. Rather than signaling the return of neurologic function, this reflex confirms corticospinal damage. It's accompanied by hyperactive DTRs, spasticity, and variable or total loss of pain and temperature sensation, proprioception, and motor function. Horner's syndrome, marked by unilateral ptosis, pupillary constriction, and facial anhidrosis, may occur with lower cervical cord injury.

♦ ***Spinal paralytic poliomyelitis.*** Unilateral or bilateral Babinski's reflex occurs 5 to 7 days after the onset of fever in this disorder. It's accompanied by progressive weakness, paresthesia, muscle tenderness, spasticity, irritability and, later, atrophy. Resistance to neck flexion is characteristic, as are Hoyne's, Kernig's, and Brudzinski's signs.

♦ ***Syringomyelia.*** In this disorder, bilateral Babinski's reflex occurs with muscle atrophy and weakness that may progress to paralysis. It's accompanied by spasticity, ataxia and, occasionally, deep pain. DTRs may be hypoactive or hyperactive. Cranial nerve dysfunction, such as dysphagia and dysarthria, commonly appears late in the disorder.

Special considerations

Babinski's reflex usually occurs with incoordination, weakness, and spasticity, all of which increase the patient's risk of injury. To prevent injury, assist the patient with activity and keep his environment free of obstructions.

Diagnostic tests may include a computed tomography scan or magnetic resonance imaging of the brain or spine, angiography or myelography and, possibly, a lumbar puncture to clarify or confirm the cause of Babinski's reflex. Prepare the patient as necessary.

Pediatric pointers

Babinski's reflex is a normal finding in infants up to 24 months old, reflecting immaturity of the corticospinal tract. After age 2, Babinski's reflex is pathologic and may result from hydrocephalus or any of the causes more commonly seen in adults.

BACK PAIN

Back pain affects an estimated 80% of the population; in fact, it's the second leading reason — after the common cold — for lost time from work. Although this symptom may herald a spondylogenic disorder, it may also result from genitourinary, GI, cardiovascular, or neoplastic disorders. Postural imbalance associated with pregnancy may also cause back pain. The most common cause is simple back strain from a particular or repetitive injury.

The onset, location, and distribution of pain and its response to activity and rest provide important clues about the causative disorder. Pain may be acute or chronic, constant or intermittent. It may remain localized in the back or radiate along the spine or down one or both legs. Pain may be exacerbated by activity—usually bending, stooping, or lifting—and alleviated by rest, or it may be unaffected by both.

Intrinsic back pain results from muscle spasm, nerve root irritation, fracture, or a combination of these mechanisms. It usually occurs in the lower back, or lumbosacral area. Back pain may also be referred from the abdomen or flank, possibly signaling a life-threatening perforated ulcer, acute pancreatitis, or dissecting abdominal aortic aneurysm.

Emergency interventions

If the patient reports *acute, severe back pain,* quickly take his vital signs; then perform a rapid evaluation to rule out life-threatening causes such as abdominal aortic aneurysm. Ask him when the pain began. Can he relate it to any causes? For example, did the pain occur after eating? After falling on the ice? Have the patient describe the pain. Is it burning, stabbing, throbbing, or aching? Is it constant or intermittent? Does it radiate to the buttocks or legs? Does he have any leg weakness? Or, does the pain seem to originate in the abdomen and radiate to the back? Has he had a pain like this before? What makes it better or worse? Is it affected by activity or rest? Is it worse in the morning or evening? Does it wake him up? Typically, visceral referred back pain is unaffected by activity and rest. In contrast, pain of musculoskeletal origin worsens with activity and improves with rest. Pain of neoplastic origin can be quite severe, unrelenting, and unresponsive to attempts to relieve it. It's commonly exacerbated by any activity.

If the patient describes *deep lumbar or thoracic pain unaffected by activity,* palpate for a pulsating epigastric mass. If this sign is present, suspect dissecting abdominal aortic aneurysm. Obtain an emergency ultrasound and withhold food and fluid in anticipation of possible emergency surgery. Start I.V. fluid replacement and oxygen administration.

If the patient describes severe epigastric pain that radiates through the abdomen to the back, assess for absent bowel sounds and for abdominal rigidity and tenderness. If these occur, suspect perforated ulcer or acute pancreatitis. Start an I.V. for fluids and drugs, administer oxygen, and withhold food. You may insert a nasogastric tube to check stomach contents to rule out an acute gastric bleed.

History and physical examination

If life-threatening causes of back pain are ruled out, continue with a more complete history and physical examination. Be alert to the patient's expressions of pain as you do so. Obtain a medical history, including past injuries and illnesses, and a family history. Ask about diet and alcohol intake. Also, take a drug history, including past and present prescriptions and over-the-counter drugs.

Next, perform a thorough physical examination. Observe skin color, especially in the patient's legs, and palpate skin temperature. Palpate femoral, popliteal, posterior tibial, and pedal pulses. Ask about unusual sensations in the legs, such as numbness and tingling. Observe the patient's posture if pain doesn't prohibit standing. Does he stand erect or tend to lean toward one side? Observe the level of the shoulders and pelvis and the curvature of the back. Ask the patient to bend forward, backward, and from side to side while you palpate for paravertebral muscle spasms. Note rotation of the spine on the trunk. Palpate the dorsolumbar spine for point tenderness. Then ask the patient to walk—first on his heels, then on his toes; protect him from falling as he does so. Weakness may reflect a muscular disorder or spinal nerve root irritation. Place the patient in a sitting position to evaluate and compare patellar tendon (knee), Achilles tendon, and Babinski's reflexes. Evaluate the strength of the extensor hallucis longus by asking the patient to hold up his big toe against resistance. Measure leg length and hamstring and quadriceps muscles bilaterally. Note a difference of more than 1 cm in muscle size, especially in the calf.

To reproduce leg and back pain, position the patient supine on the examining table. Grasp his heel and slowly lift his leg. If he feels pain, note its exact location and the angle between the table and his leg when it occurs. Repeat this maneuver with the opposite leg. Pain along the sciatic nerve may indicate disk herniation or sciatica. Also, note the range of motion of the hip and knee.

Palpate the flanks and percuss with the fingertips or perform fist percussion to elicit costovertebral angle tenderness.

Common medical causes

♦ ***Abdominal aortic aneurysm (dissecting).*** Life-threatening dissection of this aneurysm may initially cause low or middle back pain or dull abdominal pain. More commonly, it causes constant upper abdominal pain. A pulsating abdominal mass may be palpated in the epigastrium; after rupture, however, it no longer pulses. Dissection can also cause mottled skin below the waist, absent femoral and pedal pulses, lower blood pressure in the legs than in the arms, mild to moderate tenderness with guarding, and abdominal rigidity. Signs of shock, such as cool, clammy skin, appear if blood loss is significant.

♦ ***Ankylosing spondylitis.*** This chronic, progressive disorder causes sacroiliac pain, which radiates up the spine and is aggravated by lateral pressure on the pelvis. The pain is usually most severe in the morning or after a period of inactivity and isn't relieved by rest. Abnormal rigidity of the lumbar spine with forward flexion is also characteristic. This disorder can cause local tenderness, fatigue, fever, anorexia, weight loss, and iritis.

♦ ***Appendicitis.*** In this life-threatening disorder, a vague and dull discomfort in the epigastric or umbilical region classically but not always migrates to McBurney's point in the right lower quadrant. In retrocecal appendicitis, pain may also radiate to the back. The shift in pain is preceded by anorexia and nausea and is accompanied by fever, occasional vomiting, abdominal tenderness (especially over McBurney's point), and rebound tenderness. Some patients also have painful, urgent urination.

♦ ***Cholecystitis.*** This disorder causes severe pain in the right upper quadrant of the abdomen that may radiate to the right shoulder blade, chest, back, or the right "purse strap" location. It may arise suddenly or increase gradually over several hours, and patients usually have a history of similar pain after a high-fat meal. Accompanying signs and symptoms include anorexia, fever, nausea, vomiting, right-upper-quadrant tenderness, abdominal rigidity, pallor, and diaphoresis.

♦ ***Chordoma.*** A slowly developing malignant tumor, chordoma causes persistent pain in the lower back, sacrum, and coccyx. As the tumor expands, pain may be accompanied by constipation and bowel and bladder incontinence.

♦ ***Endometriosis.*** This disorder causes deep sacral pain and severe, cramping pain in the lower abdomen. The pain worsens just before or during menstruation and may be aggravated by defecation. It's accompanied by constipation, abdominal tenderness, dysmenorrhea, and dyspareunia.

♦ ***Intervertebral disk rupture.*** This disorder causes gradual or sudden lower back pain with or without leg pain (sciatica). It rarely causes leg pain alone. Pain usually begins in the back and radiates to the buttocks and leg. The pain is exacerbated by activity, coughing, and sneezing and is eased by rest. It's accompanied by paresthesia (most commonly, numbness or tingling in the lower leg and foot), paravertebral muscle spasm, and decreased reflexes on the affected side. This disorder also affects posture and gait. The patient's spine is slightly flexed, and he leans toward the painful side. He walks slowly and rises from a sitting to a standing position with extreme difficulty.

♦ ***Lumbosacral sprain.*** This disorder causes aching, localized pain, and tenderness associated with muscle spasm on lateral motion. The recumbent patient typically flexes his knees and hips to help ease pain. Flexion of the spine intensifies pain. The pain worsens with movement and is relieved by rest.

♦ ***Metastatic tumors.*** These tumors commonly spread to the spine, causing lower back pain in at least 25% of patients. Typically, the pain begins abruptly, is accompanied by cramping muscular pain (usually worse at night), and isn't relieved by rest.

♦ ***Myeloma.*** Back pain caused by this primary malignant tumor frequently begins abruptly and worsens with exercise. It may be accompanied by arthritic symptoms, such as achiness, joint swelling, and tenderness. Other clinical effects include fever, malaise, peripheral paresthesia, and weight loss.

♦ ***Pancreatitis (acute).*** This life-threatening disorder usually causes fulminating, continuous upper abdominal pain that may radiate to both flanks and to the back. To relieve this pain, the patient may bend forward, draw his knees to his chest, or move restlessly about.

Early associated signs and symptoms include abdominal tenderness, nausea, vomiting, fever, pallor, tachycardia and, in some patients, abdominal guarding, rigidity, rebound tenderness, and hypoactive bowel sounds. A late sign may be jaundice. Occurring as inflammation subsides, Turner's sign (ecchymosis of the abdomen or flank) or Cullen's sign (bluish discoloration of skin around the umbilicus and in both flanks) signals hemorrhagic pancreatitis.

♦ ***Perforated ulcer.*** In some patients, perforation of a duodenal or gastric ulcer causes sudden, prostrating epigastric pain that may radiate throughout the abdomen and to the back. This life-threatening disorder also causes boardlike abdominal rigidity, tenderness with guarding, generalized rebound tenderness, the absence of bowel sounds, and grunting, shallow respirations. Associated signs commonly include fever, tachycardia, and hypotension.

♦ ***Prostatic carcinoma.*** Chronic aching back pain may be the only symptom of prostate cancer. This disorder may also cause hematuria and decrease the urine stream.

♦ ***Pyelonephritis (acute).*** This disorder causes progressive flank and lower abdominal pain accompanied by back pain or tenderness (especially over the costovertebral angle). Other signs and symptoms include high fever and chills, nausea and vomiting, flank and abdominal tenderness, and urinary frequency and urgency.

♦ ***Renal calculi.*** The colicky pain of this disorder usually results from irritation of the ureteral lining, which increases the frequency and force of peristaltic contractions. The pain travels from the costovertebral angle to the flank, suprapubic region, and external genitalia. Its intensity varies but may become excruciating if calculi travel down a ureter. If calculi are in the renal pelvis and calyces, dull and constant flank pain may occur. Renal calculi also cause nausea, vomiting, urinary urgency (if a calculus lodges near the bladder), hematuria, and agitation due to pain. Pain resolves or significantly decreases after calculi move to the bladder. Encourage the patient to recover the calculi for analysis by straining his urine.

♦ ***Spinal neoplasm (benign).*** This disorder typically causes severe, localized back pain.

♦ ***Spinal stenosis.*** Resembling a ruptured intervertebral disk, this disorder causes back pain with or without sciatica. Frequently, sciatica affects both legs. The pain may radiate to the toes and may progress to numbness or weakness unless the patient rests.

♦ ***Spondylolisthesis.*** A major structural disorder characterized by forward slippage of one vertebra onto another, spondylolisthesis may be asymptomatic or may cause lower back pain with or without nerve root involvement. Associated symptoms of nerve root involvement include paresthesia, buttock pain, and pain radiating down the leg. Palpation of the lumbar spine may reveal a "step-off" of the spinous process. Flexion of the spine may be limited.

♦ ***Transverse process fracture.*** This fracture causes severe localized back pain with muscle spasm and hematoma.

♦ ***Vertebral compression fracture.*** Initially, this fracture may be painless. Several weeks later, it causes back pain aggravated by weight bearing and local tenderness. Fracture of a thoracic vertebra may cause referred pain in the lumbar area.

♦ ***Vertebral osteomyelitis.*** Initially, this disorder causes insidious back pain. As it progresses, the pain may become constant, more pronounced at night, and aggravated by spinal movement. Accompanying symptoms include vertebral and hamstring spasms, tenderness of the spinous processes, fever, and malaise.

♦ ***Vertebral osteoporosis.*** This disorder causes chronic, aching back pain that is aggravated by activity and somewhat relieved by rest. Tenderness may also occur.

Other causes

♦ ***Neurologic tests.*** Lumbar puncture and myelography can cause transient back pain.

Special considerations

If back pain suggests a life-threatening cause, monitor the patient closely. Be alert for increasing pain, altered neurovascular status in the legs, loss of bowel or bladder control, altered vital signs, diaphoresis, and cyanosis.

Until a tentative diagnosis is made, withhold analgesics, which may mask symptoms. Also withhold food and fluids in case surgery is necessary. Make the patient as comfortable as possible by elevating the head of the bed and placing a pillow under his knees. Encourage relaxation techniques such as deep breathing. Prepare the patient for a rectal or pelvic examination. He also may require routine blood tests, urinalysis, computed tomography scan, appropriate biopsies, and X-rays of the chest, abdomen, and spine.

Refer the patient to a brace specialist for a properly fitted corset or lumbosacral support. Instruct him not to wear this in bed. He may also require heat or cold therapy, a backboard, a convoluted foam mattress, or pelvic traction. Explain these pain-relief measures to the patient. Teach the patient about alternatives to analgesic drugs, such as biofeedback and transcutaneous electrical nerve stimulation. Refer the patient to other professionals, such as a physical therapist, an occupational therapist, or a psychologist, if indicated.

Pediatric pointers

Because a child may have difficulty describing back pain, be alert for nonverbal clues, such as wincing or refusal to walk. Closely observe family dynamics during history taking for clues suggesting child abuse.

Back pain in the child may stem from intervertebral disk inflammation (diskitis), neoplasms, idiopathic juvenile osteoporosis, and spondylolisthesis. Disk herniation typically doesn't cause back pain. Scoliosis rarely causes back pain.

Geriatric pointers

Suspect metastatic cancer, especially of the prostate, in older patients with a recent onset of back pain that usually isn't relieved by rest and worsens at night.

BATTLE'S SIGN

Battle's sign — ecchymosis over the mastoid process of the temporal bone — is commonly the only outward sign of a basilar skull fracture. In fact, this type of fracture may go undetected even by skull X-rays. If left untreated, it can be fatal because of associated injury to the nearby cranial nerves and brain stem as well as to blood vessels and the meninges.

Appearing behind one or both ears, Battle's sign is easily overlooked or even hidden by the patient's hair. During emergency care of a trauma victim, it may be overshadowed by imminently life-threatening or more apparent injuries.

A force that's strong enough to fracture the base of the skull causes Battle's sign by damaging supporting tissues of the mastoid area and causing seepage of blood from the fracture site to the mastoid. Battle's sign usually develops 24 to 36 hours after the fracture and may persist for several days to weeks.

History and physical examination

Perform a complete neurologic examination. Begin with the history. Ask the patient about recent trauma to the head. Did the patient sustain a severe blow to the head? Was he involved in a motor vehicle accident? Note level of consciousness as the patient responds. Does the patient respond quickly or slowly? Are his answers appropriate or does he appear confused?

Check the patient's vital signs; be alert for widening pulse pressure and bradycardia, signs of increased intracranial pressure. Assess cranial nerve function in nerves II, III, IV, VI, VII, and VIII. Evaluate pupillary size and response to light as well as motor and verbal responses. Relate these data to the Glasgow Coma Scale. Also note cerebrospinal fluid (CSF) leakage from the nose or ears. Ask about postnasal drip, which may reflect CSF drainage down the throat. Look for the halo sign — a bloodstain encircled by a yellowish ring — on bed linens or dressings. To confirm that drainage is CSF, test it with a Dextrostix; CSF is positive for glucose, whereas mucus isn't. Follow up the neurologic examination with a complete physical examination to detect other injuries associated with basilar skull fracture.

Common medical causes

♦ ***Basilar skull fracture.*** Battle's sign may be the only outward sign of this fracture, or it may be accompanied by periorbital ecchymosis (raccoon eyes), conjunctival hemorrhage, nystagmus, ocular deviation, epistaxis, anosmia, a bulging tympanic membrane (from CSF or blood accumulation), visible fracture lines on the external auditory canal, tinnitus, impaired hearing, facial paralysis, or vertigo.

Special considerations

Expect the patient with basilar skull fracture to be on bed rest for several days to weeks. Keep him flat to decrease pressure on dural tears and to minimize CSF leakage. Monitor neurologic status closely. Avoid nasogastric intubation and nasopharyngeal suction, both of which may cause cerebral infection. Also, caution the patient against blowing his nose, which may worsen a dural tear.

The patient may need skull X-rays and a computed tomography scan to help confirm basilar skull fracture and to evaluate the severity of head injury. Typically, basilar skull fracture and any associated dural tears heal spontaneously within several days to weeks. However, if the patient has a large dural tear, a craniotomy may be necessary to repair the tear with a graft patch.

Pediatric pointers
Children who are victims of abuse frequently sustain basilar skull fractures from severe blows to the head. As in adults, Battle's sign may be the only outward sign of fracture and, perhaps, the only clue to child abuse. If you suspect child abuse, follow hospital protocol for reporting the incident.

Biot's respirations
[Ataxic respirations]

A late and ominous sign of neurologic deterioration, Biot's respirations are characterized by irregular and unpredictable rate, rhythm, and depth. This rare breathing pattern may appear abruptly and may reflect increased pressure on the medulla coinciding with brain stem compression.

Emergency interventions
Observe the patient's breathing pattern for several minutes to avoid confusing Biot's respirations with other respiratory patterns. (See *Identifying Biot's respirations.*) Prepare to intubate the patient and provide mechanical ventilation. Next, take vital signs, noting especially increased systolic pressure.

Common medical causes
◆ ***Brain stem compression.*** Biot's respirations are characteristic in this neurologic emergency. Rapidly enlarging lesions may cause ataxic respirations and commonly lead to complete respiratory arrest.

Special considerations
Monitor vital signs frequently. Elevate the head of the patient's bed 30 degrees to help reduce intracranial pressure. Prepare the patient for emergency surgery to relieve pressure on the brain stem. Computed tomography scans or magnetic resonance imaging may confirm the cause of brain stem compression.

Because Biot's respirations typically reflect a grave prognosis, give the patient's family information and emotional support.

Identifying Biot's respirations

Biot's respirations, also known as ataxic respirations, have a completely irregular pattern. Both shallow and deep breaths occur randomly, and there are haphazard, irregular pauses. The respiratory rate tends to be slow and may progressively decelerate to apnea.

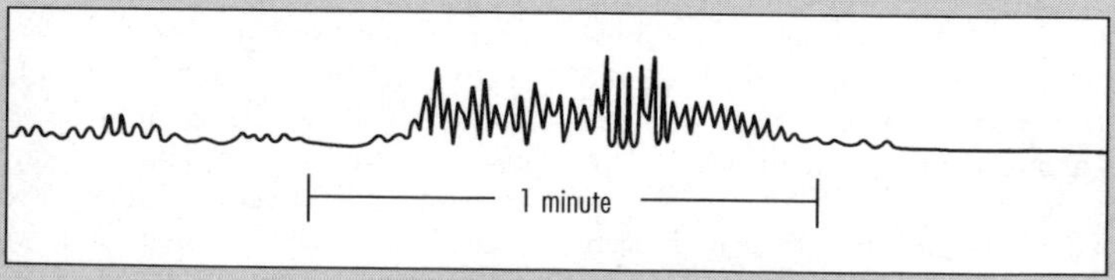

Pediatric pointers
Biot's respirations are rarely seen in children.

Bladder distention

Bladder distention — abnormal enlargement of the bladder — results from an inability to excrete urine, which results in its accumulation. Distention can be caused by mechanical and anatomic obstructions, neuromuscular disorders, and the use of certain drugs. Relatively common in all ages and both sexes, it occurs most frequently in older men with prostate disorders.

Distention usually develops gradually but occasionally has a sudden onset. Gradual distention usually remains asymptomatic until stretching of the bladder causes discomfort. Acute distention causes suprapubic fullness, pressure, and pain. If severe distention isn't corrected promptly by catheterization or massage, the bladder expands upward within the abdomen, its walls become thin, and renal function can be impaired.

Bladder distention is aggravated by intake of caffeine, alcohol, large quantities of fluid, and diuretics. (See *Bladder distention: Common causes and associated findings*, pages 70 and 71.)

Emergency interventions
If the patient has severe distention, insert an indwelling urinary catheter to help relieve discomfort and prevent bladder rupture.

History and physical examination
If distention isn't severe, begin by reviewing the patient's voiding patterns. Find out the time and amount of his last voiding and the amount of fluid consumed since then. Ask if he has difficulty urinating. Does he use Valsalva's or Credé's maneuver to initiate urination? Does he urinate with urgency or without warning? Is urination painful or irritating? Ask about the force and continuity of his urine stream and whether he feels that his bladder is empty after voiding.

Explore the patient's history for urinary tract obstruction or infections; venereal disease; neurologic, intestinal, or pelvic surgery; lower abdominal or urinary tract trauma; and systemic or neurologic disorders. Note his drug history, including use of over-the-counter preparations.

Take the patient's vital signs, and percuss and palpate the bladder. (Remember that an empty bladder can't be palpated through the abdominal wall.) Inspect the urethral meatus and measure its diameter. Describe the appearance and amount of any discharge. Finally, test for perineal sensation and anal sphincter tone; in male patients, examine the prostate gland.

Common medical causes
◆ ***Benign prostatic hyperplasia.*** Bladder distention usually develops gradually as the prostate enlarges but, occasionally, its onset is acute. Initially, the patient experiences urinary hesitancy, straining, and frequency; reduced force of and inability to stop urine stream; nocturia; and postvoiding dribbling. As the disorder progresses, it causes prostate enlargement, sensations of suprapubic fullness and incomplete bladder emptying, perineal pain, constipation, and hematuria.

◆ ***Bladder calculi.*** This disorder may cause bladder distention, but more commonly it causes pain as its only symptom. The pain is usually referred to the tip of the penis, the vulvar area, the lower back, or the heel of the foot. It worsens during walking or exercise and abates when the patient lies down. It can be accompanied by urinary frequency and urgency, terminal hematuria, and dysuria.

Bladder distention: Common causes and associated findings

CAUSES	MAJOR ASSOCIATED SIGNS AND SYMPTOMS											
	Ataxia	Constipation	Dysuria	Fatigue	Fever	Hematuria	Muscle weakness	Myalgia	Nausea	Nocturia	Pain, buttock and sacral	Pain, flank
Benign prostatic hyperplasia		♦				♦				♦		
Bladder calculi			♦			♦						
Bladder neoplasms			♦			♦				♦	♦	♦
Multiple sclerosis	♦						♦					
Prostatic neoplasms		♦	♦	♦						♦		
Prostatitis (acute)			♦	♦	♦	♦		♦	♦			
Prostatitis (chronic)			♦			♦					♦	
Urethral calculi											♦	
Urethral strictures			♦									

Pain is usually most severe when micturition ceases.

♦ ***Bladder neoplasms.*** By blocking the urethral orifice, neoplasms can cause bladder distention. Associated signs and symptoms include hematuria (most common); urinary frequency and urgency; nocturia; dysuria; pyuria; pain in the bladder, rectum, pelvis, flank, back, or legs; vomiting; diarrhea; and sleeplessness. A mass may be palpable on bimanual examination.

♦ ***Multiple sclerosis.*** In this neuromuscular disorder, urine retention and bladder distention result from interruption of upper motor neuron control of the bladder. Associated signs and symptoms include optic neuritis, paresthesia, impaired position and vibratory senses, diplopia, nystagmus, dizziness, abnormal reflexes, dysarthria, muscle weakness, emotional lability, Lhermitte's sign (transient, electric-like shocks that spread down the body when the head is flexed), Babinski's reflex, and ataxia.

♦ ***Prostatic neoplasm.*** This disease eventually causes bladder distention in approximately 25% of patients. The usual clinical features include dysuria, urinary frequency and urgency, nocturia, weight loss, fatigue, perineal pain, constipation, and induration of the prostate or a rigid, irregular prostate on digital rectal examination. For some patients, urine retention and bladder distention are the only signs.

♦ ***Prostatitis.*** In *acute prostatitis,* bladder distention occurs rapidly with per-

caused vascular clots. Check for a history of acute pancreatitis, diverticulitis, or gynecologic infection, which may have led to intra-abdominal infection and bowel dysfunction. Be sure to ask about previous toxic conditions, such as uremia, and about spinal cord injury, which can lead to paralytic ileus.

If the patient's pain isn't severe or accompanied by life-threatening signs, obtain a detailed medical and surgical history and perform a complete physical examination followed by an abdominal assessment and pelvic examination.

Start your assessment by inspecting abdominal contour. Stoop at the recumbent patient's side and then at the foot of his bed to detect localized or generalized distention. Percuss and palpate the abdomen gently. Listen for dullness over fluid-filled areas and tympany over pockets of gas. Palpate for abdominal rigidity and guarding, which suggest peritoneal irritation that can lead to paralytic ileus.

EXAMINATION TIP

Are bowel sounds really absent?

Before concluding that your patient has absent bowel sounds, ask yourself these three questions.

1. *Did you use the diaphragm of your stethoscope to auscultate for the bowel sounds?*
The diaphragm detects high-frequency sounds, such as bowel sounds, whereas the bell detects low-frequency sounds, such as a vascular bruit or a venous hum.

2. *Did you listen in the same spot for at least 5 minutes for the presence of bowel sounds?*
Normally, bowel sounds occur every 5 to 15 seconds, but the duration of a single sound may be less than 1 second.

3. *Did you listen for bowel sounds in all quadrants?*
Bowel sounds may be absent in one quadrant but present in another.

Common medical causes

♦ ***Complete mechanical intestinal obstruction.*** Absent bowel sounds follow a period of hyperactive bowel sounds in this potentially life-threatening disorder. This silence accompanies acute, colicky abdominal pain that arises in the quadrant of obstruction and may radiate to the flank or lumbar regions. Associated signs and symptoms include abdominal distention and bloating, constipation, and nausea and vomiting (the higher the blockage, the earlier and more severe the vomiting). In late stages, signs of shock may occur with fever, rebound tenderness, and abdominal rigidity.

♦ ***Mesenteric artery occlusion.*** In this life-threatening disorder, bowel sounds disappear after a brief period of hyperactive sounds. Sudden, severe midepigastric or periumbilical pain occurs next, followed by abdominal distention and possible bruits, vomiting, constipation, and signs of shock. Fever is common. Abdominal rigidity may appear late.

♦ ***Paralytic (adynamic) ileus.*** The cardinal sign is absent bowel sounds. In addition to abdominal distention, associated signs and symptoms of paralytic ileus include generalized discomfort and constipation or passage of small, liquid stools. If paralytic ileus follows acute abdominal infection or bowel surgery, the patient may also experience fever and abdominal pain.

Other causes

♦ ***Abdominal surgery.*** Bowel sounds are normally absent after abdominal surgery—the result of anesthetic use and surgical manipulation.

Special considerations

After you've inserted a nasogastric tube or an intestinal tube, elevate the head of the patient's bed at least 30 degrees, and turn the patient to facilitate passage of the tube through the GI tract. Remember not to tape an intestinal tube to the patient's face. Ensure tube patency by checking for drainage and for properly functioning suction devices, and irrigate accordingly.

Continue I.V. fluids and electrolytes, and make sure that you send a serum specimen to the laboratory for electrolyte analysis at least once a day. The patient may need X-ray studies and further blood work to determine the cause of absent bowel sounds.

After mechanical obstruction and intra-abdominal sepsis have been ruled out as the cause of absent bowel sounds, give the patient drugs to control pain and stimulate peristalsis.

Pediatric pointers

Absent bowel sounds in children may result from Hirschsprung's disease or intussusception, both of which can lead to life-threatening obstruction.

Geriatric pointers

Older patients with a bowel obstruction that doesn't respond to decompression should be considered for early surgical intervention to avoid the risk of bowel infarct.

BOWEL SOUNDS, HYPERACTIVE

Sometimes audible without a stethoscope, hyperactive bowel sounds reflect increased intestinal motility (peristalsis) and are commonly referred to as *borborygmus.* They're commonly characterized as rapid, rushing, gurgling waves of sounds. (See *Hyperactive bowel sounds: Common causes and associated findings.*) They may stem from life-threatening bowel obstruction or GI hemorrhage as well as GI infection, inflammatory bowel disease (which usually follows a chronic course), food allergies, or stress.

Emergency interventions

After detecting hyperactive bowel sounds, quickly check vital signs and ask the patient about associated symptoms, such as abdominal pain, vomiting, and diarrhea. If he reports cramping abdominal pain or vomiting, continue to auscultate for bowel sounds. If bowel sounds stop abruptly, suspect complete bowel obstruction and prepare to assist with GI suction and decompression and to give I.V. fluids and electrolytes. Prepare the patient for surgery and withhold food and drink.

If he has diarrhea, record its frequency, amount, color, and consistency. If you detect excessive watery diarrhea or bleeding, prepare to administer antidiarrheal drugs, I.V. fluids and electrolytes, and possibly blood transfusions.

History and physical examination

If you have ruled out life-threatening conditions, obtain a detailed medical and surgical history. Ask the patient if he has had a hernia or abdominal surgery because these may cause mechanical intestinal obstruction. Does he have a history of inflammatory bowel disease? Also, ask about recent eruptions of gastroenteritis among family members, friends, or co-workers. If the patient has traveled recently, even within the United States, was he aware of any endemic illnesses?

In addition, determine whether stress may have contributed to the patient's problem. Ask about food allergies and recent ingestion of unusual foods or fluids. Check for fever, which suggests infection. Having already auscultated, now

Hyperactive bowel sounds: Common causes and associated findings

S&S

CAUSES	Abdominal distention	Abdominal pain	Anorexia	Constipation	Diarrhea	Fever	Nausea	Perianal lesions	Rectal bleeding	Tenesmus	Vomiting	Weight change
	MAJOR ASSOCIATED SIGNS AND SYMPTOMS											
Crohn's disease	♦	♦	♦		♦	♦		♦				♦
Food hypersensitivity					♦		♦				♦	
Gastroenteritis		♦			♦	♦	♦				♦	
GI hemorrhage	♦	♦			♦				♦			
Mechanical intestinal obstruction	♦	♦		♦			♦				♦	
Ulcerative colitis (acute)			♦		♦	♦				♦		♦

gently inspect, percuss, and palpate the abdomen.

Common medical causes

♦ ***Crohn's disease.*** Hyperactive bowel sounds usually arise insidiously. Associated signs and symptoms include diarrhea, cramping abdominal pain that may be relieved by defecation, anorexia, low-grade fever, abdominal distention and tenderness and, commonly, a fixed mass in the right lower quadrant. Perianal and vaginal lesions are common. Muscle wasting, weight loss, and signs of dehydration may occur as Crohn's disease progresses.

♦ ***Food hypersensitivity.*** Malabsorption — typically lactose intolerance — may cause hyperactive bowel sounds. Associated findings include diarrhea and, possibly, nausea and vomiting, angioedema, and urticaria.

♦ ***Gastroenteritis.*** Hyperactive bowel sounds may follow sudden nausea and vomiting and accompany "explosive" diarrhea. Abdominal cramping or pain is common, commonly after a peristaltic wave. Fever may occur, depending on the causative organism.

♦ ***GI hemorrhage.*** Hyperactive bowel sounds provide the most immediate indication of persistent upper GI bleeding. Other findings may include hematemesis, coffee-ground vomitus, abdominal distention, bloody diarrhea, rectal passage of bright red clots and jellylike material or melena, and pain during bleeding. Decreased urine output, tachycardia, and hypotension follow blood loss.

♦ ***Mechanical intestinal obstruction.*** Hyperactive bowel sounds occur simultaneously with cramping abdominal pain every few minutes in this potentially life-threatening disorder; bowel sounds may later become hypoactive and then disappear. In *small-bowel* obstruction, nausea and vomiting occur earlier and with greater severity than in *large-bowel* obstruction. In *complete* bowel obstruction, hyperactive sounds are also accompanied by abdominal distention and constipation, although the part of the bowel distal to the obstruction may continue to empty for up to 3 days.

♦ ***Ulcerative colitis (acute).*** Hyperactive bowel sounds arise abruptly in this disorder and are accompanied by bloody diarrhea, anorexia, abdominal pain, nausea and vomiting, fever, and tenesmus. Weight loss, arthralgias, and arthritis may occur.

Special considerations

Prepare the patient for diagnostic tests. These may include endoscopy to view a suspected lesion, barium X-rays, or stool analysis.

Pediatric pointers

Hyperactive bowel sounds in children usually result from gastroenteritis, erratic eating habits, excessive ingestion of certain foods (such as unripened fruit), or food allergy.

BOWEL SOUNDS, HYPOACTIVE

Hypoactive bowel sounds, detected by auscultation, are diminished in regularity, tone, and loudness from normal bowel sounds. In themselves, hypoactive bowel sounds don't herald an emergency; in fact, they're considered normal during sleep. However, they may portend absent bowel sounds, which can indicate a life-threatening disorder.

Hypoactive bowel sounds result from decreased peristalsis, which, in turn, can result from a developing bowel obstruction. The obstruction may be mechanical (as from hernia, tumor, or twisting), vascular (as from embolism or thrombosis), or neurogenic (as from mechanical, ischemic, or toxic impairment of bowel innervation). Hypoactive bowel sounds can also result from the use of certain drugs, abdominal surgery, and radiation therapy.

History and physical examination

After detecting hypoactive bowel sounds, look for related symptoms. Ask the patient about the location, onset, duration, frequency, and severity of any pain. Cramping or colicky abdominal pain usually indicates a mechanical bowel obstruction, whereas diffuse abdominal pain usually indicates intestinal distention related to paralytic ileus.

Ask the patient about any recent vomiting: When did it begin? How often does it occur? Does the vomitus look bloody? Also, ask about any changes in bowel habits: Does he have a history of constipation? When was the last time he had a bowel movement or expelled gas?

Obtain a detailed medical and surgical history of any conditions that may cause mechanical bowel obstruction, such as an abdominal tumor or hernia. Does the patient have a history of severe pain; trauma; conditions that can cause paralytic ileus, such as pancreatitis; bowel inflammation or gynecologic infection, which may cause peritonitis; or toxic conditions, such as uremia? Has he recently had radiation therapy or abdominal surgery or ingested drugs such as opiates, which can decrease peristalsis and cause hypoactive bowel sounds?

Once the history is complete, perform a careful physical examination. Inspect the abdomen for distention, noting surgical incisions and obvious masses. Gently percuss and palpate the abdomen for masses, gas, fluid, tenderness, and rigidity. Measure abdominal girth to detect any subsequent increase in distention. Also check for poor skin turgor, hypotension, narrowed pulse pressure, and other signs of dehydration and electrolyte imbalance, which may result from paralytic ileus.

Common medical causes

◆ ***Mechanical intestinal obstruction.*** Bowel sounds may become hypoactive after a period of hyperactivity. The patient may also have acute colicky abdominal pain in the quadrant of obstruction, possibly radiating to the flank or lumbar region; nausea and vomiting (the higher the obstruction, the earlier and more severe the vomiting); constipation; and abdominal distention and bloating. If the obstruction becomes complete, signs of shock may occur.

◆ ***Mesenteric artery occlusion.*** After a brief period of hyperactivity, bowel sounds become hypoactive and then quickly disappear, signifying a life-threatening crisis. Associated signs and symptoms include fever; history of colicky abdominal pain leading to sudden and severe midepigastric or periumbilical pain, followed by abdominal distention and possible bruits; vomiting; constipation; and signs of shock. Abdominal rigidity may appear late.

◆ ***Paralytic (adynamic) ileus.*** Bowel sounds are hypoactive and may become absent. Associated signs and symptoms include abdominal distention, generalized discomfort, and constipation or passage of flatus and small, liquid stools. If the disorder follows acute abdominal infection, fever and abdominal pain may occur.

Other causes

◆ ***Drugs.*** Certain classes of drugs reduce intestinal motility and thus produce hypoactive bowel sounds. These include opiates, such as codeine; anticholinergics, such as propantheline bromide; phenothiazines, such as chlorpromazine; and vinca alkaloids, such as vincristine. General or spinal anesthetics produce transient hypoactive sounds.

◆ ***Radiation therapy.*** Hypoactive bowel sounds and abdominal tenderness may occur after irradiation of the abdomen.

◆ ***Surgery.*** Hypoactive bowel sounds may occur after manipulation of the bowel. Motility and bowel sounds in the small intestine usually resume within 24 hours; colonic bowel sounds, in 3 to 5 days.

Special considerations

Frequently evaluate the patient with hypoactive bowel sounds for indications of shock (thirst; anxiety; restlessness; tachycardia; cool, clammy skin; weak, thready pulse), which can develop if peristalsis continues to diminish and fluid is lost from the circulation.

Be alert for sudden absence of bowel sounds, especially in postoperative and hypokalemic patients because those patients are at increased risk for paralytic ileus. Monitor the patient's vital signs and auscultate for bowel sounds every 2 to 4 hours.

Severe pain, abdominal rigidity, guarding, and fever, accompanied by hypoactive bowel sounds, may indicate paralytic ileus from peritonitis. If these signs occur, prepare for emergency interventions (see "Bowel sounds, absent").

The patient with hypoactive bowel sounds may require GI suction and decompression, using a nasogastric or intestinal tube. If so, be sure to restrict the patient's oral intake. Then elevate the head of the bed at least 30 degrees, and turn the patient to facilitate passage of the tube through the GI tract. Remember not to tape an intestinal tube to the patient's face. Ensure tube patency by watching for drainage and for properly functioning suction devices. Irrigate the tube and closely monitor drainage.

Continue I.V. fluids and electrolytes, and send a serum specimen to the laboratory for electrolyte analysis at least once a day. Recognize that the patient may need X-ray studies, endoscopic procedures, and further blood work to determine the cause of hypoactive bowel sounds.

Provide comfort measures as needed. Semi-Fowler's position offers the best relief for the patient with paralytic ileus. Sometimes, ambulating the patient can reactivate the sluggish bowel. However, if the patient can't tolerate ambulation, range-of-motion exercises or turning from side to side may stimulate peristalsis. Also, turning from side to side helps move gas through the intestines.

Pediatric pointers

Hyperactive bowel sounds in a child may simply be due to bowel distention from excessive swallowing of air while the child was eating or crying. However, be sure to observe the child for further signs of illness. As with an adult, sluggish bowel sounds in a child may signal the onset of paralytic ileus or peritonitis.

Bradycardia

Bradycardia refers to a heart rate of less than 60 beats/minute. It occurs normally during sleep and in young adults, trained athletes, and elderly people. It's also a normal response to vagal stimulation caused by coughing, vomiting, or straining during defecation. When bradycardia results from these causes, the heart rate rarely drops below 40 beats/minute. However, when it results from pathologic causes (such as cardiovascular disorders), the heart rate may be slower.

By itself, bradycardia is a nonspecific sign. But, in conjunction with such symptoms as chest pain, dizziness, syncope, or shortness of breath, it can signal a life-threatening disorder.

History and physical examination

After detecting bradycardia, check for related signs of life-threatening disorders. (See *Managing severe bradycardia.*) If the patient's bradycardia isn't accompanied by untoward signs, ask the patient if he or a family member has a history of a slow pulse rate, which may be inherited. Also, find out if he has an underlying metabolic disorder, such as hypothyroidism, that can precipitate bradycardia. Ask which medications he's taking and if he's complying with the prescribed schedule and dosage.

Common medical causes

♦ ***Cardiac arrhythmia.*** Depending on the type of arrhythmia and the patient's tolerance of it, bradycardia may be transient or sustained, benign or life-threatening. Related findings may include hypotension, palpitations, dizziness, weakness, syncope, and fatigue.

♦ ***Cardiomyopathy.*** This potentially life-threatening disorder may cause transient or sustained bradycardia and is usually associated with tachycardia. Other findings include dizziness, syncope, edema, fatigue, jugular vein distention, orthopnea, dyspnea, and peripheral cyanosis.

♦ ***Hypothermia.*** Bradycardia usually appears when core temperature drops below 89.6° F (32° C). It's accompanied by shivering, peripheral cyanosis, muscle rigidity, bradypnea, and confusion leading to stupor.

♦ ***Hypothyroidism.*** This disorder causes severe bradycardia along with fatigue, constipation, unexplained weight gain, and sensitivity to cold. Related signs include cool, dry, thick skin; sparse, dry hair; facial swelling; periorbital edema; thick, brittle nails; and confusion that progresses to stupor.

♦ ***Myocardial infarction (MI).*** Sinus bradycardia is the most common arrhythmia associated with acute MI. Accompanying signs and symptoms of MI include an aching, burning, or viselike pressure in the chest that may radiate to the jaw, shoulder, arm, back, or epigastric area; nausea and vomiting; cool, clammy, and pale or cyanotic skin; anxiety; and dyspnea. Blood pressure may

EMERGENCY INTERVENTIONS

Managing severe bradycardia

Bradycardia can signal a life-threatening disorder when accompanied by pain, shortness of breath, dizziness, syncope, or other symptoms; prolonged exposure to cold; or head or neck trauma. In such patients, quickly take vital signs. Connect the patient to a cardiac monitor, and insert an I.V. line. Depending on the cause of bradycardia, you'll need to administer fluids, atropine, steroids, or thyroid medication. If indicated, insert an indwelling urinary catheter. Intubation, mechanical ventilation, or placement of a pacemaker may be necessary if the patient's respiratory rate falls.

If appropriate, perform a focused evaluation to help locate the cause of bradycardia. For example, ask about pain. Viselike pressure or crushing or burning chest pain that radiates to the arms, back, or jaw may indicate acute myocardial infarction (MI); a severe headache may signal increased intracranial pressure. Also, ask about nausea, vomiting, or shortness of breath — symptoms associated with acute MI and cardiomyopathy. Observe the patient for peripheral cyanosis, edema, or neck vein distention, which may indicate cardiomyopathy. Look for a thyroidectomy scar because severe bradycardia may reflect hypothyroidism caused by failure to take thyroid hormone replacement.

If the cause of bradycardia is evident, provide supportive care. For example, keep the hypothermic patient warm by applying blankets, and monitor his core temperature until it reaches 99° F (37.2° C); stabilize the head and neck of a trauma patient until cervical spinal injury is ruled out.

be elevated or depressed. Auscultation may reveal abnormal heart sounds.

Other causes

- ***Diagnostic tests.*** Cardiac catheterization and electrophysiologic studies can induce temporary bradycardia.
- ***Drugs.*** Beta-adrenergics and some calcium channel blockers, cardiac glycosides, topical miotics (such as pilocarpine), protamine sulfate, quinidine and other antiarrhythmics, and sympatholytics may cause transient bradycardia. Failure to take thyroid replacements may cause bradycardia.
- ***Invasive treatments.*** Suctioning can induce hypoxia and vagal stimulation, causing bradycardia. Edema or damage to conduction tissues during cardiac surgery can cause bradycardia.

Special considerations

Continue to monitor vital signs frequently. Be especially alert for changes in cardiac rhythm, respiratory rate, and level of consciousness.

Prepare the patient for laboratory tests, which can include complete blood count; cardiac enzyme, serum electrolyte, blood glucose, and thyroid function tests; arterial blood gas analysis; blood urea nitrogen levels; and a 12-lead electrocardiogram. If appropriate, prepare the patient for 24-hour Holter monitoring.

Pediatric pointers

Heart rates are normally higher in children than in adults. Fetal bradycardia — a heart rate of less than 120 beats/minute — may occur during prolonged labor or complications of delivery, such as compression of the umbilicus, partial abruptio placentae, and placenta previa. Intermittent bradycardia, sometimes accompanied by apnea, commonly occurs in premature infants. Bradycardia rarely occurs in full-term infants or children. However, it can result from congenital heart defects, acute glomerulonephritis, and transient or complete heart block associated with cardiac catheterization or cardiac surgery.

Geriatric pointers

Sinus node dysfunction is the most common bradyarrhythmia encountered among the elderly. It may present as fatigue, exercise intolerance, dizziness, or syncope. If the patient is asymptomatic, no intervention is necessary. Symptomatic patients, however, require careful scrutiny of their medications. Beta-blockers, verapamil, diazepam, sympatholytic and antihypertensive medications, and some antiarrhythmics have been implicated; symptoms may clear when these drugs are discontinued. Pacing is usually indicated in patients with symptomatic bradycardia lacking a correctable cause.

Bradypnea

Commonly preceding life-threatening apnea or respiratory arrest, bradypnea is a pattern of regular respirations with a rate of fewer than 12 breaths/minute. This sign results from neurologic and metabolic disorders and drug overdose, which depress the brain's respiratory control centers. (See *Neurologic control of breathing.*)

Emergency interventions

Depending on the degree of central nervous system (CNS) depression, the patient with severe bradypnea may require constant stimulation to breathe. If the patient seems excessively sleepy, try to arouse him by shaking and instructing him to breathe. Quickly take the patient's vital signs. Assess his neurologic status by checking pupil size and reactions and by evaluating his level of consciousness (LOC) and his ability to move his extremities.

Place the patient on an apnea monitor, keep emergency airway equipment available, and be prepared to assist with intubation and mechanical ventilation if spontaneous respirations cease. To prevent aspiration, position the patient on his side or keep the head elevated 30 degrees higher than the rest of the body, and clear his airway with suction or finger sweeps, if necessary.

History and physical examination

Obtain a brief history from the patient, if possible, or whoever accompanied him to the hospital. Ask if he may have taken a drug overdose and, if so, try to determine what drugs he took, how much, when, and by what route. Check his arms for needle marks, indicating possible drug abuse. You may need to administer I.V. naloxone, a narcotic antagonist.

If you rule out a drug overdose, ask about chronic illnesses, such as diabetes and renal failure. Check for a medical identification bracelet or an I.D. card that identifies an underlying condition. Also, ask whether the patient has a history of head trauma, brain tumor, neurologic infection, or stroke.

Common medical causes

♦ ***Diabetic ketoacidosis.*** Bradypnea occurs late in severe, uncontrolled diabetes. Patients with severe ketoacidosis may manifest Kussmaul's respirations. Associated signs and symptoms include decreased LOC, fatigue, weakness, fruity breath odor, and oliguria.

♦ ***Hepatic failure.*** Occurring in end-stage hepatic failure, bradypnea may be accompanied by coma, hyperactive reflexes, asterixis, Babinski's reflex, fetor hepaticus, and other signs.

♦ ***Increased intracranial pressure.*** A late sign of this life-threatening condition, bradypnea is preceded by decreased LOC,

Neurologic control of breathing

The mechanical aspects of breathing are regulated by respiratory centers, groups of discrete neurons in the medulla and pons that function as a unit. In the medullary respiratory center, neurons associated with inspiration and neurons associated with expiration interact to control respiratory rate and depth. In the pons, two additional centers interact with the medullary center to regulate rhythm: the apneustic center stimulates inspiratory neurons in the medulla to precipitate inspiration; these, in turn, stimulate the pneumotaxic center to inhibit inspiration, allowing passive expiration to occur.

Normally, the breathing mechanism is stimulated by increased carbon dioxide levels and decreased oxygen levels in the blood. Chemoreceptors in the medulla and in the carotid and aortic bodies respond to changes in partial pressure of arterial carbon dioxide ($PaCO_2$), pH, and partial pressure of arterial oxygen, signaling respiratory centers to adjust respiratory rate and depth. Respiratory depression occurs when decreased cerebral perfusion inactivates respiratory center neurons, when changes in $PaCO_2$ and arterial blood pH affect chemoreceptor responsiveness, or when neuron responsiveness to $PaCO_2$ changes is reduced—for example, in narcotic overdose.

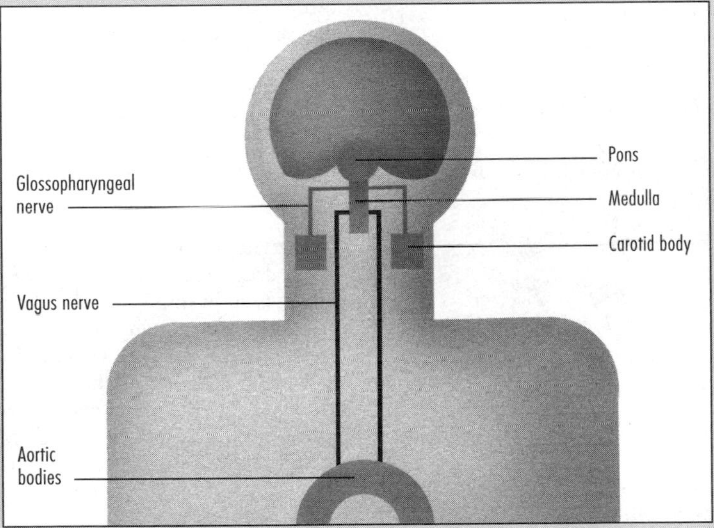

deteriorating motor function, and fixed, dilated pupils. The triad of bradypnea, bradycardia, and hypertension is a classic sign of late medullary strangulation.

◆ ***Renal failure.*** Occurring in end-stage renal failure, bradypnea may be accompanied by seizures, decreased LOC, GI bleeding, hypotension or hypertension, uremic frost, and diverse other signs.

◆ ***Respiratory failure.*** Bradypnea occurs in end-stage respiratory failure along with cyanosis, diminished breath sounds, tachycardia, mildly increased blood pressure, and decreased LOC.

Respiratory rates in children

This graph shows normal respiratory rates in children, which are higher than normal rates in adults. Accordingly, bradypnea in children is defined by the age of the child.

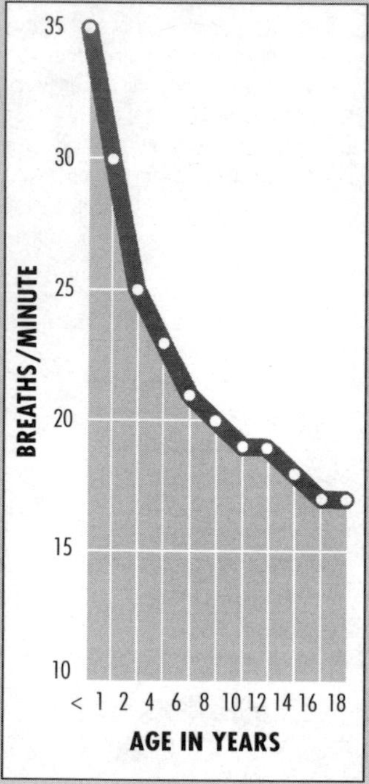

Other causes

♦ ***Drugs.*** An overdose of narcotic analgesics or, less commonly, sedatives, barbiturates, phenothiazines, or other CNS depressants can cause bradypnea. Use of any of these drugs with alcohol can also cause bradypnea.

Special considerations

Because the patient with bradypnea may develop apnea, check his respiratory status frequently and be prepared to give ventilatory support if necessary. Don't leave the patient unattended, especially if his LOC is decreased. Keep his bed in the lowest position and raise the side rails. Obtain blood for arterial blood gas analysis, electrolyte studies, and a possible drug screen. Ready the patient for chest X-rays and, possibly, a computed tomography scan of the head.

Administer drugs and oxygen. Avoid giving CNS-depressant drugs to the patient because these exacerbate bradypnea. Similarly, give oxygen judiciously to a patient with chronic carbon dioxide retention, which may occur in chronic obstructive pulmonary disease, because excess oxygen therapy can have a negative effect.

When dealing with slow breathing in hospitalized patients, always review all medications and dosages given during the past 24 hours.

Pediatric pointers

Because respiratory rates are higher in children than in adults, bradypnea in children is defined according to age. (See *Respiratory rates in children.*)

Geriatric pointers

When drugs are prescribed for older patients, keep in mind that they have a higher risk of developing bradypnea secondary to drug toxicity. That's because they commonly take several drugs that can potentiate this effect and typically have other conditions that predispose them to it. Warn older patients about this potentially life-threatening complication.

BREAST DIMPLING

Breast dimpling — the puckering or retraction of skin on the breast — results from abnormal attachment of the skin to underlying tissue. It suggests an inflammatory or malignant mass beneath the skin surface and usually represents a late sign of breast cancer; benign lesions usually don't produce this effect. Dimpling usually occurs in women over age 40 but also occasionally occurs in men.

Because breast dimpling occurs over a mass or induration, the patient usually discovers other signs before becoming aware of this sign. However, a thorough breast examination may reveal dimpling and alert the patient and nurse to a breast problem. (See *Identifying breast dimpling*.)

Identifying breast dimpling

Dimpling usually suggests an inflammatory or malignant mass beneath the skin's surface. This illustration shows breast dimpling and nipple retraction caused by a malignant mass above the areola.

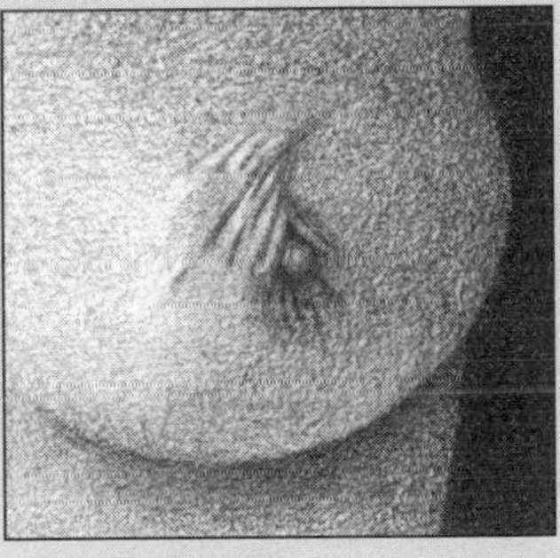

History and physical examination

Obtain a medical, reproductive, and family history, noting factors that place the patient at a high risk for breast cancer. Ask about her pregnancy history because women who didn't have a full-term pregnancy before age 30 are at higher risk for developing breast cancer. Has her mother or a sister had breast cancer? Has she herself had a previous malignancy, especially cancer in the other breast? Has she had any therapeutic or cosmetic procedures? Has she had any trauma of the breast? Ask about the patient's dietary habits because a high-fat diet predisposes women to breast cancer.

Ask the patient if she has noticed any changes in the shape of her breast. Is any area painful or tender, and is the pain cyclic? If she's lactating, has she recently experienced high fever, chills, malaise, muscle aches, fatigue, or other flulike symptoms? Can she remember sustaining any trauma to the breast?

Carefully inspect the dimpled area. Is it swollen, red, or warm to the touch? Do you see bruises or contusions? Ask the patient to tense her pectoral muscles by pressing her hips with both hands or by raising her hands over her head. Does puckering increase? Gently pull the skin upward toward the clavicle. Is dimpling exaggerated?

Observe the breast for nipple retraction. Do both nipples point in the same direction? Are the nipples flattened or inverted? Does the patient report nipple discharge? If so, ask her to describe the color and character of the discharge. Observe the contour of both breasts. Are they symmetrical?

Examine both breasts with your patient supine, sitting, and leaning forward. Does the skin move freely over both breasts? If you can palpate a lump, describe its size, location, consistency, mobility, and delineation. What relation does the lump have to breast dimpling? Gently mold the breast skin around the lump. Is dimpling exaggerated? Also examine breast and axillary lymph nodes, noting any enlargement.

Common medical causes

♦ ***Breast cancer.*** Breast dimpling is an important but somewhat late sign of breast cancer. A neoplasm that causes dimpling is usually close to the skin and at least 1 cm in diameter; it feels irregularly shaped and fixed to underlying tissue and is usually painless. Other signs of breast cancer may include peau d'orange; changes in breast symmetry or size; nipple retraction; and a unilateral, spontaneous, nonmilky nipple discharge that is serous or bloody. (A bloody nipple discharge in the presence of a lump is a classic sign of breast cancer.) Axillary lymph nodes may be enlarged. Pain may be present but isn't a reliable symptom of breast cancer. A breast ulcer may appear as a late sign.

◆ ***Fat necrosis.*** Breast dimpling from fat necrosis follows inflammation and trauma to fatty tissue of the breast (although the patient commonly can't remember such trauma). Tenderness, erythema, bruising, and contusions may occur. Other findings include a hard, indurated, poorly delineated lump, which is fibrotic and fixed to underlying tissue or overlying skin, as well as signs of nipple retraction. Fat necrosis is difficult to differentiate from breast cancer.

◆ ***Mastitis.*** Breast dimpling may signal bacterial mastitis, which usually results from duct obstruction and milk stasis during lactation. Heat, erythema, swelling, induration, pain, and tenderness usually accompany mastitis. Dimpling is more likely to occur with diffuse induration than with a single hard mass. The skin on the breast may feel fixed to underlying tissue. Other possible findings include nipple retraction, nipple cracks, a purulent discharge, and enlarged axillary lymph nodes. Flulike signs and symptoms, such as fever, malaise, fatigue, and aching, commonly occur.

Special considerations

Remember that any breast problem can arouse fears of mutilation, loss of sexuality, and death. Allow the patient to express her feelings.

Pediatric pointers

Because breast cancer, the most likely cause of dimpling, is extremely rare in children, consider trauma as a likely cause. As in adults, breast dimpling may occur in adolescents from fatty tissue necrosis due to trauma.

Geriatric pointers

Postmenopausal women may attribute breast changes to hormonal decrease and aging. Encourage continued regular breast self-examination. Ask about use of hormone replacement therapy (HRT), including herbal forms of HRT.

Breast nodule

[Breast lump]

A frequently reported gynecologic sign, a breast nodule has two chief causes: benign breast disease and cancer. Benign breast disease, the leading cause of nodules, can stem from cyst formation in obstructed and dilated lactiferous ducts, hypertrophy or tumor formation in the ductal system, and inflammation or infection.

Although fewer than 20% of breast nodules are malignant, the clinical signs of breast cancer aren't easily distinguished from those of benign breast disease. Breast cancer is a leading cause of death among women but can occur in men, with the same signs and symptoms found in women. Thus, breast nodules in both sexes should always be evaluated.

A woman who's familiar with the feel of her breasts and performs monthly breast self-examination can detect a nodule 5 mm or less in size, considerably smaller than the 1-cm nodule that's readily detectable by an experienced examiner. However, a woman may fail to report a nodule because of fear of breast cancer.

Breast cancer prevention is a mainstream focus for researchers today. Studies have shown that alternative therapies, such as diet modification with specific foods, have been linked to cancer prevention. (See *Fatty acids and cancer prevention.*)

History and physical examination
If your patient reports a lump, ask her how and when she discovered it. Does the size and tenderness of the lump vary with her menstrual cycle? Has the lump changed since she first noticed it? Has she noticed any other breast signs, such as a change in breast shape, size, or contour; a discharge; or nipple changes?

Is she lactating? Does she have fever, chills, fatigue, or other flulike symptoms? Ask her to describe any pain or tenderness associated with the lump. Is the pain in one breast only? Has she sustained recent trauma to the breast?

Explore the patient's medical and family history for factors that increase her risk of breast cancer. These include a high-fat diet, having a mother or sister with breast cancer, or having a history of cancer, especially cancer in the other breast. Other risk factors include nulliparity and a first pregnancy after age 30. Ask her about history of breast trauma or breast procedures including therapeutic, diagnostic, and cosmetic.

Next, perform a thorough breast examination. Pay special attention to the upper outer quadrant of each breast, where half the ductal tissue is located. This is the most common site of malignant breast tumors.

Carefully palpate a suspected breast nodule, noting its location, shape, size, consistency, mobility, and delineation. Does the nodule feel soft, rubbery, and elastic or hard? Is it mobile, slipping away from your fingers as you palpate it, or firmly fixed to adjacent tissue? Does the nodule seem to limit the mobility of the entire breast? Note the nodule's delineation. Are the borders clearly defined or indefinite? Or does the area feel more like a hardness or diffuse induration than a nodule with definite borders?

Do you feel one nodule or several small ones? Is the shape round, oval, lobular, or irregular? Inspect and palpate the skin over the nodule for warmth, redness, and edema. Palpate the lymph nodes of the breast and axilla for enlargement.

Observe the contour of the breasts, looking for asymmetry and irregularities. Be alert for signs of retraction, such as skin dimpling and nipple deviation, retraction, or flattening. (To exaggerate dimpling, have your patient raise her arms over her head or press her hands against her hips.) Gently pull the breast skin toward the clavicle. Is dimpling evident? Mold the breast skin and again observe for dimpling.

Be alert for a nipple discharge that's spontaneous, unilateral, and nonmilky (serous, bloody, or purulent). Be careful not to confuse it with the grayish discharge that can commonly be elicited from the nipples of a woman who has been pregnant. (See *Breast nodule: Common causes and associated findings*, page 96.)

ALTERNATIVE THERAPY

Fatty acids and cancer prevention

Omega-3 fatty acids, polyunsaturated fats thought to be essential for cell function, are believed to have some beneficial effects in preventing breast cancer. Soybeans, linseed oil, and cold-water fish, such as herring, salmon, and sardines, are rich in omega-3 fatty acids.

Common medical causes

◆ ***Areolar gland abscess.*** Tender, palpable abscesses on the periphery of the areola follow inflammation of the sebaceous glands of Montgomery. Fever may also be present.

◆ ***Breast abscess.*** A localized, hot, tender, fluctuant mass with erythema and peau d'orange typifies *acute abscess.* As-

Breast nodule: Common causes and associated findings

CAUSES	MAJOR ASSOCIATED SIGNS AND SYMPTOMS							
	Breast dimpling	Breast pain or tenderness	Erythema	Fever	Lymphadenopathy	Nipple discharge	Nipple retraction signs	Peau d'orange
Areolar gland abscess		◆		◆				
Breast abscess (acute)		◆	◆	◆				◆
Breast abscess (chronic)	◆				◆		◆	◆
Breast cancer	◆					◆	◆	◆
Mastitis	◆	◆	◆	◆			◆	◆
Proliferative breast disease		◆				◆		

sociated symptoms commonly include fever, chills, malaise, and generalized discomfort. In *chronic abscess,* the nodule is nontender, irregular, and firm and may feel like a thick wall of fibrous tissue. It's commonly accompanied by skin dimpling, peau d'orange, nipple retraction and, sometimes, axillary lymphadenopathy.

♦ ***Breast cancer.*** A hard, poorly delineated nodule that's fixed to the skin or underlying tissue suggests breast cancer. Malignant nodules commonly cause breast dimpling, nipple discharge, peau d'orange, nipple deviation or retraction, or flattening of the nipple or breast contour. Forty to fifty percent of malignant nodules occur in the upper outer quadrant.

Nodules usually occur singly, although satellite nodules may surround the main one. They're usually nontender. Nipple discharge may be serous or bloody. (A bloody nipple discharge in the presence of a nodule is a classic sign of breast cancer.) Additional findings may include edema (peau d'orange) of the skin overlying the mass, erythema, tenderness, and axillary lymphadenopathy. A breast ulcer may occur as a late sign. Breast pain, an unreliable symptom, may be present.

♦ ***Cysts.*** These individual fluid-filled sacs occuring most commonly in women ages 35 to 50 and frequently become tender and enlarged during menses. Cysts are commonly found in both breasts and can range from microscopic to, rarely, several inches across.

♦ ***Fat necrosis.*** Firm, round, painless lumps resulting from damaged and disintegrating fatty tissue. This occurs most frequently in obese women with very large breasts and is frequently the result of trauma. The skin around the lump may be red or bruised.

♦ ***Fibroadenoma.*** The extremely mobile or "slippery" feel of this benign neoplasm helps distinguish it from other breast nodules. The nodule usually occurs singly and characteristically feels firm, elastic, and round or lobular, with well-defined margins. It doesn't cause pain or tenderness, can vary from pinhead size to very large, commonly grows rapidly especially during pregnancy or lactation, and usually lies around the nipple or on the lateral side of the upper outer quadrant.

♦ ***Mastitis.*** In this disorder, breast nodules feel firm and indurated or tender, flocculent, and discrete. Gentle palpation defines the area of maximum purulent accumulation. Skin dimpling and nipple deviation, retraction, or flattening may be present, and the nipple may show a crack or abrasion. Accompanying signs and symptoms include breast warmth, erythema, tenderness, and peau d'orange, plus high fever, chills, malaise, and fatigue.

♦ ***Paget's disease.*** This slow-growing intraductal carcinoma begins as a scaling, eczematoid unilateral nipple lesion. The nipple later becomes reddened and excoriated and may eventually be completely destroyed. The process extends along the skin as well as in the ducts, usually progressing to a deep-seated mass.

♦ ***Proliferative breast disease.*** The most common cause of breast nodules, this condition produces smooth, round, slightly elastic nodules, which increase in size and tenderness just before menstruation. The nodules may occur in fine, granular clusters in both breasts or as widespread, well-defined lumps of varying sizes. A thickening of adjacent tissue may be palpable. Cystic nodules are mobile, which helps differentiate them from malignant ones. Because cystic nodules aren't fixed to underlying breast tissue, they don't cause retraction signs, such as nipple deviation or dimpling. Nipple discharge may appear in one or both breasts and can be serous or sticky brown or green discharge. Symptoms of premenstrual syndrome, including headache, irritability, bloating, nausea, vomiting, and abdominal cramping, may also be present.

♦ ***Sclerosing adenosis.*** Excessive growth of tissue in breast lobules is a benign condition that commonly causes breast pain. The changes are commonly microscopic but can cause lumps and commonly are detected as calcifications by mammogram.

Special considerations

Although many women regard a breast lump as a sign of breast cancer, most nodules are benign. Therefore, try to avoid alarming your patient further. Provide a simple explanation of your examination, and encourage the patient to express her feelings.

Prepare the patient for diagnostic tests, which may include transillumination, mammography, thermography, needle aspiration or open biopsy of the nodule for tissue examination, and cytologic examination of nipple discharge.

Postpone teaching the patient how to perform breast self-examination until she overcomes her initial anxiety at discovering a lump. Regular breast self-examination is especially important for women who have had a previous cancer, have a family history of breast cancer, are nulliparous, or had their first child after age 30.

Although most nodules occurring during lactation result from mastitis, the possibility of cancer demands careful evaluation. Advise the lactating mother with mastitis to pump her breasts to prevent further milk stasis, to discard the milk, and to substitute formula until the infection responds to antibiotics.

Pediatric pointers

Most nodules in children and adolescents reflect the normal response of breast tissue to hormonal fluctuations. For instance, the breasts of young teenage girls may normally contain cordlike nodules that become tender just before menstruation.

A transient breast nodule in young boys (as well as women between ages 20 and 30) may result from juvenile mastitis, which usually affects one breast. Signs of inflammation are present in a firm mass beneath the nipple.

Geriatric pointers

In women age 70 and older, three-quarters of all breast lumps are malignant.

BREAST PAIN

[Mastalgia]

Breast pain is the most common sign of benign breast disorder. It may occur during rest or movement and may be aggravated by manipulation or palpation. Breast pain may be unilateral or bilateral; cyclic, intermittent, or constant; and dull or sharp. It may result from surface cuts, furuncles, contusions, and similar lesions (superficial pain); nipple fissures and inflammation in the papillary ducts and areolae (severe localized pain); stromal distention in the breast parenchyma; a tumor that affects nerve endings (severe, constant pain); or inflammatory lesions that not only distend the stroma but also irritate sensory nerve endings (severe, constant pain). Breast pain may radiate to the back, the arms, and sometimes the neck.

Breast tenderness refers to pain elicited by physical contact. It may occur before menstruation and during pregnancy. Before menstruation, breast pain or tenderness stems from increased mammary blood flow due to hormonal changes. During pregnancy, breast tenderness and throbbing, tingling, or pricking sensations may occur, also from hormonal changes. In men, breast pain may stem from gynecomastia (especially during puberty and senescence), reproductive tract anomalies, and organic disease of the liver or pituitary, adrenal cortex, and thyroid glands.

History and physical examination

Begin by asking the patient to describe any breast discomfort. She may describe it as sticking, stinging, shooting, stabbing, throbbing, or burning. Determine if the pain affects one breast or both, and ask the patient to point to the painful area. Ask about onset and character. If it's intermittent, determine the relationship of pain to the phase of the menstrual cycle. Is the patient a nursing mother? If not, ask about any nipple discharge and have her describe it. Is she pregnant? Has she reached menopause? Has she recently experienced any flulike symptoms or sustained any injury to the breast? Has she noticed any change in breast shape or contour?

Instruct the patient to place her arms at her sides and inspect the breasts. Note their size, symmetry, and contour and the appearance of the skin. Remember that breast shape and size vary widely and that breasts undergo normal changes during the menstrual cycle, pregnancy, and lactation and with aging. Are the breasts red or edematous? Are the veins prominent?

Note the size, shape, and symmetry of the nipples and areolae. Do you see ecchymosis, a rash, ulceration, or a discharge? Do the nipples point in the same direction? Do you see signs of retraction, such as skin dimpling or nipple inversion or flattening? Repeat your inspection, first with the patient's arms raised above her head and then with her hands pressed against her hips and her elbows pointing out.

Palpate the breasts, first with the patient seated and then with her lying down with a pillow under her shoulder on the side being examined. Use the pads of your three central fingers to compress

Breast pain: Common causes and associated findings

CAUSES	MAJOR ASSOCIATED SIGNS AND SYMPTOMS							
	Breast nodule	Erythema	Fever	Lymphadenopathy	Nipple discharge	Nipple retraction signs	Peau d'orange	Pruritus
Areolar gland abscess	◆		◆					
Breast abscess (acute)	◆	◆	◆				◆	
Mammary duct ectasia	◆	◆		◆	◆	◆	◆	◆
Proliferative breast disease	◆				◆			
Sebaceous cyst (infected)	◆	◆					◆	

breast tissue against the chest wall. Proceed systematically in a small circular pattern from nipple to perimeter extending from sternum to axilla. Note any warmth, tenderness, nodules, masses, or irregularities. Palpate the nipple, noting tenderness and nodules, and check for discharge. Palpate axillary lymph nodes, noting any enlargement. Also take an oral temperature. (See *Breast pain: Common causes and associated findings.*)

Common medical causes

◆ ***Areolar gland abscess.*** Tender, palpable abscesses on the periphery of the areola follow inflammation of the sebaceous glands of Montgomery. Fever may also occur.

◆ ***Breast abscess (acute).*** In the affected breast, local pain, tenderness, erythema, peau d'orange, and warmth are associated with a nodule. Malaise, fever, and chills may also occur.

◆ ***Breast cyst.*** A breast cyst that enlarges rapidly may cause acute, localized, and usually unilateral pain. A palpable breast nodule may be present.

◆ ***Fat necrosis.*** Local pain and tenderness may develop in this benign disorder. A history of trauma usually is present. Associated findings include ecchymosis; erythema of the overriding skin; a firm, irregular, fixed mass; and skin retraction signs, such as skin dimpling and nipple retraction. Fat necrosis may be difficult to differentiate from cancer.

◆ ***Mammary duct ectasia.*** Burning pain and itching around the areola may occur, although ectasia is frequently asymptomatic at first. The history may include one or more episodes of inflammation with pain, tenderness, erythema, and acute fever, or with pain and tenderness alone, which develop and then subside spontaneously within 7 to 10 days. Other findings may include a rubbery, subareolar breast nodule; swelling and erythema around the nipple; nipple retraction; a bluish green discoloration or peau d'orange of the skin overlying the nodule; a thick, sticky, multicolored nipple discharge from multiple ducts; and possible axillary lymphadenopathy. A breast ulcer may occur in late stages.

♦ ***Mastitis.*** Unilateral pain may be severe, particularly when the inflammation occurs near the skin surface. Breast skin is frequently red and warm at the inflammation site; peau d'orange may be present. Palpation reveals a firm area of induration. Skin retraction signs, such as breast dimpling and nipple deviation, inversion, or flattening, may be present. Systemic signs and symptoms, such as high fever, chills, malaise, and fatigue, may also occur.

♦ ***Proliferative breast disease.*** This common cause of breast pain is associated with the development of cysts that may cause pain before menstruation and are asymptomatic afterward. Later in the course of the disorder, pain and tenderness may persist throughout the cycle. The cysts feel firm, mobile, and well defined; they are frequently bilateral and found in the upper outer quadrant of the breast but may also be unilateral and generalized. A clear, serous nipple discharge may be present in one or both breasts. Symptoms of premenstrual syndrome, including headache, irritability, bloating, nausea, vomiting, and abdominal cramping, may also be present.

♦ ***Sebaceous cyst (infected).*** Breast pain may be reported with this cutaneous cyst. Associated symptoms include a small, well-delineated nodule, localized erythema, and induration.

Special considerations

Provide emotional support for the patient and, when appropriate, emphasize the importance of monthly breast self-examination.

Prepare the patient for diagnostic tests, such as mammography, thermography, cytology of nipple discharge, biopsy, or culture of any aspirate.

Pediatric pointers

Transient gynecomastia can cause breast pain in males during puberty.

Geriatric pointers

Reports of breast pain in postmenopausal women should be evaluated immediately. Elderly patients with decreased pain perception or decreased cognitive function may not report breast pain.

BREAST ULCER

An ulcer anywhere in the breast indicates destruction of the skin and subcutaneous tissue. In women, a breast ulcer is frequently a late sign of cancer, appearing well after the confirming diagnosis. In men, in whom delayed diagnosis is common, an ulcer may be the presenting symptom. Breast ulcers can also result from trauma, infection, dermatitis, or radiation. (See *Identifying a breast ulcer.*)

History and physical examination

Begin the history by asking when the patient first noticed the ulcer and if it was preceded by other breast changes, such as nodules, edema, or nipple discharge, deviation, or retraction. Does the ulcer seem to be getting better or worse? Does it cause pain or produce drainage? Has there been any change in breast shape? Has she had a skin rash? If she has been treating the ulcer at home, find out how.

Review the patient's personal and family history for factors that indicate an increased risk of breast cancer. Determine whether the patient's mother or sister has had breast cancer. Ask the patient's age at menarche and menopause because more than 30 years of menstrual activity increases the risk of breast cancer. Also ask about pregnancy because nulliparity or birth of a first child after age 30 also increases the risk of breast cancer.

Ask about the presence of diabetes, lactation history, and use of oral antibiotics. She might be predisposed to *Candida* infections. Ask about history of breast-related procedures: diagnostic, therapeutic, or cosmetic.

Inspect the patient's breast, noting any asymmetry or flattening. Look for a rash, scaling, cracking, or red excoriation on the nipples, areola, and inframammary fold. Check especially for skin changes, such as warmth, erythema, or peau d'orange. Palpate the breast for masses, noting any induration beneath the ulcer. Then carefully palpate for tenderness or nodules around the areola and the axillary lymph nodes.

Common medical causes

♦ ***Breast cancer.*** A breast ulcer that doesn't heal within a month usually indicates cancer. Ulceration along a mastectomy scar may indicate metastatic cancer; a nodule beneath the ulcer may be a late sign of a fulminating tumor. Other signs include a palpable breast nodule, skin dimpling, nipple retraction, bloody or serous nipple discharge, erythema, peau d'orange, and enlarged axillary lymph nodes.

♦ ***Breast trauma.*** Tissue destruction with inadequate healing may produce breast ulcers. Associated signs depend on the type of trauma but may include ecchymosis, lacerations, abrasions, swelling, and hematoma.

♦ **Candida albicans *infection.*** Severe *Candida* infection can cause maceration of breast tissue followed by ulceration. Well-defined, bright red papular patches — usually with scaly borders — characterize the infection, which can develop in the breast folds. In breast-feeding women, cracked nipples predispose to infection. Women describe the pain, felt when the infant sucks, as a burning pain that penetrates into the chest wall.

♦ ***Paget's disease.*** Bright red nipple excoriation can extend to the areola and ulcerate. Serous or bloody nipple discharge and extreme nipple itching may accompany ulceration. Symptoms are usually unilateral.

Identifying a breast ulcer

Skin irritations and cancer can cause ulcers on the breast, nipple, or areola. The area of tissue destruction can vary in size.

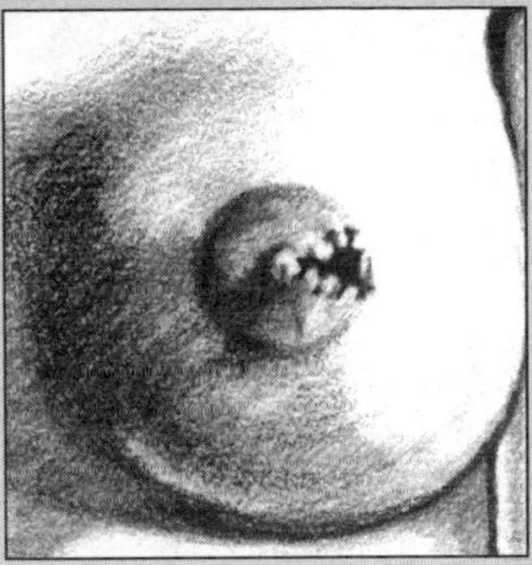

Other causes

♦ ***Radiation therapy.*** After treatment, the breasts appear "sunburned." Subsequently, the skin ulcerates and the surrounding area becomes red and tender.

Special considerations

Because breast ulcers become infected easily, teach the patient how to apply topical antifungal and antibiotic preparations. Instruct her to keep the ulcer dry and to protect the area from local irritation either with a dressing or with a properly fitting bra. If a *Candida* infection is suspected, prepare her for skin or blood cultures. When cancer is suspected, provide emotional support and prepare her for diagnostic tests, such as ultrasonography, thermography, mammography, nipple discharge cytology, and breast biopsy.

Geriatric pointers

Breast ulcers should be considered cancerous until proven otherwise. Nutrition and domestic circumstances may also need to be evaluated as contributing factors.

BREATH WITH AMMONIA ODOR

[Uremic fetor]

The odor of ammonia on the breath—described as urinous or "fishy" breath—typically occurs in end-stage chronic renal failure. This sign abates after hemodialysis and persists throughout the course of the disorder.

Ammonia breath odor reflects the long-term metabolic disturbances and biochemical abnormalities associated with uremia and end-stage chronic renal failure. It's produced by metabolic end products blown off by the lungs and the breakdown of urea in the saliva to ammonia. A specific uremic toxin hasn't yet been identified, however. In animals, breath odor analysis has revealed toxic metabolites, such as dimethylamine and trimethylamine, which contribute to the fishy odor. The source of these amines, although still unclear, may be intestinal bacteria acting on dietary chlorine.

History and physical examination

When you detect ammonia breath odor, the diagnosis of chronic renal failure will probably already be well established. But look for associated GI symptoms of chronic renal failure so that palliative care and support can be individualized.

Inspect the patient's oral cavity for bleeding, swollen gums or tongue, and ulceration with drainage. Ask the patient if he has experienced a metallic taste, loss of smell, increased thirst, heartburn, difficulty swallowing, loss of appetite at the sight of food, and early morning vomiting. Because GI bleeding is common in chronic renal failure, ask about bowel habits, noting especially melenous stools or constipation.

Take the patient's vital signs. Watch for any indications of hypertension (the patient with end-stage chronic renal failure is usually somewhat hypertensive) or hypotension. Be alert for other signs of shock (such as tachycardia, tachypnea, and cool, clammy skin) and altered mental status. Any significant changes can indicate complications, such as massive GI bleeding or pericarditis with tamponade.

Common medical causes

- ***End-stage chronic renal failure.*** Ammonia breath odor is a late finding. Accompanying signs and symptoms include anuria, skin pigmentation changes and excoriation, brown arcs under the nail margins, tissue wasting, Kussmaul's respirations, neuropathy, lethargy, somnolence, confusion, disorientation, behavior changes with irritability, and mood lability. Later neurologic signs that signal impending uremic coma include muscle twitching and fasciculation, asterixis, paresthesia, and footdrop. Cardiovascular findings may include hypertension, myocardial infarction, signs of heart failure, pericarditis, and even sudden death and stroke. GI findings include anorexia, nausea, heartburn, vomiting, constipation, hiccups, and a metallic taste, with oral manifestations such as stomatitis, gum ulceration and bleeding, and a coated tongue. The patient has an increased risk of peptic ulceration and acute pancreatitis. Weight loss is common; uremic frost, pruritus, and signs of hormonal changes, such as impotence or amenorrhea, also appear.

Special considerations

Ammonia breath odor is offensive to others, but the patient may become accustomed to it. As a result, remind him to perform frequent mouth care, particularly before meals because reducing foul mouth taste and odor may stimulate his appetite. A half-strength hydrogen peroxide mixture or lemon juice gargle helps neutralize the ammonia; the patient may also want to use commercial lozenges or breath sprays or to suck on hard candy. Advise him to use a soft toothbrush or sponge to prevent trauma. If he's unable to perform mouth care, do it for him and teach his family members how to assist him.

Maximize dietary intake by offering the patient frequent small meals of his favorite foods, within dietary limitations. Encourage him to take the ordered antacids.

Pediatric pointers

Ammonia breath odor also occurs in children with end-stage chronic renal failure. Provide hard candies to relieve bad mouth taste and odor. If the child is able to gargle, try mixing hydrogen peroxide with flavored mouthwashes.

BREATH WITH FECAL ODOR

Fecal breath odor typically accompanies fecal vomiting associated with a longstanding intestinal obstruction or gastrojejunocolic fistula. It represents an important late diagnostic clue to a potentially life-threatening GI disorder because complete obstruction of any part of the bowel, if untreated, can cause death within hours from vascular collapse and shock.

When the obstructed or adynamic intestine attempts self-decompression by regurgitating its contents, vigorous peristaltic waves propel bowel contents backward into the stomach. When the stomach fills with intestinal fluid, further reverse peristalsis results in vomiting. The odor of feculent vomitus lingers in the mouth.

Fecal breath odor may also occur in patients with a nasogastric or intestinal tube. The odor is detected only while the underlying disorder persists and abates soon after its resolution.

Emergency interventions

Because fecal breath odor signals a potentially life-threatening intestinal obstruction, you'll need to quickly evaluate your patient's condition. Monitor vital signs and be alert for signs of shock, such as hypotension, tachycardia, narrowed pulse pressure, and cool, clammy skin. Ask the patient if he's experiencing nausea or has vomited. Find out the frequency of vomiting as well as the color, odor, amount, and consistency of the vomitus. Have an emesis basin nearby to collect and accurately measure vomitus.

Anticipating possible surgery to relieve an obstruction or repair a fistula, withhold all food and fluids. Be prepared to insert a nasogastric or intestinal tube for GI tract decompression. Insert a peripheral I.V. line for vascular access, or assist with central line insertion for large-bore access and central venous pressure monitoring. Obtain a blood sample and send it to the laboratory for complete blood count and electrolyte analysis because large fluid losses and shifts can cause electrolyte imbalances. Maintain adequate hydration and support circulatory status with additional fluids. Give a physiologic solution, such as Ringer's lactate, normal saline, or Plasmanate, to prevent metabolic acidosis from gastric losses and metabolic alkalosis from intestinal fluid losses.

History and physical examination

If the patient's condition permits, ask about previous abdominal surgery because adhesions can cause an obstruction. Also ask about loss of appetite. Is the patient experiencing abdominal pain?

Fecal breath odor: Common causes and associated findings

CAUSES	MAJOR ASSOCIATED SIGNS AND SYMPTOMS								
	Abdominal distention	Abdominal pain	Anorexia	Constipation	Diarrhea	Hyperactive bowel sounds	Nausea	Vomiting	Weight loss
Distal small-bowel obstruction	♦	♦		♦	♦	♦	♦	♦	
Gastrojejunocolic fistula	♦	♦	♦		♦			♦	♦
Large-bowel obstruction	♦	♦		♦			♦	♦	

If so, have him describe its onset, duration, and location. Ask if the pain is intense, persistent, or spasmodic. Have the patient describe his normal bowel habits, noting especially constipation, diarrhea, or leakage of stool. Ask when the patient's last bowel movement occurred, and have him describe the stool's color, consistency, and amount.

Auscultate for bowel sounds — hyperactive, high-pitched sounds may indicate *impending* bowel obstruction, whereas hypoactive or absent sounds occur *late* in obstruction and paralytic ileus. Inspect the abdomen, noting contour and any surgical scars. Measure abdominal girth to provide baseline data for subsequent assessment of distention. Palpate for tenderness, distention, and rigidity. Percuss for tympany, indicating a gas-filled bowel, and dullness, indicating fluid.

Rectal and pelvic examinations should be performed. All patients with a suspected bowel obstruction should have flat and upright abdominal X-rays; some will also need a chest X-ray, sigmoidoscopy, and a barium enema. (See *Fecal breath odor: Common causes and associated findings*.)

Common medical causes

♦ ***Distal small-bowel obstruction.*** In late obstruction, nausea is present, although vomiting may be delayed. Vomitus initially consists of gastric contents, then changes to bilious contents, followed by fecal contents with resultant fecal breath odor. Accompanying symptoms may include achiness, malaise, drowsiness, and polydipsia. Bowel changes (ranging from diarrhea to constipation) are accompanied by abdominal distention, persistent epigastric or periumbilical colicky pain, and hyperactive bowel sounds and borborygmi; as the obstruction becomes complete, bowel sounds become hypoactive or absent. Fever, hypotension, tachycardia, and rebound tenderness may indicate strangulation or perforation.

♦ ***Gastrojejunocolic fistula.*** In this disorder, symptoms may be variable and intermittent because the fistula is temporarily blocked. Fecal vomiting with resulting fecal breath odor may occur, but the most common presenting sign is diarrhea, commonly accompanied by abdominal pain. Related GI findings include anorexia, weight loss, abdominal distention and, possibly, marked malabsorption.

◆ ***Large-bowel obstruction.*** Vomiting is usually absent at first, but fecal vomiting with resultant fecal breath odor occurs as a late sign. Typically, symptoms develop more slowly than in small-bowel obstruction. Colicky abdominal pain appears suddenly and is followed by continuous hypogastric pain. Marked abdominal distention and tenderness occur, and loops of large bowel may be visible on the abdominal wall. Although constipation develops, defecation may continue for up to 3 days after complete obstruction because stool remains in the bowel below the obstruction. Leakage of stool is common with partial obstruction.

Special considerations

After a nasogastric or intestinal tube has been inserted, keep the head of the bed elevated at least 30 degrees and turn the patient to facilitate passage of the intestinal tube through the GI tract. Don't tape the intestinal tube to the patient's face. Ensure tube patency by monitoring drainage and watching that suction devices function properly. Irrigate as required. Monitor GI drainage losses, and send serum specimens to the laboratory for electrolyte analysis at least once a day. Prepare the patient for diagnostic tests, such as abdominal X-rays, barium enema, and proctoscopy.

Pediatric pointers

Carefully monitor the child's fluid and electrolyte status because dehydration can occur rapidly from persistent vomiting. The absence of tears and dry or parched mucous membranes are important clinical indicators of dehydration.

Geriatric pointers

In older patients, the high risk of bowel infarct may mandate early surgical intervention if bowel obstruction does not respond to decompression.

BREATH WITH FRUITY ODOR

Fruity breath odor results from respiratory elimination of excess acetone. This sign characteristically occurs in ketoacidosis — a potentially life-threatening condition that requires immediate treatment to prevent severe dehydration, irreversible coma, and death.

Ketoacidosis results from the excessive catabolism of fats for cellular energy in the absence of usable carbohydrates. This process begins when insulin levels are insufficient to transport glucose into the cells, as in diabetes mellitus, or when glucose is unavailable and hepatic glycogen stores are depleted, as in low-carbohydrate diets and malnutrition, with or without concurrent alcohol use. After alcohol ingestion with inadequate caloric ingestion, a combination of glyconeogenesis and hepatic depletion of the coenzyme NADPH due to alcohol metabolism results in ketone accumulation. Lacking glucose, the cells burn fat faster than enzymes can handle the ketones, the acidic end products. As a result, the ketones (acetone, beta-hydroxybutyric acid, and acetoacetic acid) accumulate in the blood and urine. To compensate for increased acidity, Kussmaul's respirations expel carbon dioxide with enough acetone to flavor the breath. Eventually, this compensatory mechanism fails, producing ketoacidosis.

Emergency interventions

When you detect fruity breath odor, check for Kussmaul's respirations and examine the patient's level of consciousness (LOC). Take vital signs, including orthostatic pulse and blood pressure, if patient can tolerate it, and check skin turgor. Be alert for fruity breath odor that accompanies rapid, deep respirations, stupor, and poor skin turgor. Try to obtain a brief history, noting especially diabetes mellitus, nutritional problems such as anorexia nervosa, and fad diets with little or no carbohydrates. Obtain venous and arterial blood samples for glucose, electrolyte, acetone, complete blood count, and arterial blood gas (ABG) studies. Also obtain a urine specimen to test for glucose and acetone. Administer I.V. fluids and electrolytes to maintain hydration and electrolyte balance and, in diabetic ketoacidosis, give regular insulin to reduce blood glucose levels.

If the patient is obtunded, you'll need to insert endotracheal and nasogastric tubes; suction as needed. Insert an indwelling urinary catheter, and monitor intake and output. Insert central venous pressure and arterial lines to monitor the patient's fluid status and blood pressure. Place the patient on a cardiac monitor, monitor vital signs and neurologic status, and draw blood hourly for glucose, acetone, electrolyte, and ABG studies.

History and physical examination

If the patient isn't in severe distress, obtain a thorough history. Ask about the onset and duration of fruity breath odor. Find out about any changes in breathing pattern. Ask about increased thirst, frequent urination, weight loss, fatigue, and abdominal pain. Ask the female patient if she has had monilial vaginitis or vaginal secretions with itching. If the patient has a history of diabetes mellitus, ask about stress, infections, and noncompliance with therapy — the most common causes of ketoacidosis in known diabetics. If the patient is suspected of having anorexia nervosa, obtain a dietary and weight history.

Common medical causes

◆ ***Ketoacidosis.*** Fruity breath odor accompanies *alcoholic ketoacidosis*, which occurs most commonly in females with a history of alcohol abuse. It typically follows cessation of drinking after a marked increase in alcohol consumption has caused severe vomiting. Kussmaul's respirations begin abruptly and accompany dehydration, abdominal pain and distention, and absent bowel sounds. Blood glucose levels are normal or slightly decreased.

In *diabetic ketoacidosis*, fruity breath odor commonly occurs as ketoacidosis develops over 1 or 2 days. Other findings include polydipsia, polyuria, nocturia, weak and rapid pulse, hunger, weight loss, weakness, fatigue, nausea, vomiting, and abdominal pain. Eventually, Kussmaul's respirations, orthostatic hypotension, dehydration, tachycardia, confusion, and stupor occur. Symptoms may lead to coma. *Starvation ketoacidosis* is a potentially life-threatening disorder that has a gradual onset. Besides fruity breath odor, typical findings include signs of cachexia and dehydration, decreased LOC, bradycardia, and a history of severely limited food intake (anorexia nervosa).

Other causes

◆ ***Drugs.*** Any drug known to cause metabolic acidosis, such as nitroprusside, can result in fruity breath odor.

◆ ***Fad diets.*** Fad diets, especially those encouraging little or no carbohydrate intake, may cause fruity breath odor.

Special considerations

Provide emotional support for the patient and his family. Explain tests and treatments clearly. When the patient is more alert and his condition stabilizes, remove the nasogastric tube and start him on an appropriate diet. Switch his insulin from the I.V. to the subcutaneous route.

Pediatric pointers

Fruity breath odor in an infant or a child usually reflects uncontrolled diabetes mellitus. Ketoacidosis develops rapidly in this age-group because they have low glycogen reserves. As a result, prompt administration of insulin and correction of fluid and electrolyte imbalance are necessary to prevent shock and death.

Geriatric pointers

Elderly patients may have poor oral hygiene, increased dental caries, decreased salivary function with dryness, and poor dietary intake. In addition, they are frequently taking multiple medications. Consider all of these factors when evaluating an elderly patient with mouth odor.

BRUDZINSKI'S SIGN

A positive Brudzinski's sign (flexion of the hips and knees in response to passive flexion of the neck) signals meningeal irritation. Passive flexion of the neck stretches the nerve roots, causing pain and involuntary flexion of the knees and hips.

Brudzinski's sign is a common and important early indicator of life-threatening meningitis and subarachnoid hemorrhage. It can be elicited in children as well as adults, although more reliable indicators of meningeal irritation exist for infants.

Testing for Brudzinski's sign isn't part of the routine examination, unless meningeal irritation is suspected. (See *Testing for Brudzinski's sign*, page 108.)

Emergency interventions

If the patient is alert, ask him about headache, neck pain, nausea, and visual disturbances (blurred or double vision and photophobia) — all symptoms of increased intracranial pressure (ICP). Next, observe for signs of increased ICP, such as altered level of consciousness (restlessness, irritability, confusion, lethargy, personality changes, and coma), pupillary changes, bradycardia, widened pulse pressure, Cheyne-Stokes or Kussmaul's respirations, vomiting, and moderate fever.

Keep artificial airways, intubation equipment, an a handheld resuscitation bag, and suction equipment on hand because your patient's condition may deteriorate suddenly. Elevate the head of the patient's bed 30 to 60 degrees to promote venous drainage. Administer an osmotic diuretic such as mannitol to reduce cerebral edema.

Monitor ICP and be alert for a continuous increase. You may have to provide mechanical ventilation and to administer barbiturates and additional doses of diuretics. Also, cerebrospinal fluid (CSF) may have to be drained.

History and physical examination

Continue your neurologic examination by evaluating the patient's cranial nerve function and noting any motor or sensory deficits. Also, be sure to look for Kernig's sign (resistance to knee extension after flexion of the hip), which is a further indication of meningeal irritation. In addition, you should look for signs of central nervous system infection, such as fever and nuchal rigidity.

Ask the patient or his family, if necessary, about a history of hypertension, spinal arthritis, or recent head trauma. Also ask about dental work and abscessed teeth (a possible cause of meningitis), open head injury, endocarditis, and I.V. drug abuse. Ask about sudden onset of headaches, which may be associated with subarachnoid hemorrhage.

Testing for Brudzinski's sign

Here's how to test for Brudzinski's sign when you suspect meningeal irritation.

With the patient in a supine position, place your hands behind her neck and lift her head toward her chest.

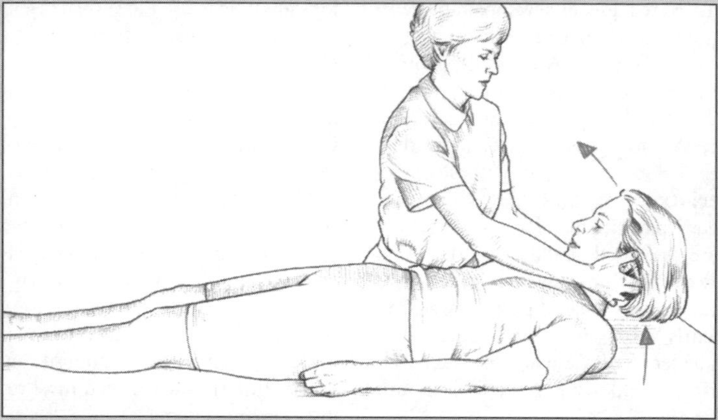

If your patient has meningeal irritation, she'll flex her hips and knees in response to the passive neck flexion.

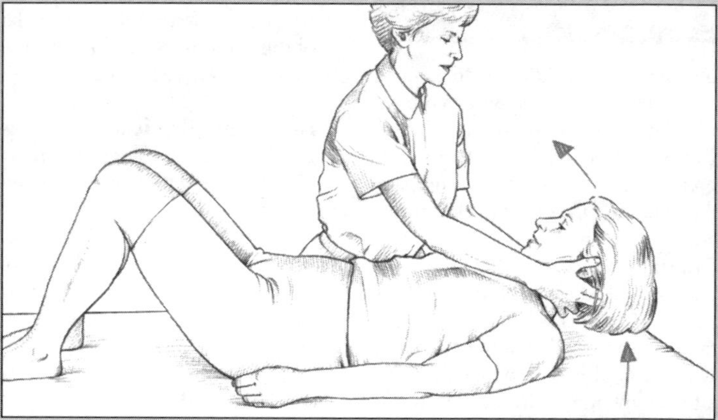

Common medical causes

◆ ***Arthritis.*** In severe spinal arthritis, a positive Brudzinski's sign can occasionally be elicited. The patient may also report back pain (especially after weight bearing) and limited mobility.

◆ ***Meningitis.*** A positive Brudzinski's sign can usually be elicited 24 hours after the onset of this life-threatening disorder. Accompanying findings may include headache, a positive Kernig's sign, nuchal rigidity, irritability or restlessness, deep stupor or coma, vertigo, fever (high or low, depending on the severity of the infection), chills, malaise, hyperalgesia, muscular hypotonia, opisthotonos, symmetrical deep tendon reflexes, papilledema, ocular and facial palsies, nausea and vomiting, photophobia, diplopia, and unequal, sluggish pupils. As ICP rises, arterial hypertension, bradycardia, widened pulse pressure, Cheyne-Stokes or Kussmaul's respirations, and coma may develop.

♦ ***Subarachnoid hemorrhage.*** Brudzinski's sign may be elicited within minutes after initial bleeding in this life-threatening disorder. Accompanying signs and symptoms include sudden onset of severe headache, nuchal rigidity, altered level of consciousness, dizziness, photophobia, cranial nerve palsies (as evidenced by ptosis, pupil dilation, and limited extraocular muscle movement), nausea and vomiting, fever, and a positive Kernig's sign. Focal signs, such as hemiparesis, vision disturbances, or aphasia, may also occur. As ICP rises, arterial hypertension, bradycardia, widened pulse pressure, Cheyne-Stokes or Kussmaul's respirations, and coma may develop.

Special considerations

The patient with a positive Brudzinski's sign is commonly critically ill and needs constant ICP monitoring and frequent neurologic checks, along with intensive assessment and monitoring of vital signs, intake and output, and cardiorespiratory status. To promote patient comfort, maintain low lights and minimal noise, and elevate the head of the bed. The patient usually won't receive narcotic analgesics because they may mask signs of increased ICP.

Prepare the patient for diagnostic tests. These may include blood, urine, and sputum cultures to identify bacteria; lumbar puncture to assess CSF and relieve pressure; and computed tomography scan, magnetic resonance imaging, cerebral angiography, and spinal X-rays to locate a hemorrhage.

Pediatric pointers

Brudzinski's sign may not be useful as an indicator of meningeal irritation in infants because more reliable signs, such as bulging fontanels, weak cry, fretfulness, vomiting, and poor feeding, appear early.

Bruits

Commonly an indicator of life-threatening or limb-threatening vascular disease, bruits are swishing sounds caused by turbulent blood flow. They're characterized by location, duration, intensity, pitch, and time of onset in the cardiac cycle. Loud bruits produce intense vibration and a palpable thrill. A thrill, however, doesn't provide any further clue to the causative disorder or to its severity.

Bruits are most significant when heard over the abdominal aorta; the renal, carotid, femoral, popliteal, and subclavian arteries; and the thyroid gland. (See *Auscultating bruits*, page 110.) They're also significant when heard consistently despite changes in patient position and when heard during diastole.

History and physical examination

If you detect bruits over the abdominal aorta, check for a pulsating mass or a bluish discoloration around the umbilicus (Cullen's sign). Either of these signs or severe, tearing pain in the abdomen, flank, or lower back may signal life-threatening dissection of an aortic aneurysm. Also check peripheral pulses, comparing intensity in the upper versus lower extremities.

If you suspect dissection, monitor the patient's vital signs constantly, and withhold food and fluids until a definitive diagnosis is made. Watch for signs of hy-

EXAMINATION TIP

Auscultating bruits

To detect a bruit, an abnormal sound caused by turbulent blood flow in the vessels, assess the arteries. Use the bell of the stethoscope to auscultate the carotid, femoral, and popliteal arteries on both sides of the trachea, as shown. To evaluate the femoral and popliteal arteries, place the bell of the stethoscope over the pulse sites that were palpated earlier in the assessment. Finally, auscultate the abdominal artery by listening at the epigastric area. Normally, auscultation should detect no vascular sounds.

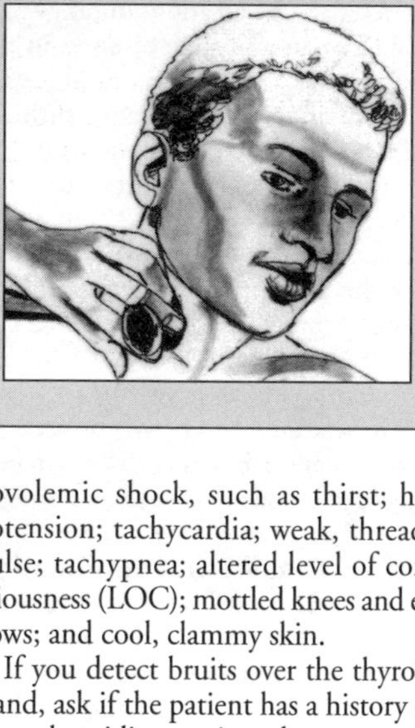

povolemic shock, such as thirst; hypotension; tachycardia; weak, thready pulse; tachypnea; altered level of consciousness (LOC); mottled knees and elbows; and cool, clammy skin.

If you detect bruits over the thyroid gland, ask if the patient has a history of hyperthyroidism or signs that suggest it, such as nervousness, tremors, weight loss, palpitations, heat intolerance or, in females, amenorrhea. Watch for symptoms of life-threatening thyroid storm, such as tremor, restlessness, diarrhea, abdominal pain, and hepatomegaly.

If you detect carotid artery bruits, be alert for signs and symptoms of a transient ischemic attack (TIA), including dizziness, diplopia, slurred speech, flashing lights, and syncope. These findings may indicate an impending cerebrovascular accident (CVA). Be sure to evaluate the patient frequently for changes in LOC and muscle function.

If you detect bruits over the femoral, popliteal, or subclavian arteries, watch for signs of decreased or absent peripheral circulation — edema, weakness, and paresthesia. Does the patient have a history of intermittent claudication? Frequently check distal pulses and skin color and temperature. Also watch for sudden absence of pulse, pallor, or coolness, which may indicate a threat to the affected limb. If you detect a bruit, be sure to check for further vascular damage and perform a thorough cardiac assessment.

Common medical causes

♦ ***Abdominal aortic aneurysm.*** A pulsating periumbilical mass accompanied by a systolic bruit over the aorta characterizes this disorder. Associated findings may include a rigid, tender abdomen; mottled skin; diminished peripheral pulses; and claudication. Sharp, tearing pain in the abdomen, flank, or lower back signals imminent dissection.

♦ ***Abdominal aortic atherosclerosis.*** Loud systolic bruits in the epigastric and midabdominal areas are common. They may be accompanied by leg weakness, numbness, paresthesia, or paralysis; leg pain; and decreased or absent femoral, popliteal, and pedal pulses. Abdominal pain is rarely present.

♦ ***Anemia.*** Increased cardiac output causes increased blood flow. In severe anemia, short systolic bruits may be heard over both carotid arteries and may be accompanied by headache, fatigue, dizziness, pallor, jaundice, palpitations, mild tachycardia, dyspnea, nausea, anorexia, and glossitis.

♦ ***Carotid artery stenosis.*** Systolic bruits can be heard over one or both carotid arteries. Other signs and symptoms may be absent. However, dizziness, vertigo, headache, syncope, aphasia, dysarthria, sudden vision loss, hemiparesis, or hemiparalysis signals TIA and may herald CVA.

♦ ***Carotid cavernous fistula.*** Continuous bruits heard over the eyeballs and temples are characteristic, as are vision disturbances and protruding, pulsating eyeballs.

♦ ***Peripheral vascular disease.*** This condition characteristically causes bruits over the femoral artery and other arteries in the legs. It can also cause diminished or absent femoral, popliteal, or pedal pulses; intermittent claudication; numbness, weakness, pain, and cramping in the legs, feet, and hips; and cool, shiny skin and hair loss on the affected extremity. It also predisposes the patient to lower extremity ulcers that heal with difficulty.

♦ ***Renal artery stenosis.*** Systolic bruits commonly are heard over the abdominal midline and flank on the affected side. Hypertension commonly accompanies stenosis; headache, palpitations, tachycardia, anxiety, dizziness, retinopathy, hematuria, and mental sluggishness may also appear.

♦ ***Thyrotoxicosis.*** A systolic bruit is commonly heard over the thyroid gland. Accompanying signs and symptoms appear in all body systems, but the most characteristic ones include thyroid enlargement, fatigue, nervousness, tachycardia, heat intolerance, sweating, tremor, diarrhea, and weight loss despite increased appetite. Exophthalmos may also be present.

Special considerations

Because bruits can signal a life-threatening vascular disorder, frequently check the patient's vital signs and auscultate over the affected arteries. Be especially alert for bruits that become louder or develop a diastolic component.

As needed, administer medications, such as vasodilators, anticoagulants, antiplatelets, or antihypertensives. Prepare the patient for diagnostic tests, such as blood studies, radiographs, an electrocardiogram, cardiac catheterization, and ultrasonography.

Pediatric pointers

Bruits are common in young children but are usually of little significance; for example, cranial bruits are normal until age 4. However, certain bruits may be significant. Because birthmarks commonly accompany congenital arteriovenous fistulas, carefully auscultate for bruits in a child with port-wine spots or cavernous or diffuse hemangiomas.

Geriatric pointers

Elderly people with atherosclerosis can present with bruits heard over several arteries. Those related to carotid artery stenosis are particularly important because of the high incidence of associated stroke. Close follow-up is mandatory, as is prompt surgical referral when indicated.

BUTTERFLY RASH

The presence of a butterfly rash is commonly a sign of systemic lupus erythematosus (SLE), but it can also signal dermatologic disorders. Typically, butterfly rash appears in a malar distribution across the nose and cheeks. (See *Identifying butterfly rash,* page 113.) Similar rashes may appear on the neck, scalp, and other areas. Butterfly rash is sometimes mistaken for sunburn because it can be provoked or aggravated by ultraviolet rays, but it has more substance, is more sharply demarcated, and has a thicker feel in relation to surrounding skin.

History and physical examination

Ask the patient when he first noticed the butterfly rash and if he has recently been exposed to the sun. Has he noticed a rash elsewhere on his body? Also, ask about

Butterfly rash: Common causes and associated findings

CAUSES	Acne	Alopecia	Erythema	Maculopapular lesions	Malaise	Mucous membrane lesions	Photosensitivity	Plaques	Pruritus	Scaling	Telangiectases
	MAJOR ASSOCIATED SIGNS AND SYMPTOMS										
Discoid lupus erythematosus		◆	◆			◆	◆	◆		◆	◆
Erysipelas					◆						
Rosacea			◆	◆							◆
Seborrheic dermatitis	◆			◆					◆		
Systemic lupus erythematosus		◆	◆		◆						◆

recent weight or hair loss. Does he have a family history of lupus? Is he taking hydralazine or procainamide (common causes of drug-induced lupus erythematosus)?

Inspect the rash, noting any macules, papules, pustules, and scaling. Is the rash edematous? Are areas of hypopigmentation or hyperpigmentation present? Look for blisters or ulcers in the mouth, and note any inflamed lesions. Check for rashes elsewhere on the body. (See *Butterfly rash: Common causes and associated findings.*)

Common medical causes

♦ ***Erysipelas.*** In this streptococcal infection, butterfly rash appears as warm, indurated, tender, pruritic, edematous, and erythematous plaques, enlarging peripherally with sharply elevated margins; vesicles and bullae form. Commonly, the rash appears abruptly and covers the bridge of the nose and one or both cheeks, halting at the hairline of the scalp or beard. However, the rash may also appear on the hands and genitals. Associated signs and symptoms include fever, malaise, headache, vomiting and sore throat and, in some patients, cervical lymphadenopathy.

♦ ***Rosacea.*** Initially, butterfly rash may appear as a prominent, nonscaling, intermittent erythema limited to the lower half of the nose or including the chin, cheeks, and central forehead. As rosacea develops, the duration of the rash increases; instead of disappearing after each episode, the rash varies in intensity and is commonly accompanied by telangiectasia. In advanced rosacea, the skin is oily, with papules, pustules, nodules, and telangiectasis restricted to the central oval of the face. In men with severe rosacea, butterfly rash may be accompanied by rhinophyma — a thickened, lobulated overgrowth of sebaceous glands and epithelial connective tissue on the lower half of the nose and, possibly, the adjacent cheeks.

♦ ***Seborrheic dermatitis.*** Butterfly rash appears as greasy, scaling, slightly yellow macules and papules of varying size on the cheeks and the bridge of the nose, in a "butterfly" pattern. The scalp, beard, eyebrows, portions of the forehead above the bridge of the nose, nasolabial fold, or trunk may also be involved. Associated signs and symptoms may include crusts and fissures (particularly when the external ear and scalp are involved), pruritus, redness, blepharitis, styes, and oily skin. Severe seborrheic dermatitis of the face occurs in acquired immunodeficiency syndrome.

♦ ***Systemic lupus erythematosus.*** Occurring in about 40% of patients with this connective tissue disorder, butterfly rash appears as a red, commonly scaly, sharply demarcated macular eruption. The rash may be transient in acute SLE or may progress slowly to include the forehead, chin, the area around the ears, and other exposed areas. Common associated skin findings include photosensitivity; scaling; patchy alopecia; mucous membrane lesions; mottled erythema of the palms and fingers; periungual erythema with edema; reddish purple macular lesions on the volar surfaces of the fingers; telangiectasia of the base of the nails or eyelids; purpura; petechiae; and ecchymoses.

Butterfly rash may also be accompanied by joint pain, stiffness, and deformities, particularly ulnar deviation of the fingers and subluxation of the proximal interphalangeal joints. Related findings include periorbital and facial edema, dyspnea, low-grade fever, malaise, weakness, fatigue, weight loss, anorexia, nausea, vomiting, lymphadenopathy, and hepatosplenomegaly.

Other causes

♦ ***Drugs.*** Hydralazine and procainamide can cause an SLE-like syndrome.

Identifying butterfly rash

In classic butterfly rash, lesions appear on the cheeks and the bridge of the nose, creating a characteristic butterfly pattern. The rash may vary in severity from malar erythema to discoid lesions (plaques).

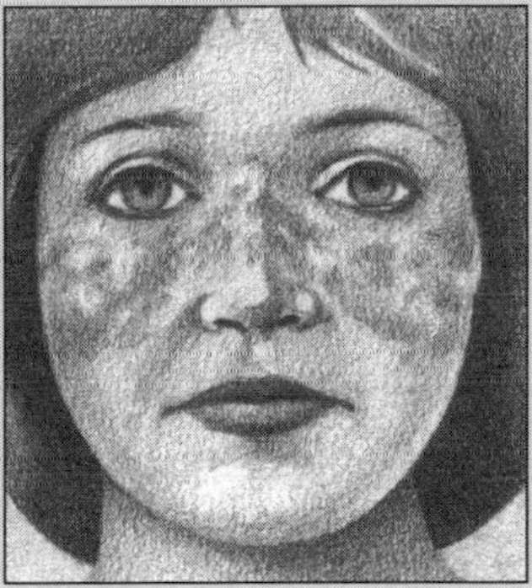

Special considerations

Prepare the patient for immunologic studies, complete blood count, and possibly liver studies. Obtain a urine specimen, if needed. Withhold photosensitizing drugs, such as phenothiazines, sulfonamides, sulfonylureas, and thiazide diuretics. Instruct the patient to avoid exposure to the sun or to use a sunscreen. Suggest that she use hypoallergenic makeup to help conceal facial lesions.

Pediatric pointers

Rare in pediatric patients, a butterfly rash may occur as part of an infectious disease such as erythema infectiosum, or "slapped cheek syndrome."

C

Capillary refill time, prolonged

Capillary refill time is the duration required for color to return to the nail bed of a finger or toe after application of slight pressure that causes blanching. This duration reflects the quality of peripheral vasomotor function. Normal capillary refill time is less than 3 seconds.

Prolonged refill time isn't diagnostic of any disorder but must be evaluated with other signs and symptoms. However, this sign usually signals obstructive peripheral arterial disease or decreased cardiac output.

Capillary refill time is typically tested during a routine cardiovascular assessment. It isn't tested in suspected life-threatening disorders because other, more characteristic signs and symptoms appear earlier.

History and physical examination

If you detect prolonged capillary refill time, take the patient's vital signs and check pulses in the affected limb. Does the limb feel cold or look cyanotic? Does the patient report pain or any unusual sensations in his fingers or toes, especially after exposure to cold?

Take a brief medical history, noting especially previous peripheral vascular disease. Find out what medications the patient is taking.

Common medical causes

♦ ***Aortic aneurysm (dissecting).*** Capillary refill time is prolonged in the fingers and toes of a patient with a dissecting aneurysm in the thoracic aorta, and is prolonged in the toes only when the dissecting aneurysm is in the abdominal aorta. Common accompanying signs and symptoms include a pulsating abdominal mass, systolic bruit, and substernal back or abdominal pain.

♦ ***Aortic arch syndrome.*** Prolonged capillary refill time in the fingers occurs early in this syndrome. Carotid pulses are absent, and radial pulses may be unequal. Signs and symptoms that usually precede loss of pulses include fever, night sweats, arthralgia, weight loss, anorexia, nausea, malaise, skin rash, splenomegaly, and pallor.

♦ ***Arterial occlusion (acute).*** Prolonged capillary refill time occurs early in the affected limb. Arterial pulses are usually absent distal to the obstruction; the affected limb appears cool and pale or cyanotic. Intermittent claudication, moderate to severe pain, numbness, and paresthesia or paralysis of the affected limb may occur.

♦ ***Buerger's disease.*** Capillary refill time is prolonged in the toes. On exposure to low temperatures, the feet become cold, cyanotic, and numb; later, they become hot, redden, and tingle. Other findings include intermittent claudication of the instep, weak peripheral pulses and, in later stages, ulceration, muscle atrophy, and gangrene. If the disease affects the hands, prolonged capillary refill may accompany painful fingertip ulcerations.

♦ ***Cardiac tamponade.*** Prolonged capillary refill time is a late sign of decreased cardiac output. Associated signs include tachycardia, cyanosis, dyspnea, neck vein distention, and hypotension.

♦ ***Hypothermia.*** Prolonged capillary refill time may appear early as a compensatory response. Associated signs and symptoms depend on the degree of hypothermia and may include some combination of shivering, fatigue, weakness, decreased level of consciousness, slurred speech, ataxia, muscle stiffness or rigidity, tachycardia or bradycardia, hyporeflexia or areflexia, diuresis, oliguria, bradypnea, decreased blood pressure, and cold, pale skin.

♦ ***Peripheral arterial trauma.*** Any trauma to a peripheral artery that reduces distal blood flow also prolongs capillary refill time in the affected extremity. Related findings in that extremity include bruising or pulsating bleeding, weakened pulse, cyanosis, paresthesia, sensory loss, and cool, pale skin.

♦ ***Raynaud's disease.*** Capillary refill time is prolonged in the fingers, the usual site of this disease's characteristic episodic arterial vasospasm. Exposure to cold or stress causes the sequence of blanching, cyanosis, and erythema before fingers return to normal temperature. Warmth relieves symptoms, which may include paresthesia. Chronic disease may cause trophic changes, such as sclerodactyly, ulcerations, or chronic paronychia.

♦ ***Volkmann's contracture.*** Prolonged capillary refill time results from this contracture's characteristic vasospasm. Associated signs include loss of mobility and loss of strength in the affected extremity.

Other causes

♦ ***Diagnostic tests.*** Cardiac catheterization can cause arterial hematoma or clot formation and prolonged capillary refill time.

♦ ***Drugs.*** Drugs that cause vasoconstriction (particularly alpha adrenergics) prolong capillary refill time.

♦ ***Treatments.*** An arterial or umbilical line (which can cause arterial hematoma and obstructed distal blood flow) or an improperly fitting cast (which constricts circulation) can prolong capillary refill time.

Special considerations

Frequently assess the patient's vital signs, level of consciousness, and affected extremity, and report any changes, such as progressive cyanosis or loss of an existing pulse. Prepare the patient for diagnostic tests, which may include arteriography or Doppler ultrasonography, to help confirm or rule out arterial occlusion.

Pediatric pointers

Capillary refill time may be prolonged in newborns with acrocyanosis, but this is a normal finding. Typically, prolonged capillary refill time is associated with the same disorders in children as in adults. However, its most common pediatric cause is cardiac surgery, such as repair of congenital heart defects.

CARPOPEDAL SPASM

Carpopedal spasm is a significantly noticeable, painful contraction of the muscles in the hands and feet. (See *Recognizing carpopedal spasm,* page 116.) It's an important sign of tetany, a potentially life-threatening condition characterized by increased neuromuscular excitation and sustained muscle contraction and commonly associated with hypocalcemia.

Carpopedal spasm requires prompt evaluation and intervention. If the primary event is not treated promptly, the

Recognizing carpopedal spasm

In the hand, carpopedal spasm begins with adduction of the thumb over the palm, followed by flexion of the metacarpophalangeal joints, extension of the interphalangeal joints (fingers together), adduction of the hyperextended fingers, and flexion of the wrist and elbow joints. Similar effects occur in the joints of the feet.

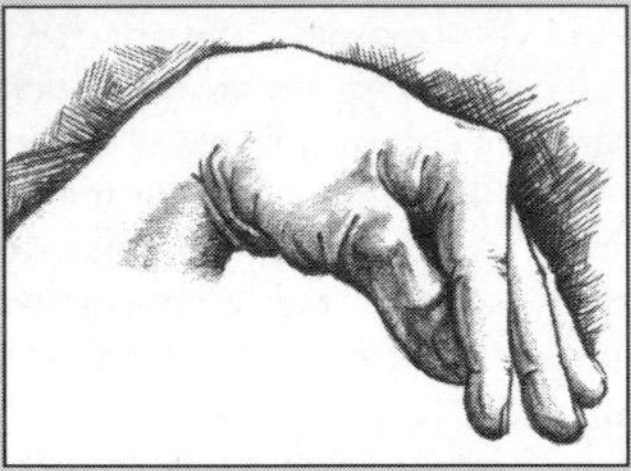

patient can develop laryngospasm, seizures, cardiac arrhythmias, or cardiac or respiratory arrest.

Emergency interventions

If you detect carpopedal spasm, quickly examine the patient for signs of respiratory distress (laryngospasm, stridor, loud crowing noises, cyanosis) or cardiac arrhythmias, both of which suggest hypocalcemia. Obtain blood specimens for electrolyte analysis (especially calcium), and perform an electrocardiogram. Connect the patient to a monitor to detect arrhythmias. Administer an I.V. calcium preparation, and provide emergency respiratory and cardiac support. If calcium infusion doesn't control seizures, administer a sedative, such as chloral hydrate or phenobarbital.

History and physical examination

If the patient isn't in distress, obtain a detailed history. Ask about the onset and duration of the spasms and the degree of pain they cause. Also ask about related signs of hypocalcemia, such as numbness and tingling of the fingertips and feet; other muscle cramps or spasms; and nausea, vomiting, and abdominal pain. Check for previous neck surgery, calcium or magnesium deficiency, tetanus exposure without previous vaccination, and hypoparathyroidism.

During the history, form a general impression of the patient's mental status and behavior. If possible, ask family members or friends if they've noticed changes in the patient's behavior.

Inspect the patient's skin and fingernails, noting any dryness or scaling and ridged, brittle nails.

Common medical causes

♦ ***Hypocalcemia.*** Carpopedal spasm is an early sign of hypocalcemia. It's usually accompanied by paresthesia of the fingers, toes, and perioral area; muscle weakness, twitching, and cramping; hyperreflexia; chorea; fatigue; and palpitations. Positive Chvostek's and Trousseau's signs can be elicited. Laryngospasm, stridor, and seizures may occur in severe hypocalcemia.

Chronic hypocalcemia may be accompanied by mental status changes; cramps; dry, scaly skin; brittle nails; and thin, patchy hair and eyebrows.

♦ ***Tetanus.*** This infectious disease develops when *Clostridium tetani* enters a wound in a nonimmunized person. The patient develops muscle spasms and painful seizures. Difficulty swallowing and a low-grade fever are also present. If the patient is not treated or treatment is delayed, the mortality rate is high.

Other causes

♦ ***Treatments.*** Multiple blood transfusions and parathyroidectomy may cause hypocalcemia, resulting in carpopedal spasm. Surgical procedures that impair calcium absorption, such as ileostomy formation and gastric resection with gastrojejunostomy, may also cause hypocalcemia.

Special considerations

Carpopedal spasm can cause severe pain and anxiety, leading to hyperventilation. If this occurs, help the patient slow his breathing by providing a relaxing touch, a reassuring attitude, and clear directions about what he should do. Provide a quiet, dark environment to reduce his anxiety. Have the patient slowly breathe into a paper bag. A hyperventilating patient may not be obviously hyperventilating. You can confirm hyperventilation with an arterial blood gas analysis.

Prepare the patient for laboratory tests, such as complete blood count and serum calcium, phosphorus, and parathyroid hormone studies.

Pediatric pointers

Idiopathic hypoparathyroidism is a common cause of hypocalcemia in children. Carefully monitor children with this condition because carpopedal spasm may herald the onset of epileptiform seizures or generalized tetany followed by prolonged tonic spasms.

Geriatric pointers

Always ask elderly patients about their immunization record. Suspect tetanus in anyone who presents with carpopedal spasm, difficulty swallowing, and seizures. Such patients may have incomplete immunizations or may not have had a recent booster shot. Always ask about any recent wound, no matter how inconsequential it may seem.

CAT'S CRY

In an infant, this mewing, kittenlike sound is the primary indicator of cri du chat (also known as cat's cry) syndrome. This syndrome affects 1 in 50,000 neonates — more often females — and causes profound mental retardation, failure to thrive and, frequently, death before age 1. The chromosomal defect responsible (deletion of the short arm of chromosome 5) usually appears spontaneously but may be inherited from a carrier parent. The characteristic cry is thought to result from abnormal laryngeal development.

Emergency interventions

Suspect cri du chat syndrome if you detect cat's cry in a neonate. Be alert for signs of respiratory distress, such as nasal flaring; irregular, shallow respirations; cyanosis; and a respiratory rate over 60 breaths/minute. Be prepared to suction the infant and to administer warmed oxygen. Keep emergency resuscitation equipment nearby because bradycardia may develop.

History and physical examination

Perform a physical examination and note any abnormalities. If you detect cat's cry in an older infant, ask the parents when it developed. Sudden onset of an abnormal cry in an infant with a previously normal, vigorous cry suggests other disorders. (See "Cry, high-pitched," page 165.)

Common medical causes

- ***Cri du chat syndrome.*** A kittenlike cry begins at birth or shortly thereafter. It's accompanied by profound mental retardation, microcephaly, low birth weight, hypotonia, failure to thrive, and feeding difficulties. Typically, the infant has a round face with wide-set eyes; strabismus; a broad-based nose with oblique or down-sloping epicanthal folds; abnormally shaped, low-set ears; and an unusually small jaw. He may also have a short neck, webbed fingers, and a simian crease.

Special considerations

Connect the infant to an apnea monitor, and check for signs of respiratory distress. Keep suction equipment and warmed oxygen available. Watch for signs of increased intracranial pressure. Obtain a blood sample for chromosomal analysis. Prepare the infant for a computed tomography scan to rule out other causes of microcephaly and for an ear, nose, and throat examination to evaluate vocal cords.

Because the infant with cri du chat usually eats poorly, monitor intake, output, and weight. Instruct the parents to offer small, frequent feedings.

CHEST EXPANSION, ASYMMETRICAL

Asymmetrical chest expansion is the uneven extension of portions of the chest wall during inspiration. During normal inspiration, the thorax uniformly expands upward and outward, then on expiration, contracts downward and inward. When this process is disrupted, breathing becomes uncoordinated, resulting in asymmetrical chest expansion.

Asymmetrical chest expansion may develop suddenly or gradually and may affect one or both sides of the chest wall. It may occur as delayed expiration (chest lag); as abnormal movement during inspiration (for example, intercostal retractions, paradoxical movement, or chest-abdomen asynchrony); or as unilateral absence of movement. This sign usually results from pleural disorders, such as life-threatening hemothorax or tension pneumothorax. (See *Recognizing life-threatening causes of asymmetrical chest expansion.*) It can also reflect a musculoskeletal or urologic disorder, airway obstruction, or trauma. Regardless of its underlying cause, asymmetrical chest expansion causes rapid and shallow or deep respirations that increase the work of breathing.

Emergency interventions

If you detect asymmetrical chest expansion, first consider traumatic injury to the patient's ribs or sternum, which can cause flail chest, a life-threatening emergency characterized by paradoxical chest movement. Quickly take the patient's vital signs and look for signs of acute respiratory distress — rapid and shallow respirations, tachycardia, and cyanosis. Use tape or sandbags to temporarily splint the unstable flail segment.

Depending on the severity of respiratory distress, administer oxygen by nasal cannula, mask, or mechanical ventilator. Insert an I.V. line to allow fluid replacement and administration of pain medication. Draw a blood sample from the patient for arterial blood gas analysis, and connect the patient to a cardiac monitor.

Although asymmetrical chest expansion may result from hemothorax, tension pneumothorax, bronchial obstruction, or other life-threatening causes, it's not a cardinal sign of these disorders. Because any form of asymmetrical chest expansion can compromise the patient's respiratory status, don't leave the patient unattended; be alert for signs of respiratory distress.

History and physical examination

If you don't suspect flail chest, and if the patient isn't experiencing acute respiratory distress, obtain a brief history. Asymmetrical chest expansion often results from mechanical airflow obstruction, so find out if the patient is experiencing dyspnea or pain during breathing. If so, does he feel short of breath constantly or intermittently? Does the pain worsen his feeling of breathlessness? Does repositioning, coughing, or any other activity relieve or worsen the patient's dyspnea or pain? Is the pain more noticeable during inspiration or expiration? Can he inhale deeply?

Recognizing life-threatening causes of asymmetrical chest expansion

Asymmetrical chest expansion can result from several life-threatening disorders. Two common causes — bronchial obstruction and flail chest — produce distinctive chest wall movements that provide important clues about the underlying disorder.

BRONCHIAL OBSTRUCTION

Only the unaffected portion of the chest wall expands during inspiration. Intercostal bulging during expiration may indicate that the air is trapped in the chest.

INSPIRATION

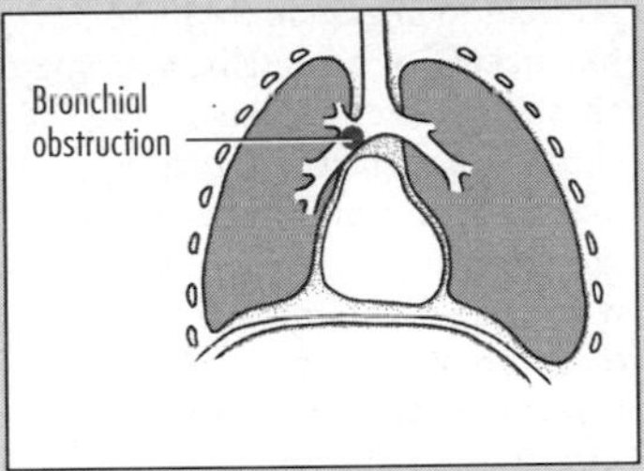

EXPIRATION

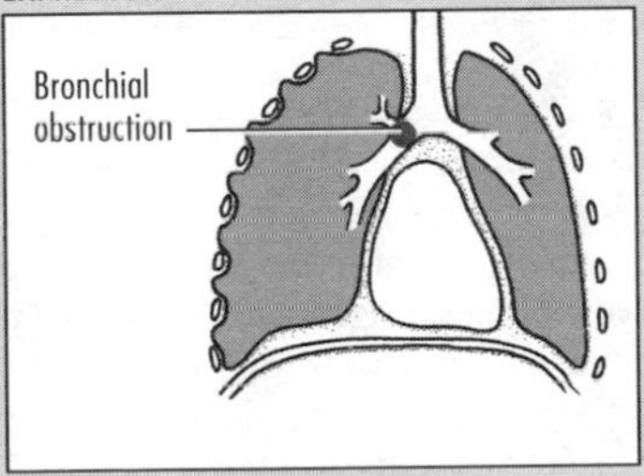

FLAIL CHEST

In this disruption of the thorax caused by multiple rib fractures, the unstable portion of the chest wall collapses inward at inspiration and balloons outward at expiration.

INSPIRATION

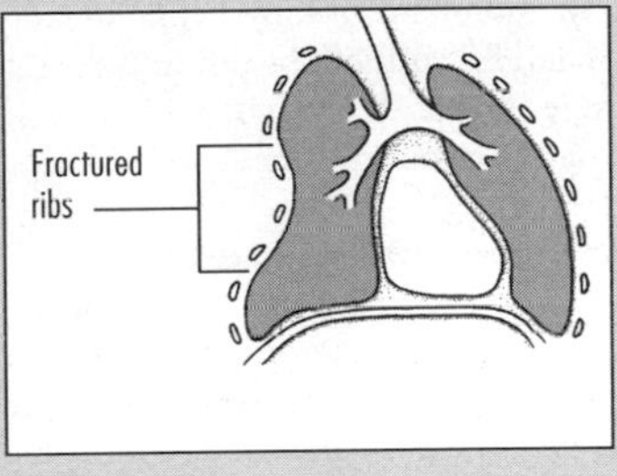

EXPIRATION

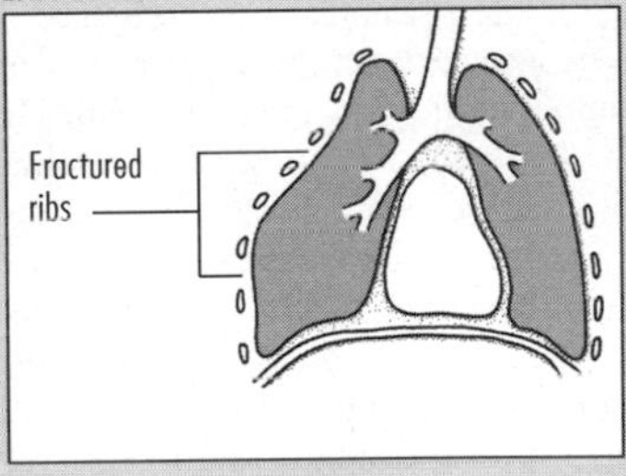

Ask if the patient has a history of pulmonary or systemic illness, such as frequent upper respiratory infections, asthma, tuberculosis, pneumonia, or cancer. Has he had thoracic surgery? (This typically causes asymmetrical chest expansion on the affected side.) Also, ask about blunt or penetrating chest trauma, which may have caused pulmonary injury. And obtain an occupational history to find out if the patient may have inhaled toxic fumes or aspirated a toxic substance.

Next, perform a physical examination. Begin by gently palpating the trachea for midline positioning. (Deviation of the trachea usually indicates an acute problem requiring immediate intervention.) Then examine the posterior chest wall for areas of tenderness or deformity. To evaluate the extent of asymmetrical chest expansion, place your hands — fingers together and thumbs abducted toward the spine — flat on both sections of the lower posterior chest wall. Position your thumbs at the 10th rib, and grasp the lateral rib cage with your hands. As the patient inhales, note the uneven separation of your thumbs, and gauge the distance between them. Then repeat this technique on the upper posterior chest wall. Next, use the ulnar surface of your hand to palpate for vocal or tactile fremitus on both sides of the chest. To check for vocal fremitus, ask the patient to repeat "99" as you proceed. Note any asymmetrical vibrations and areas of enhanced, diminished, or absent fremitus. Then percuss and auscultate to detect air and fluid in the lungs and pleural spaces. Finally, auscultate all lung fields for normal and adventitious breath sounds. Examine the patient's anterior chest wall, using the same assessment techniques.

Common medical causes

♦ ***Flail chest.*** In this life-threatening injury to the ribs or sternum, the unstable portion of the chest wall collapses inward during inspiration and balloons outward during expiration (paradoxical movement). The patient may have ecchymoses, severe localized pain, and other signs of traumatic injury to the chest wall. He may also exhibit rapid, shallow respirations, tachycardia, and cyanosis.

♦ ***Kyphoscoliosis.*** Abnormal curvature of the thoracic spine in the anteroposterior direction (kyphosis) or the lateral direction (scoliosis) gradually compresses one lung and distends the other. This causes decreased chest wall movement on the compressed-lung side and expands the intercostal muscles during inspiration on the opposite side. It can also cause ineffective coughing, dyspnea, back pain, and fatigue.

♦ ***Myasthenia gravis.*** Progressive loss of ventilatory muscle function causes asynchrony of the chest and abdomen during inspiration ("abdominal paradox"), which can lead to onset of acute respiratory distress. Typically, the patient's shallow respirations and increased muscle weakness cause severe dyspnea, tachypnea, and possible apnea.

♦ ***Pleural effusion.*** Chest lag at end inspiration occurs gradually in this life-threatening accumulation of fluid, blood, or pus in the pleural space. Usually, some combination of dyspnea, tachypnea, and tachycardia precedes chest lag; the patient may also have pleuritic pain that worsens with coughing or deep breathing. The area of the effusion is delineated by dullness on percussion, decreased or absent breath sounds, and decreased tactile fremitus. Fever appears if infection causes the effusion.

♦ ***Pneumonia.*** Depending on whether fluid consolidation in the lungs develops unilaterally or bilaterally, asymmetrical chest expansion occurs as inspiratory chest lag or as chest-abdomen asynchrony. The patient typically has fever, chills, tachycardia, tachypnea, and dyspnea with crackles, rhonchi, and chest pain that worsens during deep breathing. He may also have a productive cough with rust-colored sputum. Egophony and bronchophony (or whispered pectoriloquy) may occur if consolidation is present.

♦ ***Pulmonary embolism.*** This acute, life-threatening disorder causes chest lag; sudden, stabbing chest pain; and tachycardia. The patient usually has severe dyspnea, blood-tinged sputum, pleural friction rub, and acute anxiety.

Other causes

♦ ***Treatments.*** Asymmetrical chest expansion can result from pneumonectomy or surgical removal of several ribs. Chest lag or absence of chest movement may also result from intubation of a mainstem bronchus, a serious complication typically due to incorrect insertion of an endotracheal tube or movement of the tube while it's in the trachea.

Special considerations

If you're caring for an intubated patient, regularly auscultate breath sounds in the lung peripheries to help detect a misplaced tube. If this occurs, prepare the patient for a chest X-ray to allow rapid repositioning of the tube. Because asymmetrical chest expansion increases the work of breathing, supplemental oxygen is usually given during acute events.

Pediatric pointers

Children are more likely than adults to require mainstem bronchus (especially left bronchus) intubation. A child's breath sounds are frequently referred from one lung to the other because of the small size of the thoracic cage, so use chest wall expansion as an indicator of correct tube position. Children with acute respiratory illnesses such as bronchiolitis, asthma, or croup also develop asymmetrical chest expansion, paradoxical breathing, and retractions.

Congenital abnormalities, such as cerebral palsy and diaphragmatic hernia, can also cause asymmetrical chest expansion. In cerebral palsy, asymmetrical facial muscles usually accompany chest-abdomen asynchrony. In life-threatening diaphragmatic hernia, asymmetrical expansion usually occurs on the left side of the chest.

Geriatric pointers

Asymmetrical chest expansion may be more difficult to detect in this population because of the structural deformities associated with aging.

CHEST PAIN

Chest pain usually results from disorders that affect thoracic or abdominal organs — the heart, pleurae, lungs, esophagus, rib cage, gallbladder, pancreas, or stomach. An important indicator of several acute and life-threatening cardiopulmonary and GI disorders, chest pain can also result from musculoskeletal and hematologic disorders, anxiety, and drug therapy.

Chest pain can arise suddenly or gradually, and its cause may be difficult to ascertain initially. The pain can radiate to the arms, neck, jaw, or back. It can be steady or intermittent, mild or acute. And it can range in character from a sharp shooting sensation to a feeling of heaviness, fullness, or even indigestion. It can be provoked or aggravated by stress, anxiety, exertion, deep breathing, or eating certain foods.

Emergency interventions

Ask the patient when his chest pain began. Did it develop suddenly or gradually? Is it more severe or frequent now than when it first started? Does anything relieve the pain? Ask the patient about associated symptoms. Sudden, severe chest pain requires prompt evaluation and treatment because it may herald a life-threatening disorder. (See *Managing severe chest pain,* pages 122 and 123.)

History and physical examination

If the chest pain isn't severe, proceed with the history. Ask if the patient feels diffuse pain or can point to the painful area. Sometimes a patient won't perceive the sensation he's feeling as pain, so ask whether he has any discomfort radiating to his neck, jaw, arms, or back. If he does, ask him to describe it. Is it a dull, aching, pressurelike sensation? A sharp, stabbing, knifelike pain? Does he feel it on the surface or deep inside? Find out whether it's constant or intermittent. If it's intermittent, how long does it last? Ask if movement, exertion, breathing, position changes, or eating certain foods worsens or helps relieve the pain. Does anything in particular seem to bring it on?

Review the patient's history for cardiac or pulmonary disease, chest trauma, intestinal disease, or sickle cell anemia. Find out what medications he's taking, if any, and ask about recent dosage or schedule changes.

(Text continues on page 124.)

EMERGENCY INTERVENTIONS

Managing severe chest pain

Sudden, severe chest pain may result from several life-threatening disorders. Your evaluation and interventions will vary, depending on the pain's location and character. The flowchart below will help you establish priorities for managing this emergency successfully.

Patient reports sudden onset of pleuritic chest pain, which he characterizes as crushing, shooting, and deep.

Assess for diaphoresis, dyspnea, hemoptysis, and tachycardia.

If you detect these signs and symptoms, suspect *pulmonary embolism.*

Patient reports sudden onset of tearing, ripping, stabbing chest pain, with syncope and hemiplegia.

Assess for differences in blood pressure between legs and arms, as well as weak or absent femoral or pedal pulses.

If you detect these signs, suspect *dissecting aortic aneurysm.*

What to do: Quickly take the patient's vital signs. Obtain a 12-lead electrocardiogram. Insert an I.V. line to administer fluids and drugs, and give oxygen. Check the patient's vital signs frequently to detect changes from baseline. Begin cardiac monitoring to detect arrhythmias. As appropriate, prepare the patient for emergency surgery.

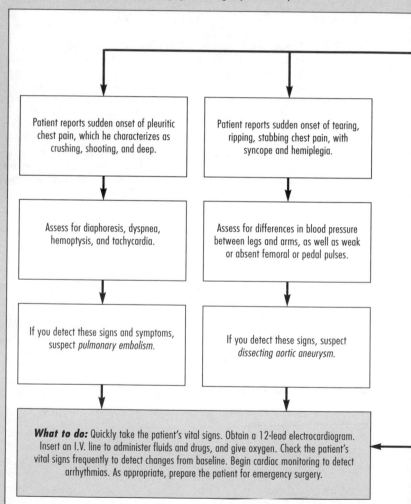

ASK THE PATIENT TO CHARACTERIZE HIS CHEST PAIN.

Patient reports sudden onset of severe substernal pain that radiates to his left arm, jaw, neck, or shoulder blades; he describes the pain as a squeezing, viselike, burning sensation.

Assess for pallor, diaphoresis, nausea, vomiting, apprehension, weakness, fatigue, and dyspnea.

If you detect these signs and symptoms, suspect *myocardial infarction.*

Patient reports sudden onset of diffuse chest tightness.

Assess for wheezing, dry cough, dyspnea, tachycardia, and hyperventilation.

If you detect these signs and symptoms, suspect an *acute asthmatic attack.*

What to do: Try to calm the patient to slow his respiratory rate. Ask the patient if he's ever had this pain before and, if so, what (if anything) eased it. Give oxygen and insert an I.V. line to administer fluids and drugs. Expect to give epinephrine and a bronchodilator and to begin respiratory therapy.

Take the patient's vital signs, noting tachypnea, fever, tachycardia, pulsus paradoxus, and hypertension or hypotension. Also look for jugular vein distention and peripheral edema. Observe the patient's breathing pattern, and inspect his chest for asymmetrical expansion. Auscultate his lungs for pleural friction rub, crackles, rhonchi, wheezing, or diminished or absent breath sounds. Next, auscultate for murmurs, clicks, gallops, or pericardial friction rub. Palpate for lifts, heaves, thrills, gallops, tactile fremitus, and abdominal mass or tenderness. (See *Chest pain: Common causes and associated findings,* pages 126 and 127.)

Common medical causes

♦ ***Angina.*** The patient with *angina pectoris* may experience a feeling of tightness or pressure in the chest that he describes as pain or a sensation of indigestion or expansion. The pain usually occurs in the retrosternal region over a palm-sized or larger area. It may radiate to the neck, jaw, and arms — classically, to the inner aspect of the left arm. Anginal pain tends to begin gradually, build to its maximum, then slowly subside. Provoked by exertion, emotional stress, or a heavy meal, the pain typically lasts 2 to 10 minutes (usually no longer than 20 minutes). Associated findings may include dyspnea, nausea, vomiting, tachycardia, dizziness, diaphoresis, belching, or palpitations. You may hear an atrial gallop (S_4) or murmur during an anginal episode.

In *Prinzmetal's angina,* caused by vasospasm of coronary vessels, chest pain typically occurs when the patient is at rest — or it may awaken him. It may be accompanied by shortness of breath, nausea, vomiting, dizziness, and palpitations. During an attack, you may hear an atrial gallop.

♦ ***Anxiety.*** Acute anxiety — or, more commonly, panic attacks — can cause intermittent, sharp, stabbing pain, often behind the left breast. This pain isn't related to exertion and lasts only a few seconds, but the patient may experience a precordial ache or a sensation of heaviness that lasts for hours or days. Associated signs and symptoms may include precordial tenderness, palpitations, fatigue, headache, insomnia, breathlessness, nausea, vomiting, diarrhea, and tremors. Panic attacks may be associated with agoraphobia — fear of leaving home or being in open places with other people.

♦ ***Aortic aneurysm (dissecting).*** The chest pain associated with this life-threatening disorder usually begins suddenly and is most severe at its onset. The patient describes an excruciating tearing, ripping, stabbing pain in his chest and neck that radiates to his upper back, abdomen, and lower back. He may also have abdominal tenderness; a palpable abdominal mass; tachycardia; murmurs; syncope; blindness; loss of consciousness; weakness or transient paralysis of the arms or legs; a systolic bruit; systemic hypotension; asymmetrical brachial pulses; lower blood pressure in the legs than in the arms; or weak or absent femoral or pedal pulses. His skin is pale, cool, diaphoretic, and mottled below the waist. Capillary refill time is prolonged in the toes, and palpation reveals decreased pulsation in one or both carotid arteries.

♦ ***Asthma.*** In a life-threatening asthma attack, diffuse and painful chest tightness arises suddenly with a dry cough and mild wheezing, which progress to a productive cough, audible wheezing, and severe dyspnea. Related respiratory findings include rhonchi, crackles, prolonged expirations, intercostal and supraclavicular retractions on inspiration, accessory muscle use, flaring nostrils, and tachypnea. Other clinical features are anxiety, tachycardia, diaphoresis, flushing, and cyanosis.

♦ ***Bronchitis.*** In its acute form, this disorder causes a burning chest pain or a sensation of substernal tightness. It also causes a cough, initially dry but later productive, that worsens the chest pain. Other findings include: low-grade fever, chills, sore throat, tachycardia, muscle and back pain, rhonchi, crackles, and wheezing. Severe bronchitis causes fever of 101° to 102° F (38.3° to 38.8° C) and possible bronchospasm with worsening wheezing and increased coughing.

♦ ***Cholecystitis.*** This disorder typically causes abrupt epigastric or right upper quadrant pain, which may be sharp or intensely aching. Steady or intermittent pain may radiate to the back or the right shoulder. Commonly associated findings include nausea, vomiting, fever, diaphoresis, and chills. Palpation of the right upper quadrant may reveal an abdominal mass, rigidity, distention, and tenderness. Murphy's sign — inspiratory arrest elicited when the examiner palpates the right upper quadrant as the patient takes a deep breath — may also occur.

♦ ***Interstitial lung disease.*** As this disease advances, the patient may experience pleuritic chest pain with progressive dyspnea, cellophane-type crackles, nonproductive cough, fatigue, weight loss, decreased exercise tolerance, clubbing, and cyanosis.

♦ ***Lung abscess.*** Pleuritic chest pain develops insidiously in this disorder with a pleural friction rub and a cough that raises copious amounts of purulent, foul-smelling, blood-tinged sputum. The affected side is dull to percussion, and decreased breath sounds and crackles may be heard. The patient also displays diaphoresis, anorexia, weight loss, fever, chills, fatigue, weakness, dyspnea, and clubbing.

♦ ***Lung cancer.*** The chest pain associated with lung cancer is often described as an intermittent aching felt deep within the chest. If the tumor metastasizes to the ribs or vertebrae, the pain becomes localized, continuous, and gnawing. Associated findings may include cough (sometimes bloody), wheezing, dyspnea, fatigue, anorexia, weight loss, or fever.

♦ ***Mitral valve prolapse.*** Most patients with mitral valve prolapse are asymptomatic, but some may experience sharp, stabbing precordial chest pain or precordial ache. The pain can last for seconds or for hours, and occasionally mimics the pain of ischemic heart disease. The characteristic sign of mitral prolapse is a midsystolic click followed by a systolic murmur at the apex. The patient may experience cardiac awareness, migraine headache, dizziness, weakness, episodic severe fatigue, dyspnea, tachycardia, mood swings, and palpitations.

♦ ***Myocardial infarction (MI).*** The chest pain in an MI lasts from 15 minutes to hours. Typically a crushing substernal pain, unrelieved by rest or nitroglycerin, it may radiate to the patient's left arm, jaw, neck, or shoulder blades. Other possible findings include pallor, clammy skin, dyspnea, diaphoresis, nausea, vomiting, anxiety, restlessness, a feeling of impending doom, hypotension or hypertension, an atrial gallop, murmurs, and crackles.

♦ ***Pancreatitis.*** In its acute form, this disorder usually causes intense epigastric pain that radiates to the back and worsens when the patient is supine. Nausea, vomiting, fever, abdominal tenderness and rigidity, diminished bowel sounds, and crackles at the lung bases may also occur. A patient with severe pancreatitis may be extremely restless and have mottled skin, tachycardia, and cold, sweaty extremities. Fulminant pancreatitis causes massive hemorrhage, resulting in shock and coma.

♦ ***Peptic ulcer.*** In this disorder, sharp and burning pain usually arises in the epigastric region. This pain characteristically arises hours after food intake, often during the night. It lasts longer than angina-like pain and is relieved by food or antacids. Other findings may include nausea, vomiting (sometimes with blood), melena, and epigastric tenderness.

Chest pain: Common causes and associated findings

CAUSES	MAJOR ASSOCIATED SIGNS AND SYMPTOMS												
	Abdominal mass	Abdominal tenderness	Atrial gallop	Breath sounds, decreased	Cough	Crackles	Cyanosis	Diaphoresis	Dizziness	Dyspnea	Fever	Hemoptysis	Murmur
Angina pectoris			◆					◆	◆	◆			◆
Aortic aneurysm (dissecting)	◆	◆						◆					◆
Asthma					◆	◆	◆	◆		◆			
Bronchitis					◆	◆					◆		
Cholecystitis	◆	◆						◆			◆		
Interstitial lung disease					◆	◆	◆			◆			
Lung abscess				◆	◆	◆		◆		◆	◆	◆	
Lung cancer					◆					◆	◆	◆	
Mitral valve prolapse									◆	◆			◆
Myocardial infarction			◆			◆		◆		◆	◆		◆
Pancreatitis		◆				◆					◆		
Peptic ulcer		◆											
Pericarditis										◆	◆		
Pleurisy				◆		◆	◆			◆	◆		
Pneumonia				◆	◆	◆	◆	◆		◆	◆		
Pneumothorax				◆	◆		◆			◆			
Pulmonary embolism					◆	◆	◆	◆		◆	◆	◆	

♦ ***Pericarditis.*** This disorder causes precordial or retrosternal pain aggravated by deep breathing, coughing, position changes and, occasionally, by swallowing. The pain is commonly sharp or cutting and radiates to the shoulder and neck. Associated signs and symptoms may include pericardial friction rub, fever,

	Nausea or vomiting	Pericardial friction rub	Pleural friction rub	Skin mottling	Syncope	Tachycardia	Tachypnea	Wheezing
	♦					♦		
				♦	♦	♦		
						♦	♦	♦
						♦		♦
	♦							
			♦					
								♦
						♦		
	♦							
	♦			♦		♦		
	♦							
		♦				♦		
			♦				♦	
						♦	♦	
						♦	♦	
			♦			♦	♦	♦

tachycardia, and dyspnea. Pericarditis usually follows a viral illness, but several other causes should be considered, including myocardial infarction.

♦ ***Pleurisy.*** The chest pain of pleurisy arises abruptly and reaches maximum intensity within a few hours. The pain is sharp, even knifelike, usually unilateral, and located in the lower and lateral aspects of the chest. Deep breathing, coughing, or thoracic movement characteristically aggravates it. Auscultation over the painful area may reveal decreased breath sounds, inspiratory crackles, and a pleural friction rub. Dyspnea; rapid, shallow breathing; cyanosis; fever; and fatigue may also occur.

♦ ***Pneumonia.*** This disorder causes pleuritic chest pain that increases with deep inspiration and is accompanied by shaking chills and fever. The patient has a dry cough that later becomes productive. Other signs and symptoms may include crackles, rhonchi, tachycardia, tachypnea, myalgias, fatigue, headache, dyspnea, abdominal pain, anorexia, cyanosis, decreased breath sounds, or diaphoresis.

♦ ***Pneumothorax.*** Spontaneous pneumothorax, a life-threatening disorder, causes sudden sharp chest pain that's severe, often unilateral, and rarely localized; it increases with chest movement. When the pain is centrally located and radiates to the neck, it may mimic that of an MI. After the pain's onset, dyspnea and cyanosis progressively worsen. Breath sounds are decreased or absent on the affected side; hyperresonance or tympany, subcutaneous crepitation, or decreased vocal fremitus may be heard. Asymmetrical chest expansion, accessory muscle use, nonproductive cough, tachypnea, tachycardia, anxiety, and restlessness are other common findings.

♦ ***Pulmonary embolism.*** This disorder causes chest pain or a choking sensation. Typically, the patient first experiences sudden dyspnea with intense angina-like or pleuritic pain aggravated by deep breathing and thoracic movement. Other findings may include tachycardia, tachypnea, cough (nonproductive or producing blood-tinged sputum), low-grade fever, restlessness, diaphoresis, crackles, pleural friction rub, diffuse wheezing, dullness to percussion, signs of circulatory collapse (weak, rapid pulse; hypotension), pulsus paradoxus, signs of cerebral ischemia (transient unconsciousness, coma, seizures), signs of hypoxia (restlessness), and — particularly in the elderly — hemiplegia and other focal neurologic deficits. Less-common signs include massive hemoptysis, chest splinting, and leg edema. A patient with a large embolus may have cyanosis and distended neck veins.

♦ ***Sickle cell crisis.*** Chest pain associated with sickle cell crisis typically has a bizarre distribution. It may start as a vague pain, often in the back, hands, or feet. As the pain worsens, it becomes generalized or localized to the abdomen or chest, causing severe pleuritic pain. The presence of chest pain and dyspneic breathing requires prompt intervention. The patient may also have abdominal distention and rigidity, fever, or jaundice.

♦ ***Thoracic outlet syndrome.*** Often causing paresthesia in the ulnar distribution of the arm, this syndrome can be confused with angina, especially when it affects the left arm. The patient usually experiences angina-like pain after lifting his arms above his head, working with his hands above his shoulders, or lifting a weight. The pain disappears as soon as he lowers his arms. Other signs and symptoms may include pale skin and a difference in blood pressure between both arms.

♦ ***Tuberculosis.*** In a patient with this disorder, pleuritic chest pain and fine crackles occur after coughing. Associated signs and symptoms may include night sweats, anorexia, weight loss, fever, malaise, dyspnea, easy fatigability, mild to severe productive cough, occasional hemoptysis, dullness to percussion, increased tactile fremitus, or amphoric breath sounds.

Other causes

♦ ***Chinese restaurant syndrome.*** This benign condition — a reaction to excessive ingestion of monosodium glutamate, a common additive in Chinese foods — mimics the signs of acute MI. The patient may report retrosternal burning, ache, or pressure; a burning sensation over his arms, legs, and face; a sensation of facial pressure; headache; shortness of breath; and tachycardia.

♦ ***Drugs.*** Abrupt withdrawal of beta blockers can cause rebound angina in patients with coronary heart disease — especially those who have received high doses for a prolonged period.

Special considerations

As needed, prepare the patient for cardiopulmonary studies, such as an electrocardiogram and a lung scan. Perform venipuncture to collect a serum sample for cardiac enzymes and other studies. Explain the purpose and procedure of each diagnostic test to the patient to help alleviate anxiety. Also explain the purpose of any prescribed medications, and make sure the patient understands the dosage, schedule, and possible adverse effects.

A patient with chest pain may deny his discomfort, so stress the importance of reporting symptoms to allow adjustment of his treatment.

Pediatric pointers

Even children old enough to talk may have difficulty describing chest pain, so be alert for nonverbal clues, such as restlessness, facial grimaces, or holding the painful area. Ask the child to point to the painful area and then to where the pain goes (to find out if it's radiating). Determine the pain's severity by asking the parents if the pain interferes with the child's normal activities and behavior.

Geriatric pointers

Because older people have a higher risk of developing life-threatening conditions such as MI, angina, and aortic dissection, you must carefully evaluate chest pain in this population.

CHEYNE-STOKES RESPIRATIONS

The most common pattern of periodic breathing, Cheyne-Stokes respirations are characterized by a waxing and waning period of hyperpnea that alternates with a shorter period of apnea. This pattern can occur normally in patients with heart or lung disease. It may also indicate increased intracranial pressure from a deep cerebral or brain stem lesion, or a metabolic disturbance in the brain.

Cheyne-Stokes respirations may indicate a major change in the patient's condition — usually for the worse. For example, in a patient who has had head trauma or brain surgery, Cheyne-Stokes respirations may signal increasing intracranial pressure (ICP).

Emergency interventions

If you detect Cheyne-Stokes respirations in a patient with a history of head trauma, recent brain surgery, or another brain insult, quickly take his vital signs. Keep his head elevated 30 degrees, and perform a rapid neurologic examination to obtain baseline data. Reevaluate the patient's neurologic status frequently. If ICP continues to rise, you'll detect changes in the patient's level of consciousness (LOC), pupillary reactions, and ability to move his extremities. ICP monitoring is indicated.

Time the periods of hyperpnea and apnea for 3 or 4 minutes to evaluate respirations and to obtain baseline data. Be alert for prolonged periods of apnea. Frequently check blood pressure; also check skin color to detect signs of hypoxemia. Maintain airway patency and administer oxygen as needed. If the patient's condition worsens, endotracheal intubation may be necessary.

History

If the patient's condition permits, obtain a brief history. Ask especially about drug use — large doses of narcotics, hypnotics, or barbiturates can precipitate Cheyne-Stokes respirations.

Common medical causes

◆ ***Heart failure.*** In left ventricular failure, Cheyne-Stokes respirations may occur with exertional dyspnea and orthopnea. Related findings include fatigue, weakness, tachycardia, tachypnea, and crackles. The patient may also have a cough, generally nonproductive but occasionally producing clear or blood-tinged sputum.

◆ ***Hypertensive encephalopathy.*** In this life-threatening disorder, severe hypertension precedes Cheyne-Stokes respirations. The patient's LOC is decreased, and he may experience vomiting or seizures, severe headaches, visual disturbances (including transient blindness), and transient paralysis.

◆ ***Increased ICP.*** As ICP rises, Cheyne-Stokes is the first irregular respiratory pattern to occur. It's preceded by decreased LOC and is accompanied by hypertension, headache, vomiting, impaired or unequal motor movement, and visual disturbances (blurring, diplopia, photophobia, and pupillary changes). In late stages of increased ICP, bradycardia and widened pulse pressure occur.

◆ ***Renal failure.*** In end-stage chronic renal failure, Cheyne-Stokes respirations may occur with bleeding gums, oral lesions, ammonia breath odor, and marked changes in every body system.

Other causes

◆ ***Drugs.*** Large doses of hypnotics, narcotics, or barbiturates can precipitate Cheyne-Stokes respirations.

Special considerations
When evaluating Cheyne-Stokes respirations, be careful not to mistake periods of hypoventilation or decreased tidal volume for complete apnea.

Pediatric pointers
Cheyne-Stokes respirations rarely occur in children, except during late heart failure.

Geriatric pointers
Cheyne-Stokes respirations can occur normally in elderly patients during sleep.

CHILLS
[Rigors]

Chills are extreme, involuntary muscle contractions with characteristic paroxysms of violent shivering and teeth chattering. Commonly accompanied by fever, chills tend to arise suddenly, usually heralding the onset of infection. Certain diseases, such as pneumococcal pneumonia, usually cause only a single, shaking chill. Other diseases, such as malaria, cause intermittent chills with recurring high fever. Still others cause continuous chills for up to 1 hour, precipitating a high fever. (See *Why chills accompany fever.*)

Chills can also result from lymphomas, transfusion reactions, and certain drugs. Chills without fever occur as a normal response to exposure to cold.

History and physical examination
Ask the patient when the chills began and if they're continuous or intermittent. Because fever often accompanies or follows chills, take his rectal temperature to obtain a baseline reading. Then check his temperature often to monitor fluctuations and to determine his temperature curve. Typically, a localized infection causes sudden onset of shaking chills, sweats, and high fever. A systemic infection causes intermittent chills with recurring episodes of high fever or continuous chills that may last up to 1 hour and precipitate a high fever.

Ask about related signs and symptoms, such as headache, dysuria, diarrhea, confusion, abdominal pain, cough, sore throat, or nausea. Does the patient have any known allergies, an infection, or a recent history of an infectious disorder? Find out what medications he's taking and if any drug has improved or worsened his symptoms. Has he received any treatment that may predispose him to an infection (such as chemotherapy)? Ask about recent exposure to farm animals, guinea pigs, hamsters, dogs, and such birds as pigeons, parrots, and parakeets. Also ask about recent insect or animal bites, travel to foreign countries, and contact with persons who have an active infection.

Common medical causes
♦ ***Acquired immunodeficiency syndrome.*** This fatal disease is caused by infection with human immunodeficiency virus transmitted by blood or semen. The patient usually develops lymphadenopathy and may also experience fatigue, anorexia and weight loss, diarrhea, diaphoresis, skin disorders, or signs of upper respiratory infection. Opportunistic infections can cause serious disease in these patients.

♦ ***Cholangitis.*** Charcot's triad — chills with spiking fever, abdominal pain, and jaundice — characterizes sudden obstruction of the common bile duct. The patient may have associated pruritus, weakness, and fatigue.

♦ ***Gram-negative bacteremia.*** This infection causes sudden chills and fever, nausea, vomiting, diarrhea, and prostration.

♦ ***Hepatic abscess.*** This infection usually arises abruptly, with chills, fever, nausea, vomiting, diarrhea, anorexia, and severe upper abdominal tenderness and

Why chills accompany fever

Fever usually occurs when exogenous pyrogens activate endogenous pyrogens to reset the body's thermostat to a higher level. At this higher thermostatic set point, the body feels cold and responds through several compensatory mechanisms, including rhythmic muscle contractions or chills. These muscle contractions in turn generate body heat and help produce fever. This flowchart outlines the events that link chills to fever.

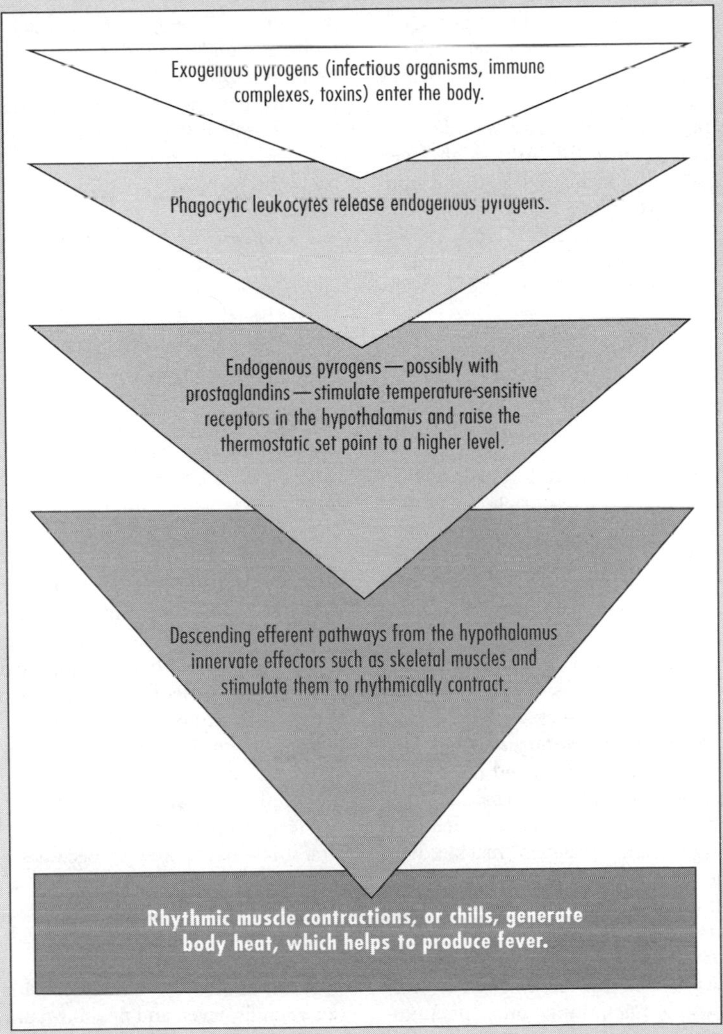

Exogenous pyrogens (infectious organisms, immune complexes, toxins) enter the body.
Phagocytic leukocytes release endogenous pyrogens.
Endogenous pyrogens—possibly with prostaglandins—stimulate temperature-sensitive receptors in the hypothalamus and raise the thermostatic set point to a higher level.
Descending efferent pathways from the hypothalamus innervate effectors such as skeletal muscles and stimulate them to rhythmically contract.
Rhythmic muscle contractions, or chills, generate body heat, which helps to produce fever.

pain that may radiate to the right shoulder.

♦ ***Infective endocarditis.*** This infection causes abrupt onset of intermittent, shaking chills with fever after the disease has been present for some time. Petechiae commonly develop, and the patient may also have Janeway lesions on his hands and feet and Osler's nodes on his palms and soles. Associated findings include murmur, hematuria, eye hemorrhage, Roth's spots, and signs of cardiac failure (dyspnea, peripheral edema).

♦ ***Influenza.*** Initially, this disorder causes abrupt onset of chills, high fever, malaise, headache, myalgia, and nonproductive cough. Some patients may also suddenly develop rhinitis, rhinorrhea, laryngitis, conjunctivitis, hoarseness, and sore throat. Chills generally subside after the first few days, but intermittent fever, weakness, and cough may persist for up to 1 week.

♦ ***Malaria.*** The paroxysmal cycle of malaria begins with a period of chills lasting 1 to 2 hours. This is followed by a high fever lasting 3 to 4 hours, and then 2 to 4 hours of profuse diaphoresis. Paroxysms occur every 48 to 72 hours when caused by *Plasmodium malariae* and every 48 hours when caused by *P. vivax* or *P. ovale.* In benign malaria, the paroxysms may be interspersed with periods of well-being. The patient also has a headache, muscle pain, and possibly hepatosplenomegaly.

♦ ***Pelvic inflammatory disease.*** This infection causes chills and fever with, typically, lower abdominal pain and tenderness; profuse, purulent vaginal discharge; or abnormal menstrual bleeding. The patient may also develop nausea and vomiting, an abdominal mass, and dysuria.

♦ ***Pneumonia.*** A single shaking chill usually heralds the sudden onset of pneumococcal pneumonia; other pneumonias characteristically cause intermittent chills. In any type of pneumonia, related findings may include fever, productive cough with bloody sputum, pleuritic chest pain, dyspnea, tachypnea, or tachycardia. The patient may be cyanotic and diaphoretic, with bronchial breath sounds and crackles, rhonchi, increased tactile fremitus, dullness on percussion, or grunting respirations. He may also experience achiness, anorexia, fatigue, or headache.

♦ ***Puerperal or postabortal sepsis.*** Chills and high fever occur as early as 6 hours or as late as 10 days postpartum or postabortion. The patient may also have a purulent vaginal discharge, an enlarged and tender uterus, abdominal pain, backache, or possibly nausea, vomiting, or diarrhea.

♦ ***Pyelonephritis.*** In acute pyelonephritis, the patient develops chills, high fever, and possibly nausea and vomiting over several hours to days. He generally also has anorexia, fatigue, myalgia, flank pain, costovertebral angle tenderness, hematuria or cloudy urine, and urinary frequency, urgency, and burning.

♦ ***Renal abscess.*** This abscess initially causes sudden chills and fever. Later effects include flank pain, costovertebral angle tenderness, abdominal muscle spasm, and transient hematuria.

♦ ***Rocky Mountain spotted fever.*** This disorder begins with sudden onset of chills, fever, malaise, excruciating headache, and muscle, bone, and joint pain. Typically, the patient's tongue is covered with a thick white coating that gradually turns brown. After 2 to 6 days of fever and occasional chills, a macular or maculopapular rash appears on the hands and feet and then becomes generalized; after a few days, the rash becomes petechial.

♦ ***Septic arthritis.*** Chills and fever accompany the characteristic red, swollen, and painful joints of this disorder.

♦ ***Septic shock.*** Initially, septic shock causes chills, fever, and possibly nausea, vomiting, and diarrhea. The patient's skin is typically flushed, warm, and dry; his blood pressure is low; also, he has tachycardia and tachypnea. As septic shock progresses, the patient's arms and legs become cool and cyanotic, and he develops oliguria, thirst, anxiety, restlessness, confusion, and hypotension. Later, his skin becomes cold and clammy; his pulse, rapid and thready. He further develops severe hypotension, persistent oliguria or anuria, signs of respiratory failure, and coma.

♦ ***Sinusitis.*** In acute sinusitis, chills occur with fever and headache, and pain, tenderness, and occasional swelling over the affected sinuses. Maxillary sinusitis causes pain over the cheeks and upper teeth; ethmoid sinusitis, pain over the eyes; frontal sinusitis, pain over the eyebrows; and sphenoid sinusitis, pain behind the eyes. The primary indicator of sinusitis is nasal discharge, which is often bloody for 24 to 48 hours before it gradually becomes purulent.

♦ ***Snake bite.*** Most pit viper bites that result in envenomization cause chills, typically with fever. Other systemic signs and symptoms may include sweating, weakness, dizziness, fainting, hypotension, nausea, vomiting, diarrhea, or thirst. The area around the snake bite may be marked by immediate swelling and tenderness, pain, ecchymoses, petechiae, blebs, bloody discharge, or local necrosis. The patient may have difficulty speaking, blurred vision, or paralysis. He may also show bleeding tendencies and signs of respiratory distress and shock.

♦ ***Violin spider bite.*** This bite causes chills, fever, malaise, weakness, nausea, vomiting, and joint pain within 24 to 48 hours. The patient may also develop a rash or delirium.

Other causes

♦ ***Drugs.*** Amphotericin B heads the list of common drugs associated with chills. Phenytoin is also a common cause of drug-induced fever that can produce chills; other potentially causative drugs include I.V. bleomycin and oral antipyretics administered intermittently.

♦ ***I.V. therapy.*** Infection at the I.V. insertion site (superficial phlebitis) can cause chills, high fever, and local redness, warmth, induration, and tenderness.

♦ ***Transfusion reaction.*** Hemolytic reaction may cause chills during the transfusion or immediately afterward. A nonhemolytic febrile reaction may also cause chills.

Special considerations

Check the patient's vital signs often, especially if his chills result from a known or suspected infection. Be alert for such signs of progressive septic shock as hypotension, tachycardia, and tachypnea. If appropriate, obtain samples of blood, sputum, or wound drainage for culture to determine the causative organism. Give antibiotics. Radiographic studies or serum and urine samples may be required.

Because chills are an involuntary response to an increased body temperature set by the hypothalamic thermostat, blankets won't stop a patient's chills or shivering. Keep his room temperature as even as possible, provide adequate hydration and nutrients, and give antipyretics to help control fever. Irregular use of antipyretics can trigger compensatory chills.

Pediatric pointers

Chills don't occur in infants because they have poorly developed shivering mechanisms. In addition, most classic febrile childhood infections, such as measles and mumps, don't typically cause chills. However, older children and teenagers may have chills with mycoplasmal pneumonia and acute pyogenic osteomyelitis.

Geriatric pointers

Chills in an elderly patient usually indicate an underlying infection, such as urinary tract infection, pneumonia (commonly associated with aspiration of gastric contents), diverticulitis, or skin breakdown in pressure areas. Also, consider an ischemic bowel in an elderly patient with fever, chills, and abdominal pain. The geriatric patient presents with a lesser fever than does a younger patient with the same disorder.

Chvostek's sign

Chvostek's sign is an abnormal spasm of facial muscles that's elicited by lightly tapping the patient's facial nerve near his lower jaw. (See *Eliciting Chvostek's sign.*) This sign usually suggests hypocalcemia, but it is a normal finding in about 25% of patients. Typically, it precedes other signs of hypocalcemia and persists until the onset of tetany. It can't be elicited during tetany because of strong muscle contractions.

Normally, eliciting Chvostek's sign is attempted only in patients with suspected hypocalcemic disorders. Because the parathyroid gland regulates calcium balance, Chvostek's sign may also be tested in patients before neck surgery to obtain a baseline.

Eliciting Chvostek's sign

Begin by telling the patient to relax his facial muscles. Then stand directly in front of him, and tap the facial nerve either just anterior to the earlobe and below the zygomatic arch, or between the zygomatic arch and the corner of his mouth. A positive response varies from twitching of the lip at the corner of the mouth to spasm of all facial muscles, depending on the severity of hypocalcemia.

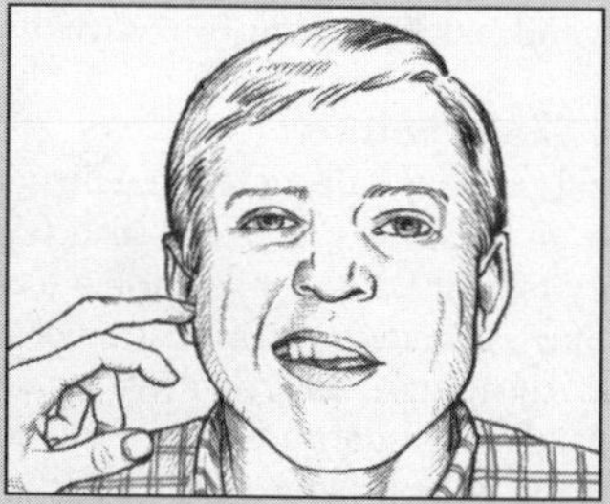

Emergency interventions

Test for Trousseau's sign, a reliable indicator of hypocalcemia. Closely monitor the patient for signs of tetany, such as carpopedal spasms or circumoral and extremity paresthesia.

Be prepared to act rapidly if a seizure occurs. Perform an electrocardiogram to observe for changes associated with hypocalcemia that can predispose the patient to arrhythmias. Place the patient on a cardiac monitor.

History

Obtain a brief history. Find out if the patient has had the parathyroid glands surgically removed, or if he has a history of hypoparathyroidism, hypomagnesemia, or malabsorption disorder. Ask him or his family if they've noticed any mental changes, such as depression or slowed responses, which can accompany chronic hypocalcemia.

Common medical causes

♦ ***Hypocalcemia.*** The degree of muscle spasm elicited reflects the patient's serum calcium level. Initially, hypocalcemia causes paresthesia in the fingers, toes, and circumoral area that progresses to muscle tension and carpopedal spasms. The patient may also complain of muscle weakness, fatigue, or palpitations. Muscle twitching, hyperactive deep tendon reflexes, choreiform movements, or muscle cramps may also occur. The patient with chronic hypocalcemia may have mental status changes; diplopia; difficulty swallowing; abdominal cramps; dry, scaly skin; brittle nails; or thin, patchy scalp and eyebrow hair.

Other causes

♦ ***Blood transfusion.*** A massive transfusion can lower serum calcium levels and allow Chvostek's sign to be elicited.

Special considerations

Collect blood samples for serial calcium studies to evaluate the severity of hypocalcemia and the effectiveness of therapy. Such therapy involves oral or I.V. calcium supplements. Also, look for Chvostek's sign when evaluating a patient postoperatively.

Pediatric pointers

Because Chvostek's sign may be positive in healthy infants, it isn't elicited to detect neonatal tetany.

CLUBBING

A nonspecific sign of pulmonary and cyanotic cardiovascular disorders, clubbing is the painless, usually bilateral increase in soft tissue around the terminal phalanges of the fingers or toes. It doesn't involve changes in the underlying bone. In early clubbing, the normal 160-degree angle between the nail and the nail base approximates 180 degrees. As clubbing progresses, this angle widens and the base of the nail becomes visibly swollen. In late clubbing, the angle at which the nail meets the now-convex nail base extends more than halfway up the nail.

History and physical examination

You'll probably detect clubbing while evaluating other signs of known pulmonary or cardiovascular disease. Review the patient's current plan of treatment because clubbing may resolve with correction of the underlying disorder. Also, evaluate the extent of clubbing in both the fingers and the toes. (See *Evaluating clubbed fingers.*)

Common medical causes

♦ ***Bronchiectasis.*** Clubbing occurs commonly in the late stage of this disorder. You may also see this classic sign: a cough that produces copious, foul-smelling, and mucopurulent sputum. Hemoptysis and coarse crackles over the affected area, heard during inspiration, are also characteristic. The patient may complain of weight loss, fatigue, weakness, or dysp-

EXAMINATION TIP

Evaluating clubbed fingers

To quickly examine a patient's fingers for early clubbing, gently palpate the bases of his nails. Normally, they feel firm, but in early clubbing, nail bases feel springy when palpated. To evaluate late clubbing, have the patient place the first phalanges of the forefingers together, as shown. Normal nail bases are concave and create a small space when the first phalanges are opposed (as shown below).

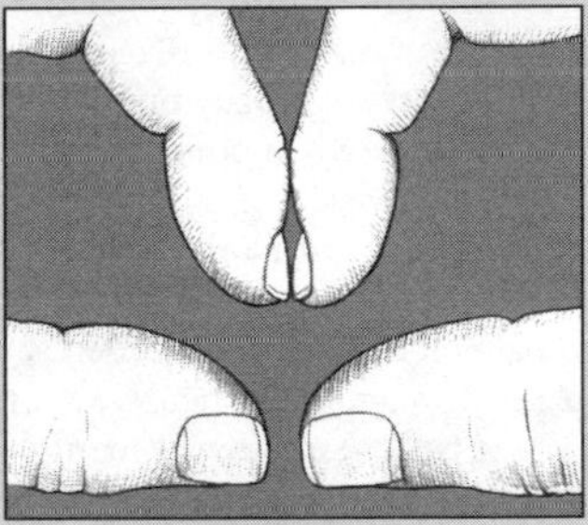

In late clubbing, however, the now-convex nail bases can touch without leaving a space (as shown below).

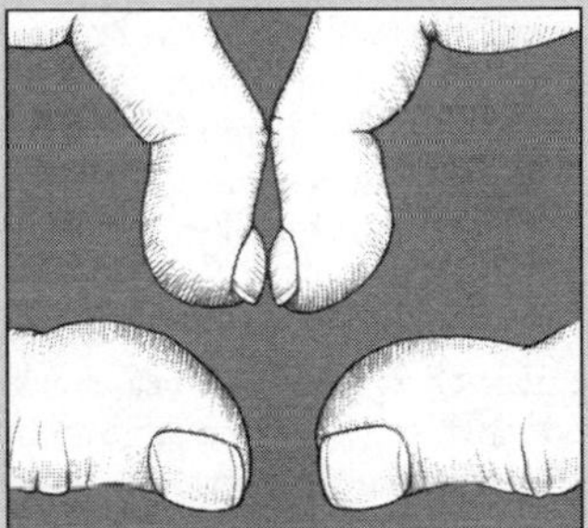

nea on exertion. He may also have rhonchi, fever, malaise, or halitosis.

◆ ***Bronchitis.*** In chronic bronchitis, clubbing may occur as a late sign and is unrelated to the severity of the disease. The patient has a chronic productive cough and may display barrel chest, dyspnea, wheezing, increased use of accessory muscles, cyanosis, tachypnea, crackles, scattered rhonchi, or prolonged expiration.

◆ ***Endocarditis.*** In subacute infective endocarditis, clubbing may be accompanied by fever, anorexia, pallor, weakness, night sweats, fatigue, tachycardia, and weight loss. The patient may also develop arthralgia, petechiae, Osler's nodes, splinter hemorrhages, Janeway lesions, splenomegaly, or Roth's spots. Cardiac murmurs are usually present.

◆ ***Heart failure.*** Clubbing occurs as a late sign with wheezing, dyspnea, and fatigue. Other findings may include neck vein distention, hepatomegaly, tachypnea, palpitations, dependent edema, unexplained weight gain, nausea, anorexia, chest tightness, slowed mental response, hypotension, diaphoresis, narrow pulse pressure, pallor, oliguria, a gallop rhythm (S_3), or crackles on inspiration.

◆ ***Interstitial fibrosis.*** Clubbing occurs in almost all patients with advanced interstitial fibrosis. Typically, the patient also develops intermittent chest pain, dyspnea, crackles, hypoxemia, fatigue, weight loss, and possible cyanosis.

◆ ***Lung abscess.*** Initially, this disorder causes clubbing, which may reverse with resolution of the abscess. It can also cause pleuritic chest pain; dyspnea; crackles; productive cough with a large amount of purulent, foul-smelling, often bloody sputum; or halitosis. The patient may also experience weakness, fatigue, anorexia, headache, malaise, weight loss, or fever with chills. You may hear decreased breath sounds.

◆ ***Lung or pleural cancer.*** Clubbing is a common finding in patients with these cancers. Associated findings may include hemoptysis, dyspnea, wheezing, chest pain, weight loss, anorexia, fatigue, or fever.

Special considerations

Don't mistake curved nails — a normal variation — for clubbing. How? Always remember that the angle between the nail and its base remains normal in curved nails, but not with clubbing.

Pediatric pointers

In children, clubbing occurs most often in cyanotic congenital heart disease and cystic fibrosis. Surgical correction of heart defects may reverse clubbing.

Geriatric pointers

Arthritic deformities of the fingers or toes may disguise the presence of clubbing.

COGWHEEL RIGIDITY

Cogwheel rigidity is a cardinal sign of Parkinson's disease marked by muscle rigidity that reacts with superimposed ratchetlike movements when the muscle is passively stretched. This sign can be elicited by stabilizing the patient's forearm and then moving his wrist through the range of motion. (Cogwheel rigidity usually appears in the arms but can sometimes be elicited in the ankle.) These characteristic movements are thought to be a combination of rigidity and tremor.

History and physical examination

After you've elicited cogwheel rigidity, take the patient's history to determine when he first noticed associated signs of Parkinson's disease. For example, has he experienced tremors? Did he notice tremors of his hands first? Does he have "pill-rolling" hand movements? When did he first notice that his movements were becoming slower? How long has he been experiencing stiffness in his arms and legs? Has his handwriting gotten smaller? While taking the history, observe for signs of pronounced parkinsonism, such as drooling, masklike facies, dysphagia, monotone speech, and altered gait.

Find out what medications the patient is taking, and ask if they've helped relieve some of his symptoms. If he's taking levodopa and his symptoms have worsened, find out if he has exceeded the prescribed dosage. If you suspect an overdosage, withhold the drug. If the patient has been taking a phenothiazine or another antipsychotic drug and has no history of Parkinson's disease, he may be having an adverse reaction to his medication. Withhold the drug, as appropriate.

Common medical causes

♦ ***Parkinson's disease.*** In this disorder, cogwheel rigidity occurs with an insidious tremor, which usually begins in the fingers (unilateral pill-roll tremor), increases during stress or anxiety, and decreases with purposeful movement and sleep.

Bradykinesia (slowness of voluntary movements and speech) also occurs. The patient walks with short, shuffling steps; his gait lacks normal parallel motion and may be retropulsive or propulsive. He has a monotonal way of speaking and a masklike facial expression. He may also experience drooling, dysphagia, dysarthria, and loss of postural control, causing him to walk with his body bent forward. An oculogyric crisis (eyes fixed upward and involuntary tonic movements) or blepharospasm (complete eyelid closure) may also occur.

Other causes

♦ ***Drugs.*** Phenothiazines and other antipsychotics, such as haloperidol, thiothixene, chlorpromazine. fluphenazine, and loxapine, can cause cogwheel rigidity. Metoclopramide infrequently causes it.

Special considerations

If the patient has associated muscular dysfunction, assist him with ambulation, feeding, and other activities of daily living, as needed. Provide symptomatic care as appropriate. For example, administer stool softeners if the patient develops constipation, and offer a soft diet with small, frequent feedings if he experiences dysphagia. Refer the patient to the National Parkinson Foundation or the American Parkinson Disease Association, both of which provide educational materials and support.

Pediatric pointers

Cogwheel rigidity doesn't occur in children.

CONFUSION

An umbrella term for puzzling or inappropriate behavior or responses, confusion is the inability to think quickly and coherently. Depending on its cause, confusion may arise suddenly or gradually and may be temporary or irreversible. Aggravated by stress and sensory deprivation, confusion often occurs in hospitalized patients — especially the elderly, in whom it may be mistaken for senility.

When severe confusion arises suddenly and the patient also has hallucinations and psychomotor hyperactivity, his condition is classified as *delirium.* Long-term, progressive confusion with deterioration of all cognitive functions is classified as *dementia.*

Confusion can result from fluid and electrolyte imbalance or hypoxemia due to pulmonary disorders. It can also have a metabolic, neurologic, cardiovascular, cerebrovascular, or nutritional origin; it can result from a severe systemic infection or from the effects of toxins, drugs, or alcohol. Confusion may signal worsening of an underlying and perhaps irreversible disease.

ALTERNATIVE THERAPY

Music therapy for Alzheimer's patients

Based on the theory that sound waves affect brain frequencies, muscle tension, breathing, and other body processes, music therapy is currently being used to treat patients with Alzheimer's disease. Music is an external sensory stimulant for Alzheimer's patients, who may not be able to communicate through words or movement. It is thought to tap into remote memories, provide emotional comfort, and improve communication through rhythm.

History and physical examination

When you take his history, ask the patient to describe what's bothering him. He may not report confusion as his chief complaint but may complain of memory loss, persistent apprehension, or inability to concentrate. He may be unable to respond logically to direct questions. Check with a family member or friend about onset and frequency. Find out, too, if the patient has a history of head trauma or a cardiopulmonary, metabolic, cerebrovascular, or neurologic disorder. What medication is he taking, if any? Ask about any changes in eating or sleeping habits and in drug or alcohol use.

Perform an assessment to detect systemic disorders. Check vital signs and assess for changes in blood pressure, temperature, and pulse. Next, perform a neurologic assessment to establish the patient's level of consciousness.

Common medical causes

♦ ***Brain tumor.*** In the early stages of brain tumor, confusion is usually mild and difficult to detect. As the tumor impinges on cerebral structures, however, confusion worsens and the patient may exhibit personality changes, bizarre behavior, sensory and motor deficits, visual field deficits, and aphasia.

♦ ***Dementia.*** This group of progressive brain diseases — such as Alzheimer's disease — eventually causes severe and irreversible confusion with memory loss and intellectual deterioration. (See *Music therapy for Alzheimer's patients.*) Disorientation, tremors, or gait disturbances may also occur.

♦ ***Fluid and electrolyte imbalance.*** The extent of imbalance determines the severity of the patient's confusion. Typically, he'll show signs of dehydration, such as lassitude, poor skin turgor, dry skin and mucous membranes, and oliguria. He may also develop hypotension and a low-grade fever.

♦ ***Head trauma.*** Concussion, contusion, and brain hemorrhage may cause confusion at the time of injury, shortly afterward, or months or even years afterward. The patient may be delirious or may have periodic loss of consciousness. Vomiting, severe headache, pupillary changes, and sensory and motor deficits are also common.

♦ ***Heatstroke.*** This disorder causes pronounced confusion that gradually worsens as body temperature rises. Initially, the patient may be irritable and dizzy; later, he may become delirious, have seizures, and lose consciousness.

♦ ***Hypoglycemia.*** Hypoglycemia results when serum glucose is metabolized too rapidly, when glucose is released into the circulation too slowly, or when excessive insulin is released by the pancreas. When blood glucose is less than 50 mm/dl, symptoms may include confusion, nervousness, trembling, tachycardia, cold and clammy skin, or headache.

♦ ***Hypothermia.*** Confusion may be an early sign of this disorder. Typically, the patient displays slurred speech, cold and pale skin, hyperactive deep tendon reflexes, rapid pulse, and decreased blood pressure and respirations. As his body temperature continues to drop, his confusion progresses to stupor and coma, his muscles develop rigidity, and his respiratory rate decreases.

♦ ***Hypoxemia.*** Acute pulmonary disorders that result in hypoxemia cause confusion that can range from mild disorientation to delirium. Chronic pulmonary disorders can cause persistent confusion.

♦ ***Infection.*** Severe generalized infection, such as sepsis, often causes delirium. Central nervous system (CNS) infections, such as meningitis, cause varying degrees of confusion with headache and nuchal rigidity.

♦ ***Low-perfusion states.*** Mild confusion is an early symptom of decreased cerebral perfusion. Associated findings usually include hypotension, tachycardia or bradycardia, irregular pulse, ventricular gallop, edema, and cyanosis.

♦ ***Nutritional deficiencies.*** Inadequate dietary intake of thiamin, niacin, or vitamin B causes insidious, progressive confusion and possible mental deterioration.

♦ ***Seizure disorders.*** Mild to moderate confusion may immediately follow any type of seizure. The confusion usually disappears within several hours.

Other causes

♦ ***Alcohol.*** Intoxication causes confusion and stupor, and alcohol withdrawal may cause delirium and seizures.

♦ ***Drugs.*** Large doses of a CNS depressant cause confusion that can persist for several days after the drug is discontinued. Narcotic or barbiturate withdrawal also causes acute confusion, possibly with delirium. Other drugs that commonly cause confusion include lidocaine, digitalis, indomethacin, cycloserine, chloroquine, atropine, and cimetidine.

♦ **Herb alert** Herbal medicines such as St. John's wort can cause confusion, especially when taken in conjunction with antidepressants or other serotonergic drugs.

Special considerations

Never leave a confused patient unattended, to prevent injury to himself and others, but apply restraints only if necessary. Keep the patient calm and quiet, and plan uninterrupted rest periods. To help him stay oriented, keep a large calendar and a clock visible, and make a list of his activities with specific dates and times. Always reintroduce yourself to the patient each time you enter his room.

Pediatric pointers

Confusion can't be determined in infants and very young children. However, older children with acute febrile illnesses commonly display transient delirium or acute confusion.

Geriatric pointers

Confusion is more common in the elderly and routinely occurs in hospitalized patients. Depending on the cause, it may appear suddenly or gradually. Confusion is often exacerbated by stress.

CONSTIPATION

Constipation is small, infrequent, or difficult bowel movements. Because normal bowel movements can vary in frequency and from person to person, constipation must be determined in relation to the patient's normal elimination pattern. Constipation may be a minor annoyance or, uncommonly, a sign of a life-threatening disorder, such as acute intestinal obstruction. Untreated, constipation can lead to headache, anorexia, and abdominal discomfort and can adversely affect the patient's lifestyle and well-being.

Constipation most often occurs when the urge to defecate is suppressed and the muscles associated with bowel movements remain contracted. Because the autonomic nervous system controls bowel movements — by sensing rectal distention from fecal contents and by stimulating the external sphincter — any factor that influences this system may cause bowel dysfunction. (See *How habits and stress cause constipation.*)

History and physical examination
Ask the patient to describe the frequency of his bowel movements and the size, amount, and consistency of his stools. How long has he had constipation? Acute constipation usually has an organic cause, such as an anal or rectal disorder. In a patient over age 45, recent onset of constipation may be an early sign of colorectal cancer. Conversely, chronic constipation typically has a functional cause and may be related to stress.

Does the patient have pain related to constipation? If so, when did he first notice the pain, and where is it? Cramping abdominal pain and distention suggest obstipation — extreme, persistent constipation due to intestinal tract obstruction. Ask the patient if defecation worsens or helps relieve the pain. Defecation usually worsens pain but may relieve it in disorders such as irritable bowel syndrome.

Ask the patient to describe a typical day's menu; estimate his daily fiber and fluid intake. Also ask him about any changes in eating habits, medication or alcohol use, or physical activity. Has he experienced recent emotional distress? Has constipation affected his family life or social contacts? Also, ask about his job. A sedentary or stressful job can contribute to constipation.

Find out whether the patient has a history of GI, rectoanal, neurologic, or metabolic disorders; abdominal surgery; or radiation therapy. Then ask about the medications he's taking, including over-the-counter preparations, such as laxatives, mineral oil, stool softeners, opiates, narcotics, or enemas.

Inspect the abdomen for distention and scars from previous surgery. Then auscultate for bowel sounds and characterize their motility. Percuss all four quadrants, and gently palpate for abdominal tenderness, a palpable mass, and hepatomegaly. Next, examine the patient's rectum. Spread his buttocks to expose the anus, and inspect for inflammation, lesions, scars, fissures, and external hemorrhoids. Use a disposable glove and lubricant to palpate the anal sphincter for laxity or stricture and for rectal masses and fecal impaction. Finally, obtain a stool sample and test it for occult blood.

As you assess the patient, remember that constipation can result from several life-threatening disorders, such as acute intestinal obstruction and mesenteric artery ischemia, but it doesn't herald these conditions.

Common medical causes

♦ ***Anal fissure.*** A crack or laceration in the lining of the anal wall can cause acute constipation, usually due to the patient's fear of the severe tearing or burning pain associated with bowel movements. He may notice a few drops of blood streaking toilet tissue or his underwear.

♦ ***Anorectal abscess.*** In this disorder, constipation occurs with severe, throbbing, localized pain and tenderness at the abscess site. The patient may also have localized inflammation, swelling, or purulent drainage and may complain of fever and malaise.

♦ ***Cirrhosis.*** In the early stages of cirrhosis, the patient experiences constipation with nausea and vomiting, and a dull pain in the right upper quadrant. Other early findings include indigestion, anorexia, fatigue, malaise, flatulence, hepatomegaly, and possibly splenomegaly and diarrhea.

♦ ***Diabetic neuropathy.*** This neuropathy causes episodic constipation or diarrhea. Other signs and symptoms may include dysphagia, orthostatic hypotension, syncope, or painless bladder distention with overflow incontinence. A male patient may also experience impotence and retrograde ejaculation.

How habits and stress cause constipation

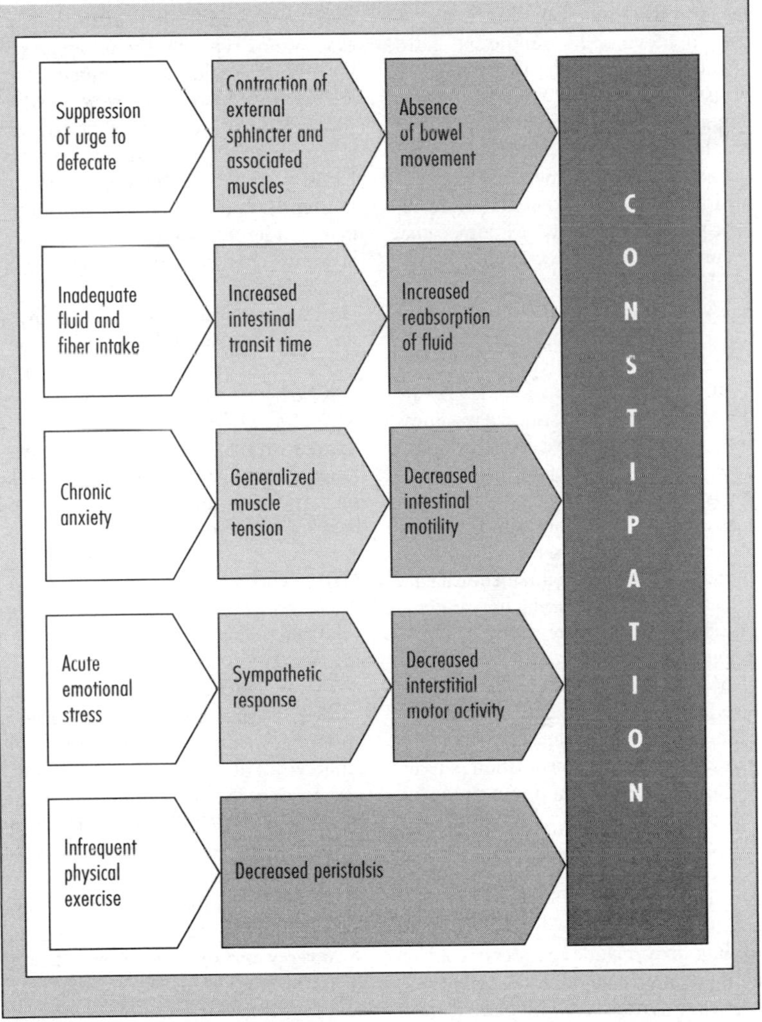

◆ ***Diverticulitis.*** In this disorder, constipation or diarrhea occurs with left lower quadrant pain and tenderness and possibly a palpable, tender, firm, fixed abdominal mass. The patient may develop mild nausea, flatulence, or a low-grade fever.

◆ ***Hemorrhoids.*** Thrombosed hemorrhoids cause constipation as the patient tries to avoid the severe pain of defecation. The hemorrhoids may bleed during defecation.

◆ ***Hepatic porphyria.*** Abdominal pain, which may be severe, colicky, localized, or generalized, precedes constipation in hepatic porphyria. The patient may also develop fever, sinus tachycardia, labile hypertension, excessive diaphoresis, severe vomiting, photophobia, urine retention, nervousness or restlessness, disorientation, or possibly visual hallucinations. Deep tendon reflexes may be diminished or absent. Some patients have skin lesions that cause itching, burning, erythema, altered pigmentation, or edema in areas exposed to light. Severe hepatic porphyria can cause delirium, coma, seizures, paraplegia, or complete flaccid quadriplegia.

♦ ***Hypercalcemia.*** In this disorder, constipation usually occurs with anorexia, nausea, vomiting, polyuria, and polydipsia. The patient may also display arrhythmias, bone pain, muscle weakness and atrophy, hypoactive deep tendon reflexes, or personality changes.

♦ ***Hypothyroidism.*** Constipation occurs early and insidiously in hypothyroidism, with fatigue, sensitivity to cold, anorexia with weight gain, menorrhagia, decreased memory, hearing impairment, muscle cramps, or paresthesia.

♦ ***Intestinal obstruction.*** Constipation associated with this disorder varies in severity and onset, depending on the location and extent of the obstruction. In partial obstruction, constipation may alternate with leakage of liquid stools. In complete obstruction, obstipation may occur. Constipation can be the earliest sign of partial colon obstruction, but it usually occurs later if the level of the obstruction is more proximal. Associated findings may include episodes of colicky abdominal pain, abdominal distention, nausea, or vomiting. The patient may also develop hyperactive bowel sounds, visible peristaltic waves, a palpable abdominal mass, or abdominal tenderness.

♦ ***Irritable bowel syndrome.*** This common syndrome usually causes chronic constipation, although some patients have intermittent, watery diarrhea and others, alternating constipation and diarrhea. Stress may trigger nausea and abdominal distention and tenderness, but defecation usually relieves these symptoms. Patients often have an intense urge to defecate and feelings of incomplete evacuation. Typically, the stools are scybalous and contain visible mucus.

♦ ***Mesenteric artery ischemia.*** This life-threatening disorder causes sudden constipation with failure to expel stool or flatus. Initially, the abdomen is soft and nontender but soon severe abdominal pain, tenderness, vomiting, and anorexia occur. Later, the patient may develop abdominal guarding, rigidity, and distention; tachycardia; syncope; tachypnea; fever; or signs of shock, such as cool, clammy skin and hypotension. A bruit may be heard.

♦ ***Spinal cord lesion.*** Constipation may occur with urine retention, sexual dysfunction, pain, and possibly motor weakness, paralysis, or sensory impairment below the level of the lesion.

Other causes

♦ ***Diagnostic tests.*** Constipation can result from retention of barium given during certain GI studies.

♦ ***Drugs.*** Patients often experience constipation when taking narcotic analgesics and other medications. These drugs include vinca alkaloids, calcium channel blockers, antacids containing aluminum or calcium, anticholinergics, and drugs with anticholinergic effects (such as tricyclic antidepressants). Patients also may experience constipation from excessive use of laxatives or enemas.

♦ ***Surgery and radiation therapy.*** Constipation can result from anorectal surgery, which may traumatize nerves, or from abdominal irradiation, which may cause intestinal stricture.

Special considerations

As indicated, prepare the patient for diagnostic tests, such as proctosigmoidoscopy, colonoscopy, barium enema, plain abdominal films, and an upper GI series. If the patient is on bed rest, reposition him frequently, and help him perform active or passive exercises, as indicated. Teach abdominal toning exercises if the patient's abdominal muscles are weak and relaxation techniques to help him reduce stress related to constipation.

Pediatric pointers

The high content of casein and calcium in cow's milk can cause hard stools and possible constipation in bottle-fed infants. Other causes of constipation in infants include inadequate fluid intake, Hirschsprung's disease, and anal fissures. In older children, constipation usually results from inadequate fiber intake and excessive intake of milk; it can also result from bowel spasm, mechanical obstruction, hypothyroidism, reluctance to stop playing for bathroom breaks, or the lack of privacy in some school bathrooms.

Geriatric pointers

Acute constipation in elderly patients is usually associated with underlying structural abnormalities. Chronic constipation, however, is chiefly caused by lifelong bowel and dietary habits and laxative use.

CORNEAL REFLEX, ABSENT

The corneal reflex is tested bilaterally by drawing a fine-pointed wisp of sterile cotton from a corner of each eye to the cornea. Normally, even though only one eye is tested at a time, the patient blinks bilaterally each time either cornea is touched — this is the corneal reflex. When this reflex is absent, neither eyelid closes when the cornea of one is touched. (See *Eliciting the corneal reflex.*)

The afferent fibers for this reflex are in the ophthalmic branch of the trigeminal nerve (cranial nerve [CN] V); the efferent fibers, in the facial nerve (CN VII). Unilateral or bilateral absence of the corneal reflex may result from damage to these nerves.

Eliciting the corneal reflex

To elicit the corneal reflex, have the patient turn her eyes away from you to avoid involuntary blinking during the procedure. Then approach the patient from the opposite side, out of her line of vision, and brush the middle of the cornea lightly with a fine wisp of sterile cotton. Repeat the procedure on the other eye.

Note: If the patient can see you coming, he will blink anyway.

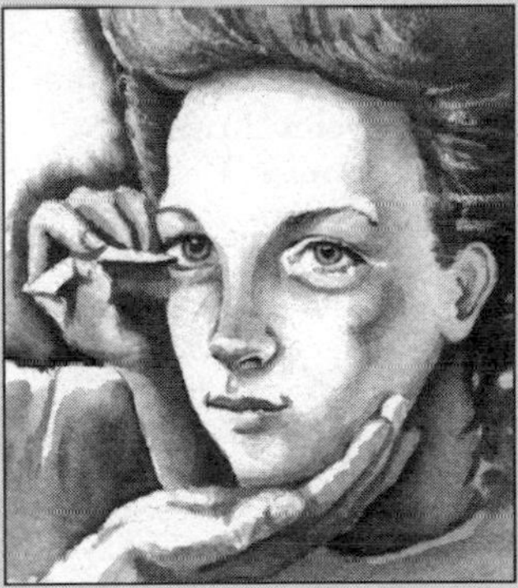

History and physical examination

If you're unable to elicit the corneal reflex, look for other signs of trigeminal nerve dysfunction. To test the three sensory portions of the nerve, touch each side of the patient's face on the brow, cheek, and jaw with a cotton wisp, and ask him to compare the sensations. The reflex may be absent or reduced if the patient often wears contact lenses. Thus a weakened blink due to facial weakness (CN VII paralysis) should be distinguished from a depressed corneal response.

If you suspect facial nerve involvement, note if both the upper face (brow and eyes) and the lower face (cheek, mouth, and chin) are weak bilaterally. Lower-motor-neuron facial weakness affects the face on the same side as the lesion, whereas upper-motor-neuron weakness affects the side opposite the lesion, and predominantly the lower facial muscles.

Because an absent corneal reflex may signify such progressive neurologic disorders as Guillain-Barré syndrome, ask the patient about associated symptoms such as facial pain, dysphagia, limb weakness, and facial hemianesthesia/hypesthesia.

Common medical causes

♦ ***Acoustic neuroma.*** This tumor affects the trigeminal nerve, causing a diminished or absent corneal reflex, tinnitus, and unilateral hearing impairment. Facial palsy and anesthesia, palate weakness, and signs of cerebellar dysfunction (for example, ataxia, nystagmus) may result if the tumor impinges on the adjacent cranial nerves, brain stem, and cerebellum.

♦ ***Bell's palsy.*** A common cause of diminished or absent corneal reflex, Bell's palsy causes paralysis of CN VII. It can also cause complete hemifacial weakness or paralysis and drooling on the affected side. The affected side also sags and appears masklike. The eye on this side can't be shut, and it tears constantly. The patient may also have numbness of the ear, face, neck, or tongue and hyperacusis.

♦ ***Brain stem infarction or injury.*** An absent corneal reflex can occur on the side opposite the lesion when infarction or injury affects CN V or VII, or their connection in the central trigeminal tract. Associated findings may include decreased level of consciousness, dysphagia, dysarthria, contralateral limb weakness, or early signs of increased intracranial pressure, such as headache and vomiting.

In massive brain stem infarction or injury, the patient also displays respiratory changes, such as apneustic breathing or periods of apnea; bilateral pupillary dilation or constriction with decreased responsiveness to light; rising systolic blood pressure; widening pulse pressure; bradycardia; and coma.

♦ ***Guillain-Barré syndrome.*** In this polyneuropathic disorder, a diminished or absent corneal reflex accompanies ipsilateral loss of facial muscle control. Muscle weakness, the dominant neurologic sign of this disorder, typically starts in the legs, then extends to the arms and facial nerves within 72 hours. Other possible findings include dysarthria, dysphagia, paresthesia, respiratory muscle paralysis, respiratory insufficiency, orthostatic hypotension, incontinence, diaphoresis, and tachycardia.

♦ ***Herpes zoster infection (shingles).*** This infection in the sensory nerves leads to pain and vesicular rash in the affected dermatome and absent corneal reflex.

Special considerations

When the corneal reflex is absent, take measures to protect the patient's affected eye from injury, such as lubricating the eye with artificial tears to prevent drying. Cover the cornea with a shield and avoid excessive corneal reflex testing. Also, because this test is often unnerving, it is better to tell the patient first what you are going to do. Prepare the patient for cranial X-rays or a computed tomography scan.

Pediatric pointers

Brain stem lesions and injuries are the most common causes of absent corneal reflexes in children; Guillain-Barré syndrome and trigeminal neuralgia occur less often. Infants, especially those born prematurely, may have an absent corneal reflex caused by anoxic damage to the brain stem.

Costovertebral angle tenderness

Costovertebral angle tenderness is an elicited symptom that indicates sudden distention of the renal capsule. It almost always accompanies unelicited, dull, constant flank pain in the costovertebral angle (CVA) just lateral to the sacrospinalis muscle and below the 12th rib. This associated pain typically travels anteriorly in the subcostal region toward the umbilicus.

Percussing the costovertebral angle elicits CVA tenderness, if present. (See *Eliciting CVA tenderness,* page 146.) A patient who doesn't have this symptom perceives a thudding, jarring, or pressurelike sensation when tested, but no pain. A patient with a disorder that distends the renal capsule experiences intense pain as the renal capsule stretches and stimulates the afferent nerves, which emanate from the spinal cord at levels T11 through L2 and innervate the kidney.

History and physical examination

After detecting CVA tenderness, determine the possible extent of renal damage. First, find out if the patient has other symptoms of renal or urologic dysfunction. Ask about voiding habits: How frequently does he urinate, and in what amounts? Has he noticed any change in intake or output? If so, when did he notice the change? (Ask about fluid intake before judging his output as abnormal.) Does he have nocturia? Ask about pain or burning during urination, or difficulty starting a stream. Does the patient strain to urinate without being able to do so (tenesmus)? Ask about urine color; brown or bright red urine may contain blood.

Explore other signs and symptoms. For example, if the patient is experiencing pain in his flank, abdomen, or back, when did he first notice the pain? How severe is it, and where is it located? Find out if the patient or a family member has a history of urinary tract infections, congenital anomalies, calculi, or other obstructive nephropathies or uropathies. Also, ask about a history of renovascular disorders, such as occlusion of the renal arteries or veins.

Perform a brief physical examination. Begin by taking the patient's vital signs. Fever and chills in a patient with CVA tenderness may indicate acute pyelonephritis. If the patient has hypertension and bradycardia, be alert for other autonomic effects of renal pain, such as diaphoresis and pallor. Inspect, auscultate, and gently palpate the abdomen for clues to the underlying cause of CVA tenderness. Be alert for abdominal distention, hypoactive bowel sounds, and palpable masses.

Common medical causes

- ***Calculi.*** Infundibular and ureteropelvic or ureteral calculi cause CVA tenderness and waves of waxing and waning flank pain that may radiate to the groin, testicles, suprapubic area, or labia. The patient may also develop nausea, vomiting, severe abdominal pain, abdominal distention, and decreased bowel sounds.
- ***Perirenal abscess.*** Causing exquisite CVA tenderness, this disorder may also cause severe unilateral flank pain, dysuria, persistent high fever, chills, erythema of the skin, and sometimes a palpable abdominal mass.
- ***Pyelonephritis (acute).*** Perhaps the most common cause of CVA tenderness, acute pyelonephritis is often accompanied by persistent high fever, chills, flank pain, anorexia, nausea and vomiting, weakness, dysuria, hematuria, nocturia, urinary urgency and frequency, and tenesmus.
- ***Renal artery occlusion.*** In this disorder, the patient experiences flank pain as well as CVA tenderness. Other findings may include severe, continuous up-

Eliciting CVA tenderness

To elicit costovertebral angle (CVA) tenderness, have the patient sit upright facing away from you, or have him lie prone. Place the palm of your left hand over the left costovertebral angle, then strike the back of your left hand with the ulnar surface of your right fist (as shown). Repeat this percussion technique over the right costovertebral angle. A patient with CVA tenderness will experience intense pain.

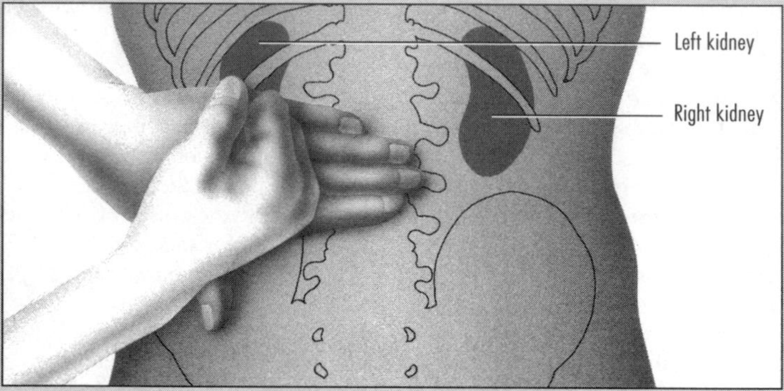

per abdominal pain; nausea; vomiting; decreased bowel sounds; and high fever.

◆ ***Renal vein occlusion.*** The patient with this disorder has CVA tenderness and flank pain. He also may have sudden, severe back pain; fever; oliguria; edema; or hematuria.

Special considerations

Administer pain medication, and continue to monitor the patient's vital signs and intake and output. Collect blood and urine samples, and then prepare the patient for radiologic studies, such as excretory urography, renal arteriography, or computed tomography scan.

Pediatric pointers

An infant with a disorder that distends the renal capsule won't exhibit CVA tenderness. Instead, he'll display nonspecific signs, such as vomiting, diarrhea, decreased appetite, fever, irritability, poor skin perfusion, or yellow to gray skin color. In older children, however, CVA tenderness has the same diagnostic significance as in adults. Vaginal discharge, vulval soreness, or pruritus may occur in girls.

Geriatric pointers

Advanced age and cognitive impairment reduce an elderly patient's ability to perceive pain or to describe its intensity.

Cough, barking

Resonant, brassy, and harsh, a barking cough is part of a complex of signs and symptoms that characterize croup syndrome, a group of pediatric disorders marked by varying degrees of respiratory distress. Croup syndrome is most common in boys and is most prevalent in the fall. It may recur in the same child.

A barking cough indicates edema of the larynx and surrounding tissue. Because children's airways are smaller in diameter than those of adults, edema can rapidly lead to airway occlusion — a life-threatening emergency.

Emergency interventions

Quickly evaluate the child's respiratory status. Then take his vital signs. Be particularly alert for tachycardia and signs of hypoxemia. Also, check for a decreased level of consciousness. Try to determine if the child was playing with a small object that he may have aspirated.

Check for cyanosis in the lips and nail beds. Observe for sternal or intercostal retractions or nasal flaring. Next, note the depth and rate of respirations; they may become increasingly shallow as respiratory distress increases. Observe the child's body position. Is he sitting up, leaning forward, struggling to breathe? Observe his activity level and facial expression. As respiratory distress increases from airway edema, the child becomes restless and has a frightened, wide-eyed expression. As air hunger continues, the child becomes lethargic and difficult to arouse.

If the child shows signs of severe respiratory distress, try to calm him, maintain airway patency, and provide oxygen. Endotracheal intubation or a tracheotomy may be necessary.

History

Ask the child's parents when the barking cough began and what other signs and symptoms accompanied it. When did the child first appear to be ill? Has he had previous episodes of croup syndrome? Did his condition improve on exposure to cold air?

Spasmodic croup and epiglottitis both typically occur in the middle of the night; the child with spasmodic croup has no fever, but the child with epiglottitis has a high fever of sudden onset. An upper respiratory tract infection typically is followed by laryngotracheobronchitis.

Common medical causes

♦ ***Epiglottiditis.*** This life-threatening disorder has become less common since the use of influenza vaccines. It occurs nocturnally, heralded by a barking cough and a high fever. The child is hoarse, dysphagic, dyspneic, and restless and appears extremely ill and panicky. The cough may progress to severe respiratory distress with sternal and intercostal retractions, nasal flaring, cyanosis, or tachycardia. The child struggles to get sufficient air as epiglottic edema increases. Epiglottitis is a true medical emergency.

♦ ***Laryngotracheobronchitis (acute).*** Also known as viral croup, this infection is most common in children between 9 and 18 months old and usually occurs in the fall and early winter. It initially causes low to moderate fever, runny nose, poor appetite, and infrequent cough. When the infection descends into the laryngotracheal area, barking cough, hoarseness, and inspiratory stridor occur.

As respiratory distress progresses, substernal and intercostal retractions occur with tachycardia and shallow, rapid respirations. Sleeping in a dry room worsens these signs. The patient becomes restless and irritable, pale and cyanotic.

♦ ***Spasmodic croup.*** Acute spasmodic croup usually occurs during sleep with abrupt onset of a barking cough that awakens the child. Typically, he doesn't have a fever but may be hoarse, restless, or dyspneic. As his respiratory distress worsens, the child may exhibit sternal and intercostal retractions, nasal flaring, tachycardia, cyanosis, and an anxious, frantic appearance. The symptoms usually subside within a few hours, but attacks tend to recur.

Special considerations

Don't attempt to inspect the throat of a child with a barking cough unless intubation equipment is available. If the child is not in severe respiratory distress, a lateral neck X-ray may be done to visualize any epiglottal edema; a chest X-ray may also be done to rule out lower respiratory tract infection. Depending on the child's age and degree of respiratory distress, oxygen may be administered. Rapid-acting epinephrine and steroids should be considered.

Observe the child frequently, and monitor the oxygen level if used. Provide the child with periods of rest with minimal interruptions. Maintain a calm, quiet environment and offer reassurance. Encourage the parents to stay with the child to help alleviate stress.

Teach the parents how to evaluate and treat recurrent episodes of croup syndrome. For example, creating steam by running hot water in a sink or shower and sitting with the child in the closed bathroom may help relieve attacks. The child may also benefit from being taken outside (properly dressed) to breathe cold night air.

COUGH, NONPRODUCTIVE

A nonproductive cough is a noisy, forceful expulsion of air from the lungs that doesn't yield sputum or blood. It's one of the most common complaints of patients with respiratory disorders.

Coughing is a necessary protective mechanism that clears airway passages. However, a nonproductive cough is ineffective and may interfere with the patient's normal daily activities. It may also cause damage, such as airway collapse or rupture of alveoli or blebs.

The cough reflex generally occurs when mechanical, chemical, thermal, inflammatory, or psychogenic stimuli activate cough receptors. (See *Reviewing the cough mechanism.*) However, external pressure — for example, from subdiaphragmatic irritation or a mediastinal tumor — can also induce it, as can voluntary expiration of air, which occasionally occurs as a nervous habit. Certain drugs, such as angiotensin-converting enzyme (ACE) inhibitors, may also cause a nonproductive cough.

A nonproductive cough may occur in paroxysms and can worsen by becoming more frequent. An acute cough has a sudden onset and may be self-limiting; a cough that persists beyond 1 month is considered chronic. Cigarette smoking is the most common cause of a chronic cough.

Someone with a chronic nonproductive cough may downplay or overlook it or accept it as normal. In fact, he generally won't seek medical attention unless he has other symptoms.

History and physical examination

Ask the patient when his cough began and whether any body position, time of day, or specific activity affects it. How does the cough sound — harsh, brassy, dry, hacking? Try to determine if the cough is related to smoking or a chemical irritant. If the patient smokes or has smoked, note the number of packs smoked daily multiplied by years ("pack-years"). Also, ask if any family members in the house smoke. Next, ask about the frequency and intensity of coughing. If he has any pain associated with coughing, breathing, or activity, when did it begin? Where is it located?

Ask the patient about recent illness (especially cardiovascular or pulmonary disorders), surgery, or trauma. Also ask about hypersensitivity to drugs, foods, pets, dust, or pollen. Find out what medications the patient takes, if any, and ask about recent changes in schedules or dosages. Also ask about recent changes in his appetite, weight, exercise tolerance, or energy level and recent exposure to irritating fumes, chemicals, or smoke.

As you're taking his history, observe the patient's general appearance and manner: Is he agitated, restless, or lethargic; pale, diaphoretic, or flushed; anxious,

Reviewing the cough mechanism

Cough receptors are thought to be located in the nose, sinuses, auditory canals, nasopharynx, larynx, trachea, bronchi, pleurae, diaphragm, and possibly pericardium and GI tract. Once a cough receptor is stimulated, the vagus and glossopharyngeal nerves transmit the impulse to the "cough center" in the medulla. From there, the impulse is transmitted to the larynx and to the intercostal and abdominal muscles. Deep inspiration (illustration at top left) is followed by closure of the glottis relaxation of the diaphragm, and contraction of the abdominal and intercostal muscles (illustration at top right). The resulting increased pressure in the lungs opens the glottis to release the forceful, noisy expiration known as a cough (bottom illustration).

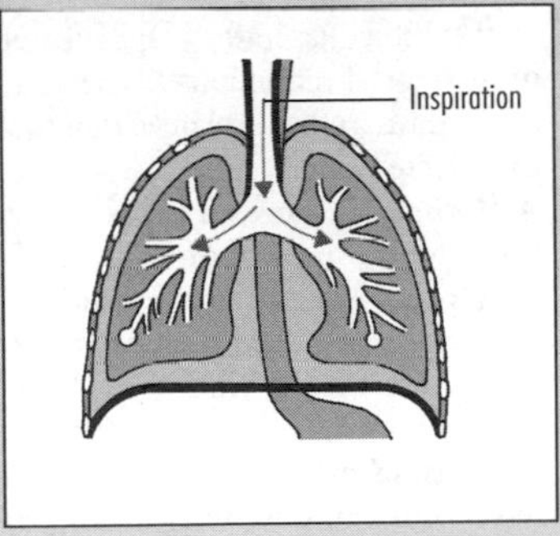

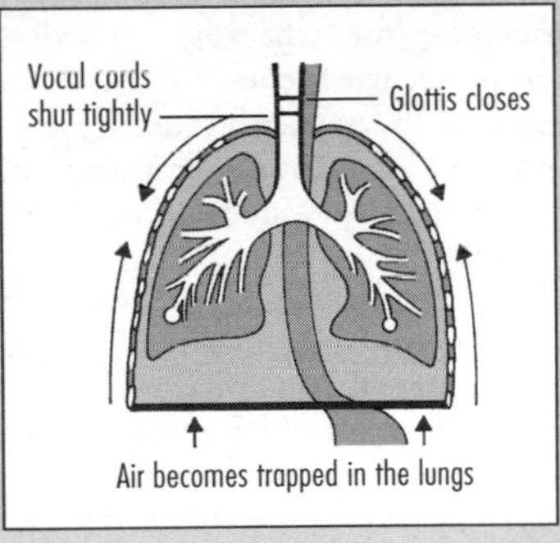

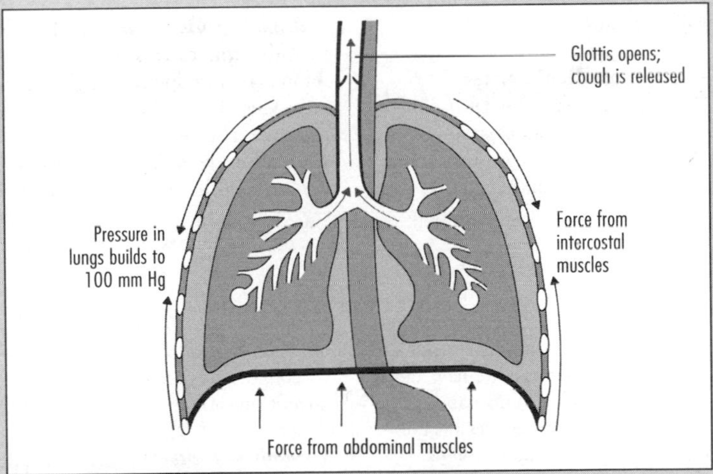

confused, or nervous? Also, note whether he's cyanotic or has clubbed fingers or peripheral edema.

Next, perform a physical examination. Start by taking the patient's vital signs. Check the depth and rhythm of his respirations, and note if wheezing or "crowing" noises occur with breathing. Feel the patient's skin: Is it cold or warm, clammy or dry? Check his nose and mouth for congestion, inflammation, drainage, and signs of infection. Inspect his neck for distended veins and tracheal deviation, and palpate for masses or enlarged lymph nodes.

Examine his chest, observing its configuration and looking for abnormal chest wall motion. Do you note any retractions or use of accessory muscles? Percuss for dullness, tympany, or flatness. Auscultate for wheezing, crackles, rhonchi, pleural friction rubs, and decreased or absent breath sounds. Finally, examine his abdomen for distention, tenderness, masses, and abnormal bowel sounds.

Because tuberculosis (TB) causes a cough, ask patients at risk for TB — the foreign-born, those in contact with acute TB, and those with high-risk behaviors (multiple sex partners, homeless, prisoners, drug and alcohol abusers, patients in mental institutions) — about potential TB exposure.

Common medical causes

♦ ***Airway occlusion.*** Partial occlusion of the upper airway causes sudden onset of dry, paroxysmal coughing. The patient gags, wheezes, and is hoarse, with stridor, tachycardia, and decreased breath sounds.

♦ ***Aortic aneurysm (thoracic).*** This disorder causes a brassy cough with dyspnea, hoarseness, wheezing, and a substernal ache in the shoulders, lower back, or abdomen. The patient may also have facial or neck edema, neck vein distention, dysphagia, prominent veins over his chest, stridor, or paresthesia or neuralgia.

♦ ***Asthma.*** An attack often occurs at night with exercise or exposure to inhaled irritants. It may start with a nonproductive cough and mild wheezing and progress to severe dyspnea, audible wheezing, chest tightness, and a cough that causes thick mucus. Other signs may include apprehension, rhonchi, prolonged expirations, intercostal and supraclavicular retractions on inspiration, accessory muscle use, flaring nostrils, tachypnea, tachycardia, diaphoresis, or flushing or cyanosis.

♦ ***Atelectasis.*** As lung tissue collapses, it stimulates cough receptors, causing a nonproductive cough. The patient may also have pleuritic chest pain, anxiety, dyspnea, tachypnea, or tachycardia. His skin may be cyanotic and diaphoretic, his breath sounds may be decreased, his chest may be dull on percussion, and he may exhibit inspiratory lag, substernal or intercostal retractions, decreased vocal fremitus, or tracheal deviation toward the affected side.

♦ ***Bronchitis (chronic).*** This disorder starts with a nonproductive, hacking cough that later becomes productive. Other possible findings include prolonged expiration, wheezing, dyspnea, accessory muscle use, barrel chest, cyanosis, tachypnea, crackles, and scattered rhonchi. Clubbing can occur in late stages.

♦ ***Bronchogenic carcinoma.*** The earliest indicators of this disease can be a chronic, nonproductive cough, dyspnea, and vague chest pain. The patient may also wheeze.

♦ ***Common cold.*** This disorder generally starts with a nonproductive, hacking cough and progresses to some mix of sneezing, headaches, malaise, fatigue, rhinorrhea, myalgia, arthralgia, nasal congestion, and sore throat.

♦ ***Esophageal achalasia.*** In this disorder, regurgitation and aspiration cause a dry cough. The patient may also have recurrent pulmonary infections and dysphagia.

♦ ***Esophageal diverticula.*** The patient with this disorder has a nocturnal nonproductive cough, regurgitation and aspiration, dyspepsia, and dysphagia. His neck may appcar swollen and have a gurgling sound. He may also exhibit halitosis and weight loss.

♦ ***Esophageal occlusion.*** This is marked by immediate nonproductive coughing and gagging, with a sensation of something stuck in the throat. Other possible findings include neck or chest pain, dysphagia, and inability to swallow.

♦ ***Hantavirus pulmonary syndrome.*** A nonproductive cough is common in this disorder, which is marked by noncardiogenic pulmonary edema. Other findings include headache, myalgia, fever, nausea, and vomiting.

♦ ***Hypersensitivity pneumonitis.*** In this disorder, an acute nonproductive cough, fever, dyspnea, and malaise usually occur 5 to 6 hours after exposure to an antigen.

♦ ***Interstitial lung disease.*** A patient with this disorder has a nonproductive cough and progressive dyspnea. He may also be cyanotic and have clubbing, fine crackles, fatigue, variable chest pain, or weight loss.

♦ ***Laryngeal tumor.*** A mild, nonproductive cough, minor throat discomfort, and hoarseness are early signs of this disorder. Later, dysphagia, dyspnea, cervical lymphadenopathy, stridor, and earache may occur.

♦ ***Laryngitis.*** In its acute form, this disorder causes a nonproductive cough with localized pain (especially when the patient is swallowing or speaking), as well as fever and malaise. Hoarseness can range from mild to complete loss of voice.

♦ ***Lung abscess.*** This disorder typically begins with nonproductive coughing, weakness, dyspnea, and pleuritic chest pain. The patient may also exhibit diaphoresis, fever, headache, malaise, fatigue, crackles, decreased breath sounds, anorexia, and weight loss. Later, his cough causes large amounts of purulent, foul-smelling, possibly bloody sputum.

♦ ***Pleural effusion.*** A nonproductive cough with dyspnea, pleuritic chest pain, and decreased chest motion are characteristic of this disorder. Other findings include pleural friction rub, tachycardia, tachypnea, egophony, flatness on percussion, decreased or absent breath sounds, or decreased tactile fremitus.

♦ ***Pneumonia.*** *Bacterial pneumonia* usually starts with a nonproductive, hacking, painful cough that rapidly becomes productive. Other possible findings include shaking chills, headache, high fever, dyspnea, pleuritic chest pain, tachypnea, tachycardia, grunting respirations, nasal flaring, decreased breath sounds, fine crackles, rhonchi, and cyanosis. The patient's chest may be dull on percussion.

In *mycoplasmal pneumonia,* a nonproductive cough arises 2 to 3 days after onset of malaise, headache, and sore throat. The cough can be paroxysmal, causing substernal chest pain. Fever commonly occurs, but the patient doesn't appear seriously ill.

Viral pneumonia causes a nonproductive, hacking cough and gradual onset of malaise, headache, anorexia, and low-grade fever.

♦ ***Pneumothorax.*** This life-threatening disorder causes a dry cough and signs of respiratory distress, such as severe dyspnea, tachycardia, tachypnea, and cyanosis. The patient experiences sudden, sharp chest pain that worsens with chest movement as well as subcutaneous crepitation, hyperresonance or tympany, decreased vocal fremitus, and decreased or absent breath sounds on the affected side.

♦ ***Pulmonary edema.*** This disorder initially causes a dry cough, exertional dyspnea, paroxysmal nocturnal dyspnea, orthopnea, tachycardia, tachypnea, dependent crackles, and ventricular gallop. If pulmonary edema is severe, the patient's respirations become more rapid and labored, with diffuse crackles and coughing that produces frothy, bloody sputum.

♦ ***Pulmonary embolism.*** Life-threatening pulmonary embolism may suddenly cause a dry cough with dyspnea and pleuritic or anginal chest pain. More often, though, the cough produces blood-tinged sputum. Tachycardia and low-grade fever are also common; less common signs and symptoms include massive hemoptysis, chest splinting, leg edema, and (with a large embolus) cyanosis, syncope, and distended neck veins. The patient may also have a pleural friction rub, diffuse wheezing, dullness on percussion, or decreased breath sounds.

♦ ***Sarcoidosis.*** In this disorder, a nonproductive cough is accompanied by dyspnea, substernal pain, and malaise. The patient may also develop fatigue, arthralgia, myalgia, weight loss, tachypnea, crackles, lymphadenopathy, hepatosplenomegaly, skin lesions, visual impairment, difficulty swallowing, or arrhythmias.

♦ ***Tracheobronchitis (acute).*** Initially, this disorder causes a dry cough that later becomes productive as secretions increase. Chills, sore throat, slight fever, muscle and back pain, and substernal tightness generally precede the cough's onset. Rhonchi and wheezes are usually heard. Severe illness causes a fever of 101° to 102° F (38.3° to 38.9° C) and possibly bronchospasm, with severe wheezing and increased coughing.

Other causes

♦ ***Diagnostic tests.*** Pulmonary function tests and bronchoscopy may stimulate cough receptors and trigger coughing.

♦ ***Treatments.*** Irritation of the carina during suctioning, or deep endotracheal or tracheal tube placement can trigger a paroxysmal or hacking cough. Intermittent positive-pressure breathing can also cause a nonproductive cough. Some inhalants, such as pentamidine, may stimulate coughing.

Special considerations

A nonproductive, paroxysmal cough may induce life-threatening bronchospasm. The patient may need a bronchodilator to relieve the bronchospasm and open his airways. Unless he has chronic obstructive pulmonary disease, you may have to give antitussives and sedatives to suppress the cough.

To relieve mucous membrane inflammation and dryness, humidify the air in the patient's room, or instruct him to use a humidifier at home. Tell him to avoid using aerosols, powders, or other respiratory irritants — especially cigarettes. And make sure the patient receives adequate fluids and nutrition.

As indicated, prepare the patient for diagnostic tests, such as X-rays, a lung scan, bronchoscopy, or pulmonary function tests.

Pediatric pointers

A nonproductive cough can be difficult to evaluate in infants and young children because it can't be induced and must be observed.

Sudden onset of paroxysmal nonproductive coughing may indicate aspiration of a foreign body — a common danger in children, especially those between 6 months and 4 years old. Nonproductive coughing can also result from several disorders that affect infants and children. In *asthma,* a characteristic nonproductive "tight" cough can arise suddenly or insidiously as an attack begins. The cough usually becomes productive toward the end of the attack. In *bacterial pneumonia,* a nonproductive, hacking cough arises suddenly and becomes productive within 2 or 3 days. *Acute bronchiolitis* has a peak incidence at age 6, with paroxysms of nonproductive coughing that become more frequent as the disease progresses. *Acute otitis media,* which frequently occurs in infants and young children because of their short eustachian tubes, also causes nonproductive coughing.

Typically, a child with *measles* has a slight, nonproductive, hacking cough that increases in severity. The earliest sign of *cystic fibrosis* may be a nonproductive, paroxysmal cough from retained secretions. Life-threatening *pertussis* causes a cough that becomes paroxysmal, with an inspiratory "whoop" or crowing sound. *Airway hyperactivity* causes a chronic nonproductive cough that increases with exercise or exposure to cold air. And *psychogenic coughing* may occur when the child is under stress, emotionally stimulated, or seeking attention.

Geriatric pointers

Always ask elderly patients about nonproductive coughing because it may be an indication of serious acute or chronic illness.

COUGH, PRODUCTIVE

Productive coughing is the body's mechanism for clearing airway passages of accumulated secretions that normal mucociliary action doesn't remove. It's a sudden, forceful, noisy expulsion from the lungs of air that contains sputum or blood (or both). (The sputum's color, consistency, and odor provide important clues about the patient's condition.) It can occur as a single cough or as paroxysmal coughing, and it can be voluntarily induced, although it's usually a reflexive response to stimulation of the airway mucosa.

Productive coughing often results from an acute or chronic infection that causes inflammation, edema, and increased mucus production in the airways. Inhalation of antigenic or irritating substances or foreign bodies also can cause a productive cough. The most common cause of chronic productive coughing is chronic bronchitis secondary to cigarette smoking, which causes mucoid sputum ranging in color from clear to yellow to brown.

Many patients minimize or overlook a chronic productive cough or accept it as normal. Such patients may not seek medical attention until an associated problem — such as dyspnea, hemoptysis, chest pain, weight loss, or recurrent respiratory infections — develops. The delay can have serious consequences because productive coughing is associated with several serious disorders requiring medical treatment.

Emergency interventions

A patient with a productive cough can develop acute respiratory distress from thick or excessive secretions, bronchospasm, or fatigue, so examine him before you take his history. Take vital signs and check the rate, depth, and rhythm of respirations. Keep his airway patent, and be prepared to provide supplemental oxygen if he becomes restless or confused, or if his respirations become shallow, irregular, rapid, or slow. Look for stridor, wheezing, choking, or gurgling. Be alert for nasal flaring and cyanosis.

A productive cough may signal a severe life-threatening disorder. For example, coughing due to pulmonary edema causes thin, frothy, pink sputum, and coughing due to an asthmatic attack causes thick, mucoid sputum.

History and physical examination

When the patient's condition permits, ask when the cough began, and find out how much sputum he's coughing up each day. The normal tracheobronchial tree can produce up to 3 oz (90 ml) of sputum per day. At what time of day does he cough up the most sputum? Does his sputum production have any relationship to what or when he eats, or to his activities or environment? Ask him if he has noticed an increase in sputum production since his coughing began. This may result from external stimuli or from such internal causes as chronic bronchial infection or a lung abscess. Also ask about the color, odor, and consistency of the sputum. Blood-tinged or rust-colored sputum may result from trauma due to coughing or from an underlying condition, such as a pulmonary infection or a tumor. Foul-smelling sputum may result from an anaerobic infection, such as bronchiectasis, bronchitis, or lung abscess.

How does the cough sound? A hacking cough results from laryngeal involvement, whereas a "brassy" cough indicates major airway involvement. Does the patient feel any pain associated with his productive cough? If so, ask about its location and severity and whether it radiates to other areas. Does coughing, changing body position, or inspiration increase or help relieve his pain?

Next, ask the patient about cigarette, drug, and alcohol use and whether his weight or appetite has changed. Find out if he has a history of asthma, allergies, or respiratory disorders, and ask about recent illnesses, surgery, or trauma. What medications is he taking? Does he work around chemicals or respiratory irritants, such as silicone?

Examine the patient's mouth and nose for congestion, drainage, or inflammation. Note breath odor: Halitosis can be a sign of pulmonary infection. Inspect his neck for distended veins, and palpate for tenderness and masses or enlarged lymph nodes. Observe his chest for accessory muscle use, retractions, and uneven chest expansion, and percuss for dullness, tympany, or flatness. Finally, auscultate for pleural friction rub and abnormal breath sounds — rhonchi, crackles, or wheezes. (See *Productive cough: Common causes and associated findings.*)

Common medical causes

♦ ***Actinomycosis.*** This disorder begins with a cough that produces purulent sputum. Fever, weight loss, fatigue, weakness, dyspnea, night sweats, pleuritic chest pain, and hemoptysis may also occur.

♦ ***Aspiration pneumonitis.*** This disorder causes coughing that produces pink, frothy, possibly purulent sputum. The patient also has marked dyspnea, fever, tachypnea, tachycardia, wheezing, or cyanosis.

♦ ***Bronchiectasis.*** The chronic cough of this disorder produces copious, mucopurulent sputum that has characteristic layering (top, frothy; middle, clear; bottom, dense with purulent particles). The patient has halitosis: His sputum may smell foul or sickeningly sweet. Other characteristic findings include hemoptysis, persistent coarse crackles over the affected lung area, occasional wheezing, rhonchi, exertional dyspnea, weight loss, fatigue, malaise, weakness, recurrent fever, or late-stage finger clubbing.

♦ ***Bronchitis (chronic).*** This disorder is characterized by a productive cough. It produces mucoid sputum that becomes purulent. Secondary infection can also produce mucopurulent sputum, which may become blood-tinged and foul smelling.

The patient also exhibits prolonged expirations, increased use of accessory muscles for breathing, barrel chest, tachypnea, cyanosis, wheezing, exertional dyspnea, scattered rhonchi, coarse crackles (which can be precipitated by coughing), or late-stage clubbing.

♦ ***Chemical pneumonitis.*** This disorder produces a cough with purulent sputum. It can also cause dyspnea, wheezing, orthopnea, fever, malaise, or crackles; mucous membrane irritation of the conjunctivae, throat, and nose; laryngitis; or rhinitis. Signs and symptoms may increase for 24 to 48 hours after exposure, then resolve; if severe, however, they may recur 2 to 5 weeks later.

♦ ***Common cold.*** When this disorder causes productive coughing, the sputum is mucoid or mucopurulent. Early indications of the common cold include a dry, hacking cough, sneezing, headache, malaise, fatigue, rhinorrhea (watery to tenacious, mucopurulent secretions), nasal congestion, sore throat, myalgia, or arthralgia.

♦ ***Lung abscess (ruptured).*** The cardinal sign of ruptured lung abscess is coughing that produces copious amounts of purulent, foul-smelling, possibly blood-tinged sputum. A ruptured abscess can also cause diaphoresis, anorexia, clubbing, weight loss, weakness, fatigue, fever with chills, dyspnea, headache, malaise, pleuritic chest pain, halitosis, inspiratory crackles, or tubular or amphoric breath sounds. The patient's chest is dull on percussion on the affected side.

Productive cough: Common causes and associated findings

S&S

CAUSES	MAJOR ASSOCIATED SIGNS AND SYMPTOMS												
	Chest pain	Crackles	Cyanosis	Decreased breath sounds	Dyspnea	Fatigue	Fever	Rhonchi	Sore throat	Tachycardia	Tachypnea	Weight loss	Wheezing
Actinomycosis	◆				◆	◆	◆					◆	
Aspiration pneumonia		◆	◆		◆	◆	◆	◆		◆	◆		◆
Bronchiectasis		◆			◆	◆	◆	◆				◆	◆
Bronchitis (chronic)		◆	◆		◆			◆			◆		◆
Chemical pneumonitis		◆			◆		◆	◆					◆
Common cold						◆	◆		◆	◆			
Lung abscess (ruptured)	◆	◆			◆	◆	◆					◆	
Lung cancer	◆				◆	◆	◆					◆	◆
Nocardiosis	◆			◆		◆	◆					◆	
North American blastomycosis	◆					◆	◆					◆	
Pneumonia (bacterial)	◆	◆	◆		◆	◆	◆	◆			◆		
Pneumonia (mycoplasmal)	◆	◆				◆	◆		◆	◆			
Psittacosis	◆	◆					◆				◆		
Pulmonary coccidioidomycosis	◆						◆	◆	◆				◆
Pulmonary edema		◆	◆		◆	◆	◆				◆		
Pulmonary embolism	◆	◆	◆		◆		◆			◆	◆		◆

(continued)

Productive cough: Common causes and associated findings *(continued)*

CAUSES	MAJOR ASSOCIATED SIGNS AND SYMPTOMS: Chest pain	Crackles	Cyanosis	Decreased breath sounds	Dyspnea	Fatigue	Fever	Rhonchi	Sore throat	Tachycardia	Tachypnea	Weight loss	Wheezing
Pulmonary tuberculosis	♦	♦			♦	♦	♦	♦				♦	
Silicosis		♦			♦	♦					♦	♦	
Tracheobronchitis	♦	♦					♦	♦	♦				♦

♦ ***Lung cancer.*** One of the earliest signs of bronchogenic carcinoma is a chronic cough that produces small amounts of purulent (or mucopurulent), blood-streaked sputum. In a patient with bronchoalveolar cancer, however, coughing produces large amounts of frothy sputum. Other signs and symptoms include dyspnea, anorexia, fatigue, weight loss, chest pain, fever, diaphoresis, wheezing, or clubbing.

♦ ***Nocardiosis.*** This disorder causes a productive cough (with purulent, thick, tenacious, and possibly blood-tinged sputum) and fever that may last several months. Other findings include night sweats, pleuritic pain, anorexia, malaise, fatigue, weight loss, or diminished or absent breath sounds. The patient's chest is dull on percussion.

♦ ***North American blastomycosis.*** In this chronic disorder, coughing is dry and hacking, or produces bloody or purulent sputum. Other findings include pleuritic chest pain, fever, chills, anorexia, weight loss, malaise, fatigue, night sweats, cutaneous lesions (small, painless, nonpruritic macules or papules), or prostration.

♦ ***Pneumonia.*** *Bacterial pneumonia* initially causes a dry cough that becomes productive. Rust-colored sputum occurs in pneumococcal pneumonia; "brick red" or "currant jelly" sputum in *Klebsiella* pneumonia; salmon-colored sputum in staphylococcal pneumonia; and mucopurulent sputum in streptococcal pneumonia. Associated signs and symptoms develop suddenly: shaking chills, high fever, myalgia, headache, pleuritic chest pain that increases with chest movement, tachypnea, tachycardia, dyspnea, cyanosis, diaphoresis, decreased breath sounds, fine crackles, or rhonchi.

Mycoplasmal pneumonia may cause a cough that produces scant blood-flecked sputum. Most common, however, is a nonproductive cough that starts 2 to 3 days after the onset of malaise, headache, fever, and sore throat. Paroxysmal coughing causes substernal chest pain. Patients may develop crackles but generally don't appear seriously ill.

♦ ***Psittacosis.*** As this disorder progresses, the characteristic hacking cough, nonproductive at first, may later produce a small amount of mucoid, blood-streaked sputum. The infection may begin abruptly, with chills, fever, headache, myalgia, and prostration. Other signs and symptoms may include tachypnea, fine crackles, chest pain (rare), epistaxis, photophobia, abdominal distention and tenderness, nausea, vomiting, or a faint macular rash. Severe infection may cause stupor, delirium, or coma.

♦ ***Pulmonary coccidioidomycosis.*** This disorder causes a nonproductive or slightly productive cough with fever, occasional chills, pleuritic chest pain, sore throat, headache, backache, malaise, marked weakness, anorexia, hemoptysis, or an itchy macular rash. Rhonchi and wheezing may be heard. The disease may spread to other areas, causing arthralgia, swelling of the knees and ankles, or erythema nodosum or erythema multiforme.

♦ ***Pulmonary edema.*** When severe, this life-threatening disorder causes a cough that produces frothy, bloody sputum. Early signs and symptoms include dyspnea on exertion; paroxysmal nocturnal dyspnea, followed by orthopnea; and coughing, which may be nonproductive initially. Other clinical features include fever, fatigue, tachycardia, tachypnea, dependent crackles, or ventricular gallop. As the patient's respirations become increasingly rapid and labored, he develops more diffuse crackles and the productive cough, worsening tachycardia, or possibly arrhythmias. His skin becomes cold, clammy, and cyanotic; his blood pressure falls; and his pulse becomes thready.

♦ ***Pulmonary embolism.*** This life-threatening disorder causes a cough that may be nonproductive or may produce blood-tinged sputum. Usually, the first symptom of pulmonary embolism is severe dyspnea, which may be accompanied by anginal or pleuritic chest pain. The patient experiences marked anxiety, a low-grade fever, tachycardia, tachypnea, and diaphoresis. Less-common signs include massive hemoptysis, chest splinting, leg edema, or (with a large embolus) cyanosis, syncope, or distended neck veins. The patient may also have a pleural friction rub, diffuse wheezing, crackles, chest dullness on percussion, decreased breath sounds, or signs of circulatory collapse.

♦ ***Pulmonary tuberculosis.*** This disorder causes a mild to severe productive cough with some combination of hemoptysis, malaise, dyspnea, and pleuritic chest pain. Sputum may be scant and mucoid or copious and purulent. Typically, the patient experiences night sweats, easy fatigability, and weight loss. His breath sounds are amphoric. He may have chest dullness on percussion and, after coughing, increased tactile fremitus with crackles.

♦ ***Silicosis.*** Productive cough with mucopurulent sputum is the earliest sign of this disorder. The patient also has exertional dyspnea, tachypnea, weight loss, fatigue, general weakness, or recurrent respiratory infections. Auscultation reveals end-inspiratory fine crackles at the lung bases.

♦ ***Tracheobronchitis.*** Inflammation initially causes a nonproductive cough that later — following the onset of chills, sore throat, slight fever, muscle and back pain, and substernal tightness — becomes productive as secretions increase. Sputum is mucoid, mucopurulent, or purulent. The patient may have rhonchi and wheezes; he may also develop crackles. Severe tracheobronchitis may cause fever of 101° to 102° F (38.3° to 38.9° C) and bronchospasm.

Other causes

♦ ***Diagnostic tests.*** Bronchoscopy and pulmonary function tests may increase productive coughing.

♦ ***Drugs.*** Expectorants, of course, increase productive coughing. These include ammonium chloride, calcium iodide, guaifenesin, iodinated glycerol, potassium iodide, and terpin hydrate.

♦ ***Respiratory therapy.*** Intermittent positive-pressure breathing, nebulizer therapy, and incentive spirometry often loosen secretions and cause or increase productive coughing.

Special considerations

Avoid taking measures to suppress a productive cough because retention of sputum may interfere with alveolar aeration or impair pulmonary resistance to infection. Expect to give mucolytics and expectorants, and increase the patient's intake of oral fluids to thin his secretions and enhance their flow. In addition, you may give a bronchodilator to relieve bronchospasms and to open airways. Antibiotics may be ordered to treat underlying infection.

Humidify the air around the patient; this relieves mucous membrane inflammation and helps loosen dried secretions. Provide pulmonary physiotherapy, such as postural drainage with vibration and percussion, to loosen secretions. Aerosol therapy may be necessary.

Provide the patient with uninterrupted rest periods. Keep him from using respiratory irritants. If he's confined to bed rest, change his position often to promote drainage of secretions.

Prepare the patient for diagnostic tests, such as chest X-ray, bronchoscopy, lung scan, and pulmonary function tests. Collect sputum samples for culture and sensitivity testing.

Pediatric pointers

Because his airway is narrow, a child with a productive cough can quickly develop airway occlusion and respiratory distress from thick or excessive secretions. Causes of productive cough in children include asthma, bronchiectasis, bronchitis, acute bronchiolitis, cystic fibrosis, and pertussis.

When caring for a child with a productive cough, administer expectorants. To soothe inflamed mucous membranes and prevent drying of secretions, provide humidified air or oxygen. Remember, high humidity can induce bronchospasm in a hyperactive child or cause overhydration in an infant.

Geriatric pointers

Always ask elderly patients about a productive cough because this sign may indicate a serious acute or chronic illness.

CRACKLES

[Rales, crepitations]

A common finding in certain cardiovascular and pulmonary disorders, crackles are nonmusical clicking or rattling noises heard during auscultation of breath sounds. They usually occur during inspiration and recur constantly from one respiratory cycle to the next. They can be unilateral or bilateral, moist or dry. They're characterized by their pitch, loudness, location, persistence, and timing during the respiratory cycle.

Crackles indicate abnormal movement of air through fluid-filled airways. They can be irregularly dispersed, as in pneumonia, or localized, as in bronchiectasis. A few basilar crackles can be heard in normal lungs after prolonged shallow breathing; these normal crackles clear with a few deep breaths. Usually, though, crackles indicate the degree of an underlying illness. When crackles result from a generalized disorder, they usually occur in the less distended and more dependent areas of the lungs, such as the lung bases when the patient is standing. Crackles due to air passing through inflammatory exudate may not be audible if the involved portion of the lung isn't being ventilated because of shallow respirations. (See *How crackles occur.*)

Emergency interventions

Quickly take the patient's vital signs and examine him for signs of respiratory distress or airway obstruction. Check the depth and rhythm of respirations. Is he struggling to breathe? Check for increased accessory muscle use and chest wall motion, retractions, stridor, or nasal flaring. Pro-

How crackles occur

Crackles occur when air passes through fluid-filled airways, causing collapsed alveoli to pop open as airway pressure equalizes. They can also occur when membranes lining the chest cavity and the lungs become inflamed. The illustrations below show a normal alveolus and two pathologic alveolar changes that cause crackles.

NORMAL ALVEOLUS

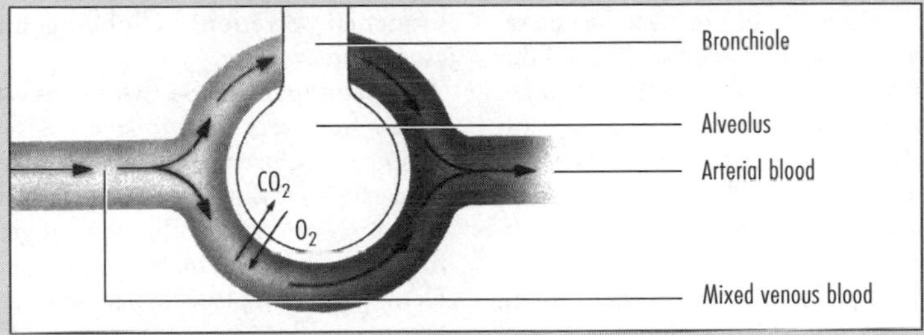

ALVEOLUS IN PULMONARY EDEMA

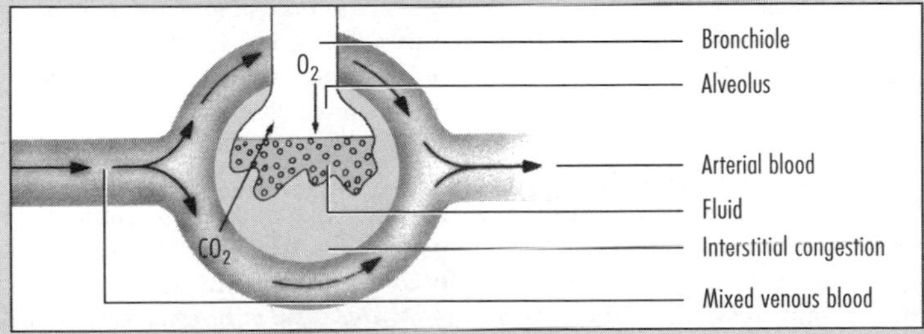

ALVEOLUS IN INFLAMMATION

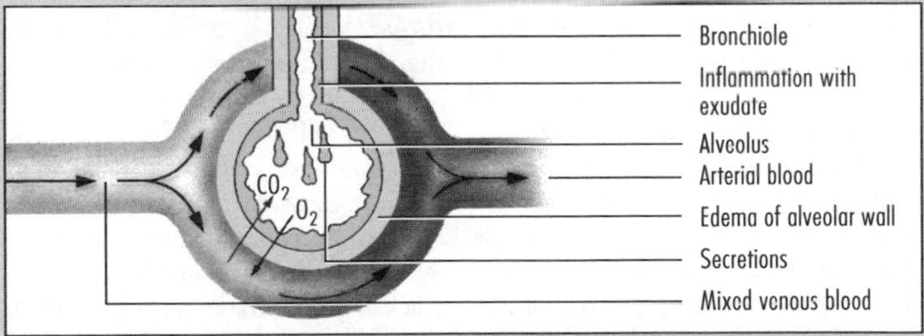

vide supplemental oxygen. Endotracheal intubation may be necessary.

History and physical examination

If the patient also has a cough, ask when it began and if it's constant or intermittent. Find out what the cough sounds like and whether he's coughing up sputum or blood. If the cough is productive, determine the sputum's consistency, amount, odor, and color.

Ask the patient if he has any pain. If so, where is it located? When did he first notice it? Does it radiate to other areas?

Also ask the patient if movement, coughing, or breathing worsens or helps relieve his pain. Note the patient's position: Is he lying still or moving about restlessly?

Obtain a brief medical history. Does the patient have cancer or any known respiratory or cardiovascular problems? Ask if he has had any recent surgery, trauma, or illness and whether he smokes or drinks alcohol. Is he experiencing hoarseness or difficulty swallowing? Find out which medications he's taking. Also ask about recent weight loss, anorexia, nausea, vomiting, fatigue, weakness, vertigo, and syncope. Has the patient been exposed to irritants, such as vapors, fumes, or smoke?

Next, perform a physical examination. Examine the patient's nose and mouth for signs of infection, such as inflammation or increased secretions. Note his breath odor: Halitosis could indicate pulmonary infection. Check his neck for masses, tenderness, swelling, lymphadenopathy, and venous distention.

Inspect the patient's chest for abnormal configuration or uneven expansion. Percuss for dullness, tympany, or flatness. Auscultate his lungs for other abnormal, diminished, or absent breath sounds. Listen to his heart for abnormal sounds, and check his hands and feet for edema or clubbing. (See *Crackles: Common causes and associated findings.*)

Common medical causes

♦ ***Adult respiratory distress syndrome (ARDS).*** This life-threatening disorder causes diffuse, fine to coarse crackles usually heard in the dependent portions of the lungs. It also causes cyanosis, nasal flaring, tachypnea, tachycardia, grunting respirations, rhonchi, dyspnea, anxiety, or decreased level of consciousness.

♦ ***Bronchiectasis.*** In this disorder, persistent, coarse crackles are heard over the affected area of the lung. They're accompanied by a chronic cough that causes copious amounts of mucopurulent sputum. Other characteristics include halitosis, occasional wheezes, exertional dyspnea, rhonchi, weight loss, fatigue, malaise, weakness, recurrent fever, or late-stage clubbing.

♦ ***Bronchitis (chronic).*** This disorder causes coarse crackles that are usually heard at the lung bases. Prolonged expirations, wheezing, rhonchi, exertional dyspnea, tachypnea, or persistent, productive cough occurs because of increased bronchial secretions. Clubbing and cyanosis may occur.

♦ ***Legionnaires' disease.*** Symptoms vary widely from very mild to severe. Usual symptoms include malaise, muscle aches, headache, confusion, fever, chills, cough, and often sputum production ranging from scant to thin to thick and purulent. Hemoptysis and pleuritic pain may also be present. Breath sounds may include only crackles or signs of consolidation.

♦ ***Pneumonia.*** *Bacterial pneumonia* causes diffuse fine crackles, sudden onset of shaking chills, high fever, tachypnea, pleuritic chest pain, grunting respirations, nasal flaring, decreased breath sounds, myalgias, headache, tachycardia, dyspnea, diaphoresis, or rhonchi. The patient also has a dry cough that later becomes productive.

Mycoplasmal pneumonia causes medium to fine crackles together with a harsh nonproductive cough, malaise, sore throat, headache, or fever. The patient may have blood-flecked sputum.

Viral pneumonia causes gradually developing, diffuse crackles. The patient may also have a nonproductive cough, malaise, headache, anorexia, low-grade fever, or decreased breath sounds.

♦ ***Pulmonary edema.*** Moist, bubbling crackles on inspiration are one of the first signs of this life-threatening disorder. Other early findings include dyspnea on exertion; paroxysmal nocturnal dyspnea, then orthopnea; and coughing, which may be initially nonproductive but later causes pink frothy sputum. Related clinical effects include tachycardia, tachypnea, and S_3 gallop. As the condition worsens, the patient's respirations become increasingly rapid and labored,

Crackles: Common causes and associated findings

CAUSES	MAJOR ASSOCIATED SIGNS AND SYMPTOMS												
	Chest pain	Cough	Cyanosis	Dyspnea	Fatigue	Fever	Hemoptysis	Rhonchi	Tachycardia	Tachypnea	Vomiting	Weakness	Weight loss
Adult respiratory distress syndrome			◆	◆				◆	◆	◆			
Bronchiectasis		◆		◆	◆	◆		◆				◆	◆
Bronchitis (chronic)		◆	◆	◆			◆	◆		◆			
Legionnaires' disease	◆	◆		◆	◆	◆	◆		◆	◆	◆	◆	
Pneumonia (bacterial)	◆	◆		◆	◆	◆		◆	◆	◆			
Pneumonia (mycoplasmal)		◆				◆	◆			◆			
Pneumonia (viral)		◆				◆				◆			
Pulmonary edema		◆	◆	◆			◆		◆	◆			
Pulmonary embolism	◆	◆	◆	◆		◆	◆		◆	◆			
Pulmonary tuberculosis	◆	◆		◆	◆	◆	◆					◆	◆
Tracheobronchitis	◆	◆				◆		◆					

he develops more diffuse crackles, worsening tachycardia, hypotension, a rapid and thready pulse, cyanosis, and cold, clammy skin.

◆ ***Pulmonary embolism.*** This life-threatening disorder can cause fine to coarse crackles and a cough that may be dry or produce blood-tinged sputum. Usually, the first sign of pulmonary embolism is severe dyspnea, which may be accompanied by anginal or pleuritic chest pain. The patient has marked anxiety, a low-grade fever, tachycardia, tachypnea, or diaphoresis. Less-common signs include massive hemoptysis, chest splinting, leg edema, and with a large embolus, cyanosis, syncope, and distended neck veins. The patient may also have a pleural friction rub, diffuse wheezing, chest dullness on percussion, decreased breath sounds, or signs of circulatory collapse.

◆ ***Pulmonary tuberculosis.*** In this disorder, fine crackles occur after coughing. The patient has some combination of hemoptysis, malaise, dyspnea, and pleuritic chest pain. Sputum may be scant and mucoid or copious and purulent.

Typically, the patient experiences night sweats, easy fatigue, weakness, or weight loss. His breath sounds are amphoric.

♦ ***Tracheobronchitis.*** In its acute form, this disorder causes moist or coarse crackles with a productive cough, chills, sore throat, slight fever, muscle and back pain, and substernal tightness. The patient typically has rhonchi and wheezes. Severe tracheobronchitis may cause moderate fever and bronchospasm.

Special considerations

To keep the patient's airway patent and to facilitate breathing, elevate the head of his bed. To liquefy thick secretions and relieve mucous membrane inflammation, administer fluids, humidified air, or oxygen. Diuretics may be needed if crackles result from cardiogenic pulmonary edema. Turn the patient every 1 to 2 hours, and encourage him to breathe deeply.

Plan daily uninterrupted rest periods to help the patient relax and sleep. Prepare the patient for diagnostic tests, such as chest X-rays, lung scan, and sputum analysis.

Pediatric pointers

Crackles in an infant or child may indicate a serious cardiovascular or respiratory disorder. Pneumonias cause diffuse, sudden crackles in children. Esophageal atresia and tracheoesophageal fistula can cause bubbling, moist crackles due to aspiration of food or secretions into the lungs — especially in newborn infants. Pulmonary edema causes fine crackles at the bases of the lungs, and bronchiectasis causes moist crackles. Cystic fibrosis causes widespread, fine to coarse inspiratory crackles and wheezing in infants. And sickle cell anemia may cause crackles when it causes pulmonary infarction or infection.

Geriatric pointers

Crackles that clear after deep breathing may indicate mild basilar atelectasis. In older patients, auscultate lung bases before and after auscultating apices.

CREPITATION, BONY

[Bony crepitus]

Bony crepitation is a palpable vibration or an audible crunching sound that results when one bone grates against another. This sign often reflects a fracture, but it can happen when bones that have been stripped of their protective articular cartilage grind against each other as they articulate — for example, in advanced arthritic or degenerative joint disorders.

Eliciting bony crepitation can help confirm diagnosis of a fracture, but it can also cause further soft-tissue, nerve, or vessel injury. What's more, rubbing fractured bone ends together can convert a closed fracture into an open one if a bone end penetrates the skin. So, after initial detection of crepitation in a patient with a fracture, avoid eliciting this sign.

History and physical examination

If you detect bony crepitation in a patient with a suspected fracture, ask if he feels any pain and if he can point to the painful area. To prevent lacerating nerves, blood vessels, or other structures, immobilize the affected area by applying a splint that includes the joints above and below the affected area. Elevate the affected area, if possible, and apply cold packs. Inspect for abrasions or lacerations. Find out how and when the injury occurred. Palpate pulses distal to the injury site; check the skin for pallor or coolness. Test motor and sensory function distal to the injury site.

If the patient doesn't have a suspected fracture, ask about a history of osteoarthritis or rheumatoid arthritis. Which medications does he take? Has any medication helped ease arthritic discomfort? Take the patient's vital signs and test joint range of motion.

Common medical causes

♦ ***Fracture.*** Besides bony crepitation, a fracture causes acute local pain, hematoma, edema, and decreased range of motion. Other findings may include deformity, point tenderness, discoloration of the limb, or loss of limb function. Neurovascular damage may cause prolonged capillary refill time, diminished or absent pulses, mottled cyanosis, paresthesia, or decreased sensation (all distal to the fracture site). An open fracture, of course, causes an obvious skin wound.

♦ ***Osteoarthritis.*** In advanced cases of this disorder, range-of-motion testing may elicit joint crepitation. Soft fine crepitus on palpation suggests roughening of the articular cartilage; coarse grating, badly damaged cartilage. The cardinal symptom of osteoarthritis is joint pain, especially during motion and weight bearing. Other findings include joint stiffness that typically occurs after resting and subsides within a few minutes after the patient begins moving.

♦ ***Rheumatoid arthritis.*** In advanced cases of this disorder, bony crepitation is heard when the affected joint is rotated. However, rheumatoid arthritis usually develops insidiously, producing nonspecific signs and symptoms, such as fatigue, malaise, anorexia, persistent low-grade fever, weight loss, lymphadenopathy, or vague arthralgias and myalgias. Later, more specific and localized articular signs develop, frequently at the proximal finger joints. These signs usually occur bilaterally and symmetrically and may extend to the wrists, knees, elbows, or ankles. The affected joints stiffen after inactivity. The patient also has increased warmth, swelling, and tenderness of affected joints as well as limited range of motion.

Special considerations

If a fracture is suspected, prepare the patient for X-rays of the affected area, and reexamine his neurovascular status frequently. Keep the affected part immobilized and elevated until treatment begins. Give analgesics to relieve pain.

Pediatric pointers

Bony crepitation in a child usually occurs after a fracture. Obtain an accurate history of the injury, and be alert for the possibility of child abuse. In a teenager, bony crepitation and pain in the patellofemoral joint help diagnose chondromalacia of the patella.

Geriatric pointers

Degenerative joint changes, which have usually begun by age 20 or 30, progress more rapidly after age 40 and occur primarily in weight-bearing joints, such as the lumbar spine, hips, knees, and ankles.

CREPITATION, SUBCUTANEOUS

[Subcutaneous crepitus]

When bubbles of air or other gases (such as carbon dioxide) are trapped in subcutaneous tissue, palpation or stroking of the skin causes a crackling sound called subcutaneous crepitation. The bubbles feel like small, unstable nodules and aren't painful, even though subcutaneous crepitation is often associated with painful disorders. Usually, the affected tissue is visibly swollen; this can lead to life-threatening airway occlusion if the swelling affects the neck or upper chest.

The air or gas bubbles enter the tissues through open wounds, from the action of anaerobic microorganisms, or from traumatic or spontaneous rupture or perforation of pulmonary or GI organs.

History and physical examination

Because subcutaneous crepitation can indicate a life-threatening disorder, you'll need to perform a rapid initial evaluation and intervene if necessary. (See *Managing subcutaneous crepitation.*)

When the patient's condition permits, palpate the affected skin to evaluate the location and extent of subcutaneous crepitation and to obtain baseline information. Repalpate frequently to determine if the subcutaneous crepitation is increasing. Ask the patient if he's experiencing any pain or having difficulty breathing. If he's in pain, find out where the pain is located, how severe it is, and when it began. Ask about recent thoracic surgery, diagnostic tests, and respiratory therapy, or a history of trauma or chronic pulmonary disease.

Common medical causes

♦ ***Gas gangrene.*** Subcutaneous crepitation is the hallmark of this rare but often fatal infection, caused by anaerobic microorganisms. It's accompanied by local pain, swelling, and discoloration, with formation of bullae and necrosis. The skin over the wound may rupture, revealing dark red or black necrotic muscle and producing foul-smelling, watery or frothy discharge. Related findings include tachycardia, tachypnea, moderate fever, cyanosis, and lassitude.

♦ ***Orbital fracture.*** This fracture allows air from the nasal sinuses to escape into subcutaneous tissue, causing subcutaneous crepitation of the eyelid and orbit. The most common sign of orbital fracture is periorbital ecchymosis. Visual acuity is usually normal, although a swollen lid may prevent accurate testing. The patient has facial edema, diplopia, a hyphema (blood in the anterior chamber of the eye) and, occasionally, a dilated or unreactive pupil on the affected side. Extraocular movements may also be affected.

♦ ***Pneumothorax.*** Pneumothorax may cause subcutaneous crepitation in the upper chest and neck. In many cases, the patient has chest pain that is unilateral, is rarely localized initially, and increases on inspiration. Dyspnea, anxiety, restlessness, tachypnea, cyanosis, tachycardia, accessory muscle use, asymmetrical chest expansion, or a nonproductive cough can also occur. On the affected side, breath sounds are absent or decreased, percussion sounds are hyperresonant or tympanic, and decreased vocal fremitus may be present.

♦ ***Rupture of the esophagus.*** A ruptured esophagus usually causes subcutaneous crepitation in the neck, chest wall, or supraclavicular fossa, although this sign doesn't always occur. The patient with rupture of the *cervical esophagus* has excruciating pain in the neck or supraclavicular area, his neck is resistant to passive motion, and he has local tenderness, soft-tissue swelling, dysphagia, odynophagia, or orthostatic vertigo.

Life-threatening rupture of the *intrathoracic esophagus* can cause mediastinal emphysema confirmed by a positive Hamman's sign. The patient has severe retrosternal, epigastric, neck, or scapular pain and swelling of the chest wall and neck. He may also display dyspnea, tachypnea, asymmetrical chest expansion, nasal flaring, cyanosis, diaphoresis, tachycardia, hypotension, dysphagia, or fever.

♦ ***Rupture of the trachea or major bronchus.*** This life-threatening injury causes abrupt subcutaneous crepitation of the neck and anterior chest wall. The patient has severe dyspnea with nasal flaring, tachycardia, accessory muscle use, hypotension, cyanosis, extreme anxiety, and possibly hemoptysis and mediastinal emphysema, with a positive Hamman's sign.

Other causes

♦ ***Diagnostic tests.*** Endoscopic tests, such as bronchoscopy and upper GI tract endoscopy, can cause rupture or perfo-

Managing subcutaneous crepitation

Subcutaneous crepitation occurs when air or gas bubbles escape into tissues. It may signal life-threatening rupture of an air-filled or gas-producing organ, or a fulminating anaerobic infection.

ORGAN RUPTURE

If the patient shows signs of respiratory distress — such as severe dyspnea, tachypnea, accessory muscle use, nasal flaring, air hunger, or tachycardia — quickly test for Hamman's sign to detect trapped air bubbles in the mediastinum.

To test for Hamman's sign, help the patient assume a left-lateral recumbent position. Then place your stethoscope over the precordium. If you hear a loud crunching sound that synchronizes with his heartbeat, the patient has a positive Hamman's sign.

Depending on which organ is ruptured, be prepared for endotracheal intubation, an emergency tracheotomy, or chest tube insertion. Start administering supplemental oxygen immediately. Start an I.V. to administer fluids and medication, and connect the patient to a cardiac monitor.

ANAEROBIC INFECTION

If the patient has an open wound with a foul odor and local swelling and discoloration, you must act quickly. Take the patient's vital signs, checking especially for fever, tachycardia, hypotension, and tachypnea. Next, start an I.V. line to administer fluids and medication, and provide supplemental oxygen.

In addition, be prepared for emergency surgery to drain and debride the wound. If the patient's condition is life-threatening, you may need to prepare him for transfer to a facility with a hyperbaric chamber.

ration of respiratory or GI organs, producing subcutaneous crepitation.

◆ ***Respiratory treatments.*** Mechanical ventilation and intermittent positive-pressure breathing can rupture alveoli, causing subcutaneous crepitation.

◆ ***Thoracic surgery.*** If air escapes into the tissue in the area of the incision, subcutaneous crepitation can occur.

Special considerations

Monitor the patient's vital signs frequently, especially respirations. Because excessive swelling from subcutaneous crepitation in the neck and upper chest can cause airway obstruction, be alert for signs of respiratory distress, such as dyspnea. Tell the patient that the affected tissues will eventually absorb the air or gas bubbles, so the subcutaneous crepitation will decrease.

Pediatric pointers

Children may develop subcutaneous crepitation in the neck from ingestion of corrosive substances that perforate the esophagus.

CRY, HIGH-PITCHED

[Cerebral cry]

A high-pitched cry is a brief, sharp, piercing vocal sound produced by a neonate or infant. Whether acute or chronic, this cry is a late sign of increased intracranial pressure (ICP). The acute onset of a high-pitched cry demands emergency treatment to prevent permanent brain damage or death.

Any change in the volume of one of the brain's components — brain tissue, cerebrospinal fluid, and blood — may cause increased ICP. In neonates, increased ICP may result from intracranial bleeding associated with birth trauma or from congenital malformations, such as craniostenosis or Arnold-Chiari syndrome. In fact, a high-pitched cry may be an early sign of congenital malformation. In infants, increased ICP may result from meningitis, head trauma, or child abuse.

History and physical examination
Take the infant's vital signs, and then obtain a brief history. Did the infant fall recently or experience even minor head trauma? Be sure to ask the mother about any changes in his behavior during the past 24 hours. Has he seemed restless or unlike himself? Has his sucking reflex diminished? Does he cry when moved? Suspect child abuse if the infant's history is inconsistent with physical findings.

Next, perform a neurologic examination. Remember that neurologic responses in neonates and young infants are primarily reflex responses. Determine the infant's level of consciousness. Is he awake, irritable, or lethargic? Does he reach for an attractive object or turn toward the sound of a rattle? Observe his posture. Is he in the normal flexed position or in extension or opisthotonos? Examine muscle tone and observe for signs of seizure, such as tremors and twitching.

Examine the size and shape of the infant's head. Is the anterior fontanel bulging? Measure the infant's head circumference, and check pupillary size and response to light. Unilateral or bilateral dilation and a sluggish response to light may accompany increased ICP. Finally, test the infant's reflexes; expect Moro's reflex to be diminished if 4 months or younger.

After completing your examination, elevate the infant's head 20 to 30 degrees to promote cerebral venous drainage and decrease ICP. Start an I.V. line, and give diuretics and corticosteroids to decrease ICP. Be sure to keep endotracheal intubation equipment close by to secure an airway if needed.

Common medical causes
♦ ***Increased ICP.*** A high-pitched cry is a late sign of increased ICP. Typically, the infant also displays bulging fontanels, increased head circumference, and widened sutures. Later signs and symptoms of increasing ICP include seizures, bradycardia, possible vomiting, dilated pupils, decreased level of consciousness, increased systolic blood pressure, widened pulse pressure, or altered respiratory pattern.

Special considerations
The infant with increased ICP requires specialized care and monitoring in the intensive care unit. For example, you'll need to monitor his vital signs and neurologic status to detect subtle changes in his condition. Also monitor intake and output. Monitor ICP, restrict fluids, and administer diuretics and corticosteroids. For an infant with severely increased ICP, endotracheal intubation and mechanical hyperventilation may be needed to decrease serum carbon dioxide levels and constrict cerebral blood vessels. Or, barbiturate coma or hypothermia therapy may be needed to decrease the infant's metabolic rate.

Remember to avoid jostling the infant, which may aggravate increased ICP. Comfort him and maintain a calm, quiet environment because the infant's crying or exposure to environmental stimuli may also worsen increased ICP.

Cyanosis

Cyanosis — a bluish or bluish black discoloration of the skin and mucous membranes — results from excessive concentration of deoxygenated hemoglobin in the blood. This common sign may develop abruptly or gradually. It can be classified as central or peripheral, although the two types may coexist.

Central cyanosis reflects inadequate oxygenation of arterial blood caused by right-to-left cardiac shunting, pulmonary disease, or hematologic disorders. It is noted on the lips, around the mouth, and on mucous membranes in the mouth. As hypoxemia worsens, the cyanosis may become peripheral as well.

Peripheral cyanosis reflects sluggish peripheral circulation caused by vasoconstriction, reduced cardiac output, or vascular occlusion. It may be widespread or may occur locally in one extremity; however, it doesn't affect mucous membranes. Typically, peripheral cyanosis appears on exposed areas, such as the fingers, nail beds, feet, nose, and ears.

Although cyanosis is an important sign of cardiovascular and pulmonary disorders, it isn't always an accurate gauge of oxygenation. Several factors contribute to its development: hemoglobin concentration and oxygen saturation, cardiac output, and partial pressure of arterial oxygen (PaO_2). Cyanosis usually does not occur until the oxygen saturation of hemoglobin falls below 80%. Severe cyanosis is quite obvious, whereas mild cyanosis is more difficult to detect, even in natural, bright light. In dark-skinned patients, cyanosis is most apparent in the mucous membranes and nail beds.

Transient, nonpathologic cyanosis may result from environmental factors. For example, peripheral cyanosis, especially in infants, may result from cutaneous vasoconstriction following brief exposure to cold air or water. Central cyanosis may result from reduced PaO_2 at high altitudes.

Emergency interventions

It's important to distinguish between peripheral and central cyanosis because central cyanosis is a sign of inadequate oxygenation of the blood, which may be life-threatening.

Cyanosis may occur with any cardiac or pulmonary condition that becomes severe enough to interfere with adequate oxygenation of the blood. It is important to remember that cyanosis is a late sign of hypoxia and often does not appear until hypoxemia is quite severe.

If you see central cyanosis, perform a rapid evaluation. Take immediate steps to maintain an airway, assist breathing, provide oxygen, and monitor circulation. If the patient displays sudden, localized cyanosis and other signs of arterial occlusion, protect the affected limb from injury; however, do not massage the limb.

History and physical examination

If cyanosis accompanies less-acute conditions, perform a thorough examination. Begin with a history, focusing on cardiac, pulmonary, and hematologic disorders. Ask about previous surgery. Then begin the physical examination by taking vital signs. Inspect the skin and mucous membranes to determine the extent of cyanosis. Ask the patient when he first noticed the cyanosis. Does it subside and recur? Is it aggravated by cold, smoking, or stress? Alleviated by massage or rewarming? Check the skin for coolness, pallor, redness, pain, and ulceration. Also, note clubbing.

Next, evaluate the patient's level of consciousness. Ask about headaches, dizziness, or blurred vision. Then test his motor strength. Ask about pain in the arms and legs (especially with walking) and about abnormal sensations, such as numbness, tingling, and coldness.

Ask about chest pain and its severity. Can the patient identify any aggravating and alleviating factors? Palpate peripheral pulses and test capillary refill time. Also note edema. Auscultate heart rate and rhythm, noting especially gallops and murmurs. Also auscultate the abdominal aorta and femoral arteries to detect any bruits.

Does the patient have a cough? Is it productive? If so, have the patient describe the sputum. Evaluate respiratory rate and rhythm. Check for nasal flaring and use of accessory muscles. Ask about sleep apnea. Does the patient sleep with his head propped up on pillows? Inspect for asymmetrical chest expansion or barrel chest. Percuss the lungs for dullness or hyperresonance, and auscultate for decreased or adventitious breath sounds.

Inspect the abdomen for ascites, and test for shifting dullness or fluid wave. Percuss and palpate for liver enlargement and tenderness. Also, ask about nausea, anorexia, and weight loss.

Common medical causes

♦ ***Arteriosclerotic occlusive disease (chronic).*** In this disorder, peripheral cyanosis occurs in the legs whenever they're in a dependent position. Associated signs and symptoms include intermittent claudication and burning pain at rest, paresthesia, pallor, muscle atrophy, weak leg pulses, or impotence. Late signs are leg ulcers and gangrene.

♦ ***Bronchiectasis.*** This disorder causes chronic central cyanosis. Its classic sign, though, is chronic productive cough with copious, foul-smelling, mucopurulent sputum or hemoptysis. Auscultation reveals rhonchi and coarse crackles during inspiration. Other features are dyspnea, recurrent fever and chills, weight loss, malaise, and clubbing.

♦ ***Buerger's disease.*** In this disorder, exposure to cold initially causes the feet to become cold, cyanotic, and numb; later, they redden, become hot, and tingle. Intermittent claudication of the instep is characteristic; it's aggravated by exercise and smoking and relieved by rest. Associated clinical features include weak peripheral pulses and, in later stages, ulceration, muscle atrophy, or gangrene.

♦ ***Chronic obstructive pulmonary disease (COPD).*** Central cyanosis occurs in advanced stages of COPD and may be aggravated by exertion. Associated signs and symptoms include exertional dyspnea, productive cough with thick sputum, anorexia, weight loss, pursed-lip breathing, barrel chest, tachypnea, and use of accessory muscles. Auscultation may reveal wheezing or rhonchi, or diminished breath sounds. Percussion may reveal hyperresonant lung fields.

♦ ***Deep vein thrombosis.*** In this disorder, acute peripheral cyanosis occurs in the affected extremity associated with tenderness, painful movement, edema, warmth, or prominent superficial veins. Homans' sign can also be elicited.

♦ ***Heart failure.*** In left-sided heart failure that has progressed to pulmonary edema, central cyanosis occurs with tachycardia, fatigue, dyspnea, cold intolerance, orthopnea, cough, ventricular or atrial gallop, bibasilar crackles, or diffuse apical impulse.

♦ ***Lung cancer.*** Central cyanosis may occur in this condition accompanied by fever, weakness, weight loss, anorexia, dyspnea, chest pain, cough, hemoptysis, or wheezing.

♦ ***Peripheral arterial occlusion (acute).*** This disorder causes acute cyanosis of one arm or leg or, occasionally, of both legs. The cyanosis is accompanied by sharp or aching pain that worsens when the patient moves. The patient also exhibits paresthesia, weakness, and pale, cool skin in the affected extremity. Examination reveals decreased or absent pulse and prolonged capillary refill time. This situation requires immediate intervention to prevent loss of the extremity.

♦ ***Pneumonia.*** In pneumonia, acute central cyanosis is usually preceded by fever, shaking chills, cough with purulent sputum, crackles and rhonchi, and pleuritic chest pain that's exacerbated by deep inspiration. Associated signs and symptoms may include tachycardia, dyspnea, tachypnea, diminished breath sounds, diaphoresis, myalgia, fatigue, headache, or anorexia.

♦ ***Pneumothorax.*** A cardinal sign of pneumothorax, acute cyanosis is accompanied by sharp chest pain that's exacerbated by movement, deep breathing, and coughing; asymmetrical chest wall expansion; and shortness of breath. The patient may also exhibit rapid, shallow respirations; weak, rapid pulse; pallor; neck vein distention; anxiety; or absence of breath sounds over the affected lung.

◆ ***Polycythemia vera.*** A ruddy complexion that can appear cyanotic is characteristic in this chronic myeloproliferative disorder. Other findings are hepatosplenomegaly, headache, dizziness, fatigue, aquagenic pruritus, blurred vision, chest pain, intermittent claudication, or coagulation defects.

◆ ***Pulmonary edema.*** In this disorder, acute central cyanosis occurs with dyspnea; orthopnea; frothy, blood-tinged sputum; tachycardia; tachypnea; dependent crackles; ventricular gallop; cold, clammy skin; hypotension; weak, thready pulse; and confusion.

◆ ***Pulmonary embolism.*** Acute central cyanosis occurs when a large embolus causes significant obstruction of the pulmonary circulation. Syncope and neck vein distention may also occur. Other common signs and symptoms include dyspnea, chest pain, tachycardia, pulsus paradoxus, dry cough or productive cough with blood-tinged sputum, low-grade fever, restlessness, or diaphoresis.

◆ ***Raynaud's disease.*** In *Raynaud's disease,* exposure to cold or stress causes the fingers or hands first to blanch and turn cold, then to become cyanotic, and finally to redden with return of normal temperature. Numbness and tingling may also occur. *Raynaud's phenomenon* describes the same presentation when associated with other disorders, such as rheumatoid arthritis, scleroderma, or lupus erythematosus.

◆ ***Shock.*** In this disorder, acute peripheral cyanosis develops in the hands and feet, which may also be cold, clammy, and pale. Other characteristic clinical features include lethargy, confusion, prolonged capillary refill time, and a rapid, weak pulse. Tachypnea, hyperpnea, and hypotension may also be present.

◆ ***Sleep apnea.*** When chronic and severe, sleep apnea causes pulmonary hypertension and cor pulmonale (right-sided heart failure), both of which can lead to chronic cyanosis.

Special considerations

Provide supplemental oxygen to relieve shortness of breath and to decrease cyanosis. However, deliver small doses (2 L/minute) to patients with COPD, who may retain carbon dioxide. Position the patient comfortably to ease breathing. As needed, administer diuretics, bronchodilators, antibiotics, or cardiac drugs. Make sure the patient gets sufficient rest between activities to prevent dyspnea.

Prepare the patient for such tests as arterial blood gas analysis and complete blood count to determine the cause of cyanosis.

Pediatric pointers

Many pulmonary disorders responsible for cyanosis in adults also cause cyanosis in children. In addition, central cyanosis in children may result from cystic fibrosis, asthma, airway obstruction by a foreign body, acute laryngotracheobronchitis, or epiglottitis. It may also result from congenital heart defects, such as transposition of the great vessels, that cause right-to-left intracardiac shunting.

In children, circumoral cyanosis may precede generalized cyanosis. Excessive crying or exposure to cold can cause acrocyanosis (also called "glove and boot" cyanosis) in infants. Exercise and agitation enhance cyanosis, so provide comfort and regular rest periods. Also, administer supplemental oxygen during cyanotic episodes.

Geriatric pointers

Because elderly patients have reduced tissue perfusion, peripheral cyanosis can present with a slight decrease in cardiac output or systemic blood pressure.

D

DECEREBRATE POSTURE

[Decerebrate rigidity, abnormal extensor reflex]

Decerebrate posture is an ominous sign seen in persons with severe damage to the upper brain stem. The arms are adducted and extended, the wrists pronated, the fingers flexed; the legs are stiffly extended, with plantar flexion of the feet, and in severe cases, the back is acutely arched (opisthotonos). Upper brain stem damage may result from primary lesions, such as infarction, hemorrhage, or tumor; metabolic encephalopathy; head injury; or compression associated with increased intracranial pressure (ICP).

Decerebrate posture may be elicited by noxious stimuli or may occur spontaneously. It may be unilateral or bilateral. In concurrent brain stem and cerebral damage, decerebrate posture may affect only the arms, while the legs may remain flaccid. Or, decerebrate posture may affect one side of the body and decorticate posture the other. The two postures may also alternate as the patient's neurologic status fluctuates. Generally, the duration of each posturing episode correlates with the severity of brain stem damage. (See *Comparing decerebrate and decorticate postures.*)

Emergency interventions

Your first priority is to ensure a patent airway. Insert an artificial airway, elevate the head of the bed, and turn the patient's head to the side to prevent aspiration. (Don't disrupt spinal alignment if you suspect spinal cord injury.) Suction the airway as necessary.

Next, examine spontaneous respirations. Give supplemental oxygen and ventilate the patient with a handheld resuscitation bag, if necessary. Intubation and mechanical ventilation may be indicated. Keep emergency resuscitation equipment handy. Be sure to check the patient's chart for a no-code order.

History and physical examination

After taking vital signs, determine the patient's level of consciousness (LOC). Use the Glasgow Coma Scale as a reference. Then evaluate the pupils for size, equality, and response to light. Test deep tendon and cranial nerve reflexes, and check for doll's eye sign.

Next, explore the history of the patient's coma. If you're unable to obtain this information, look for clues to the causative disorder, such as hepatomegaly, cyanosis, diabetic skin changes, needle tracks, or obvious trauma. If a family member is available, find out when the patient's LOC began deteriorating. Did it occur abruptly? What did the patient complain of before he lost consciousness? Does he have a history of diabetes, liver

Comparing decerebrate and decorticate postures

Decerebrate posture results from damage to the upper brain stem. In this posture, the arms are adducted and extended, the wrists pronated, and the fingers flexed. The legs are stiffly extended with plantar flexion of the feet.

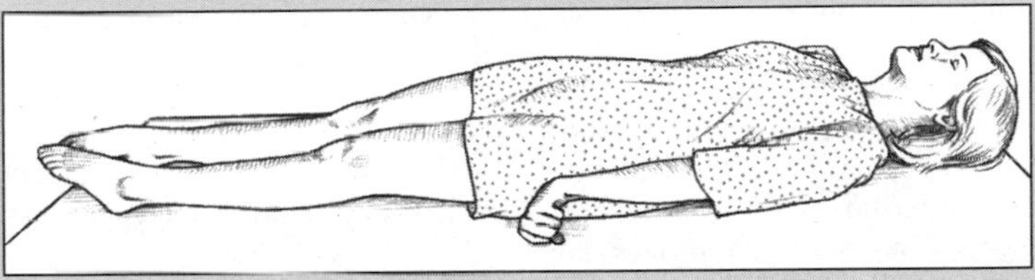

Decorticate posture results from damage to one or both corticospinal tracts. In this posture, the arms are adducted and flexed, with the wrists and fingers flexed on the chest. The legs are stiffly extended and internally rotated with plantar flexion of the feet.

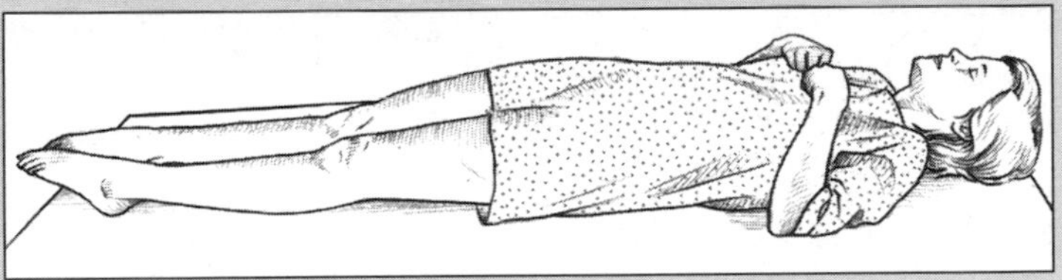

disease, cancer, blood clots, or aneurysm? Ask about any accident or trauma responsible for the coma.

Common medical causes

♦ ***Brain stem infarction.*** When this primary lesion causes a coma, decerebrate posture may occur. Decerebrate posture in upper extremities with flaccid lower extremities indicates more extensive brain damage. Associated signs and symptoms vary with the severity of the infarct and may include cranial nerve palsies, bilateral cerebellar ataxia, or sensory loss. In a deep coma, all normal reflexes are usually lost, resulting in absence of doll's eye sign, a positive Babinski's reflex, and flaccidity.

♦ ***Cerebral lesion.*** Whether the etiology is trauma, tumor, abscess, or infarction, any cerebral lesions that increase ICP, especially large cerebral lesions that compress the lower thalamus, may cause decerebrate posture. Typically, this posture is a late sign. Associated findings vary with the lesion's site and extent, but they commonly include coma, abnormal pupil size and response to light, and the classic triad of increased ICP — bradycardia, increasing systolic blood pressure, and widening pulse pressure.

♦ ***Hypoglycemic encephalopathy.*** Characterized by extremely low blood glucose levels, this disorder may cause decerebrate posture and coma. It also causes dilated pupils, slow respirations, and bradycardia. Muscle spasms, twitching, and seizures eventually progress to flaccidity.

♦ ***Hypoxic encephalopathy.*** In patients with severe hypoxia, brain stem compression associated with anaerobic metabolism and increased ICP may cause decerebrate posture. Other findings include coma, a positive Babinski's reflex, absence of doll's eye sign, hypoactive deep tendon reflexes and, possibly, fixed pupils and respiratory arrest.

♦ ***Pontine hemorrhage.*** Typically, this life-threatening disorder rapidly leads to decerebrate posture with coma. Accompanying signs include total paralysis, absence of doll's eye sign, a positive Babinski's reflex, and small, reactive pupils.

♦ ***Posterior fossa hemorrhage.*** The early signs and symptoms of this subtentorial lesion include vomiting, headache, vertigo, ataxia, stiff neck, drowsiness, papilledema, and cranial nerve palsies. The patient eventually slips into coma with decerebrate posture and, possibly, respiratory arrest.

Other causes

♦ ***Diagnostic tests.*** Relief of high ICP by removal of spinal fluid during a lumbar puncture may precipitate cerebral compression of the brain stem and cause decerebrate posture and coma.

Special considerations

Help prepare the patient for diagnostic tests that will determine the cause of his decerebrate posture. In addition to skull X-rays and a computed tomography scan or magnetic resonance imaging, diagnostic tests may include cerebral angiography, digital subtraction angiography, electroencephalography, brain scan, and ICP monitoring.

Monitor the patient's neurologic status and vital signs every 15 minutes or hourly. In addition, be alert for signs of increased ICP (bradycardia, increasing systolic blood pressure, and widening pulse pressure) and neurologic deterioration (altered respiratory pattern and abnormal temperature).

Inform the patient's family that decerebrate posture is a reflex response — not a voluntary response to pain or a sign of recovery. Offer emotional support.

Pediatric pointers

Children younger than age 2 may not display decerebrate posture because of nervous system immaturity. However, if such a posture does occur, it's usually the more severe opisthotonos. In fact, opisthotonos is more common in infants and young children than in adults and is usually a terminal sign. In children, the most common cause of decerebrate posture is head injury. It also occurs in Reye's syndrome — the result of increased ICP causing brain stem compression.

DECORTICATE POSTURE

[Decorticate rigidity, abnormal flexor response]

A sign of corticospinal damage, decorticate posture is less ominous than decerebrate posture but still very serious. The arms are adducted, the elbows flexed, and the wrists and fingers flexed on the chest. The legs are extended and internally rotated, with plantar flexion of the feet. This posture may occur unilaterally or bilaterally. It usually results from cerebrovascular accident (CVA) or head injury. It may be elicited by noxious stimuli or may occur spontaneously. The intensity of the required stimulus, the duration of the posture, and the frequency of spontaneous episodes vary with the severity and location of cerebral injury.

Decorticate posture carries a more favorable prognosis than decerebrate posture. However, if the causative disorder extends lower in the brain stem, decorticate posture may progress to decerebrate posture. (See *Comparing decerebrate and decorticate postures,* page 171.)

Emergency interventions

Obtain vital signs and evaluate the patient's level of consciousness (LOC). If his consciousness is impaired, insert an oropharyngeal airway, elevate the head of the bed 30 degrees, and turn the patient's head to the side to prevent aspiration (unless spinal cord injury is suspected). Evaluate the patient's respiratory rate, rhythm, and depth. Prepare to assist respirations with a handheld resuscitation bag or with intubation and mechanical ventilation, if necessary. In addition, institute seizure precautions.

History and physical examination

Test the patient's motor and sensory functions. Evaluate pupil size, equality, and response to light. Then test cranial nerve and deep tendon reflexes. Ask about headache, dizziness, nausea, abnormal vision, and numbness or tingling. When did the patient first notice these symptoms? Is his family aware of any behavior changes? Also, ask about a history of cerebrovascular disease, cancer, meningitis, encephalitis, upper respiratory tract infection, or recent trauma.

Common medical causes

- ***Brain abscess.*** Decorticate posture may occur in this infection. Accompanying findings vary with the size and location of the abscess; they may include aphasia, hemiparesis, headache, dizziness, seizures, nausea, or vomiting. Behavior changes, altered vital signs, and decreased LOC may also occur.
- ***Brain tumor.*** This disorder may cause decorticate posture that's usually bilateral — the result of increased intracranial pressure (ICP) associated with tumor growth. Related signs and symptoms include headache, behavior changes, memory loss, diplopia, blurred vision or vision loss, seizures, ataxia, dizziness, apraxia, aphasia, paresis, sensory loss, paresthesia, vomiting, papilledema, and signs of hormonal imbalance.
- ***Cerebrovascular accident.*** Typically, a CVA involving the cerebral cortex causes unilateral decorticate posture, also called spastic hemiplegia. Other clinical features include hemiplegia (contralateral to the lesion), dysarthria, dysphagia, unilateral sensory loss, apraxia, agnosia, aphasia, memory loss, decreased LOC, urine retention and incontinence, and constipation. Ocular effects include homonymous hemianopia, diplopia, and blurred vision.
- ***Head injury.*** Decorticate posture may be among the variable features of this disorder, depending on the site and severity of head injury. Associated signs and symptoms may include headache, nausea and vomiting, dizziness, irritability, decreased LOC, aphasia, hemiparesis, unilateral numbness, seizures, and pupillary dilation.

Special considerations

Assess the patient frequently to detect subtle signs of neurologic deterioration. Also, monitor neurologic status and vital signs every 30 minutes to 2 hours. Be alert for signs of increased ICP, including bradycardia, increasing systolic blood pressure, and widening pulse pressure.

Pediatric pointers

Decorticate posture is an unreliable sign before age 2 because of nervous system immaturity. In children, this posture usually results from head injury. It also occurs in Reye's syndrome.

DEEP TENDON REFLEXES, HYPERACTIVE

A hyperactive deep tendon reflex (DTR) is an abnormally brisk muscle contraction that occurs in response to a sudden stretch induced by sharply tapping the muscle's tendon of insertion. This elicited sign may be graded as brisk or pathologically hyperactive. Hyperactive DTRs are often accompanied by clonus.

The corticospinal tract and other descending tracts govern the reflex arc—the relay cycle that causes any reflex response. A corticospinal lesion above the level of the reflex arc being tested may result in hyperactive DTRs. Abnormal neuromuscular transmission at the end of the reflex arc may also cause hyperactive DTRs. For example, a deficiency of calcium or magnesium may cause hyperactive DTRs because these electrolytes regulate neuromuscular excitability. (See *Tracing the reflex arc in deep tendon reflexes,* pages 176 and 177.)

Although hyperactive DTRs frequently accompany other neurologic findings, they usually lack specific diagnostic value. For example, they're an early, cardinal sign of hypocalcemia.

History and physical examination

After eliciting hyperactive DTRs, first take the patient's history. Ask about spinal cord injury or other trauma and about prolonged exposure to cold, wind, or water. Could the patient be pregnant? A positive response to any of these questions requires prompt evaluation to rule out life-threatening autonomic hyperreflexia, tetanus, preeclampsia, or hypothermia. Ask about the onset and progression of associated signs and symptoms.

Next, perform a neurologic examination. Evaluate level of consciousness, and test motor and sensory function in the limbs. Ask about paresthesia. Check for ataxia or tremors and for speech and visual deficits. Test for Chvostek's and Trousseau's signs and for carpopedal spasm. Ask about vomiting or altered bladder habits. Be sure to take vital signs.

Common medical causes

◆ ***Amyotrophic lateral sclerosis.*** This disorder causes generalized hyperactive DTRs accompanied by weakness of the hands and forearms and spasticity of the legs. Eventually, the patient develops atrophy of the neck and tongue muscles, fasciculations, weakness of the legs, and possibly bulbar signs (for example, dysphagia, dysphonia, facial weakness, and dyspnea).

◆ ***Brain tumor.*** A cerebral tumor causes hyperactive DTRs on the side opposite the lesion. Associated signs and symptoms develop slowly and may include unilateral paresis or paralysis, anesthesia, visual field deficits, spasticity, and a positive Babinski's reflex.

◆ ***Cerebrovascular accident (CVA).*** Any CVA that affects the origin of the corticospinal tracts causes sudden onset of hyperactive DTRs on the side opposite the lesion. The patient may also have unilateral paresis or paralysis, anesthesia, visual field deficits, spasticity, or a positive Babinski's reflex.

◆ ***Hypocalcemia.*** This disorder may cause sudden or gradual onset of generalized hyperactive DTRs with paresthesia, muscle twitching and cramping, positive Chvostek's and Trousseau's signs, carpopedal spasm, and tetany.

◆ ***Hypomagnesemia.*** This disorder results in gradual onset of generalized hyperactive DTRs accompanied by muscle cramps, hypotension, tachycardia, paresthesia, ataxia, tetany, and possibly seizures.

◆ ***Hypothermia.*** Mild hypothermia (90° to 94° F [32.2° to 34.4° C]) causes generalized hyperactive DTRs. Other signs and symptoms include shivering, fatigue, weakness, lethargy, slurred speech, ataxia, muscle stiffness, tachycardia, diuresis, bradypnea, hypotension, and cold, pale skin.

◆ ***Preeclampsia.*** Occurring in pregnancy of at least 20 weeks' duration, preeclampsia may cause gradual onset of generalized hyperactive DTRs. Accompanying signs and symptoms include increased blood pressure; abnormal weight gain; edema of the face, fingers, and abdomen after bed rest; albuminuria; oliguria; severe headache; blurred or double vision; epigastric pain; nausea and vomiting; irritability; cyanosis; shortness of breath; and crackles. If preeclampsia progresses to eclampsia, the patient develops seizures.

♦ ***Spinal cord lesion.*** Incomplete spinal cord lesions cause hyperactive DTRs below the level of the lesion. When the lesion is traumatic, hyperactive DTRs follow resolution of spinal shock. In a patient with a neoplastic lesion, hyperactive DTRs gradually replace normal DTRs. Other signs and symptoms are paralysis and sensory loss below the level of the lesion, urine retention and overflow incontinence, and alternating constipation and diarrhea. A lesion above T6 may also cause autonomic hyperreflexia with diaphoresis and flushing above the level of the lesion, headache, nasal congestion, nausea, increased blood pressure, and bradycardia.

♦ ***Tetanus.*** In this disorder, sudden onset of generalized hyperactive DTRs accompanies tachycardia, diaphoresis, low-grade fever, painful and involuntary muscle contractions, trismus (lockjaw), and risus sardonicus.

Special considerations

Prepare the patient for diagnostic tests to evaluate hyperactive DTRs. These may include laboratory tests for serum calcium and magnesium, spinal X-rays, magnetic resonance imaging, computed tomography, lumbar puncture, and myelography.

If motor weakness accompanies hyperactive DTRs, perform or encourage range-of-motion exercises to preserve muscle integrity. Also, reposition the patient frequently, provide a special mattress, and massage his back to prevent skin breakdown. Administer muscle relaxants and sedatives to relieve severe muscle contractions. Keep emergency resuscitation equipment on hand. Provide a quiet, calm atmosphere to decrease neuromuscular excitability.

Pediatric pointers

Hyperreflexia may be a normal sign in neonates. After age 6, reflex responses are similar to those of adults. When testing DTRs in small children, use distraction techniques to promote reliable results.

Cerebral palsy frequently causes hyperactive DTRs in children. Reye's syndrome causes generalized hyperactive DTRs in Stage II; in Stage V, DTRs are absent. Adult causes of hyperactive DTRs may also appear in children.

Deep Tendon Reflexes, Hypoactive

A hypoactive deep tendon reflex (DTR) is an abnormally diminished muscle contraction that occurs in response to a sudden stretch induced by sharply tapping the muscle's tendon of insertion. It may be graded as minimal (+) or absent (0). Symmetrically reduced (+) reflexes may be normal.

Normally, a DTR operates via the reflex arc, which is governed by the corticospinal tract and other descending tracts. Hypoactive DTRs may result from damage to the reflex arc involving the specific muscle, the peripheral nerve, the nerve roots, or the spinal cord at that level. Hypoactive DTRs are an important sign of many disorders, especially when they appear with other neurologic signs and symptoms. (See *Documenting deep tendon reflexes,* page 178.)

History and physical examination

After eliciting hypoactive DTRs, obtain a thorough history from the patient or a family member. Have him describe current signs and symptoms in detail. Then take a family and drug history.

Next, evaluate the patient's level of consciousness. Test motor function in his limbs, and palpate for muscle atro-

(Text continues on page 178.)

Tracing the reflex arc in deep tendon reflexes

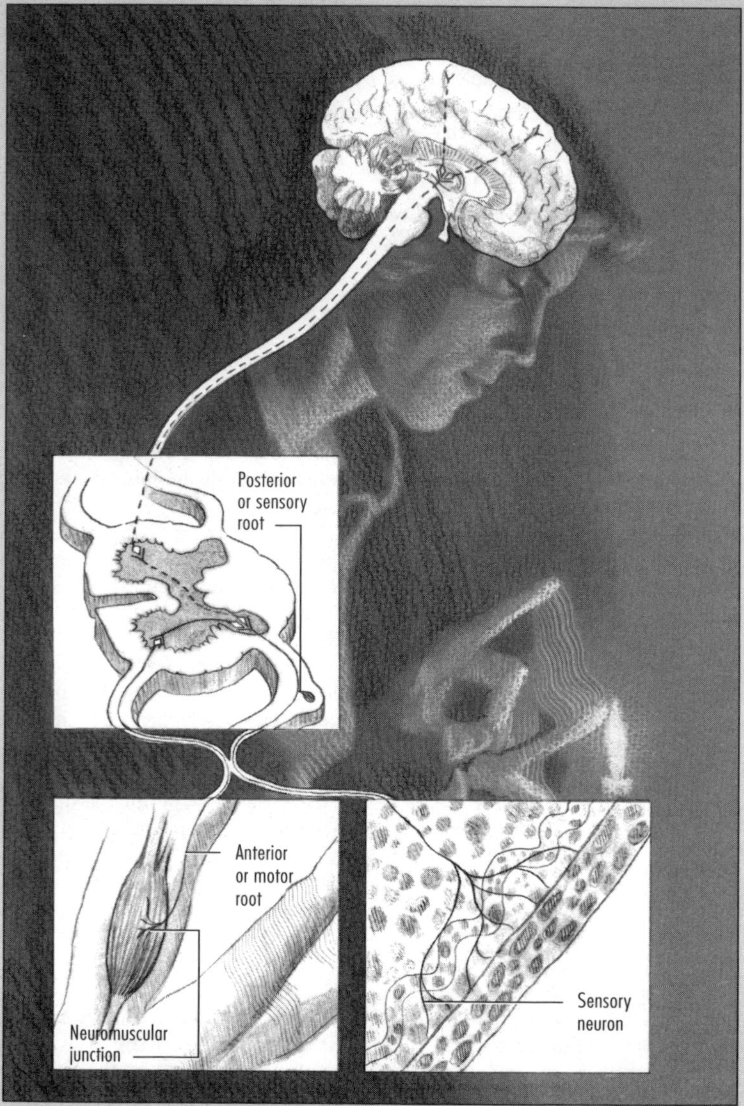

Sharply tapping a tendon initiates a sensory (afferent) impulse that travels along a peripheral nerve to a spinal nerve and then to the spinal cord. The impulse enters the spinal cord through the posterior root, synapses with a motor (efferent) neuron in the anterior horn on the same side of the spinal cord, and then is transmitted through a motor nerve fiber back to the muscle. When the impulse crosses the neuromuscular junction, the muscle contracts, completing the reflex arc.

BICEPS REFLEX
(C5-6 innervation)

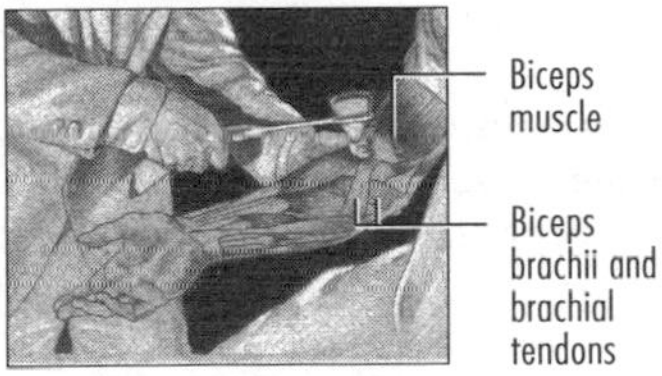

PATELLAR REFLEX
(L2, 3, 4 innervation)

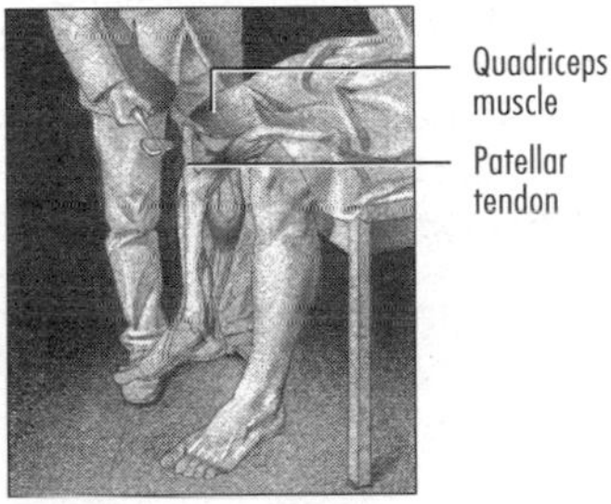

ACHILLES TENDON REFLEX
(S1-2 innervation)

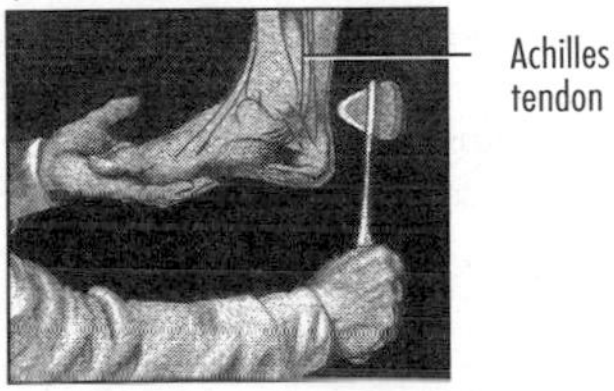

TRICEPS REFLEX
(C7-8 innervation)

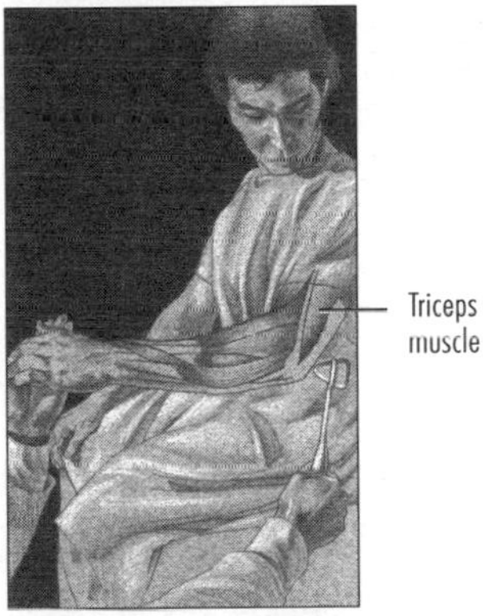

BRACHIORADIALIS REFLEX
(C5-6 innervation)

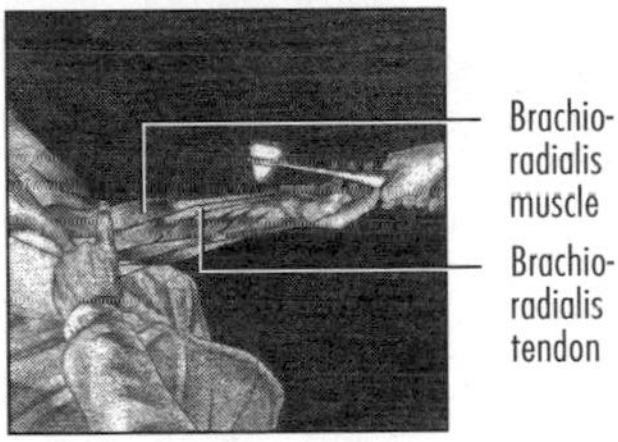

Documenting deep tendon reflexes

Record the patient's deep tendon reflex scores by drawing a stick figure and entering the grades on this scale at the proper location. The figure shown here indicates hypoactive deep tendon reflexes in the legs; other reflexes are normal.

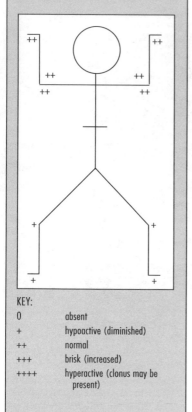

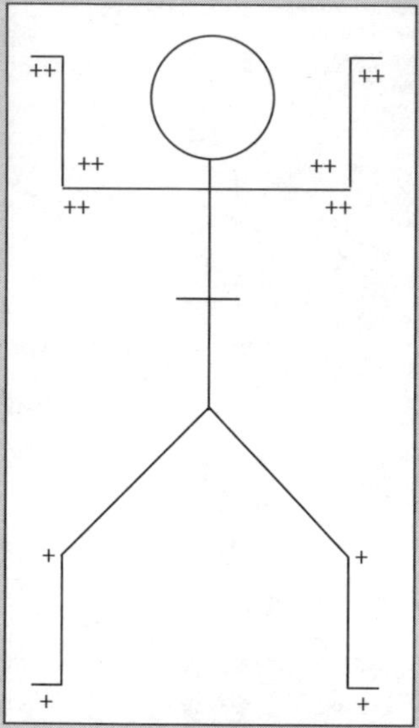

KEY:

0	absent
+	hypoactive (diminished)
++	normal
+++	brisk (increased)
++++	hyperactive (clonus may be present)

phy or increased mass. Test sensory function, including pain, touch, temperature, and vibration sense. Ask about paresthesia. To observe gait and coordination, have the patient take several steps. To check for Romberg's sign, ask him to stand with feet together and eyes closed. During conversation, evaluate speech. Observe for signs of vision or hearing loss. Abrupt onset of hypoactive DTRs accompanied by muscle weakness may occur in life-threatening Guillain-Barré syndrome, botulism, or spinal cord lesions with spinal shock.

Look for autonomic nervous system effects by taking vital signs. Also inspect the skin for pallor, dryness, flushing, or diaphoresis. Auscultate for hypoactive bowel sounds, and palpate for bladder distention. Ask about nausea, vomiting, constipation, and incontinence.

Common medical causes

♦ ***Botulism.*** In this disorder, generalized hypoactive DTRs accompany progressive descending muscle weakness. Initially, the patient usually complains of blurred and double vision and, occasionally, of anorexia, nausea, and vomiting. Other early bulbar findings include vertigo, hearing loss, dysarthria, and dysphagia. The patient may have signs of respiratory distress and severe constipation marked by hypoactive bowel sounds.

♦ ***Eaton-Lambert syndrome.*** This disorder causes generalized hypoactive DTRs. Early signs include difficulty rising from a chair, climbing stairs, and walking. The patient may complain of achiness, paresthesia, and muscle weakness that's most severe in the morning. Weakness improves with mild exercise and worsens with strenuous exercise.

♦ ***Guillain-Barré syndrome.*** This disorder, which commonly follows an upper respiratory tract infection, causes bilateral hypoactive DTRs that progress rapidly from hypotonia to areflexia in several days. Guillain-Barré syndrome typically causes muscle weakness that begins in the legs and then extends to the arms and, possibly, to the trunk and neck muscles. Occasionally, weakness may progress to total paralysis. Other clinical features include cranial nerve palsies, pain, paresthesia, and signs of brief autonomic dysfunction, such as sinus tachycardia or bradycardia, flushing, fluctuating blood pressure, and anhidrosis or episodic diaphoresis.

Usually, muscle weakness and hypoactive DTRs peak in severity within 10 to 14 days; then symptoms begin to clear. However, in severe cases, residual hypoactive DTRs and motor weakness may persist. Complete recovery may take up to 2 years.

♦ ***Peripheral neuropathy.*** Characteristic of end-stage diabetes mellitus, renal failure, and alcoholism, peripheral neuropathy results in progressive hypoactive DTRs. Other effects include motor weakness, sensory loss, paresthesia, tremors, and possible autonomic dysfunction, such as orthostatic hypotension and incontinence.

♦ ***Polymyositis.*** In this disorder, caused by inflammation of the connective tissue, hypoactive DTRs accompany muscle weakness, pain, stiffness, spasms and, possibly, increased size or atrophy. These effects are usually temporary; their locations vary with the affected muscles.

♦ ***Spinal cord lesions.*** Spinal cord injury or complete transection causes spinal shock, resulting in hypoactive DTRs (areflexia) below the level of the lesion. Associated signs and symptoms may include quadriplegia or paraplegia, flaccidity, loss of sensation below the level of the lesion, and dry, pale skin. Also characteristic are urine retention with overflow incontinence, hypoactive bowel sounds, constipation, and genital reflex loss. Hypoactive DTRs and flaccidity are usually transient; reflex activity may return within several weeks.

♦ ***Syringomyelia.*** Permanent bilateral hypoactive DTRs occur early in this slowly progressive disorder. Other clinical features are muscle weakness and atrophy; loss of sensation, usually extending in a capelike pattern over the arms, shoulders, neck, back, and occasionally the legs; deep, boring pain (despite anesthesia) in the limbs; and signs of brain stem involvement (for example, nystagmus, facial numbness, unilateral vocal cord paralysis or weakness, unilateral tongue atrophy).

Other causes

♦ ***Drugs.*** Barbiturates and paralyzing drugs, such as pancuronium and curare, may cause hypoactive DTRs.

Special considerations

Help the patient carry out his daily activities. Try to strike a balance between promoting independence and ensuring safety. Encourage him to walk with assistance. Make sure personal care articles are within easy reach, and provide an obstacle-free course from bed to bathroom.

If the patient has sensory deficits, protect him from heat or pressure injury. Test his bath water, and reposition him frequently on a soft, smooth bed surface. Keep his skin clean and dry to prevent breakdown. Perform or encourage range-of-motion exercises. Also encourage a balanced diet with increased protein.

Pediatric pointers

Hypoactive DTRs frequently occur in children with muscular dystrophy, Friedreich's ataxia, syringomyelia, or spinal cord injury. They also accompany progressive muscular atrophy. Use distraction techniques to test DTRs; assess motor function by watching the infant or child at play.

DEPRESSION

Depression is a mental state of depressed mood characterized by feelings of sadness, despair, and loss of interest or pleasure in activities. These feelings may be accompanied by somatic complaints, such as changes in appetite, sleep disturbances, restlessness or lethargy, and decreased concentration. The patient may also have thoughts of death or suicide.

Clinical depression must be distinguished from periodic bouts of dysphoria that are less persistent and severe than the clinical disorder. The criterion for major depression is one or more episodes of depressed mood, or decreased interest or ability to take pleasure in all or most activities, lasting at least 2 weeks.

Major depression strikes 10% to 15% of adults, affecting all racial, ethnic, age, and socioeconomic groups. It is twice as common in women as in men and is especially prevalent among adolescents. Depression has numerous causes, including genetic and family history, medical and psychiatric disorders, and the use of certain drugs. A complete psychiatric and physical examination should be conducted to exclude possible medical causes.

History and physical examination

During the examination, try to determine how the patient feels about herself, her family, and her environment. Your goal is to explore the nature of the depression, the extent to which other factors affect it, and the patient's coping mechanisms. Begin by asking what's bothering her. How does her current mood differ from her usual mood? Then ask her to describe the way she feels about herself. What are her plans and dreams? How realistic are they? Is she generally satisfied with what she has accomplished in her work, relationships, and other interests? Ask about any changes in her social interactions, sleep patterns, normal activities, or ability to make decisions and concentrate. Explore drug and alcohol use. Listen for clues that she may be suicidal. (See *Suicide: Caring for the high-risk patient.*)

Ask the patient about her family—its patterns of interaction and characteristic responses to success and failure. What part does she feel she plays in her family life? Find out if other family members have been depressed, and whether anyone important to the patient has been sick or has died in the past year. Finally, ask the patient about her environment. Has her lifestyle changed in the past month? Six months? Year? When she's feeling depressed, where does she go and what does she do to feel better? Find out how she feels about her role in the community and her awareness of the resources that are available to her. Try to determine if she has an adequate support network to help her cope with her depression.

Common medical causes

♦ ***Neurochemical imbalances.*** It is believed that clinical depression is caused by abnormalities in the central nervous system neurotransmitters. Specifically, low levels of serotonin and norepinephrine are related to altered mood states. This may be the result of inherited or environmental factors. Other medical conditions such as drug abuse and cerebral infarction can also lower the levels of neurotransmitters. Antidepressant drug therapy with selective serotonin reupake inhibitors or selective serotonin/norepinephrine reuptake inhibitors increases the availability of the neurotransmitter in the synaptic cleft.

♦ ***Organic disorders.*** Various organic disorders and chronic illnesses cause mild, moderate, or severe depression. Among these are *metabolic and endocrine disorders,* such as hypothyroidism, hyperthyroidism, or diabetes; *infectious diseases,* such as influenza, hepatitis, or encephalitis; *degenerative diseases,* such as Alzheimer's disease, multiple sclerosis, or multi-infarct dementia; and *neoplastic disorders.*

♦ ***Psychiatric disorders.*** *Affective disorders* are often characterized by abrupt mood swings from depression to elation (mania) or by prolonged episodes of either mood. Severe depression may last for weeks. In *cyclothymic disorders,* moderate depression usually alternates with moderate mania. Moderate depression that is more or less constant over a 2-year period often results from *dysthymic dis-*

Suicide: Caring for the high-risk patient

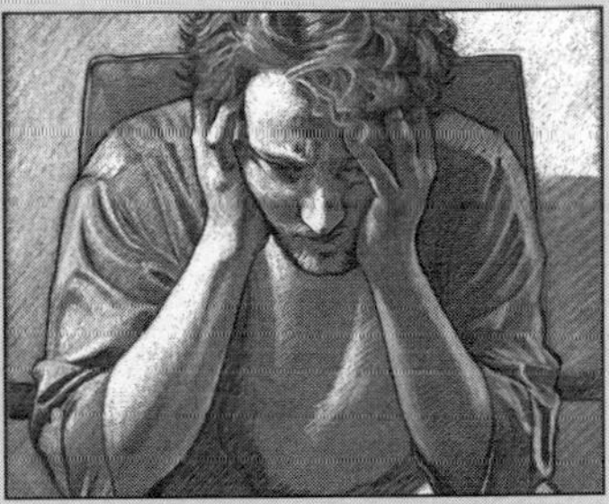

One of the most common factors contributing to suicide is hopelessness, an emotion that many depressed patients experience. As a result, you'll need to regularly assess a depressed patient for suicidal tendencies.

Usually, the patient will provide specific clues about her intentions. For example, you may notice her talking frequently about death or the futility of life, concealing potentially harmful items (such as knives and belts), giving away personal belongings, or getting her legal and financial affairs in order. If you suspect that a patient is suicidal, follow these guidelines:

◆ First, try to determine the patient's suicide potential. Find out how upset she is. Does she have a simple, straightforward suicide plan that's likely to succeed? Does she have any positive support systems — family, friends, a therapist? A patient with low to moderate suicide potential is noticeably depressed but has some form of support system. She may have thoughts of suicide, but no specific plan. A patient with high suicide potential feels profoundly hopeless and has little or no support system. She thinks about suicide frequently and has a plan that's likely to succeed.

◆ Next, observe precautions. Remove any objects she could use to harm herself, such as razors, belts, electric cords, and shoelaces. Know her whereabouts and what she's doing at all times; this may require one-on-one surveillance. Place the patient in a room that's close to your station. Always have someone accompany her when she leaves the unit.

◆ Be alert for in-hospital suicide attempts, which typically occur when there's a low staff-to-patient ratio — between shifts, during evening and night shifts, or when a critical event such as a code draws attention away from the patient.

◆ Finally, arrange for follow-up counseling. Recognize suicidal ideation and behavior as a desperate cry for help. Contact a mental health professional for a referral.

orders. In addition, depression may accompany *chronic anxiety disorders,* such as panic or obsessive-compulsive disorder.

Other causes

◆ ***Alcohol abuse.*** Intoxication or withdrawal often causes depression.

◆ ***Drugs.*** Various drugs cause depression as a side effect. Among the more common are barbiturates; chemotherapeutic drugs, such as asparaginase; anticonvulsants, such as diazepam; and antiarrhythmics, such as disopyramide. Other depression-inducing drugs include centrally acting antihypertensives, such as reserpine (common in high dosages), methyldopa, and clonidine; beta-adrenergic blockers, such as propranolol; levodopa; indomethacin; cycloserine; corticosteroids; and oral contraceptives.

Special considerations

Caring for a depressed patient takes time, tact, and energy. It also requires an awareness of your own vulnerability to feelings of despair that can stem from interacting with a depressed patient. Help the patient set realistic goals; encourage her to promote feelings of self-worth by asserting her opinions and making decisions. Try to determine her suicide po-

ALTERNATIVE THERAPY

Light therapy for depression

Because light is associated with maintenance of the body's natural rhythms, it is being used to treat a variety of disorders, including winter depression, also known as seasonal affective disorder (SAD). Although researchers disagree about the exact cause of SAD, many theorize that it results when a person receives insufficient morning light to suppress the hormone melatonin. Too much melatonin can cause depression. Bright light suppresses blood levels of melatonin.

Light therapy is the treatment of choice for patients with SAD because it is noninvasive and has a high success rate. Therapeutic response is achieved by replacing the light normally found in a long summer day with artificial light. The patient is asked to sit in front of a light box that emits intense bright light. The light enters the eye, hits the retina, and is transmitted by nerve impulses to the pineal gland, which controls melatonin secretion.

Intense bright light is the key to this treatment. Full-spectrum light is not required or recommended. Treatment duration varies from 15 minutes to 2 hours daily; relief typically begins in 3 to 4 days and is complete within 2 weeks. Sessions are usually discontinued when spring arrives with its longer days.

tential, and take steps to help ensure her safety. The patient may require close surveillance to prevent a suicide attempt. (See *Light therapy for depression.*)

Make sure the patient receives adequate nourishment and rest, and keep her environment free from stress and excessive stimulation. Arrange for ordered diagnostic tests to determine if her depression has an organic cause, and administer prescribed drugs. In addition, arrange for follow-up counseling, or contact a mental health professional for a referral.

Pediatric pointers

Because emotional lability is normal in adolescence, depression can be difficult to assess and diagnose in teenagers. Clues to underlying depression may include somatic complaints, sexual promiscuity, poor grades, withdrawing from family and friends, and abuse of alcohol or drugs.

Use of a family systems model often helps determine the cause of depression in adolescents. Once family roles are determined, family therapy or group therapy with peers may help the patient overcome her depression.

Geriatric pointers

Depressed older adults at highest risk for suicide are those who are age 85 or older, have high self-esteem, and need to be in control. Even a frail nursing home resident with these characteristics may have the strength to kill herself.

Diaphoresis

Diaphoresis is profuse sweating — at times, amounting to more than 1 L of sweat per hour. This sign represents an autonomic nervous system response to physical or psychogenic stress, fever, or high environmental temperature. Diaphoresis caused by stress may be generalized or limited to the palms of the hands, soles of the feet, and forehead; when caused by fever or high environmental temperature, it's generalized; and when caused by anxiety, it's limited to the palms, soles, and forehead.

Diaphoresis usually begins abruptly and may be accompanied by other autonomic system signs, such as tachycardia or hypertension. However, because sweat glands function immaturely in infants and are less active in the elderly, these age groups may not display diaphoresis associated with its common causes. Intermittent diaphoresis may accompany chronic disorders characterized by recurrent fever; isolated diaphoresis may mark an episode of acute pain or fever. Night sweats may characterize intermittent fever because body temperature tends to return to normal between 2 a.m. and 4 a.m. before rising again.

Diaphoresis is a normal response to high external temperature. Acclimatization usually requires several days of exposure to high temperatures; during this process, diaphoresis helps maintain normal body temperature. During menopause, diaphoresis preceded by a sensation of intense heat (a hot flash) is common. Other causes include exercise or exertion that accelerates metabolism, creating internal heat, and mild to moderate anxiety that helps initiate the fight-or-flight response. (See *Understanding diaphoresis,* pages 184 and 185.)

History and physical examination

If the patient is diaphoretic, quickly rule out the possibility of a life-threatening cause. (See *When diaphoresis spells trouble,* page 186.) Begin the history by having the patient describe his chief complaint. Then explore associated signs and symptoms. Note general fatigue and weakness. Does the patient have insomnia, headache, and changes in vision or hearing? Is he often dizzy? Does he have palpitations? Ask about pleuritic pain, cough, sputum, difficulty breathing, nausea, vomiting, abdominal pain, and altered bowel or bladder habits.

Ask the female patient about amenorrhea and any changes in her menstrual cycle. Is she menopausal? Ask about paresthesia, muscle cramps or stiffness, and joint pain. Has she noticed any changes in elimination habits? Note any weight loss or gain. Has the patient had to change her glove or shoe size lately?

Complete the history by asking about recent travel. Note recent exposure to high environmental temperatures or to pesticides. Did the patient recently experience an insect bite? Check for a history of partial gastrectomy or of drug or alcohol abuse. Finally, obtain a thorough drug history.

Next, perform a physical examination. First, determine the extent of diaphoresis by inspecting the trunk and extremities as well as the palms, soles, and forehead. Also, check the patient's clothing and bedding for dampness. Note whether diaphoresis occurs during the day or at night. Observe for flushing, abnormal skin texture or lesions, and an increased amount of coarse body hair. Note poor skin turgor and dry mucous membranes. Check for splinter hemorrhages and Plummer's nails (separation of the fingernail ends from the nail beds).

Then evaluate the patient's mental status and take vital signs. Observe for fasciculations and flaccid paralysis. Be alert for seizures. Note the patient's facial expression and examine the eyes for pupillary dilation or constriction, exophthalmos, and excessive tearing. Test visual fields. Also, check for hearing loss and for tooth or gum disease. Percuss the lungs for dullness and auscultate for crackles, diminished or bronchial breath sounds, and increased vocal fremitus. Look for decreased respiratory excursion. Palpate for lymphadenopathy and hepatosplenomegaly.

Common medical causes

◆ ***Acromegaly.*** In this slowly progressive disorder, which involves hypersecretion of growth hormone and increased metabolic rate, diaphoresis is a sensitive gauge of disease activity. The patient has a hulking appearance with an enlarged supraorbital ridge, thickened ears and nose, and thickened heel pads. Other signs and symptoms include warm, oily, thickened

Understanding diaphoresis

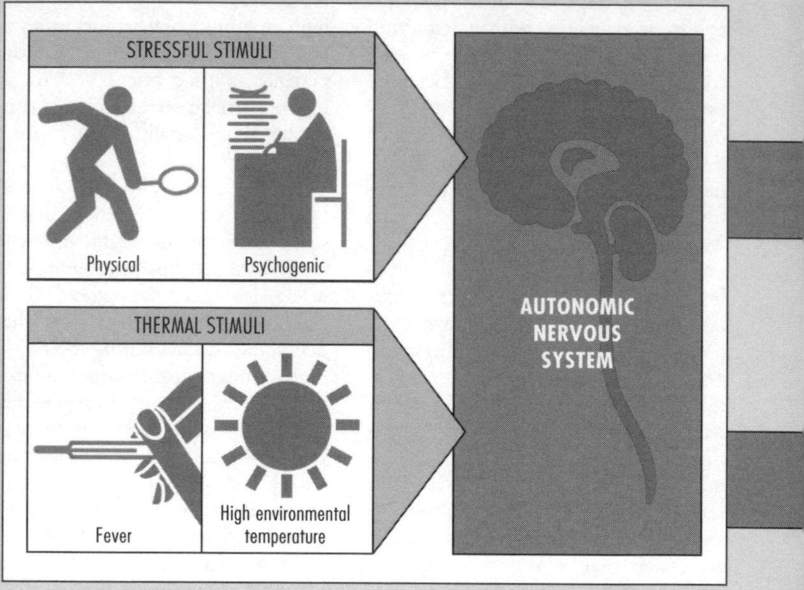

skin; enlarged hands, feet, and jaw; joint pain; weight gain; hoarseness; and increased coarse body hair. Increased blood pressure, severe headache, and visual field deficits or blindness may also occur.

♦ ***Anxiety disorders.*** Acute anxiety characterizes panic; chronic anxiety characterizes phobias, conversion disorders, obsessions, and compulsions. Whether acute or chronic, anxiety may cause sympathetic stimulation, resulting in diaphoresis. The diaphoresis is most dramatic on the palms, soles, and forehead and is accompanied by palpitations, tachycardia, tachypnea, tremors, and GI distress. Psychological symptoms — fear, difficulty concentrating, and behavior changes — also occur.

♦ ***Autonomic hyperreflexia.*** Occurring after resolution of spinal shock in a patient with spinal cord injury above T6, hyperreflexia causes profuse diaphoresis, pounding headache, blurred vision, and dramatically elevated blood pressure. Diaphoresis occurs above the level of the injury, especially on the forehead, and is accompanied by flushing. Other findings may include restlessness, nausea, nasal congestion, and bradycardia.

♦ ***Heart failure.*** Typically, diaphoresis follows fatigue, dyspnea, orthopnea, and tachycardia in left-sided heart failure, and neck vein distention and dry cough in right-sided heart failure. Other features include tachypnea, cyanosis, dependent edema, crackles, ventricular gallop, and anxiety.

♦ ***Heat exhaustion.*** Although this condition is marked by failure of heat to dissipate, it initially may cause profuse diaphoresis, fatigue, weakness, and anxiety. These symptoms may progress to circulatory collapse and shock (confusion, thready pulse, hypotension, tachy-

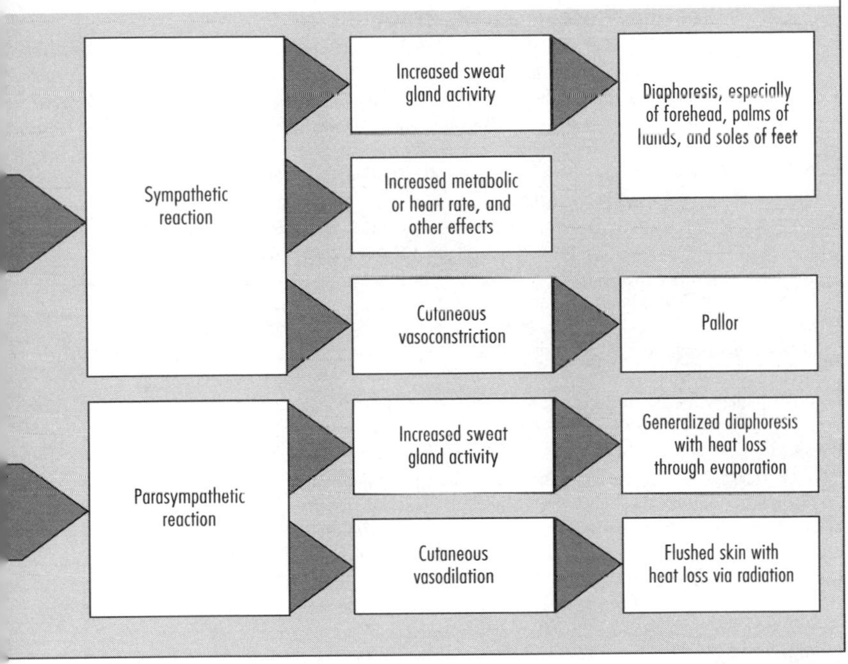

cardia, and cold, clammy skin). Other features are an ashen-gray appearance, dilated pupils, and normal or subnormal temperature.

♦ ***Hodgkin's disease.*** Especially in the elderly, early features of Hodgkin's disease may include night sweats, fever, fatigue, pruritus, and weight loss. Usually, though, this disease initially causes painless swelling of a cervical lymph node. Occasionally, a Pel-Ebstein fever pattern is present—several days or weeks of fever and chills alternating with afebrile periods with no chills. Systemic symptoms, such as weight loss, fever, and night sweats, indicate a poor prognosis. Progressive lymphadenopathy eventually causes widespread effects, such as hepatomegaly and dyspnea.

♦ ***Hypoglycemia.*** Rapidly induced hypoglycemia may cause diaphoresis accompanied by irritability, tremors, hypotension, blurred vision, tachycardia, hunger, and loss of consciousness.

♦ ***Infective endocarditis (subacute).*** Generalized night sweats occur early in this disorder. Accompanying signs and symptoms include intermittent low-grade fever, weakness, fatigue, weight loss, anorexia, and arthralgia. A sudden change in a murmur or the discovery of a new murmur is a classic sign. Petechiae and splinter hemorrhages are also common.

♦ ***Lung abscess.*** Drenching night sweats are common in this disorder. Its chief sign, though, is a cough productive of copious purulent, foul-smelling, often bloody sputum. Associated findings include fever with chills, pleuritic chest pain, dyspnea, weakness, anorexia, weight loss, headache, malaise, clubbing, tubular or amphoric breath sounds, and dullness on percussion.

EMERGENCY INTERVENTIONS

When diaphoresis spells trouble

Diaphoresis is an early sign of certain life-threatening disorders. These guidelines will help you detect such disorders promptly and intervene to minimize harm to the patient.

HYPOGLYCEMIA

If you observe diaphoresis in a patient who complains of blurred vision, be sure to ask him about increased irritability and anxiety. Has he been unusually hungry lately? Does he have tremors? Take the patient's vital signs, noting hypotension and tachycardia. Then ask about a history of insulin-dependent diabetes. If you suspect hypoglycemla, evaluate the patient's blood glucose level using a glucose reagent strip, or send a serum sample to the laboratory.

Administer I.V. glucose 50% to return the patient's glucose level to normal. Monitor his vital signs and cardiac rhythm. Ensure a patent airway, and be prepared to assist with breathing and circulation if necessary.

HEATSTROKE

If you observe profuse diaphoresis in a weak, tired, and apprehensive patient, suspect heatstroke, which can progress to circulatory collapse. Take vital signs, noting a normal or subnormal temperature. Check for ashen-gray skin and dilated pupils. Was the patient recently exposed to high temperatures and humidity? Was he wearing heavy clothing at the time? Also, ask if he uses diuretics, which interfere with normal sweating.

Take the patient to a cool room, remove his clothing, and use a fan to direct cool air over his body. Insert an I.V. line and prepare for electrolyte and fluid replacement. Monitor for signs of shock.

AUTONOMIC HYPERREFLEXIA

If you observe diaphoresis in a patient with a spinal cord injury above T6 or T7, ask if he has a pounding headache, restlessness, blurred vision, or nasal congestion. Take the patient's vital signs, noting bradycardia and extremely elevated blood pressure. If you suspect autonomic hyperreflexia, quickly rule out its common complications. Examine for eye pain associated with intraocular hemorrhage and for facial paralysis, slurred speech, or limb weakness associated with intracerebral hemorrhage.

Quickly reposition the patient to remove any pressure stimuli. Also, check for a distended bladder or fecal impaction. Remove any kinks from the urinary catheter if necessary, or administer a suppository or manually remove impacted feces. If you can't locate and relieve the causative stimulus, start an I.V. line. Prepare to administer hydralazine for hypertension.

MYOCARDIAL INFARCTION OR HEART FAILURE

If the diaphoretic patient complains of chest pain and dyspnea, suspect myocardial infarction or heart failure. Connect the patient to a cardiac monitor, ensure a patent airway, and administer supplemental oxygen. Start an I.V. line and administer analgesics. Be prepared to begin emergency resuscitation if cardiac or respiratory arrest occurs.

♦ ***Myocardial infarction.*** Diaphoresis usually accompanies acute, substernal, radiating chest pain in this life-threatening disorder. Associated signs and symptoms include anxiety, dyspnea, nausea, vomiting, tachycardia, irregular pulse, blood pressure change, fine crackles, pallor, and clammy skin.

♦ ***Pesticide poisoning.*** Among the toxic effects of pesticide poisoning are diaphoresis, nausea, vomiting, diarrhea, blurred vision, miosis, and excessive lacrimation and salivation. The patient may display fasciculations, muscle weakness, and flaccid paralysis. Signs of repiratory depression and coma may also occur.

♦ ***Pheochromocytoma.*** This disorder commonly causes diaphoresis, but its cardinal sign is persistent or paroxysmal hypertension. Other effects include headache, palpitations, tachycardia, anxiety, tremors, pallor, flushing, paresthesia, abdominal pain, tachypnea, nausea, vomiting, and orthostatic hypotension.

♦ ***Pneumonia.*** Intermittent, generalized diaphoresis accompanies fever and chills in patients with pneumonia. The patient complains of pleuritic chest pain that increases with deep inspiration. Other features include tachypnea, dyspnea, productive cough (with scant and mucoid or copious and purulent sputum), headache, fatigue, myalgia, abdominal pain, anorexia, and cyanosis. Auscultation reveals bronchial breath sounds.

♦ ***Tetanus.*** This disorder commonly causes profuse sweating accompanied by low-grade fever, tachycardia, and hyperactive deep tendon reflexes. Early restlessness, pain, and stiffness in the jaw, abdomen, and back progress to spasms associated with lockjaw, risus sardonicus, dysphagia, and opisthotonos. Laryngospasm may result in cyanosis or sudden death by asphyxiation.

♦ ***Thyrotoxicosis.*** This disorder commonly causes diaphoresis accompanied by heat intolerance, weight loss despite increased appetite, tachycardia, palpitations, an enlarged thyroid, dyspnea, nervousness, diarrhea, tremors, Plummer's nails, and possibly exophthalmos. Gallops may also occur.

♦ ***Tuberculosis.*** Although often asymptomatic in primary infection, this disorder may cause night sweats, low-grade fever, fatigue, weakness, anorexia, and weight loss. In reactivation, a productive cough with mucopurulent sputum, occasional hemoptysis, and chest pain may be present.

Other causes

♦ ***Drugs.*** Sympathomimetics, certain antipsychotics, thyroid hormone, and antipyretics may cause diaphoresis. Aspirin and acetaminophen poisoning also cause this sign.

♦ ***Dumping syndrome.*** The result of rapid emptying of gastric contents into the small intestine soon after eating in patients with partial gastrectomy, this syndrome causes diaphoresis, palpitations, profound weakness, epigastric distress, nausea, and explosive diarrhea.

♦ ***Pesticide poisoning.*** Among the toxic effects of pesticides are diaphoresis, nausea, vomiting, diarrhea, blurred vision, miosis, and excessive lacrimation and salivation. The patient may display fasciculations, muscle weakness, and flaccid paralysis. Signs of respiratory depression and coma may also occur.

Special considerations

After an episode of diaphoresis, sponge the patient's face and body and change wet clothes and sheets. To prevent skin irritation, dust skin folds in the groin and axillae and under pendulous breasts with cornstarch or powder, or tuck gauze or cloth into the folds. Encourage regular bathing.

Replace fluids and electrolytes. Regulate infusions of I.V. saline or Ringer's lactate solution, and monitor urine output. Encourage oral fluids high in electrolytes (such as Gatorade). Enforce bed rest and maintain a quiet environment. Keep the patient's room temperature moderate to prevent additional diaphoresis.

Prepare the patient for diagnostic tests, such as blood tests, cultures, chest X-rays, immunologic studies, biopsy, computed tomography scan, and audiometry.

Pediatric pointers

Diaphoresis in children often results from environmental heat or overdressing; it's usually most apparent around the head. Other causes include drug withdrawal associated with maternal addiction, heart failure, thyrotoxicosis, and the effects of such drugs as antihistamines, ephedrine, haloperidol, and thyroid hormone.

Assess fluid status carefully. Some fluid loss through diaphoresis may precipitate hypovolemia more rapidly in a child than in an adult. Monitor input and output, weigh the child daily, and note the duration of each episode of diaphoresis.

Geriatric pointers

Fever and night sweats, the hallmark of tuberculosis, may not occur in elderly patients, who instead may exhibit a change in activity or weight. Also, keep in mind that older patients may not exhibit diaphoresis because of a decreased sweating mechanism. For this reason, they're at increased risk for developing heatstroke in high temperatures.

DIARRHEA

Usually a chief sign of intestinal disorders, diarrhea is an increase in the volume of stools compared with the patient's normal bowel habits. It varies in severity and may be acute or chronic. Acute diarrhea may result from acute infection, stress, toxins, fecal impaction, or the effects of drugs. Chronic diarrhea may result from chronic infection, obstructive and inflammatory bowel disease, malabsorption syndromes, certain endocrine disorders, and the effects of GI surgery. Periodic diarrhea may result from food intolerance or from ingestion of spicy or high-fiber foods or caffeine.

One or more pathophysiologic mechanisms may contribute to diarrhea. (See *What causes diarrhea?*) The fluid and electrolyte imbalances it causes may precipitate life-threatening arrhythmias or hypovolemic shock.

Emergency interventions

If the patient's diarrhea is profuse, check for signs of shock — tachycardia, hypotension, and cool, pale, clammy skin. If you detect these signs, place the patient in the supine position and elevate his legs 20 degrees. Insert an I.V. line for fluid replacement. Monitor for electrolyte imbalances, and look for an irregular pulse, muscle weakness, anorexia, and nausea and vomiting. Keep emergency resuscitation equipment handy.

History and physical examination

If the patient is not in shock, proceed with a brief physical examination. Evaluate hydration, check skin turgor, and take blood pressure with the patient lying, sitting, and standing. Inspect the abdomen for distention and palpate for tenderness. Auscultate bowel sounds. Take the patient's temperature and note any chills. Also, look for a rash. Conduct a rectal examination and a pelvic examination if indicated.

Explore signs and symptoms associated with diarrhea. Does the patient have abdominal pain and cramps? Difficulty breathing? Is he weak or fatigued? Find out his drug history. Has he had GI surgery or radiation therapy recently? Ask the patient to briefly describe his diet. Does he have any known food allergies? Last, find out if he's under unusual stress or has recently traveled out of the country.

Common medical causes

♦ ***Carcinoid syndrome.*** In this disorder, severe diarrhea occurs with flushing — usually of the head and neck — that's often caused by emotional stimuli or the ingestion of food, hot water, or alcohol. Associated signs and symptoms include abdominal cramps, dyspnea, weight loss, anorexia, weakness, palpita-

What causes diarrhea?

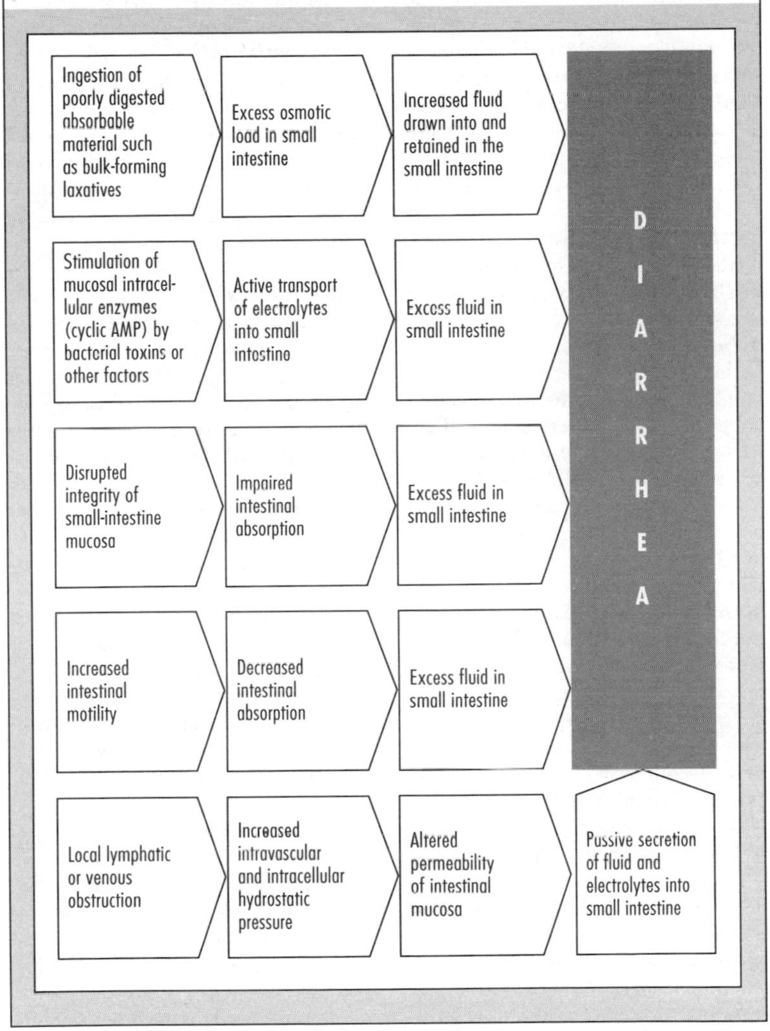

tions, valvular heart disease, and depression.

◆ **Clostridium difficile *infection.*** The patient may be asymptomatic or may have soft, unformed stools or watery diarrhea that may be foul-smelling or grossly bloody; abdominal pain, cramping, and tenderness; fever; and a white blood cell count as high as 20,000/µl. In severe cases, the patient may develop toxic megacolon, colonic perforation, or peritonitis.

◆ ***Crohn's disease.*** This recurring inflammatory disorder causes diarrhea accompanied by abdominal pain with guarding, tenderness, and nausea. The patient may also display fever, chills, weakness, anorexia, and weight loss.

♦ ***Infections.*** Acute viral, bacterial, and protozoal infections (such as cryptosporidiosis) cause the sudden onset of watery diarrhea, as well as abdominal pain, cramps, nausea, vomiting, and fever. Significant fluid and electrolyte loss may cause signs of dehydration and shock. Chronic tuberculosis and fungal and parasitic infections may cause a less severe but more persistent diarrhea, accompanied by epigastric distress, vomiting, weight loss and, possibly, passage of blood and mucus.

♦ ***Intestinal obstruction.*** Partial intestinal obstruction increases intestinal motility, resulting in diarrhea, abdominal pain with tenderness and guarding, nausea and, possibly, distention.

♦ ***Irritable bowel syndrome.*** Diarrhea alternates with constipation or normal bowel function. Related findings: abdominal pain, tenderness, and distention; dyspepsia; and nausea.

♦ ***Ischemic bowel disease.*** This life-threatening disorder causes bloody diarrhea with abdominal pain. If severe, shock may occur, mandating surgery.

♦ ***Lactose intolerance.*** Diarrhea occurs within several hours of ingesting milk or milk products. It's accompanied by cramps, abdominal pain, borborygmi, bloating, nausea, and flatus.

♦ ***Pseudomembranous enterocolitis.*** This potentially life-threatening disorder often follows antibiotic administration. It causes copious watery, green, foul-smelling, bloody diarrhea that rapidly precipitates signs of shock. Other features include colicky abdominal pain, distention, fever, and dehydration.

♦ ***Rotavirus gastroenteritis.*** This disorder frequently starts with fever, nausea, and vomiting, followed by diarrhea. The illness can range from mild to severe and lasts from 3 to 9 days. Diarrhea and vomiting may result in dehydration.

♦ ***Thyrotoxicosis.*** In this disorder, diarrhea is accompanied by nervousness, tremors, diaphoresis, weight loss despite increased appetite, dyspnea, palpitations, tachycardia, enlarged thyroid, heat intolerance and, possibly, exophthalmos.

♦ ***Ulcerative colitis.*** The hallmark of this disorder is recurrent bloody diarrhea with pus or mucus. Other features are tenesmus, hyperactive bowel sounds, cramping lower abdominal pain, low-grade fever, anorexia and, at times, nausea and vomiting. Weight loss, anemia, and weakness are late findings.

Other causes

♦ ***Drugs.*** Many antibiotics, such as ampicillin, cephalosporins, tetracyclines, and clindamycin, cause diarrhea. Other drugs that may cause diarrhea include magnesium-containing antacids, colchicine, guanethidine, lactulose, dantrolene, ethacrynic acid, mefenamic acid, methotrexate, metyrosine and, in high doses, digoxin and quinidine. Laxative abuse can cause acute or chronic diarrhea.

♦ **Herb alert** Herbal medicines, such as ginkgo biloba, ginseng, and licorice, may cause diarrhea.

♦ ***Treatments.*** Gastrectomy, gastroenterostomy, or pyloroplasty may cause diarrhea. High-dose radiation therapy may cause enteritis associated with diarrhea.

Special considerations

Administer analgesics for pain and an opiate to decrease intestinal motility. Ensure the patient's privacy during defecation, and empty bedpans promptly. Clean the perineum thoroughly, and apply ointment to prevent skin breakdown.

Stress the need for medical follow-up to patients with inflammatory bowel disease (particularly ulcerative colitis), who have an increased risk of developing colon cancer.

Pediatric pointers

Diarrhea in children frequently results from infection, although chronic diarrhea may result from malabsorption syndrome, anatomic defects, or allergies. Because dehydration and electrolyte imbalance occur rapidly in children, diarrhea can be life-threatening. Diligently monitor all episodes of diarrhea, and replace lost fluids immediately.

Geriatric pointers

In the elderly patient with new-onset segmental colitis, always consider ischemia before labeling the patient as having Crohn's disease.

Diplopia

Diplopia is double vision — seeing one object as two. This symptom results when extraocular muscles fail to work together, causing images to fall on noncorresponding parts of the retinas. Orbital lesions, head trauma, the effects of surgery, or impaired function of cranial nerves that supply extraocular muscles (oculomotor, CN III; trochlear, CN IV; abducens, CN VI) may be responsible. (See *Testing extraocular muscles,* page 192.)

Diplopia usually begins intermittently but may be constant, and it affects near or far vision, but not both. It can be classified as monocular or binocular; the latter is more common. Monocular diplopia is often a split shadow, or ghost, image. It may result from an early cataract, retinal edema or scarring, iridodialysis, a subluxated lens, a poorly fitting contact lens, or an uncorrected refractive error such as astigmatism. Binocular diplopia can be vertical, horizontal, diagonal, or torsional. It may result from ocular deviation or displacement, extraocular muscle palsies, or psychoneurosis, or it may occur after retinal surgery. Diplopia may also occur with hysteria or malingering in an otherwise healthy person.

History and physical examination

If the patient complains of double vision, first check his neurologic status. Evaluate his level of consciousness (LOC), pupil size and response to light, and motor and sensory function. Then take his vital signs. Briefly ask about associated symptoms, especially a severe headache. Find out about associated neurologic symptoms first because diplopia can accompany serious disorders.

Next, continue with a more detailed examination. Find out when the patient first noticed diplopia. Are the images side-by-side (horizontal), one above the other (vertical), or a combination? Does diplopia affect near or far vision? Does it affect certain directions of gaze? Ask if diplopia has worsened, remained the same, or subsided. Does its severity change throughout the day? Diplopia that worsens or appears in the evening may indicate myasthenia gravis. If diplopia occurs intermittently and is associated with dizziness, suspect transient ischemic attacks affecting the vertebrobasilar system. Find out if the patient can correct diplopia by tilting his head; if so, ask him to show you. If the patient has a fourth nerve lesion, tilting of the head toward the opposite shoulder causes compensatory tilting of the unaffected eye. If he has incomplete sixth nerve palsy, tilting of the head toward the side of the paralyzed muscle may relax the affected lateral rectus muscle.

Explore associated symptoms, such as eye pain. Ask about hypertension, diabetes mellitus, allergies, and thyroid, neurologic, or muscular disorders. Also, note a history of extraocular muscle disorders, trauma, or eye surgery.

Observe the patient for ocular deviation, ptosis, proptosis, lid edema, and conjunctival injection. Distinguish monocular from binocular diplopia by asking the patient to occlude one eye. If he still sees double, he has monocular diplopia. Test visual acuity and extraocular muscles. Check vital signs.

EXAMINATION TIP

Testing extraocular muscles

The coordinated action of six muscles controls eyeball movements. To test the function of each muscle and the cranial nerve (CN) that innervates it, ask the patient to look in the direction controlled by that muscle. The six directions you can test make up the *cardinal fields of gaze.* The patient's inability to turn the eye in the designated direction indicates muscle weakness or paralysis.

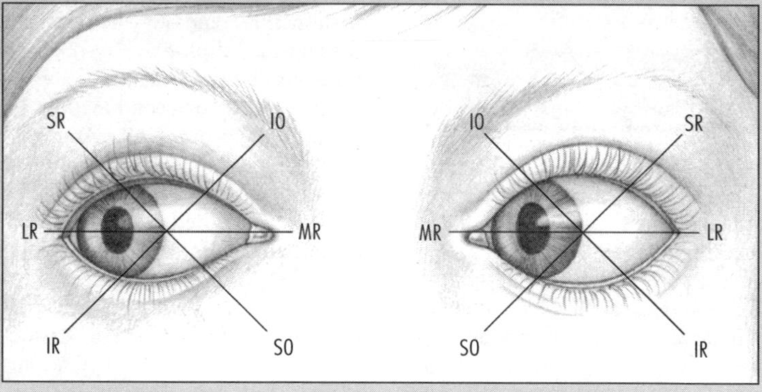

SR = superior rectus (CN III)
LR = lateral rectus (CN VI)
IR = inferior rectus (CN III)
IO = inferior oblique (CN III)
MR = medial rectus (CN III)
SO = superior oblique (CN IV)

Common medical causes

♦ ***Alcohol intoxication.*** Diplopia is a common symptom of this disorder. It's accompanied by confusion, slurred speech, halitosis, staggering gait, behavior changes, nausea, vomiting, and possibly conjunctival injection.

♦ ***Botulism.*** Hallmark signs are diplopia, dysarthria, dysphagia, and ptosis. Early findings include dry mouth, sore throat, vomiting, and diarrhea. Later, descending weakness or paralysis of extremity and trunk muscles causes hyporeflexia and dyspnea.

♦ ***Brain tumor.*** Diplopia may be an early symptom of a brain tumor. Accompanying features vary with the tumor's size and location but may include eye deviation, emotional lability, decreased LOC, headache, vomiting, petit or grand mal seizures, hearing loss, visual field deficits, abnormal pupillary responses, nystagmus, motor weakness, and paralysis.

♦ ***Cavernous sinus thrombosis.*** This disorder may cause diplopia and limited eye movement. Associated signs and symptoms include exophthalmos, orbital and lid edema, diminished or absent pupillary responses, impaired visual acuity, papilledema, and fever.

♦ ***Cerebrovascular accident.*** Diplopia characterizes this life-threatening disorder when it affects the vertebrobasilar artery. Other clinical features may include unilateral motor weakness or paralysis, ataxia, decreased LOC, dizziness, aphasia, visual field deficits, circumoral numbness, slurred speech, dysphagia, and amnesia.

♦ ***Cranial nerve paresis.*** Complete paralysis of CN III (oculomotor nerve) results in both vertical and horizontal diplopia with associated ptosis of the upper eye and an inability to rotate the eye inward, upward, or downward. The trochlear nerve (CN IV) innervates the superior oblique muscle. Complete paralysis causes vertical diplopia, and the patient may notice difficulty with downward gaze. These patients sometimes tilt the head toward the opposite shoulder to decrease the amount of diplopia. Complete paralysis of the abducens nerve (CN VI) may cause horizontal diplopia and loss of abduction.

♦ ***Diabetes mellitus.*** Among the long-term effects of this disorder may be diplopia due to isolated CN III palsy. Diplopia typically begins suddenly and may be accompanied by pain.

♦ ***Encephalitis.*** Initially, this disorder may cause a brief episode of diplopia and eye deviation. However, it usually begins with sudden onset of high fever, severe headache, and vomiting. As the inflammation progresses, the patient may display signs of meningeal irritation, decreased LOC, seizures, ataxia, and paralysis.

♦ ***Head injury.*** Potentially life-threatening head injuries may cause diplopia, depending on the site and extent of the injury. Associated signs and symptoms may include eye deviation, pupillary changes, headache, decreased LOC, altered vital signs, nausea, vomiting, and motor weakness or paralysis.

♦ ***Intracranial aneurysm.*** This life-threatening disorder initially causes diplopia and eye deviation, perhaps accompanied by ptosis and a dilated pupil on the affected side. The patient complains of a recurrent, severe, unilateral, frontal headache. After the aneurysm ruptures, the headache becomes violent. Associated signs and symptoms include neck and spinal pain and rigidity, decreased LOC, tinnitus, dizziness, nausea, vomiting, and unilateral muscle weakness or paralysis.

♦ ***Multiple sclerosis (MS).*** Diplopia, a common early symptom in MS, is usually accompanied by blurred vision and paresthesia. As MS progresses, signs and symptoms may include nystagmus, constipation, muscle weakness, paralysis, spasticity, hyperreflexia, intention tremor, gait ataxia, dysphagia, dysarthria, impotence, emotional lability, and urinary frequency, urgency, and incontinence.

♦ ***Myasthenia gravis.*** This disorder initially causes diplopia and ptosis, which worsen throughout the day. It then progressively involves other muscles, resulting in blank facial expression; nasal voice; difficulty chewing, swallowing, and making fine hand movements; and possibly signs of life-threatening respiratory muscle weakness.

♦ ***Ophthalmologic migraine.*** Occurring most often in young adults, this disorder results in diplopia that persists for days after the headache. Accompanying signs and symptoms are severe, unilateral pain; ptosis; and extraocular muscle palsies. Irritability, depression, or slight confusion may also occur.

♦ ***Orbital blowout fracture.*** This fracture usually causes monocular diplopia affecting the upward gaze. However, when marked periorbital edema is present, diplopia may affect other directions of gaze. This fracture commonly causes periorbital ecchymosis but doesn't affect visual acuity, although eyelid edema may prevent accurate testing. Subcutaneous crepitation of the eyelid and orbit is typical. Occasionally, the patient's pupil is dilated and unreactive, and he may have a hyphema.

♦ ***Orbital cellulitis.*** Inflammation of the orbital tissues and eyelids causes sudden diplopia. Other findings are eye deviation and pain, purulent drainage, lid edema, chemosis and redness, proptosis, nausea, and fever.

♦ ***Orbital tumors.*** Enlarging tumors can cause diplopia. Exophthalmos and possibly blurred vision may also occur.
♦ ***Thyrotoxicosis.*** Diplopia occurs when exophthalmos characterizes the disorder. It usually begins in the upper field of gaze because of infiltrative myopathy involving the inferior rectus muscle. It's accompanied by impaired eye movement, excessive tearing, lid edema, and possibly inability to close the lids. Other cardinal findings include tachycardia, palpitations, weight loss, diarrhea, tremors, an enlarged thyroid, dyspnea, nervousness, diaphoresis, and heat intolerance.

Other causes

♦ ***Eye surgery.*** Fibrosis associated with eye surgery may restrict eye movement, resulting in diplopia.

Special considerations

Continue to monitor vital signs and neurologic status if you suspect an acute neurologic disorder. Prepare the patient for neurologic tests, such as a computed tomography scan. Provide a safe environment. If diplopia is severe, remove sharp obstacles and assist the patient with ambulation. Institute seizure precautions, if indicated.

Pediatric pointers

Strabismus, which can be congenital or acquired at an early age, causes diplopia; however, in young children, the brain rapidly compensates for double vision by suppressing one image, so diplopia is a rare complaint. School-age children who complain of double vision require a careful examination to rule out serious disorders, such as brain tumor.

DIZZINESS

A common symptom, dizziness is a sensation of imbalance or faintness, sometimes associated with giddiness, weakness, confusion, and blurred or double vision. Episodes of dizziness are usually brief; they may be mild or severe with abrupt or gradual onset. Dizziness may be aggravated by standing up quickly and alleviated by lying down and by rest.

Dizziness typically results from inadequate blood flow and oxygen supply to the cerebrum and spinal cord. It may occur in anxiety, in respiratory and cardiovascular disorders, and in postconcussion syndrome. It's a key symptom in certain serious disorders, such as hypertension and vertebrobasilar artery insufficiency.

Dizziness is often confused with vertigo — a sensation of revolving in space or of surroundings revolving about oneself. However, unlike dizziness, vertigo is often accompanied by nausea, vomiting, nystagmus, staggering gait, and tinnitus or hearing loss. Dizziness and vertigo may occur together, as in postconcussion syndrome.

Emergency interventions

If the patient complains of dizziness, first determine its severity and onset. Ask the patient to describe it. Is the dizziness associated with headache or blurred vision? Next, take the patient's vital signs and ask about a history of high blood pressure. Tell the patient to lie down, and recheck his vital signs every 15 minutes. Start an I.V. line, and prepare to administer medications as ordered.

History and physical examination

Ask about a history of diabetes and cardiovascular disease. Is the patient taking drugs prescribed for high blood pressure? If so, when did he take his last dose?

If the patient's blood pressure is normal, obtain a more complete history. Ask about myocardial infarction, heart failure, or atherosclerosis, all of which may predispose the patient to cardiac arrhythmias, hypertension, and a transient ischemic attack (TIA). Does he have a history of anemia, chronic obstructive pulmonary disease, anxiety disorder, or head injury? Obtain a complete drug history.

Next, fully explore the patient's dizziness. How often does it occur? How long does each episode last? Does the dizziness abate spontaneously? Does it lead to loss of consciousness? Find out if dizziness is triggered by sitting or standing up suddenly or stooping over. Does being in a crowd make the patient feel dizzy? Ask about emotional stress. Has the patient been irritable or anxious lately? Does he have insomnia or difficulty concentrating? During the interview, look for fidgeting and eyelid twitching. Does the patient startle easily? Also, ask about palpitations, chest pain, diaphoresis, shortness of breath, and chronic cough.

Next, perform a physical examination. Begin with a quick neurocheck, assessing level of consciousness (LOC), motor and sensory functions, and reflexes. Then inspect for poor skin turgor and dry mucous membranes, signs of dehydration. Auscultate heart rate and rhythm. Inspect for barrel chest, clubbing, cyanosis, and use of accessory muscles. Also auscultate breath sounds. Take the patient's blood pressure while he's lying, sitting, and standing to check for orthostatic hypotension. Test capillary refill time in the extremities, and palpate for edema.

Common medical causes

◆ ***Anemia.*** Typically, this disorder causes dizziness that's aggravated by postural changes or exertion. Other clinical features include pallor, dyspnea, fatigue, tachycardia, and bounding pulse. Capillary refill time is prolonged.

◆ ***Cardiac arrhythmias.*** Dizziness lasts for several seconds or longer and may precede fainting. The patient may experience palpitations; irregular, rapid, or thready pulse; and possibly hypotension. He may also experience weakness, blurred vision, paresthesia, and confusion.

◆ ***Emphysema.*** Dizziness may follow exertion or the chronic productive cough in this disorder. Associated signs and symptoms include dyspnea, anorexia, weight loss, malaise, use of accessory muscles, pursed-lip breathing, tachypnea, peripheral cyanosis, and diminished breath sounds. Barrel chest and clubbing may be present.

◆ ***Hypertension.*** In this disorder, dizziness may precede fainting, but it may also be relieved by rest. Other common signs and symptoms include headache and blurred vision. Retinal changes include hemorrhage, sclerosis of retinal blood vessels, exudate, and papilledema.

◆ ***Hyperventilation syndrome.*** Episodes of hyperventilation cause dizziness that usually lasts a few minutes; however, if these episodes occur frequently, dizziness may persist between them. Other effects include apprehension, diaphoresis, pallor, dyspnea, chest tightness, palpitations, trembling, fatigue, and peripheral and circumoral paresthesia.

◆ ***Orthostatic hypotension.*** This condition causes dizziness that may terminate in fainting or may disappear with rest. Related findings include dim vision, spots before the eyes, pallor, diaphoresis, hypotension, tachycardia, and possibly signs of dehydration.

◆ ***Postconcussion syndrome.*** Occurring 1 to 3 weeks after a head injury, this syndrome is marked by dizziness, headache (throbbing, aching, bandlike, or stabbing), emotional lability, alcohol intolerance, fatigue, anxiety, and possibly vertigo. Dizziness and other symptoms are intensified by mental or physical stress. The syndrome may persist for years, but symptoms eventually abate.

◆ ***TIA.*** Lasting from a few seconds to 24 hours, a TIA frequently signals impending stroke and may be triggered by turning the head to the side. In addition to dizziness of varying severity, TIAs are accompanied by unilateral or bilateral diplopia, blindness or visual field deficits, ptosis, tinnitus, hearing loss, paresis, and numbness. Other possible findings include dysarthria, dysphagia, vomiting, hiccups, confusion, decreased LOC, and pallor.

Other causes

♦ ***Drugs.*** Antianxiety drugs, central nervous system depressants, narcotics, decongestants, antihistamines, antihypertensives, and vasodilators frequently cause dizziness.

♦ **Herb alert** Herbal medicines such as St. John's wort can cause dizziness. Over-the-counter diet medications that contain caffeine or ephedra (ma huang) can cause arrhythmias that result in dizziness followed by fainting.

Special considerations

Prepare the patient for diagnostic tests, such as blood studies, arteriography, computed tomography scan, electroencephalography, and magnetic resonance imaging.

Pediatric pointers

Dizziness is less common in children than in adults. Children often have difficulty describing this symptom and instead complain of tiredness, stomachache, or feeling sick. If you suspect dizziness, assess for vertigo as well. A more common symptom in children, vertigo may result from vision disorders, ear infections, and the effects of antibiotics.

DOLL'S EYE SIGN, ABSENT

[Negative oculocephalic reflex]

An indicator of brain stem dysfunction, the absence of the doll's eye sign is detected by rapid, gentle turning of the patient's head from side to side. The eyes remain fixed in midposition, instead of moving laterally toward the side opposite the direction the head is turned. (See *Testing for absent doll's eye sign.*)

The steady gaze of the eyes at rest in a fully conscious person indicates an intact cerebral cortex. The absence of doll's eye sign indicates injury to the midbrain or pons, involving cranial nerves III, VI, and VIII. It typically accompanies coma caused by lesions of the cerebellum and brain stem. This sign usually can't be relied upon in a conscious patient because he can control eye movements voluntarily. Absence of doll's eye reflex is commonly assessed in patients who are comatose with increased ICP as part of the protocol for determining brain death.

A variant of absent doll's eye sign that develops gradually is known as *abnormal doll's eye sign:* Because conjugate eye movement is lost, one eye may move laterally while the other remains fixed or moves in the opposite direction. An abnormal doll's eye sign usually accompanies metabolic coma or increased intracranial pressure (ICP). Associated brain stem dysfunction may be reversible or may progress to deeper coma with absent doll's eye sign.

Physical examination

After detecting an absent doll's eye sign, perform a neurologic examination. First, evaluate the patient's level of consciousness (LOC), using the Glasgow Coma Scale. Note decerebrate or decorticate posture. Examine the pupils for size, equality, and response to light. Check for signs of increased ICP—hypertension, rising pulse pressure, and bradycardia.

Common medical causes

♦ ***Brain stem infarction.*** This infarction causes absent doll's eye sign with coma. It also causes limb paralysis, cranial nerve palsies (facial weakness, diplopia, blindness or visual field deficits, nystagmus), bilateral cerebellar ataxia, variable sensory loss, a positive Babinski's reflex, decerebrate posture, and muscle flaccidity.

♦ ***Brain stem tumors.*** Absent doll's eye sign accompanies coma in this type of tumor. This sign may be preceded by hemiparesis, nystagmus, extraocular nerve palsies, facial pain or sensory loss, facial paralysis, diminished corneal reflex, tinnitus, hearing loss, dysphagia, drooling, vertigo, dizziness, ataxia, and vomiting.

♦ ***Central midbrain infarction.*** Accompanying absent doll's eye sign are coma, Weber's syndrome (oculomotor palsy with contralateral hemiplegia), contralateral ataxic tremor, nystagmus, and pupillary abnormalities.

♦ ***Pontine hemorrhage.*** Absent doll's eye sign and coma develop within minutes in this life-threatening disorder. Other ominous signs, such as complete paralysis, decerebrate posture, positive Babinski's reflex, and small, reactive pupils, may then rapidly progress to death.

♦ ***Posterior fossa hematoma.*** A subdural hematoma at this location typically causes absent doll's eye sign and coma. These signs may be preceded by characteristic clinical features, such as headache, vomiting, drowsiness, confusion, unequal pupils, dysphagia, cranial nerve palsies, stiff neck, and cerebellar ataxia.

Other causes

♦ ***Drugs.*** Barbiturates may cause severe central nervous system depression, resulting in coma and absent doll's eye sign.

Special considerations

Do not attempt to elicit doll's eye sign in a comatose patient with suspected cervical spine injury; doing so risks spinal cord damage. Instead, evaluate the oculovestibular reflex with the cold caloric test. Normally, instilling cold water in the ear causes the eyes to move slowly toward the irrigated ear. Cold caloric testing may also be done to confirm an absent doll's eye sign.

Testing for absent doll's eye sign

To evaluate the patient's oculocephalic reflex, hold her upper eyelids open and quickly (but gently) turn her head from side to side, noting eye movements with each head turn. In absent doll's eye sign, the eyes remain fixed in midposition.

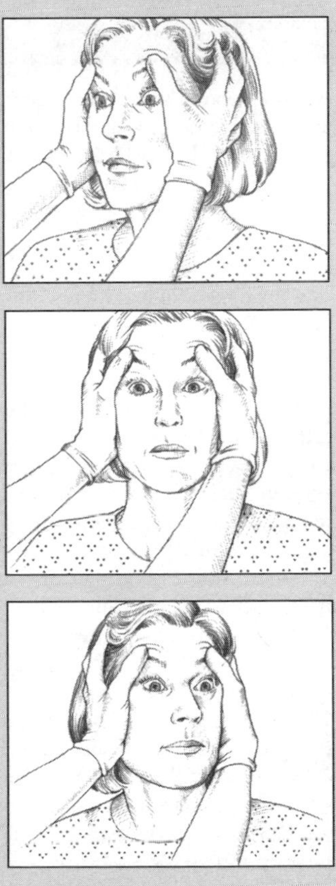

Continue to monitor vital signs and neurologic status in the patient with an absent doll's eye sign.

Pediatric pointers

Normally, the doll's eye sign is not present for the first 10 days after birth, and it may be irregular until age 2. After that, this sign reliably indicates brain stem function. Absent doll's eye sign in a child may accompany coma associated with head injury, near-drowning or near-suffocation, or brain stem astrocytoma.

DYSARTHRIA

Dysarthria, poorly articulated speech, is characterized by slurring and labored, irregular rhythm. It may be accompanied by nasal voice tone caused by palate weakness. Whether it occurs abruptly or gradually, dysarthria is usually evident in ordinary conversation. It's confirmed by asking the patient to make a few simple sounds and words, such as "ba," "sh," and "cat." However, dysarthria is occasionally confused with aphasia, loss of the ability to cause or comprehend speech.

Dysarthria results from damage to the brain stem that affects cranial nerve IX, X, or XI. Degenerative neurologic disorders commonly cause dysarthria; in fact, dysarthria is a chief sign of olivopontocerebellar degeneration. It may also result from ill-fitting dentures.

Emergency interventions

If the patient displays dysarthria, ask him about associated difficulty swallowing. Then determine respiratory rate and depth. Assess for agitation and restlessness as signs of respiratory distress. Measure vital capacity with a Wright respirometer, if available. Assess blood pressure and heart rate. Usually, tachycardia, slightly increased blood pressure, and shortness of breath are early signs of respiratory muscle weakness.

Ensure a patent airway. Place the patient in Fowler's position and suction him if necessary. Administer oxygen, and keep emergency resuscitation equipment nearby. Anticipate intubation and mechanical ventilation in a patient with progressive respiratory muscle weakness. Withhold oral fluids if the patient has associated dysphagia.

If dysarthria is not accompanied by respiratory muscle weakness and dysphagia, continue to assess for other neurologic deficits. Compare muscle strength and tone in the limbs. Then evaluate tactile sensation. Ask the patient about numbness or tingling. Test deep tendon reflexes and note gait ataxia. Next, test visual fields and ask about double vision. Check for signs of facial weakness, such as ptosis. Finally, determine level of consciousness (LOC) and mental status.

History

Explore dysarthria fully. When did it begin? Has it gotten better? Speech improves with resolution of a transient ischemic attack, but not in a completed stroke. Ask if dysarthria worsens during the day. Then obtain a drug and alcohol history. Also ask about a history of seizures. (See *Dysarthria: Common causes and associated findings,* pages 200 and 201.) It is important to obtain a timeline for when symptoms increase and what helps relieve them.

Common medical causes

♦ ***Alcoholic cerebellar degeneration.*** This disorder commonly causes chronic, progressive dysarthria along with ataxia, diplopia, ophthalmoplegia, hypotension, and altered mental status.

♦ ***Amyotrophic lateral sclerosis.*** Dysarthria occurs when this disorder affects the bulbar nuclei; it may worsen as the disease progresses. Other signs and symptoms are dysphagia; difficulty breathing; muscle atrophy and weakness, especially of the hands and feet; fasciculations; spasticity; hyperactive deep tendon reflexes in the legs; and occasionally, excessive drooling. Progressive bulbar palsy may cause crying spells or inappropriate laughter.

♦ ***Basilar artery insufficiency.*** This disorder causes random, brief episodes of bilateral brain stem dysfunction, resulting in dysarthria. Accompanying it are diplopia, vertigo, facial numbness, ataxia, paresis, and visual field loss, all of which last for minutes to hours.

♦ ***Botulism.*** The hallmark of this disorder is acute cranial nerve dysfunction causing dysarthria, dysphagia, diplopia, and ptosis. Early findings include dry mouth, sore throat, weakness, vomiting, and diarrhea. Later, descending weakness or paralysis of muscles in the extremities and trunk causes hyporeflexia and dyspnea.

♦ ***Brain stem cerebrovascular accident (CVA).*** This type of CVA is characterized by bulbar palsy, resulting in the triad of dysarthria, dysphonia, and dysphagia. The dysarthria is most severe at onset; it may diminish or disappear with rehabilitation. Other findings may include facial weakness, diplopia, hemiparesis, spasticity, drooling, dyspnea, and decreased LOC.

♦ ***Cerebral CVA.*** A massive bilateral CVA causes pseudobulbar palsy. Bilateral weakness causes dysarthria that is most severe at onset. This sign is accompanied by dysphagia, drooling, dysphonia, bilateral hemianopia, and aphasia. Sensory loss, spasticity, and hyperreflexia may also occur.

♦ ***Multiple sclerosis.*** When demyelination affects the brain stem and cerebellum, the patient displays dysarthria accompanied by nystagmus, blurred or double vision, dysphagia, ataxia, and intention tremor. Exacerbations and remissions of these symptoms are common. Other clinical features may include paresthesia, spasticity, hyperreflexia, muscle weakness or paralysis, constipation, emotional lability, and urinary frequency, urgency, and incontinence.

♦ ***Myasthenia gravis.*** This neuromuscular disorder causes dysarthria associated with a nasal voice tone. Typically, the dysarthria worsens during the day. Other findings are dysphagia, drooling, facial weakness, diplopia, ptosis, dyspnea, and muscle weakness.

♦ ***Olivopontocerebellar degeneration.*** Dysarthria, a major sign, accompanies cerebellar ataxia and spasticity.

♦ ***Parkinson's disease.*** This disorder causes dysarthria and a monotone voice. It also causes muscle rigidity, bradykinesia, involuntary tremor usually beginning in the fingers, difficulty in walking, muscle weakness, and stooped posture. Other features include masklike facies, dysphagia and, occasionally, drooling.

♦ ***Poisoning.*** Chronic *manganese* poisoning causes progressive dysarthria accompanied by weakness, fatigue, confusion, hallucinations, drooling, hand tremors, limb stiffness, spasticity, gross rhythmic movements of the trunk and head, and propulsive gait. Chronic *mercury* poisoning also causes progressive dysarthria accompanied by weakness, fatigue, depression, lethargy, irritability, confusion, ataxia, and tremors.

♦ ***Shy-Drager syndrome.*** Marked by chronic orthostatic hypotension, this syndrome eventually causes dysarthria as well as cerebellar ataxia, bradykinesia, masklike facies, dementia, impotence, and possibly stooped posture and incontinence.

Other causes

♦ ***Drugs.*** Dysarthria can occur when anticonvulsant dosage is too high. Ingestion of large doses of barbiturates may cause dysarthria.

Special considerations

Encourage the patient with dysarthria to speak slowly so that he can be understood. Give him time to express himself, and encourage him to use gestures. Dysarthria usually requires consultation with a speech pathologist. If the ability to form speech is severely affected, com-

Dysarthria: Common causes and associated findings

S&S

CAUSES	MAJOR ASSOCIATED SIGNS AND SYMPTOMS												
	Aphasia	Ataxia	Bradykinesia	Diplopia	Drooling	Dysphagia	Dyspnea	Fasciculations	Gait, propulsive	Hyperreflexia	Hypotension	LOC, decreased	Masklike facies
Alcoholic cerebellar degeneration		◆		◆							◆	◆	
Amyotrophic lateral sclerosis					◆	◆	◆	◆		◆			
Basilar artery insufficiency		◆		◆									
Botulism				◆		◆	◆						
CVA (brain stem)				◆	◆	◆	◆						
CVA (cerebral)	◆				◆	◆				◆			
Multiple sclerosis		◆		◆		◆				◆			
Myasthenia gravis				◆	◆	◆	◆						
Olivopontocerebellar degeneration		◆											
Parkinson's disease			◆		◆	◆			◆				◆

puter systems that generate a voice to faciliate communication are available.

Pediatric pointers

Dysarthria in children usually results from brain stem glioma, a slow-growing tumor that primarily affects children. It may also result from cerebral palsy.

Dysarthria may be difficult to detect, especially in an infant or a young child who hasn't perfected speech. Be sure to look for other neurologic deficits, too. Encourage speech in a child with dysarthria; a child's potential for rehabilitation is typically greater than an adult's.

DYSMENORRHEA

Dysmenorrhea affects over 50% of menstruating women and is the leading cause of absence from school and work in this population. Functional dysmenorrhea (primary) is cyclic pain associated with menses and without pathologic origin.

	Muscle atrophy	Muscle weakness	Ptosis	Spasticity	Tremor	Vertigo	Visual field deficits
	◆	◆		◆			
		◆				◆	◆
		◆	◆				
		◆		◆			
		◆		◆			
		◆		◆	◆		
		◆	◆				
				◆			
		◆			◆		

Acquired (secondary) dysmenorrhea is a symptom of pathologic changes. Dysmenorrhea may involve sharp, intermittent pain or dull, aching pain. It's usually characterized by mild to severe cramping or colicky pain in the pelvis or lower abdomen that may radiate to the thighs and lower sacrum. Pain may precede menstruation by several days or may accompany it. The pain generally peaks after 24 hours and subsides after 48 hours.

Primary dysmenorrhea is possibly due to uterine contraction and ischemia and is believed to be influenced by prostaglandins secreted by the endometrium. Secondary amenorrhea is frequently due to endometriosis but can also be the result of adenomyosis, changes that occur after procedures on the cervical os, pedunculated submucosal fibroid, extruding endometrial polyps, or pelvic inflammatory disease. (See *Drug therapy for dysmenorrhea,* page 202.)

History and physical examination

Have the patient fully describe her symptoms. Is the pain intermittent or continuous? Sharp, cramping, or aching? Ask where the pain begins, and how or if it travels or radiates. How long has she been experiencing it? When does the pain begin and end, and when is it severe? Explore associated symptoms, such as headache, nausea and vomiting, altered bowel or urinary habits, bloating, pelvic or rectal pressure, unusual fatigue, irritability, and depression.

Then obtain a menstrual, sexual, and reproductive history. Ask the patient if her menstrual flow is heavy or scant. Have her describe any vaginal discharge between menses. Does she experience pain during sexual intercourse, and does it occur with menses? Find out what relieves her cramps. Does she take pain medication? Is it effective? Note her method of contraception, and ask about a history of pelvic infection. Does she have any signs and symptoms of urinary system obstruction, such as pyuria, urine retention, or incontinence? Has she had any dignostic or therapeutic uterine procedures? Has she had any abdominal or transvaginal surgery?

Ask about use of prescription medications; a number of prescription drugs list dysmenorrhea as a known side effect (for example, cefaclor, fexofenadine, sumatriptan).

Drug therapy for dysmenorrhea

To relieve cramping and other symptoms caused by primary dysmenorrhea or an intrauterine device, the patient may receive prostaglandin inhibitors, such as aspirin, ibuprofen, indomethacin, or naproxen. These nonsteroidal anti-inflammatory drugs block prostaglandin synthesis early in the inflammatory reaction, thereby inhibiting prostaglandin action at receptor sites. These drugs also have analgesic and antipyretic effects. Make sure you and your patient are informed about the side effects and cautions associated with these drugs.

SIDE EFFECTS
Alert the patient to possible side effects of prostaglandin inhibitors. Central nervous system effects include dizziness, headache, and visual disturbances. GI effects include nausea, vomiting, heartburn, and diarrhea. Advise the patient to take the drug with milk or after meals to reduce gastric irritation.

CONTRAINDICATIONS
Because prostaglandin inhibitors are potentially teratogenic, be sure to rule out the possibility of pregnancy before starting therapy. Advise any patient who suspects she's pregnant to delay therapy until menstruation begins.

OTHER CAUTIONS
Administer prostaglandin inhibitors cautiously to patients with cardiac decompensation, hypertension, renal dysfunction, or coagulation defects and in those receiving ongoing anticoagulant therapy. Because patients who are hypersensitive to aspirin may also be hypersensitive to other prostaglandin inhibitors, watch for signs of gastric ulceration and bleeding.

Next, perform a focused physical examination. Take vital signs, noting fever and accompanying chills. Inspect the abdomen for distention, and palpate for tenderness and masses. Check for costovertebral angle tenderness.

Common medical causes

♦ ***Adenomyosis.*** In this disorder, endometrial tissue invades the myometrium, causing severe dysmenorrhea with pain radiating to the back or rectum, menorrhagia, and a symmetrically enlarged, globular uterus that is usually softer on palpation than a uterine myoma.

♦ ***Cervical stenosis.*** This structural disorder causes dysmenorrhea and scant or absent menstrual flow.

♦ ***Endometriosis.*** This disorder typically causes steady, aching pain that begins before menses and peaks at the height of menstrual flow; however, the pain may also occur between menstrual periods. The pain may arise at the endometrial deposit site or may radiate to the perineum or rectum. Associated signs and symptoms may also include premenstrual spotting, dyspareunia, infertility, nausea and vomiting, painful defecation, and rectal bleeding and hematuria during menses. A tender, fixed adnexal mass is usually palpable on bimanual examination.

♦ ***Pelvic inflammatory disease.*** Chronic infection causes dysmenorrhea accompanied by fever; malaise; foul-smelling, purulent vaginal discharge; menorrhagia; dyspareunia; severe abdominal pain; nausea and vomiting; and diarrhea. A pelvic examination may reveal cervical motion tenderness and bilateral adnexal tenderness.

♦ ***Premenstrual syndrome (PMS).*** The cramping pain of PMS usually begins with menstrual flow and persists for several hours or days, diminishing as flow increases. Common associated effects precede menses by several days to 2 weeks: abdominal bloating, breast tenderness, palpitations, diaphoresis, flushing, depression, and irritability. Other effects include nausea, vomiting, diarrhea, and headache. Because PMS usually follows an ovulatory cycle, it rarely occurs during the first 12 months of menses, which may be anovulatory.

♦ ***Primary (functional) dysmenorrhea.*** Increased prostaglandin secretion intensifies uterine contractions, apparently causing mild to severe spasmodic cramping pain in the lower abdomen, which radiates to the sacrum and inner thighs. The cramping abdominal pain peaks a few hours before menses. Patients may also experience nausea and vomiting, fatigue, diarrhea, and headache.

♦ ***Uterine leiomyomas.*** These tumors may cause constant or intermittent lower abdominal pain that worsens with menses. Associated signs and symptoms may include backache, constipation, menorrhagia, and urinary frequency or retention. Palpation may reveal the tumor mass and an enlarged uterus. The tumors are almost always nontender.

♦ ***Uterine prolapse.*** Displacement of the uterus may cause dysmenorrhea and chronic lower back pain, pelvic pressure, fatigue, leukorrhea, dyspareunia, and urinary frequency and incontinence.

Other causes

♦ ***Intrauterine devices.*** These devices may cause severe cramping and heavy menstrual flow.

Special considerations

In the past, women with dysmenorrhea were considered neurotic. Although current research suggests that prostaglandins contribute to this symptom, old attitudes persist. Encourage the patient to view dysmenorrhea as a medical problem, not as a sign of maladjustment.

Pediatric pointers

Dysmenorrhea is rare during the first year of menstruation, before the menstrual cycle becomes ovulatory. However, the incidence of dysmenorrhea is generally higher among adolescents than older women. Teach the adolescent about dysmenorrhea. Dispel myths if necessary, and inform her that this is a common event. Encourage good hygiene, nutrition, and exercise. (See *Herbal therapy for dysmenorrhea.*)

ALTERNATIVE THERAPY

Herbal therapy for dysmenorrhea

Much like the conventional drug therapy, herbal therapy uses the "active" chemicals in herbs to treat symptoms of an illness or underlying disturbances in normal physiology.

Herbs are classified according to their taste, which signifies their medical action and often their natural affinity to particular body organs. Some herbs are used to treat menstrual problems, including cramps and water retention. Herbal therapy may be used in conjunction with acupuncture.

Interest in herbal therapy is growing in the United States, possibly because of the increasing number of chronic illnesses that can't be cured by conventional treatments and the debilitating adverse effects that can occur secondary to standard drug therapy. Although herbal therapy is widely accepted and used in Europe and Asia (it's an important part of traditional Chinese medicine), much controversy surrounds its use in the United States for the following reasons:

♦ There is no licensing body for the practice of herbal medicine.

♦ The Food and Drug Administration does not regulate the production or marketing of herbs because they're considered food supplements.

♦ Herbs can't be patented because they grow naturally; consequently, pharmaceutical companies have no incentive to study their effectiveness or to develop standardized products.

Geriatric pointers
Postmenopausal women can experience similar discomfort associated with uterine bleeding induced by hormone replacement therapy.

Dyspepsia

Dyspepsia refers to an uncomfortable fullness after meals that is associated with nausea, belching, heartburn and, possibly, cramping and bloating. Frequently aggravated by spicy, fatty, or high-fiber foods and by excess caffeine intake, dyspepsia without other pathology indicates impaired digestive function.

Dyspepsia is caused by GI disorders; to a lesser extent, by cardiac, pulmonary, or renal disorders and the effects of drugs. It apparently results when abnormal gastric secretions lead to increased stomach acidity. This symptom may also result from emotional upset and overly rapid eating or improper chewing. It usually occurs a few hours after eating and lasts for a variable period of time. Its severity depends on the amount and type of food eaten and on GI motility. Additional food or antacids may relieve the discomfort.

History and physical examination
If the patient complains of dyspepsia, begin by asking him to describe it fully. How often and when does it occur, specifically in relation to meals? Do any drugs or activities relieve or aggravate it? Has he had nausea, vomiting, melena, hematemesis, cough, or chest pain? Ask what drugs he's currently taking and if he has recently had any surgery. Does he have a history of renal, cardiovascular, or pulmonary disease? Has he noticed any change in the amount or color of his urine?

Focus the physical examination on the abdomen. Inspect for distention, ascites, scars, jaundice, uremic frost, and bruising. Then auscultate for bowel sounds and characterize motility. Palpate and percuss the abdomen, noting any tenderness, pain, organ enlargement, or tympany.

Finally, examine other body systems. Ask about behavior changes, and evaluate level of consciousness. Auscultate for gallops and crackles. Percuss the lungs to detect consolidation. Note peripheral edema and any swelling of lymph nodes. (See *Dyspepsia: Common causes and associated findings.*)

Common medical causes
♦ ***Cholelithiasis.*** Dyspepsia may occur with gallstones, often after intake of fatty foods. Biliary colic, a more common symptom of gallstones, causes acute pain that may radiate to the back, shoulders, and chest. The patient may also have diaphoresis, tachycardia, chills, low-grade fever, petechiae, bleeding tendencies, jaundice with pruritus, dark urine, and clay-colored stools.

♦ ***Cirrhosis.*** In this chronic disorder, dyspepsia varies in intensity and duration and is relieved by antacids. Other GI effects are anorexia, nausea, vomiting, flatulence, diarrhea, constipation, abdominal distention, and epigastric or right upper quadrant pain. Weight loss, jaundice, hepatomegaly, ascites, dependent edema, fever, bleeding tendencies, and muscle weakness are also common. Skin changes include severe pruritus, extreme dryness, easy bruising, and lesions such as telangiectasis and palmar erythema. Gynecomastia or testicular atrophy may also occur.

♦ ***Duodenal ulcer.*** A primary symptom of duodenal ulcer, dyspepsia ranges from a vague feeling of fullness or pressure to a boring or aching sensation in the middle or right epigastrium. It usually occurs 1 to 3 hours after eating and is relieved by food or antacids. The pain may awaken the patient at night with heartburn and fluid regurgitation. Abdominal tenderness and weight gain may occur; vomiting and anorexia are rare.

♦ ***Gastric dilation (acute).*** Epigastric fullness is an early symptom of this life-

Dyspepsia: Common causes and associated findings

CAUSES	Abdominal distention	Abdominal pain	Anorexia	Bruising, easy	Chest pain	Cough	Edema	Hepatomegaly	Jaundice	Nausea/vomiting	Oliguria	Tachycardia	Weight loss
	MAJOR ASSOCIATED SIGNS AND SYMPTOMS												
Cholelithiasis		♦							♦	♦		♦	
Cirrhosis	♦	♦	♦	♦			♦	♦	♦	♦			♦
Duodenal ulcer		♦								♦			
Gastric dilation (acute)	♦									♦			
Gastric ulcer	♦	♦								♦			♦
Gastritis (chronic)		♦	♦							♦			
Heart failure		♦	♦		♦	♦	♦	♦		♦		♦	
Hepatitis			♦					♦	♦	♦			
Pulmonary embolus					♦	♦						♦	
Pulmonary tuberculosis			♦			♦							♦
Uremia		♦	♦				♦			♦	♦		

threatening disorder. Accompanying dyspepsia are nausea and vomiting, upper abdominal distention, succussion splash, and apathy. The patient may display signs and symptoms of dehydration, such as poor tissue turgor and dry mucous membranes, and of electrolyte imbalance, such as irregular pulse and muscle weakness. Gastric bleeding may cause hematemesis and melena.

♦ ***Gastric ulcer.*** Typically, dyspepsia and heartburn after eating occur early in this disorder. The cardinal symptom, though, is epigastric pain that may occur with vomiting, fullness, and abdominal distention and may not be relieved by food. Weight loss and GI bleeding are also characteristic.

♦ ***Gastritis (chronic).*** In this disorder, dyspepsia is relieved by antacids and is aggravated by spicy foods or excessive caffeine. It occurs with anorexia, a feeling of fullness, vague epigastric pain, belching, nausea, and vomiting.

♦ ***Heart failure.*** Common in right-sided heart failure, transient dyspepsia may occur with chest tightness and a constant ache or sharp pain in the right upper quadrant. Heart failure typically also causes hepatomegaly, anorexia, nausea, vomiting, bloating, ascites, tachycardia, distended neck veins, tachypnea, dyspnea, and orthopnea. Other findings include dependent edema, anxiety, fatigue, diaphoresis, hypotension, cough, crackles, ventricular and atrial gallops, nocturia, diastolic hypertension, and cool, pale skin.

♦ ***Hepatitis.*** Dyspepsia occurs in two of the three stages of hepatitis. The *preicteric* phase causes moderate to severe dyspepsia, fever, malaise, arthralgia, coryza, myalgia, nausea, vomiting, an altered sense of taste or smell, and hepatomegaly. Jaundice marks the onset of the *icteric* phase, along with continued dyspepsia and anorexia, irritability, and severe pruritus. As jaundice clears, dyspepsia and other GI effects also diminish. In the *recovery* phase, only fatigue remains.

♦ ***Pulmonary embolus.*** Sudden dyspnea characterizes this potentially fatal disorder; however, dyspepsia may manifest as oppressive, severe, substernal discomfort. Other findings include anxiety, tachycardia, tachypnea, cough, pleuritic chest pain, hemoptysis, syncope, cyanosis, distended neck veins, and hypotension.

♦ ***Pulmonary tuberculosis.*** Vague dyspepsia may occur along with anorexia, malaise, and weight loss. Common associated findings include high fever, night sweats, palpitations on mild exertion, productive cough, dyspnea, adenopathy, and occasional hemoptysis.

♦ ***Uremia.*** Of the many GI complaints associated with uremia, dyspepsia may be the earliest and most important. Others include anorexia, nausea, vomiting, bloating, diarrhea, abdominal cramps, epigastric pain, and weight gain. As the renal system deteriorates, findings may include edema, pruritus, pallor, hyperpigmentation, uremic frost, ecchymoses, sexual dysfunction, poor memory, irritability, headache, drowsiness, muscle twitching, seizures, and oliguria.

Other causes

♦ ***Drugs.*** Nonsteroidal anti-inflammatory drugs, especially aspirin, commonly cause dyspepsia. Diuretics, antibiotics, antihypertensives, and many other drugs can cause dyspepsia, depending on the patient's tolerance of the dosage.

♦ ***Surgery.*** After GI or other surgery, postoperative gastritis can cause dyspepsia, which usually disappears in a few weeks.

Special considerations

Changing the patient's position usually does not relieve dyspepsia, but providing food or antacids may. So have food available at all times, and give antacids 30 minutes before a meal or 1 hour after it. Give those drugs that can cause dyspepsia after meals, if possible.

Provide a calm environment to reduce stress, and make sure the patient gets plenty of rest. Discuss other ways to deal with stress, such as deep breathing and guided imagery. In addition, prepare the patient for endoscopy to evaluate the cause of dyspepsia.

Pediatric pointers

Dyspepsia in adolescents with peptic ulcer disease isn't relieved by food. It may occur in congenital pyloric stenosis, but projectile vomiting after meals is a more characteristic sign. It may also result from lactose intolerance.

Geriatric pointers

Most older patients with chronic pancreatitis experience less-severe pain than younger adults; some have no pain at all.

DYSPHAGIA

Dysphagia — difficulty swallowing — is a common symptom that's usually easy to localize. It may be constant or intermittent and is classified by the phase of swallowing it affects. (See *Classifying dysphagia.*) Among the factors that interfere

Classifying dysphagia

Because swallowing occurs in three distinct phases, dysphagia can be classified by the phase that it affects. Each phase suggests a specific pathology for dysphagia.

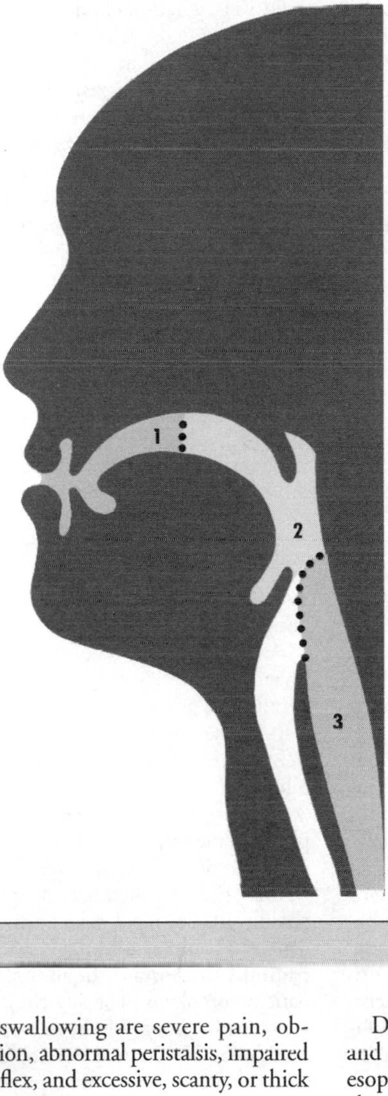

PHASE 1
Swallowing begins in the *transfer phase* with chewing and moistening of food with saliva. The tongue presses against the hard palate to transfer the chewed food to the back of the throat; the fifth cranial nerve then stimulates the swallowing reflex. *Phase 1* dysphagia typically results from a neuromuscular disorder.

PHASE 2
In the *transport phase,* the soft palate closes against the pharyngeal wall to prevent nasal regurgitation. At the same time, the larynx rises and the vocal cords close to keep food out of the lungs; breathing stops briefly as the throat muscles constrict to move food into the esophagus. *Phase 2* dysphagia usually reflects spasm or cancer.

PHASE 3
Peristalsis and gravity work together in the *entrance phase* to move food through the esophageal sphincter and into the stomach. *Phase 3* dysphagia results from lower esophageal narrowing by diverticula, esophagitis, and other disorders.

with swallowing are severe pain, obstruction, abnormal peristalsis, impaired gag reflex, and excessive, scanty, or thick oral secretions.

Dysphagia is the most common — and sometimes the *only* — symptom of esophageal disorders. However, it may also result from oropharyngeal, respiratory, neurologic, and collagen disorders or from the effects of toxins or treatments. Dysphagia increases the risk of choking and aspiration and may lead to malnutrition and dehydration.

Emergency interventions

If the patient suddenly complains of dysphagia and displays signs of respiratory distress, such as dyspnea and stridor, suspect an airway obstruction and quickly perform abdominal thrusts. Prepare to administer oxygen by mask or nasal cannula, or to assist with endotracheal intubation.

History and physical examination

If the patient's dysphagia doesn't suggest airway obstruction, begin a health history. Ask the patient if swallowing is painful. If so, is the pain constant or intermittent? Have the patient point to where dysphagia feels most intense. Does eating alleviate or aggravate the symptom? Are solids or liquids more difficult to swallow? If the answer is liquids, ask if hot, cold, and lukewarm fluids affect him differently. Does the symptom disappear after he tries to swallow a few times? Is swallowing easier if he changes position? Ask if he has recently experienced vomiting, regurgitation, weight loss, anorexia, hoarseness, dyspnea, or a cough.

To evaluate the patient's swallowing reflex, place your finger along his thyroid notch and instruct him to swallow. If you feel his larynx rise, the reflex is intact. Next, have him cough to assess his cough reflex. Check his gag reflex if you're sure he has a good swallow or cough reflex. Listen closely to his speech for signs of muscle weakness. Does he have aphasia or dysarthria? Is his voice nasal, hoarse, or breathy? Assess the patient's mouth carefully. Check for dry mucous membranes and thick, sticky secretions. Observe for tongue and facial weakness. Assess for disorientation, which may make him neglect to swallow.

Common medical causes

- ***Achalasia.*** Most common in patients ages 20 to 40, this disorder causes phase 3 dysphagia for solids and liquids. The dysphagia develops gradually and may be precipitated or exacerbated by stress. Occasionally, it's preceded by esophageal colic. Regurgitation of undigested food, especially at night, may cause wheezing, coughing, or choking as well as halitosis. Weight loss, cachexia, hematemesis, and possibly heartburn are late findings.
- ***Airway obstruction.*** Life-threatening upper airway obstruction is marked by signs of respiratory distress, such as crowing and stridor. Phase 2 dysphagia occurs with gagging and dysphonia. When hemorrhage obstructs the trachea, dysphagia is usually painless and rapid in onset. When inflammation causes the obstruction, dysphagia may be painful and develop slowly.
- ***Amyotrophic lateral sclerosis.*** Besides dysphagia, this disorder causes muscle weakness and atrophy, fasciculations, dysarthria, dyspnea, shallow respirations, tachypnea, slurred speech, hyperactive deep tendon reflexes, and emotional lability.
- ***Bulbar paralysis.*** Phase 1 dysphagia occurs with drooling, difficulty chewing, dysarthria, and nasal regurgitation. Dysphagia for both solids and liquids is painful and progressive. Accompanying features may include arm and leg spasticity, hyperreflexia, and emotional lability.
- ***Esophageal cancer.*** Phase 2 or 3 dysphagia is the earliest and most common symptom of esophageal cancer. Typically, this painless, progressive symptom is accompanied by rapid weight loss. As the cancer advances, dysphagia becomes painful and constant. In addition, the patient complains of steady chest pain, cough with hemoptysis, hoarseness, and sore throat. He also may develop nausea and vomiting, fever, hiccups, hematemesis, melena, and halitosis.

♦ ***Esophageal compression (external).*** Most often caused by a dilated carotid or aortic aneurysm, this rare condition causes phase 3 dysphagia as the primary symptom. Other features depend on the cause of the compression.

♦ ***Esophageal diverticulum.*** This disorder causes phase 3 dysphagia when the enlarged diverticulum obstructs the esophagus. Associated signs and symptoms include food regurgitation, chronic cough, hoarseness, chest pain, and halitosis.

♦ ***Esophageal obstruction by foreign body.*** Sudden onset of phase 2 or 3 dysphagia, gagging, coughing, and esophageal pain characterize this potentially life-threatening condition. Dyspnea may occur if the obstruction compresses the trachea.

♦ ***Esophageal spasm.*** The most striking symptoms of this disorder are phase 2 dysphagia for solids and liquids and dull or squeezing substernal chest pain. The pain is frequently relieved by drinking a glass of water. It may last up to an hour and may radiate to the neck, arm, back, or jaw. Bradycardia may also occur.

♦ ***Esophagitis.*** *Corrosive esophagitis,* resulting from ingestion of alkalies or acids, causes severe phase 3 dysphagia. Accompanying it are marked salivation, hematemesis, tachypnea, fever, and intense pain in the mouth and anterior chest that is aggravated by swallowing. Signs of shock, such as hypotension and tachycardia, also may occur.

Monilial esophagitis causes phase 2 dysphagia, sore throat, and possibly retrosternal pain on swallowing. In *reflux esophagitis,* phase 3 dysphagia is a late symptom that usually accompanies stricture development. The patient complains of heartburn that is aggravated by strenuous exercise, bending over, or lying down and is relieved by sitting up or taking antacids.

Other features include regurgitation; frequent, effortless vomiting; a dry, nocturnal cough; and substernal chest pain that may mimic angina pectoris. If the esophagus ulcerates, signs of bleeding, such as melena and hematemesis, may occur along with weakness and fatigue.

♦ ***Gastric carcinoma.*** Infiltration of the cardia or esophagus by gastric carcinoma causes phase 3 dysphagia along with nausea, vomiting, and pain that may radiate to the neck, back, or retrosternum. In addition, perforation causes massive bleeding with coffee-ground emesis or melena.

♦ ***Laryngeal cancer (extrinsic).*** Phase 2 dysphagia and dyspnea develop late in this disorder. Accompanying features include muffled voice, stridor, pain, halitosis, weight loss, ipsilateral otalgia, chronic cough, and cachexia. Palpation reveals enlarged cervical nodes.

♦ ***Lead poisoning.*** Painless, progressive dysphagia may result from lead poisoning. Related findings include a lead line on the gums, metallic taste, papilledema, ocular palsy, footdrop or wristdrop, and signs of hemolytic anemia, such as abdominal pain and fever. The patient may be depressed and display severe mental impairment. He may also experience seizures.

♦ ***Myasthenia gravis.*** Fatigue and progressive muscle weakness characterize this disorder and account for painless phase 1 dysphagia and possibly choking. Typically, dysphagia follows ptosis and diplopia. Other features may include masklike facies, nasal voice, frequent nasal regurgitation, and head bobbing. Shallow respirations and dyspnea may occur with respiratory muscle weakness. Signs and symptoms worsen during menses and with exposure to stress, cold, or infection.

♦ ***Oral cavity tumor.*** Painful phase 1 dysphagia develops with hoarseness and ulcerating lesions.

♦ ***Plummer-Vinson syndrome.*** This syndrome causes phase 3 dysphagia for solids in some women with severe iron deficiency anemia. Related features include upper esophageal pain; atrophy of the oral or pharyngeal mucous membranes; tooth loss; smooth, red, sore tongue; dry mouth; chills; inflamed lips; spoon-shaped nails; pallor; and splenomegaly.

♦ ***Rabies.*** Severe phase 2 dysphagia for liquids results from painful pharyngeal muscle spasms occurring late in this rare, life-threatening disorder. In fact, the patient may become dehydrated and possibly apneic. Dysphagia also causes drooling and, in 50% of patients, it's responsible for hydrophobia. Eventually, rabies causes progressive flaccid paralysis that leads to peripheral vascular collapse, coma, and death.

♦ ***Systemic lupus erythematosus.*** This disorder may cause progressive phase 2 dysphagia. However, its primary clinical features include nondeforming arthritis, a characteristic butterfly rash, and photosensitivity.

♦ ***Tetanus.*** Phase 1 dysphagia usually develops about 1 week after the patient receives a puncture wound. Other characteristics include marked muscle hypertonicity, hyperactive deep tendon reflexes, tachycardia, diaphoresis, drooling, and low-grade fever. Painful, involuntary muscle spasms account for lockjaw (trismus), risus sardonicus, opisthotonos, boardlike abdominal rigidity, and intermittent tonic seizures.

Other causes

♦ ***Radiation therapy.*** When directed against oral cancer, this therapy may cause scant salivation and temporary dysphagia.

♦ ***Surgery.*** Recent tracheostomy may cause temporary dysphagia.

Special considerations

Stimulate salivation by talking with the patient about food, adding a lemon slice or dill pickle to his tray, and providing mouth care before and after meals. Or, administer an anticholinergic or antiemetic to control excess salivation. If the patient has decreased saliva production, moisten his food with a little liquid. If he has a weak or absent cough reflex, begin tube feedings or esophageal drips of special formulas.

Consult with the dietitian to select foods with distinct temperatures and textures. Be sure to avoid sticky foods, such as bananas and peanut butter. If the patient has mucus production, avoid uncooked milk products. At mealtimes, take measures to minimize the patient's risk of choking and aspiration. Place the patient in an upright position, and have him flex his neck forward slightly and keep his chin at midline. Separate solids from liquids, which are harder to swallow.

Prepare the patient for diagnostic evaluation, including endoscopy, esophageal manometry, esophagography, and esophageal acidity testing, to pinpoint the cause of dysphagia.

Pediatric pointers

When looking for dysphagia in an infant or a small child, be sure to pay close attention to his sucking and swallowing ability. Coughing, choking, or regurgitating during feeding suggests dysphagia.

Corrosive esophagitis and esophageal obstruction by a foreign body are more common causes of dysphagia in children than in adults. However, dysphagia may also result from congenital anomalies, such as annular stenosis, dysphagia lusoria, and esophageal atresia.

Geriatric pointers

In patients over age 50, dysphagia is often the presenting symptom of head or neck cancer. The incidence of such cancers increases markedly in this age-group.

DYSPNEA

Often a symptom of cardiopulmonary dysfunction, dyspnea is the sensation of difficult or uncomfortable breathing. It's usually reported as shortness of breath.

Its severity varies greatly and is often unrelated to the severity of the underlying cause. Dyspnea may arise suddenly or slowly and may subside rapidly or persist for years.

Most people normally experience dyspnea when they overexert themselves, and its severity depends on their physical condition. In a healthy person, dyspnea is quickly relieved by rest. Pathologic causes of dyspnea include pulmonary, cardiac, neuromuscular, and allergic disorders. In addition, anxiety may cause shortness of breath.

Emergency interventions

If a patient complains of shortness of breath, quickly look for signs of respiratory distress, such as tachypnea, cyanosis, restlessness, and accessory muscle use. Prepare to administer oxygen by nasal cannula, mask, or endotracheal tube. Start an I.V. infusion and begin cardiac monitoring to detect arrhythmias. Expect to insert a chest tube for severe pneumothorax and to administer continuous positive airway pressure (CPAP), or to apply rotating tourniquets for pulmonary edema.

History and physical examination

If the patient can answer questions without increasing his distress, take a complete history. Ask if the shortness of breath began suddenly or gradually. Is it constant or intermittent? Does it occur during activity or while at rest? If the patient has had dyspneic attacks before, ask if they're increasing in severity. Can he identify what aggravates or alleviates these attacks? Does he have a productive or nonproductive cough or chest pain? Ask about recent trauma, and note a history of upper respiratory tract infections, deep vein phlebitis, or other disorders. Ask the patient if he smokes or is exposed to toxic fumes or irritants on the job. Find out if he also has orthopnea, paroxysmal nocturnal dyspnea, or progressive fatigue. (See *Dyspnea: Common causes and associated findings*, pages 212 and 213.)

Because dyspnea is subjective and exacerbated by anxiety, paitents from cultures that are highly emotional may complain of shortness of breath sooner than those who are more stoic about symptoms of illness.

During the physical examination, look for signs of chronic dyspnea, such as accessory muscle hypertrophy (especially in the shoulders and neck). Also look for pursed-lip exhalation, clubbing, peripheral edema, barrel chest, diaphoresis, and distended neck veins.

Check blood pressure and auscultate for crackles, abnormal heart sounds or rhythms, egophony, bronchophony, and whispered pectoriloquy. Finally, palpate the abdomen for hepatomegaly.

Common medical causes

♦ ***Adult respiratory distress syndrome (ARDS).*** This life-threatening form of noncardiogenic pulmonary edema usually causes acute dyspnea as the first complaint. Progressive respiratory distress then develops with restlessness, anxiety, decreased mental acuity, tachycardia, and crackles in both lung fields. Other findings may include cyanosis, tachypnea, and intercostal and suprasternal retractions. Severe ARDS can cause signs of shock, such as hypotension and cool, clammy skin.

♦ ***Amyotrophic lateral sclerosis.*** Also known as Lou Gehrig's disease, this disorder causes slow onset of dyspnea that worsens with time. Other features include dysphagia, dysarthria, muscle weakness and atrophy, fasciculations, shallow respirations, tachypnea, and emotional lability.

♦ ***Aspiration of a foreign body.*** Acute dyspnea with paroxysmal intercostal, suprasternal, and substernal retractions marks this life-threatening condition. The patient may also display accessory muscle use, inspiratory stridor, tachypnea, decreased or absent breath sounds, possibly asymmetrical chest expansion, anxiety, cyanosis, diaphoresis, and hypotension.

Dyspnea: Common causes and associated findings

S&S

CAUSES	Accessory muscle use	Blood pressure decrease	Breath sounds, decreased	Chest pain	Cough, nonproductive	Cough, productive	Crackles	Cyanosis	Diaphoresis	Edema	Fasciculations	Fever
	MAJOR ASSOCIATED SIGNS AND SYMPTOMS											
Adult respiratory distress syndrome	◆	◆					◆	◆				
Amyotrophic lateral sclerosis											◆	
Aspiration of a foreign body	◆	◆	◆		◆			◆	◆			
Asthma	◆				◆			◆	◆			
Cor pulmonale	◆					◆		◆		◆		
Emphysema	◆		◆		◆							
Flail chest	◆	◆	◆	◆				◆				
Heart failure	◆	◆			◆		◆			◆		
Myasthenia gravis												
Myocardial infarction		◆		◆					◆			
Pleural effusion			◆		◆							◆
Pneumonia			◆	◆		◆	◆	◆	◆			◆
Pulmonary edema	◆	◆			◆	◆	◆	◆	◆			
Pulmonary embolism		◆	◆	◆	◆	◆	◆	◆	◆	◆		◆
Shock		◆										

◆ ***Asthma.*** In this chronic disorder, acute dyspneic attacks occur with audible wheezing, dry cough, accessory muscle use, nasal flaring, intercostal and supraclavicular retractions, tachypnea, tachycardia, diaphoresis, prolonged expiration, flushing, and apprehension.

◆ ***Cor pulmonale.*** Chronic dyspnea begins gradually with exertion and progressively worsens until it occurs even at

Muscle weakness	Nausea	Neck vein distention	Orthopnea	Stridor	Tachycardia	Tachypnea	Weight loss
					♦	♦	
♦						♦	
				♦		♦	
					♦	♦	
		♦				♦	
						♦	♦
					♦	♦	
		♦	♦		♦	♦	
♦						♦	
	♦				♦		
					♦	♦	
					♦	♦	
		♦	♦		♦	♦	
					♦	♦	
					♦	♦	

rest. Underlying cardiac or pulmonary disease is usually present. The patient may have a chronic productive cough, wheezing, tachypnea, distended neck veins, dependent edema, and hepatomegaly. He may also experience increasing fatigue, weakness, or light-headedness.

♦ ***Emphysema.*** This chronic disorder gradually causes progressive exertional dyspnea. A history of smoking, an alpha-antitrypsin deficiency, or exposure to an occupational irritant usually accompanies barrel chest, accessory muscle hypertrophy, diminished breath sounds, anorexia, weight loss, malaise, tachypnea, pursed-lip breathing, prolonged expiration and, possibly, a chronic cough.

♦ ***Flail chest.*** Multiple rib fractures cause sudden dyspnea accompanied by paradoxical chest movement, severe chest pain, hypotension, tachypnea, tachycardia, and cyanosis. Bruising and decreased or absent breath sounds occur over the affected side.

♦ ***Heart failure.*** Dyspnea usually develops gradually in heart failure. Chronic paroxysmal nocturnal dyspnea, orthopnea, tachypnea, tachycardia, palpitations, ventricular gallop, fatigue, dependent peripheral edema, hepatomegaly, dry cough, weight gain, and loss of mental acuity may occur. With acute onset, heart failure may cause distended neck veins, bibasilar rates, oliguria, and hypotension.

♦ ***Myasthenia gravis.*** This neuromuscular disorder causes bouts of dyspnea as the respiratory muscles weaken. In myasthenic crisis, acute respiratory distress may occur, with shallow respirations and tachypnea.

♦ ***Myocardial infarction.*** Sudden dyspnea occurs with crushing substernal chest pain that may radiate to the back, neck, jaw, and arms. Other signs and symptoms include nausea, vomiting, diaphoresis, vertigo, hypertension or hypotension, tachycardia, anxiety, and pale, cool, clammy skin.

♦ ***Pleural effusion.*** Dyspnea develops slowly and becomes progressively worse with this disorder. Other findings include dry cough; dullness on percussion; egophony, bronchophony, or whispered pectoriloquy just above the fluid level;

tachycardia; tachypnea; weight loss; and decreased chest motion, tactile fremitus, and breath sounds. Fever may accompany infection.

♦ ***Pneumonia.*** Dyspnea occurs suddenly, usually accompanied by fever, shaking chills, pleuritic chest pain that worsens with deep inspiration, and a productive cough. Fatigue, headache, myalgia, anorexia, crackles, rhonchi, tachycardia, tachypnea, cyanosis, decreased breath sounds, and diaphoresis may also occur.

♦ ***Pneumothorax.*** This life-threatening disorder causes acute dyspnea unrelated to the severity of pain. Sudden, stabbing chest pain may radiate to the arms, face, back, or abdomen. Other signs include anxiety, restlessness, dry cough, cyanosis, decreased vocal fremitus, tachypnea, tympany, decreased or absent breath sounds on the affected side, asymmetrical chest expansion, splinting, and accessory muscle use. In tension pneumothorax, tracheal deviation occurs in addition to these typical findings. Decreased blood pressure and tachycardia may also occur.

♦ ***Poliomyelitis (bulbar).*** Dyspnea develops gradually and progressively worsens. Additional signs and symptoms include fever, facial weakness, dysphasia, hypoactive deep tendon reflexes, decreased mental acuity, dysphagia, nasal regurgitation, and hypopnea.

♦ ***Pulmonary edema.*** Preceded by signs of heart failure, such as distended neck veins and orthopnea, this life-threatening disorder causes acute dyspnea. Other features include tachycardia, tachypnea, crackles in both lung fields, S_3 gallop, oliguria, thready pulse, hypotension, diaphoresis, cyanosis, and marked anxiety. The patient's cough may be dry or may produce copious amounts of pink, frothy sputum.

♦ ***Pulmonary embolism.*** Acute dyspnea that is usually accompanied by sudden pleuritic chest pain characterizes this life-threatening disorder. Related findings may include tachycardia, low-grade fever, tachypnea, nonproductive or productive cough with blood-tinged sputum, pleural friction rub, crackles, diffuse wheezing, dullness on percussion, decreased breath sounds, diaphoresis, restlessness, and acute anxiety. A massive embolism may cause signs of shock, such as hypotension and cool, clammy skin.

♦ ***Shock.*** Dyspnea arises suddenly and worsens progressively in this life-threatening disorder. Related findings include severe hypotension, tachypnea, tachycardia, decreased peripheral pulses, cool and clammy skin, decreased mental acuity, restlessness, and anxiety.

♦ ***Tuberculosis.*** Dyspnea commonly occurs with chest pain, crackles, and productive cough. Other findings are night sweats, fever, anorexia and weight loss, vague dyspepsia, palpitations on mild exertion, and dullness on percussion.

Special considerations

Monitor the dyspneic patient closely. Be as calm and reassuring as possible to reduce his anxiety, and help him into a comfortable position — usually high Fowler's or forward-leaning. Support him with pillows, loosen his clothing, and administer oxygen.

Prepare the patient for diagnostic studies, such as arterial blood gas analysis and chest X-rays. Administer bronchodilators, antiarrhythmics, diuretics, and analgesics, as needed, to dilate bronchioles, correct cardiac arrhythmias, promote fluid excretion, and relieve pain.

Pediatric pointers

Normally, an infant's respirations are abdominal, gradually changing to costal by age 7. Suspect dyspnea in an infant who breathes costally, in an older child who breathes abdominally, or in any child who uses his neck or shoulder muscles to help him breathe.

Asthma, epiglottiditis, and laryngotracheobronchitis (croup) can cause severe dyspnea in a child and may even lead to respiratory or cardiovascular collapse. Expect to administer oxygen.

Geriatric pointers

Older patients with dyspnea related to chronic illness may not be aware initially of a significant change in their breathing pattern.

Dystonia

Dystonia, an abnormal prolonged twisting movement associated with extrapyramidal disease, is marked by slow, involuntary movements of large-muscle groups in the limbs, trunk, and neck. This extrapyramidal sign may involve flexion of the foot, hyperextension of the legs, extension and pronation of the arms, arching of the back, and extension and rotation of the neck (spasmodic torticollis). It's typically aggravated by walking and emotional stress and relieved by sleep. Dystonia may be intermittent — lasting just a few minutes — or continuous and painful. Occasionally, it causes permanent contractures, resulting in a grotesque posture. Although dystonia may be hereditary or idiopathic, it usually results from extrapyramidal disorders or drugs.

History and physical examination

If possible, include the patient's family in history taking; they may be more aware of behavior changes than the patient is. Begin by asking them when dystonia occurs. Is it aggravated by emotional upset? Does it disappear during sleep? Is there a family history of dystonia? Obtain a drug history, noting especially the use of phenothiazines or antipsychotics. Dystonia is a common adverse effect of these drugs, and dosage adjustments may minimize this effect.

EXAMINATION TIP

Recognizing dystonia

Dystonia, chorea, and athetosis may occur simultaneously. To differentiate these three, keep the following points in mind:

- *Dystonic movements* are slow and twisting and involve large-muscle groups in the head, neck (as shown below), trunk, and limbs. They may be intermittent or continuous.
- *Choreiform movements* are rapid, highly complex, and jerky.
- *Athetoid movements* are slow, sinuous, and writhing, but always continuous; they typically affect the hands and extremities.

DYSTONIA OF THE NECK
(Spasmodic torticollis)

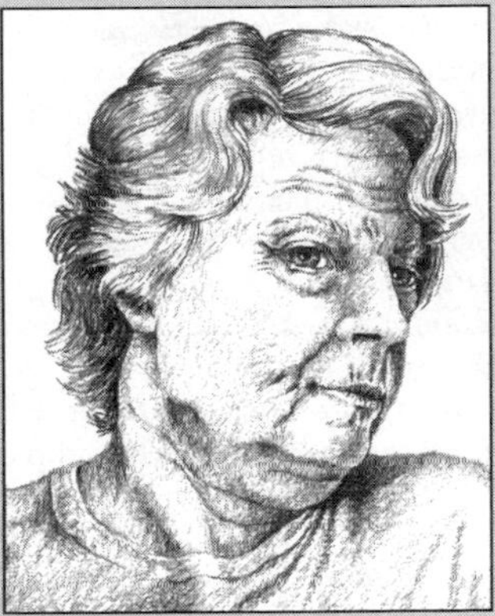

Next, examine the patient's coordination and voluntary muscle movement. Observe his gait as he walks across the room; then have him squeeze your fingers to assess muscle strength. (See *Recognizing dystonia.*) Check coordination by having him touch your fingertip and then his nose repeatedly. Follow this by testing gross motor movement of the leg: Have him place his heel on one knee, slide it down his shin, then return it to his knee. Finally, assess fine-motor movement by asking him to touch each finger to his thumb in succession.

Common medical causes

♦ ***Alzheimer's disease.*** Dystonia is a late sign of this disorder, which is marked by slowly progressive dementia. The patient typically displays decreased attention span, amnesia, agitation, an inability to carry out activities of daily living, dysarthria, and emotional lability.

♦ ***Dystonia musculorum deformans.*** Prolonged, generalized dystonia is the hallmark of this disorder, which usually develops in childhood and worsens with age. Initially, it causes foot inversion, which is followed by growth retardation and scoliosis. Late signs include twisted, bizarre postures, limb contractures, and dysarthria.

♦ ***Hallervorden-Spatz disease.*** This degenerative disease causes dystonic trunk movements accompanied by choreoathetosis, ataxia, myoclonus, and generalized rigidity. The patient also exhibits progressive intellectual decline and dysarthria.

♦ ***Huntington's disease.*** Dystonic movements mark the preterminal stage of Huntington's disease. Characterized by progressive intellectual decline, this disorder leads to dementia and emotional lability. The patient displays choreoathetosis accompanied by dysarthria, dysphagia, facial grimacing, and a wide-based, prancing gait.

♦ ***Parkinson's disease.*** Dystonic spasms are common in this disease. Other classic features include uniform or jerky rigidity, "pill-rolling" tremor, bradykinesia, dysarthria, dysphagia, drooling, mask-like facies, monotone voice, stooped posture, and propulsive gait.

♦ ***Wilson's disease.*** Progressive dystonia and chorea of the arms and legs mark this disorder. Other common signs include hoarseness, bradykinesia, behavior changes, dysphagia, drooling, dysarthria, tremors, and Kayser-Fleischer rings (rusty-brown rings at the periphery of the cornea).

Other causes

♦ ***Drugs.*** All three types of phenothiazines may cause dystonia. Piperazine phenothiazines, such as acetophenazine and carphenazine, cause this sign most frequently; aliphatics, such as chlorpromazine, cause it less often; and piperidines rarely cause it.

Haloperidol, loxapine, and other antipsychotics usually cause acute facial dystonia. So do antiemetic doses of metoclopramide, risperidone, and metyrosine, and excessive doses of levodopa.

Special considerations

Encourage the patient to obtain adequate sleep and avoid emotional upset. Avoid range-of-motion exercises, which can aggravate dystonia. If dystonia is severe, protect the patient from injury by raising and padding his bed rails. Provide an uncluttered environment if he's ambulatory.

Pediatric pointers

Children don't exhibit dystonia until after they can walk. Even so, it rarely occurs before age 10. Common causes include Fahr's syndrome, dystonia musculorum deformans, athetoid cerebral palsy, and the residual effects of anoxia at birth.

DYSURIA

Dysuria — painful or difficult urination — is often accompanied by urinary frequency, urgency, or hesitancy. This symptom usually reflects lower urinary tract infection — a common disorder, especially in women.

Dysuria results from lower urinary tract irritation or inflammation, which stimulates nerve endings in the bladder and urethra. The pain's onset provides clues to its cause; for example, pain just *before* voiding usually indicates bladder irritation or distention, whereas pain at the *start* of urination typically results from bladder outlet irritation. Pain at the *end* of voiding may signal bladder spasms; in women, it may indicate vaginal candidiasis.

History and physical examination

If the patient complains of dysuria, have him describe its severity and location. When did he first notice it? Did anything precipitate it? Does anything aggravate or alleviate it?

Next, ask about previous urinary or genital tract infections. Has the patient recently undergone invasive procedures, such as cystoscopy or urethral dilatation? Also ask if he has a history of intestinal disease. Ask the female patient about menstrual disorders and use of products that irritate the urinary tract, such as bubble bath salts, feminine deodorants, contraceptive gels, or perineal lotions. Also ask her about vaginal discharge or pruritus.

During the physical examination, inspect the urethral meatus for discharge, irritation, or other abnormalities. A pelvic or rectal examination may be necessary. (See *Dysuria: Common causes and associated medical findings,* pages 218 and 219.)

Common medical causes

♦ ***Appendicitis.*** Occasionally, this disorder causes dysuria that persists throughout voiding and is accompanied by bladder tenderness. Appendicitis is characterized by periumbilical abdominal pain that shifts to McBurney's point, anorexia, nausea, vomiting, constipation, slight fever, abdominal rigidity and rebound tenderness, and tachycardia.

♦ ***Bladder cancer.*** In this predominantly male disorder, dysuria throughout voiding is a late symptom associated with urinary frequency and urgency, nocturia, hematuria, and perineal, back, or flank pain.

Bladder cancer is twice as common in White males as Blacks. It's relatively uncommon in Asians, Hispanics, and Native Americans.

♦ ***Chemical irritants.*** Dysuria may result from irritating substances, such as bubble bath salts and feminine deodorants; it's usually most intense at the end of voiding. Spermicides may cause dysuria in both sexes. Other findings may include urinary frequency and urgency, a diminished urinary stream and, possibly, hematuria.

♦ ***Cystitis.*** Dysuria throughout voiding is common in all types of cystitis, as are urinary frequency, nocturia, straining to void, and hematuria. *Bacterial cystitis,* the most common cause of dysuria in women, may also cause urinary urgency, perineal and lower back pain, suprapubic discomfort, fatigue and, possibly, a low-grade fever. In *chronic interstitial cystitis,* dysuria is accentuated at the end of voiding. In *tubercular cystitis,* symptoms may also include urinary urgency, flank pain, fatigue, and anorexia. In *viral cystitis,* severe dysuria occurs with gross hematuria, urinary urgency, and fever.

♦ ***Paraurethral gland inflammation.*** Dysuria throughout voiding occurs with frequency and urgency, diminished urinary stream, mild perineal pain and, occasionally, hematuria.

♦ ***Prostatitis.*** *Acute* prostatitis commonly causes dysuria throughout or toward the end of voiding as well as diminished urinary stream, urinary frequency and urgency, hematuria, suprapubic fullness, fever, chills, fatigue, myalgia, nausea, vomiting, and constipation. In *chronic* prostatitis, urethral narrowing causes dysuria throughout voiding. Related effects are urinary frequency and

Dysuria: Common causes and associated findings

S&S

CAUSES	Abdominal pain	Anorexia	Back pain	Constipation	Costovertebral angle tenderness	Erythema of meatus	Fatigue	Fever	Flank pain	Hematuria	Nausea	Nocturia	Perineal pain	Straining to void
	MAJOR ASSOCIATED SIGNS AND SYMPTOMS													
Appendicitis	♦	♦		♦				♦			♦			
Bladder tumor			♦						♦	♦		♦	♦	
Chemical irritants										♦				
Cystitis (bacterial)			♦				♦	♦		♦		♦	♦	♦
Cystitis (chronic interstitial										♦		♦		♦
Cystitis (tubercular)		♦					♦		♦	♦		♦		♦
Cystitis (viral)								♦		♦		♦		♦
Paraurethral gland inflammation										♦			♦	
Prostatitis (acute)				♦			♦	♦		♦	♦		♦	
Prostatitis (chronic)			♦										♦	
Pyelonephritis		♦			♦			♦	♦	♦	♦	♦		♦
Reiter's syndrome		♦				♦		♦		♦				
Urinary obstruction														
Vaginitis										♦		♦	♦	

urgency; diminished urinary stream; perineal, back, and buttock pain; urethral discharge; and, at times, hematospermia and ejaculatory pain.

♦ ***Pyelonephritis (acute).*** More common in females, this disorder causes dysuria throughout voiding. Other features include persistent high fever with chills, costovertebral angle tenderness, unilateral or bilateral flank pain, weakness, urinary urgency and frequency, nocturia, straining on urination, and hematuria.

Suprapubic pain	Urethral discharge	Urinary frequency	Urine stream, diminished	Urinary urgency	Vaginal discharge	Vomiting	Weakness
						♦	
		♦		♦			
		♦	♦	♦			
♦		♦		♦			
		♦					
		♦		♦			
		♦		♦			
		♦	♦	♦			
		♦	♦	♦		♦	
	♦	♦	♦	♦			
		♦		♦		♦	♦
♦	♦	♦		♦			
		♦	♦	♦			
		♦		♦	♦		

Nausea, vomiting, and anorexia may also occur.

♦ ***Reiter's syndrome.*** Occurring predominantly in males, this disorder causes dysuria that occurs 1 to 2 weeks after sexual contact. Initially, the patient has a mucopurulent discharge, urinary urgency and frequency, meatal swelling and redness, suprapubic pain, anorexia, weight loss, and low-grade fever. Hematuria, conjunctivitis, arthritic symptoms, a papular rash, and oral and penile lesions may follow.

♦ ***Urinary obstruction.*** Outflow obstruction by urethral strictures or calculi causes dysuria throughout voiding. In complete obstruction, bladder distention develops and dysuria precedes voiding. Other features are diminished urinary stream, urinary frequency and urgency, and a sensation of fullness or bloating in the lower abdomen or groin.

♦ ***Vaginitis.*** Characteristically, dysuria occurs throughout voiding as urine touches inflamed or ulcerated labia. Other findings may include urinary frequency and urgency, nocturia, hematuria, perineal pain, and vaginal discharge and odor.

Other causes

♦ ***Drugs.*** Dysuria can result from monoamine oxidase inhibitors. Metyrosine can also cause transient dysuria.

Special considerations

Monitor vital signs, intake, and output. Administer prescribed drugs, and prepare the patient for such tests as urinalysis and cystoscopy.

Geriatric pointers

Be aware that elderly people tend to underreport their symptoms even though older men have an increased incidence of non-sexually related urinary tract infections and postmenopausal women have an increased incidence of noninfectious dysuria.

E

EARACHE
[Otalgia]

Earaches usually result from disorders of the external and middle ear, such as infection, obstruction, or trauma. Their severity ranges from a feeling of fullness or blockage to deep, boring pain; at times, they may be difficult to localize precisely. This common symptom may be intermittent or continuous and may develop suddenly or gradually.

History and physical examination
Ask the patient to characterize his earache. How long has he had it? Is it intermittent or continuous? Is it painful or slightly annoying? Can he localize the site of ear pain? Does he have pain in any other areas such as the jaw?

Ask about recent ear injury or other trauma. Does swimming or showering trigger ear discomfort? Is this discomfort associated with itching? If so, find out where the itching is most intense and when it began. Ask about ear drainage and, if present, have the patient characterize it. Does he hear ringing or noise in his ears? Is the ringing pulsatile? Ask about dizziness or vertigo. Does it worsen when the patient changes position? Does he have difficulty swallowing, hoarseness, neck pain, or pain when he opens his mouth?

Find out if the patient has recently had a head cold or problems with his eyes, mouth, teeth, jaws, sinuses, or throat. Disorders in these areas may refer pain to the ear along the cranial nerves.

Begin your physical examination by inspecting the external ear for redness, drainage, swelling, or deformity. Then apply pressure to the mastoid process and tragus to elicit any tenderness. Using an otoscope, examine the external auditory canal for lesions, bleeding or discharge, impacted cerumen, foreign bodies, tenderness, and swelling. Examine the tympanic membrane (TM): Is it intact? Is it pearly gray (normal)? Look for the cone of light, umbo, pars tensa, and the handle and short process of the malleus. (See *Using an otoscope correctly.*) Perform the watch tick, whispered voice, Rinne, and Weber's tests to assess for hearing loss.

Pneumatic otoscopy is the gold standard for the diagnosis of otitis media. Use it to evaluate the TM position and mobility. Decreased mobility indicates atelectasis, effusion, or perforation, and erythema can indicate infection, barotrauma, or Valsalva maneuver (for example, in a crying infant). Otitis media is uncommon in adults and suggests a secondary diagnosis, such as eustachian tube dysfunction or nasopharyngeal or middle ear tumors, especially if recurrent.

EXAMINATION TIP

Using an otoscope correctly

When the patient reports an earache, use an otoscope to inspect ear structures closely. Follow these techniques to obtain the best view and ensure patient safety.

CHILD

To inspect an infant's or a young child's ear, grasp the *lower part* of the auricle and pull it *down and back* to straighten the upward S-curve of the external canal. Then gently insert the speculum into the canal no more than ½″ (1.2 cm).

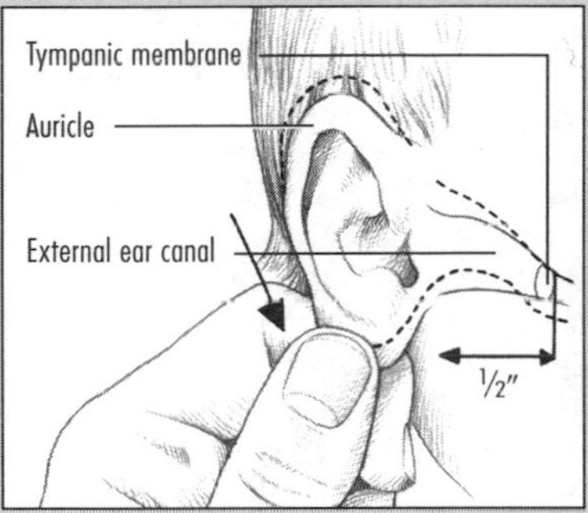

ADULT

To inspect an adult's ear, grasp the *upper part* of the auricle and pull it *up and back* to straighten the external canal. Then insert the speculum about 1″ (2.5 cm). Also, use this technique for children over age 3.

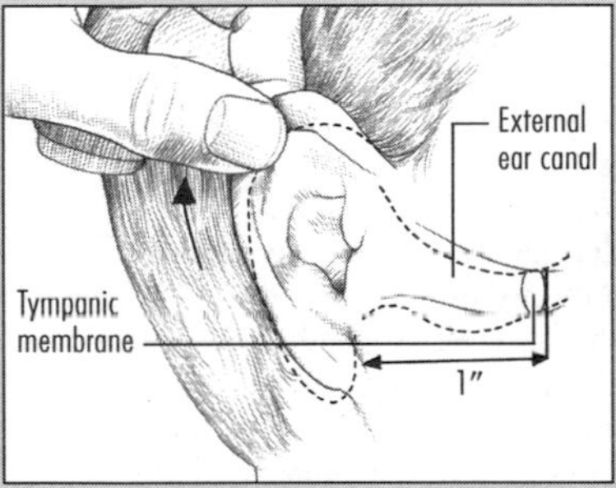

Common medical causes

♦ ***Abscess (extradural).*** Severe earache accompanied by persistent ipsilateral headache, malaise, and recurrent mild fever characterizes this serious complication of middle ear infection.

♦ ***Barotitis media.*** Failure of the eustachian tube to equalize changing pressure may lead to inflammation of the middle ear space due to negative (common) or positive (less common) pressure change between the external and middle ear spaces. It's the most common medical disorder of scuba divers and also occurs among flyers and sky divers. Symptoms may include sudden onset of ear pain, sensation of ear fullness, conductive hearing loss, dizziness, tinnitus, vertigo, nausea and vomiting, ear drum perforation, and crying (in children). Children are at greater risk than adults when flying, and they shouldn't fly with upper respiratory tract infections; chewing gum may reduce this risk.

♦ ***Cerumen impaction.*** Impacted cerumen (earwax) may cause a sensation of blockage or fullness in the ear. Additional features include partial hearing loss, itching and, possibly, dizziness.

♦ ***Herpes zoster oticus (Ramsay Hunt syndrome).*** This disorder causes burning or stabbing ear pain, commonly associated with ear vesicles. The vesicles may occur early and are transient; both patient and clinician may miss them. The patient also complains of hearing loss and vertigo. Associated signs and symptoms include transitory, ipsilateral facial paralysis; partial loss of taste; tongue vesicles; and nausea and vomiting.

♦ ***Keratosis obturans.*** Mild ear pain occurs with otorrhea and tinnitus. Inspection reveals a white glistening plug obstructing the external meatus.

♦ ***Mastoiditis (acute).*** This infection causes a dull ache behind the ear accompanied by low-grade fever (99° to 100° F [37.2° to 37.8° C]). The eardrum appears dull and edematous and may perforate; soft tissue near the eardrum may sag. A serous, mucinous, or purulent discharge may be present in the external canal.

♦ ***Ménière's disease.*** This inner ear disorder can cause a sensation of fullness in the affected ear. Its classic effects, though, include severe vertigo, tinnitus, and sensorineural hearing loss. The patient may also experience nausea and vomiting, diaphoresis, and nystagmus.

♦ ***Otitis externa.*** Earache characterizes both acute and malignant otitis externa. *Acute otitis externa* begins with mild to moderate ear pain that occurs with tragus manipulation. The pain may be accompanied by sticky yellow or purulent ear discharge, partial hearing loss, and a feeling of blockage. Later, ear pain intensifies, causing the entire side of the head to ache and throb. Examination reveals swelling of the tragus, external meatus, and external canal; eardrum erythema; and lymphadenopathy. The patient also complains of dizziness and malaise. The infection is localized, and systemic manifestations such as fever or chills are absent.

Malignant otitis externa refers to a progressive and necrotizing Pseudomonas infection of the ear. It abruptly causes ear pain that's aggravated by moving the auricle or tragus. The pain is accompanied by intense itching, purulent ear discharge, fever, parotid gland swelling, and trismus. Examination reveals a swollen external canal with exposed cartilage and temporal bone. Cranial nerve palsy may also occur.

♦ ***Otitis media (acute).*** This middle ear inflammation may be serous or suppurative. *Acute serous otitis media* may cause a feeling of fullness in the ear, hearing loss, and a vague sensation of top-heaviness. The eardrum may be slightly retracted, amber colored, and marked by air bubbles and a meniscus, or it may be blue-black from hemorrhage.

Severe, deep, throbbing ear pain, hearing loss, and fever that may reach 102° F (38.9° C) characterize *acute suppurative otitis media.* The pain increases steadily over several hours or days and may be aggravated by pressure on the mastoid antrum. Perforation of the eardrum is possible. Before rupture, the eardrum appears bulging and fiery red. Rupture causes purulent drainage and relieves the pain.

Chronic otitis media usually isn't painful except during exacerbations. Persistent pain and discharge from the ear suggest osteomyelitis of the skull base or cancer.

Special considerations

Administer analgesics and apply heat to relieve discomfort. Instill eardrops, if necessary. Teach the patient how to instill drops if they're prescribed for home use.

Pediatric pointers

Common causes of earache in children are acute otitis media and insertion of foreign bodies that become lodged or infected. In a young child, crying or ear-tugging are nonverbal clues to earache.

To examine the child's ears, place him supine with his arms extended and held securely by his parent. Then hold the otoscope with the handle pointing toward the top of the child's head, and use one or two fingers to brace it. Because an ear examination may upset the child with an earache, save it for the end of your physical examination.

EDEMA, GENERALIZED

A common sign in severely ill patients, generalized edema is the excessive accumulation of interstitial fluid throughout the body. Its severity varies widely; slight edema may be difficult to detect, especially if the patient is obese; massive edema is immediately apparent.

Generalized edema is typically chronic and progressive. It may result from cardiac, renal, endocrine, or hepatic disorders as well as from severe burns, malnutrition, or the effects of certain drugs and treatments.

Common factors responsible for edema are hypoalbuminemia and excess sodium ingestion or retention, both of which influence plasma osmotic pressure. (See *Understanding fluid balance,* page 224.) Cyclic edema associated with increased aldosterone secretion may occur in premenopausal women.

Emergency interventions

Quickly determine the edema's severity, including the degree of pitting. (See *Edema: pitting or nonpitting?* page 225.) If the patient has severe edema, promptly take his vital signs, and check for distended neck veins and cyanotic lips. Auscultate the lungs and heart. Be alert for signs of cardiac failure or pulmonary congestion, such as pulmonary crackles or ventricular gallop (S_3 or S_4) . Unless the patient is hypotensive, place him in a sitting position to make breathing easier. Prepare to administer oxygen and intravenous diuretics. Have emergency resuscitation equipment nearby.

History and physical examination

When the patient's condition permits, obtain a complete medical history. First, note when the edema began. Does it move throughout the course of the day—for example, from the upper extremities to the lower, periorbitally, or within the sacral area? Is the edema worse in the morning or at the end of the day? Is it affected by position changes? Is it accompanied by shortness of breath or pain in the arms or legs? Find out how much weight the patient has gained and over what period of time. Has his urine output changed?

Next, ask about previous burns or cardiac, renal, hepatic, endocrine, or GI disorders. Have the patient describe his diet so you can assess for protein malnutrition. Explore his drug history and note recent I.V. therapy.

Begin the physical examination by comparing the arms and legs for symmetrical edema. Also, note ecchymoses and cyanosis. Assess the back, sacrum, and hips of the bedridden patient for dependent edema. Palpate peripheral pulses, noting whether hands and feet feel cold. Finally, perform a complete cardiac and respiratory assessment.

Common medical causes

- ***Angioneurotic edema.*** Recurrent attacks of acute, painless, pitting edema affect the skin and mucous membranes, especially those of the respiratory tract. Abdominal pain, nausea, vomiting, and diarrhea accompany visceral edema; dyspnea and stridor accompany life-threatening laryngeal edema.
- ***Burns.*** Edema and associated tissue damage vary with the severity of the burn. Severe generalized edema (4+) may occur within 2 days of a major burn; localized edema may occur with a less severe burn.

Understanding fluid balance

Normally, fluid moves freely between the interstitial and intravascular spaces to maintain homeostasis. Four basic pressures control fluid shifts across the capillary membrane that separates these spaces:
- ♦ capillary hydrostatic pressure — internal fluid pressure on the capillary membrane
- ♦ interstitial fluid pressure — external fluid pressure on the capillary membrane
- ♦ plasma osmotic pressure — fluid-attracting pressure from protein concentration in the capillary
- ♦ interstitial osmotic pressure — fluid-attracting pressure from protein concentration outside the capillary.

Here's how these pressures maintain homeostasis. Normally, capillary hydrostatic pressure is greater than plasma osmotic pressure at the capillary's arterial end, so it forces fluid out of the capillary. At the capillary's venous end, the reverse is true: The higher plasma osmotic pressure draws fluid into the capillary. Normally, the lymphatic system transports excess interstitial fluid back to the intravascular space. Edema results when this balance is upset by increased capillary permeability, lymphatic obstruction, persistently increased capillary hydrostatic pressure, decreased plasma osmotic or interstitial fluid pressure, or dilation of precapillary sphincters.

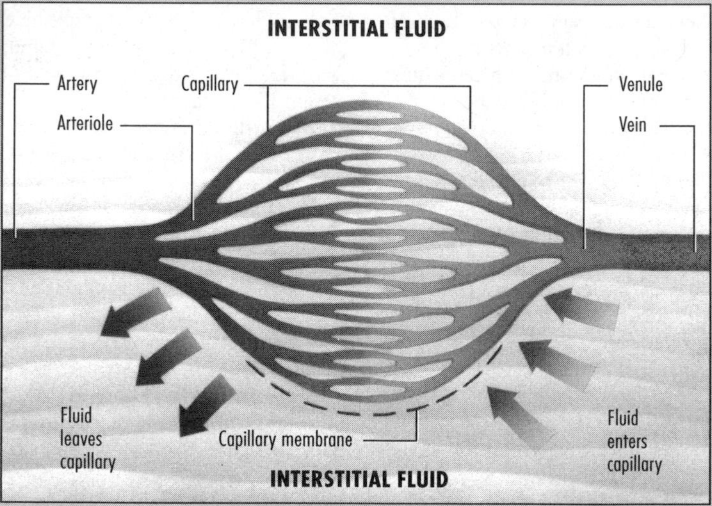

♦ ***Heart failure.*** Severe, generalized pitting edema — occasionally anasarca — may follow leg edema late in this disorder. The edema may abate after exercise or elevation of the limbs and is typically worse at the end of the day. Among other classic late findings are hemoptysis, cyanosis, marked hepatomegaly, clubbing, crackles, and a ventricular gallop. Typically, the patient has some combination of tachypnea, palpitations, hypotension, weight gain despite anorexia, nausea, slowed mental response, diaphoresis, and pallor. Dyspnea, orthopnea, tachycardia, and fatigue typify left-sided heart failure; distended neck veins, enlarged liver, and peripheral edema typify right-sided heart failure.

♦ ***Myxedema.*** In this severe form of hypothyroidism, generalized nonpitting

EXAMINATION TIP

Edema: pitting or nonpitting?

To differentiate pitting from nonpitting edema, press your finger against a swollen area for 5 seconds, then quickly remove it.

In *pitting edema,* pressure forces fluid into the underlying tissues, causing an indentation that slowly fills. To determine the severity of pitting edema, estimate the indentation's depth in centimeters: 1+ (1 cm), 2+ (2 cm), 3+ (3 cm), or 4+ (4 cm).

In *nonpitting edema,* pressure leaves no indentation because fluid has coagulated in the tissues. Typically, the skin feels unusually firm.

PITTING EDEMA (4+)

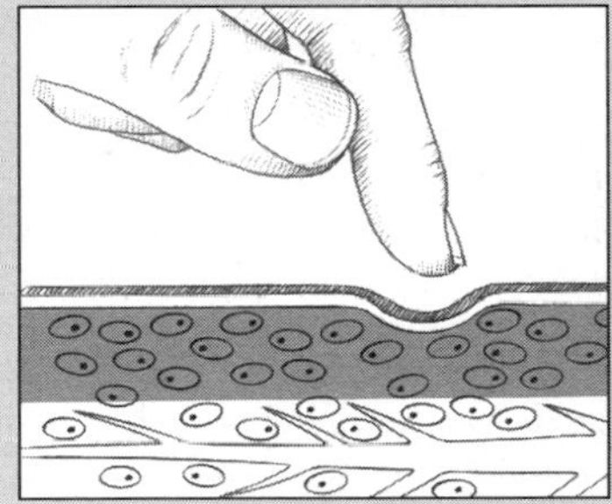

NONPITTING EDEMA

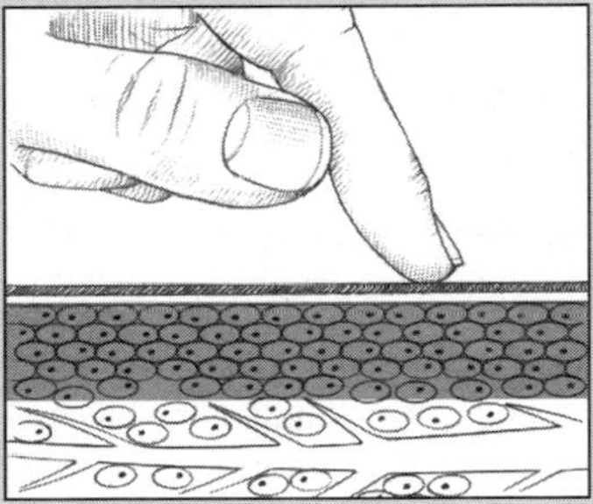

edema is accompanied by dry, waxy, pale skin. Observation also reveals masklike facies, hair loss or coarsening, and psychomotor slowing. Associated findings include hoarseness, weight gain, fatigue, cold intolerance, bradycardia, hypoventilation, constipation, abdominal distention, menorrhagia, impotence, and infertility.

◆ ***Nephrotic syndrome.*** Although this syndrome is characterized by generalized pitting edema, edema is initially localized around the eyes. In severe cases, anasarca develops, increasing body weight by up to 50%. Other common signs and symptoms are ascites, anorexia, fatigue, malaise, depression, and pallor.

◆ ***Pericardial effusion.*** In this disorder, generalized pitting edema may be most prominent in the arms and legs. It may be accompanied by chest pain, dyspnea, orthopnea, nonproductive cough, pericardial friction rub, distended neck veins, dysphagia, and fever.

◆ ***Pericarditis (chronic constrictive).*** Resembling right-sided heart failure, this disorder usually begins with pitting edema of the arms and legs that may progress to generalized edema. Other signs and symptoms may include ascites, Kussmaul's sign, dyspnea, fatigue, weakness, abdominal distention, and hepatomegaly.

◆ ***Renal failure.*** In *acute renal failure,* generalized pitting edema occurs as a late sign. In *chronic renal failure,* edema is less likely to become generalized; its severity depends on the degree of fluid overload. Both forms of renal failure cause oliguria, anorexia, nausea and vomiting, drowsiness, confusion, hypertension, dyspnea, crackles, dizziness, and pallor.

Other causes

◆ ***Drugs.*** Any drug that causes sodium retention may aggravate or cause generalized edema. Some examples are antihypertensives, corticosteroids, androgenic and anabolic steroids, estrogens, and nonsteroidal anti-inflammatory drugs, such as phenylbutazone, ibuprofen, and naproxen.

♦ ***Treatments.*** I.V. saline solution infusions and parenteral feedings may cause sodium and fluid overload, resulting in generalized edema, especially in patients with cardiac or renal disease.

Special considerations

Position the patient with his limbs above heart level to promote drainage. Periodically reposition him to avoid pressure ulcers. If the patient develops dyspnea, lower his limbs, elevate the head of the bed, and administer oxygen. Prevent skin breakdown in these areas by placing a pressure mattress, lamb's wool pad, or flotation ring on the patient's bed. Restrict fluids and sodium, and administer diuretics or I.V. albumin.

Monitor intake, output, and daily weight. Also monitor serum electrolyte levels — especially sodium and albumin. Prepare the patient for blood and urine tests, X-rays, echocardiography, or an electrocardiogram.

Pediatric pointers

Renal failure in children commonly causes generalized edema. Monitor fluid balance closely. Remember that fever or diaphoresis can lead to fluid loss, so promote fluid intake.

Kwashiorkor — protein-deficiency malnutrition — is more common in children than in adults and causes anasarca.

Geriatric pointers

Elderly patients are more likely to develop edema for several reasons, including decreased cardiac and renal function and, in some cases, poor nutritional status. Use caution when giving older patients I.V. fluids or medications that can raise sodium levels and thereby increase fluid retention.

EDEMA OF THE ARM

The result of excess interstitial fluid in the arm, this edema may be unilateral or bilateral and may develop gradually or abruptly. It may be aggravated by immobility and alleviated by arm elevation and exercise.

Arm edema signals a localized fluid imbalance between the vascular and interstitial spaces. (See *Understanding fluid balance,* page 224.) It commonly results from trauma, venous disorders, toxins, or certain treatments.

History and physical examination

One of the first questions to ask is "'How long has your arm been swollen?'" Then find out if the patient also has arm pain, numbness, or tingling. Does exercise or arm elevation decrease the edema? Ask about recent arm injury, such as burns or insect stings. Also, note recent I.V. therapy, surgery, or radiation therapy for breast cancer.

Determine the edema's severity by comparing the size and symmetry of both arms. Use a tape measure to determine the exact girth. Be sure to note whether the edema is unilateral or bilateral, and test for pitting. (See *Edema: pitting or nonpitting?* page 225.) Next, examine and compare the color and temperature of both arms. Look for erythema and ecchymoses and for wounds that suggest injury. Palpate and compare radial and brachial pulses. Finally, look for arm tenderness and decreased mobility. If you detect signs of neurovascular compromise, elevate the arm.

Common medical causes

♦ ***Angioneurotic edema.*** This common reaction is characterized by sudden onset of painless, nonpruritic edema affecting the hands, feet, eyelids, lips, face, neck, genitalia, or viscera. Although these swellings usually don't itch, they may burn and tingle. If edema spreads to the larynx, signs of respiratory distress may occur.

♦ ***Arm trauma.*** Shortly after a crush injury, severe edema may affect the entire arm. Ecchymoses or superficial bleeding, pain or numbness, and paralysis may occur.

♦ ***Burns.*** Two days or less after injury, arm burns may cause mild to severe edema, pain, and tissue damage.

♦ ***Envenomation.*** Envenomation by snakes, aquatic animals, or insects may cause edema that begins around the bite or sting and quickly spreads to the entire arm. Pain, erythema, and pruritus at the site are common; paresthesia occurs occasionally. Later, the patient may develop generalized signs and symptoms, such as nausea, vomiting, weakness, muscle cramps, fever, chills, hypotension, headache or, in severe cases, dyspnea, seizures, or paralysis.

♦ ***Superior vena cava syndrome.*** Bilateral arm edema usually progresses slowly and is accompanied by edema of the face and neck and dilated veins in these edematous areas. The patient may report headache, vertigo, or visual disturbances.

♦ ***Thrombophlebitis.*** This disorder may cause arm edema, pain, and warmth. *Deep vein thrombophlebitis* can also cause cyanosis, fever, chills, and malaise; *superficial thrombophlebitis* also causes redness, tenderness, and induration along the vein.

Other causes

♦ ***Treatments.*** Localized arm edema may result from infiltration of I.V. fluid into the interstitial tissue. A radical or modified radical mastectomy that disrupts lymphatic drainage may cause edema of the entire arm, as can axillary lymph node dissection performed with lumpectomy. Also, radiation therapy for breast cancer may cause arm edema immediately after treatment or months later.

Special considerations

Treatment of the patient with arm edema varies according to the underlying cause. General care measures include elevation of the arm, frequent repositioning, and appropriate use of bandages and dressings to promote drainage and circulation. Be sure to provide patients with meticulous skin care to prevent breakdown and formation of pressure ulcers. In addition, give analgesics and anticoagulants as needed.

Pediatric pointers

Arm edema rarely occurs in children, except as part of generalized edema, but it may result from trauma, such as burns and crush injuries.

EDEMA OF THE FACE

Facial edema refers to either localized swelling—around the eyes, for instance—or more generalized swelling that may extend to the neck and upper arms. Occasionally painful, this sign may develop gradually or abruptly. Sometimes it precedes onset of peripheral or generalized edema. Mild edema may be difficult to detect; the patient or someone who's familiar with his appearance may report it before a clinician notices it.

Facial edema results from disruption of the hydrostatic and osmotic pressures that govern fluid movement between the arteries, veins, and lymphatics. (See *Understanding fluid balance,* page 224.) Possible causes include venous, inflammatory, and certain systemic disorders; trauma; allergy; malnutrition; or the effects of certain drugs, tests, and treatments.

Emergency interventions

If the patient has facial edema associated with burns or if he reports recent exposure to an allergen, quickly evaluate his respiratory status. Edema may also affect his upper airway, causing life-threatening obstruction. If you detect audible wheezing, inspiratory stridor, or other signs of respiratory distress, administer epinephrine.

Recognizing angioneurotic edema

Most dramatic in the lips, eyelids, and tongue, angioneurotic edema commonly results from an allergic reaction. It's characterized by rapid onset of painless, nonpitting, subcutaneous swelling that usually resolves in 1 to 2 days. This type of edema may also involve the hands, feet, genitalia, and viscera; laryngeal edema may cause life-threatening airway obstruction.

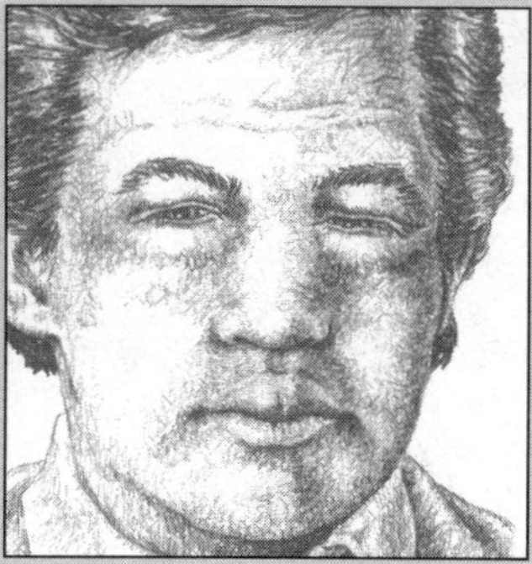

In severe distress — absent breath sounds and cyanosis — tracheal intubation, cricothyroidotomy, or tracheotomy may be required. Always administer oxygen.

History and physical examination

If the patient isn't in severe distress, take his health history. Ask if facial edema developed suddenly or gradually. Is it more prominent in the early morning, or does it worsen throughout the day? Has the patient noticed any weight gain? If so, how much and over what length of time? Has he noticed a change in his urine color or output? In his appetite? Take a drug history, and ask about recent facial trauma.

Begin the physical examination by characterizing the edema. Is it localized to one part of the face, or does it affect the entire face or other parts of the body? Determine if the edema is pitting or nonpitting, and grade its severity. (See *Edema: pitting or nonpitting?* page 225.) Next, take vital signs and assess neurologic status. Examine the oral cavity to evaluate dental hygiene and look for signs of infection. Inspect the oropharynx and look for soft-tissue swelling. (See *Recognizing angioneurotic edema.*)

Common medical causes

♦ ***Cavernous sinus thrombosis.*** This rare but serious disorder may begin with unilateral edema that quickly progresses to bilateral edema of the forehead, base of the nose, and eyelids. It may also cause chills, fever, headache, nausea, lethargy, exophthalmos, and eye pain.

♦ ***Chalazion.*** A chalazion causes localized swelling and tenderness of the affected eyelid, accompanied by a small red lump on the conjunctival surface.

♦ ***Conjunctivitis.*** This inflammation causes eyelid edema, excessive tearing, and itchy, burning eyes. Inspection reveals a thick purulent discharge, crusty eyelids, and conjunctival injection. Corneal involvement causes photophobia and pain.

♦ ***Dacryoadenitis.*** Severe periorbital swelling characterizes this disorder, which may also cause conjunctival injection, purulent discharge, and temporal pain.

♦ ***Dacryocystitis.*** Lacrimal sac inflammation causes prominent eyelid edema and constant tearing. In acute cases, pain and tenderness near the tear sac accompany purulent discharge.

♦ ***Facial burns.*** Burns may cause extensive edema that impairs respiration. Additional findings may include singed nasal hairs, red mucosa, sooty sputum, and signs of respiratory distress such as inspiratory stridor.

♦ ***Herpes zoster ophthalmicus (shingles).*** In this disorder, edematous and red eyelids are usually accompanied by excessive tearing and a serous discharge.

Severe unilateral facial pain may occur several days before vesicles erupt.

◆ ***Myxedema.*** This disorder eventually causes generalized facial edema, waxy dry skin, hair loss or coarsening, and other signs of hypothyroidism.

◆ ***Nephrotic syndrome.*** Commonly the first sign of nephrotic syndrome, periorbital edema precedes dependent and abdominal edema. Associated findings include weight gain, nausea, anorexia, lethargy, fatigue, and pallor.

◆ ***Orbital cellulitis.*** Sudden onset of periorbital edema marks this inflammatory disorder. It may be accompanied by a unilateral purulent discharge, hyperemia, exophthalmos, conjunctival injection, impaired extraocular movements, fever, and extreme orbital pain.

◆ ***Preeclampsia.*** Edema of the face, hands, and ankles is an early sign of this disorder of pregnancy. Other characteristics include excessive weight gain, severe headache, blurred vision, hypertension, and midepigastric pain.

◆ ***Rhinitis (allergic).*** In this disorder, red and edematous eyelids are accompanied by paroxysmal sneezing, itchy nose and eyes, and profuse, watery rhinorrhea. The patient may also develop nasal congestion, excessive tearing, headache, sinus pain, and sometimes malaise and fever.

◆ ***Sinusitis.*** *Frontal sinusitis* causes edema of the forehead and eyelids. *Maxillary sinusitis* causes edema in the maxillary area as well as malaise, gingival swelling, and trismus. Both types are also accompanied by facial pain, fever, nasal congestion, purulent nasal discharge, and red, swollen nasal mucosa.

◆ ***Trachoma.*** In this disorder, edema affects the eyelid and conjunctiva and is accompanied by eye pain, excessive tearing, photophobia, and eye discharge. Examination reveals an inflamed preauricular node and visible conjunctival follicles.

◆ ***Trichinosis.*** This relatively rare infectious disorder causes sudden onset of eyelid edema with fever (102° to 104° F [38.9° to 40° C]), conjunctivitis, muscle pain, itching and burning skin, sweating, skin lesions, and delirium.

Other causes

◆ ***Diagnostic tests.*** An allergic reaction to contrast media used in radiologic tests may cause facial edema.

◆ ***Drugs.*** Long-term use of glucocorticoids may cause facial edema. Any drug that causes an allergic reaction (aspirin, antipyretics, penicillin, and sulfa preparations, for example) may have the same effect.

◆ **Herb alert** Ingestion of the fruit pulp of *Ginkgo biloba* can cause severe erythema and edema and rapid formation of vesicles. Feverfew and *Chrysanthemum parthenium* can cause swelling of the lips, irritation of the tongue, and mouth ulcers. Licorice may cause facial edema and water retention or bloating, especially if ingested before menses.

◆ ***Surgery and transfusion.*** Cranial, nasal, or jaw surgery may cause facial edema, as may a blood transfusion that causes an allergic reaction.

Special considerations

Administer analgesics for pain, and apply creams to reduce itching. Unless contraindicated, apply cold compresses to the patient's eyes to decrease edema. Elevate the head of the bed to help drain the accumulated fluid. Urine and blood tests are commonly ordered to help diagnose the cause of facial edema.

Pediatric pointers

Normally, periorbital tissue pressure is lower in a child than in an adult. As a result, children are more likely to develop periorbital edema. In fact, periorbital edema is more common than peripheral edema in children with such disorders as heart failure and acute glomerulonephritis. Pertussis may also cause periorbital edema.

EDEMA OF THE LEG

This common sign results when excess interstitial fluid accumulates in one or both legs. It may affect just the foot and ankle or extend to the thigh and may be slight or dramatic, pitting or nonpitting.

Leg edema may result from venous disorders, trauma, and certain bone and cardiac disorders that disturb normal fluid balance. (See *Understanding fluid balance,* page 224.) However, several nonpathologic mechanisms may also cause mild leg edema occasionally. For example, prolonged sitting, standing, or immobility may cause bilateral orthostatic edema. This pitting edema usually affects the foot and disappears with rest and leg elevation. Increased venous pressure late in pregnancy may cause ankle edema.

History and physical examination

First ask how long the patient has had the edema. Did it develop suddenly or gradually? Does it decrease if he elevates his legs? Is it painful when touched or when he walks? Is it worse in the morning, or does it get progressively worse during the day? Ask about a recent leg injury or any recent surgery or illness that may have immobilized the patient. Does he have a history of cardiovascular disease? Finally, obtain a drug history.

Begin the physical examination by examining each leg for pitting edema. (See *Edema: pitting or nonpitting?* page 225.) Because leg edema can compromise arterial blood flow, palpate peripheral pulses to detect insufficiency. Observe leg color, and look for unusual vein patterns. Then palpate for warmth, tenderness, and cords, and gently squeeze the calf muscle against the tibia to check for deep pain. If leg edema is unilateral, try to elicit Homans' sign by dorsiflexing the foot; calf pain is the positive finding. Finally, note skin thickening or ulceration in the edematous areas.

Common medical causes

♦ ***Burns.*** Two days or less after injury, leg burns may cause mild to severe edema, pain, and tissue damage.

♦ ***Envenomation.*** Mild to severe localized edema may develop suddenly at the site of a bite or sting, with erythema, pain, urticaria, pruritus, or a burning sensation.

♦ ***Heart failure.*** Bilateral leg edema is an early sign of right-sided heart failure. Other effects may include weight gain despite anorexia, nausea, chest tightness, hypotension, pallor, tachypnea, palpitations, ventricular gallop, and inspiratory crackles. Pitting ankle edema, hepatomegaly, hemoptysis, and cyanosis signal more advanced heart failure.

♦ ***Leg trauma.*** Mild to severe localized edema may form around the trauma site.

♦ ***Osteomyelitis.*** When this bone infection affects the lower leg, it usually causes localized, mild to moderate edema that may spread to the adjacent joint. Edema typically follows fever, localized tenderness, and pain that increases with leg movement.

♦ ***Thrombophlebitis.*** Both deep and superficial vein thrombosis may cause unilateral mild to moderate edema. *Deep vein thrombophlebitis* may be asymptomatic or may cause mild to severe pain, warmth, and cyanosis in the affected leg as well as fever, chills, and malaise. *Superficial thrombophlebitis* typically causes pain, warmth, redness, tenderness, and induration along the affected vein.

♦ ***Venous insufficiency (chronic).*** Moderate to severe, unilateral or bilateral leg edema occurs in this disorder. Initially, the edema is soft and pitting; later, it becomes hard as tissues thicken. Other signs include darkened skin and painless, easily infected stasis ulcers around the ankle.

Other causes

♦ ***Coronary artery bypass surgery.*** Unilateral venous insufficiency may follow saphenous vein retrieval.

◆ ***Diagnostic tests.*** Venography is a rare cause of leg edema.

Special considerations

Provide analgesics as needed. Have the patient avoid prolonged sitting or standing, and elevate his legs as necessary. A compression boot (Unna's boot) may be used to help reduce edema. Monitor the patient's intake and output, and check weight and leg circumference daily to detect any change in the edema. Prepare him for diagnostic tests, such as blood and urine studies and X-rays.

Pediatric pointers

Uncommon in children, leg edema may result from osteomyelitis, leg trauma or, rarely, heart failure.

ENURESIS

Enuresis usually refers to nighttime urinary incontinence in a girl older than age 5 or a boy older than age 6; it's more common in boys. This sign rarely continues into adulthood. It may be classified as primary or secondary. A child who has never achieved bladder control is said to have *primary enuresis;* one who achieved bladder control for at least 3 months but lost it has *secondary enuresis.*

Among factors that may contribute to enuresis are delayed development of detrusor muscle control, unusually deep or sound sleep, organic disorders (such as urinary tract infection or obstruction), and psychological stress. Probably the most important factor, psychological stress commonly results from the birth of a sibling, the death of a parent or loved one, or premature, rigorous toilet training. The child may be too embarrassed or ashamed to discuss his bed-wetting, which intensifies psychological stress and makes enuresis more likely — thus creating a vicious cycle.

History and physical examination

When taking a history, include the parents as well as the child. First, determine the number of nights each week or month that the child wets the bed. Is there a family history of enuresis? Ask about the child's daily fluid intake. Does he drink much after supper? What are his typical sleep and voiding patterns? Has the child ever had control of his bladder? If so, try to pinpoint what may have precipitated enuresis, such as an organic disorder or psychological stress. Does the bed-wetting occur both at home and away from home? Ask the parents how they have tried to manage the problem, and have them describe the child's toilet training. Observe the child's and parents' attitudes toward bed-wetting. Finally, ask the child if it hurts when he urinates.

Next, perform a physical examination to detect signs of neurologic or urinary tract disorders. Observe the child's gait to assess for motor dysfunction, and test sensory function in his legs. Inspect the urethral meatus for erythema, and obtain a urine specimen. A rectal examination to evaluate sphincter control may be required.

Common medical causes

◆ ***Detrusor muscle hyperactivity.*** Involuntary detrusor muscle contractions may cause primary or secondary enuresis associated with urinary urgency, frequency, and incontinence. Signs and symptoms of urinary tract infection are also common.

◆ ***Urinary tract infection.*** In children, most urinary tract infections cause secondary enuresis. Associated features include urinary frequency and urgency, dysuria, straining to urinate, and hematuria. Lower back pain, fatigue, and suprapubic discomfort may also occur.

◆ ***Urinary tract obstruction.*** Although daytime incontinence is more common, this disorder may cause primary or secondary enuresis. It may also cause flank and lower back pain; upper abdominal distention; urinary frequency, urgency, hesitancy, and dribbling; dysuria; diminished urinary stream; hematuria; or variable urine output.

Special considerations

Provide emotional support to the child and his family. Encourage the parents to accept and support the child. Tell them how to manage enuresis at home.

If the child has detrusor muscle hyperactivity, bladder training may help control enuresis. An alarm device may be useful for a child older than age 8. This moisture-sensitive device fits in his mattress and triggers an alarm when made wet, waking the child. This device conditions him to avoid bed-wetting and should be used only if enuresis is having adverse psychological effects on the child. Pharmacologic treatment with imipramine, desmopressin, or an anticholinergic may be helpful.

EPISTAXIS

A common sign, epistaxis (nosebleed) can be spontaneous or induced from the front or back of the nose. Most nosebleeds occur in the anterior-inferior nasal septum (Kiesselbach's area), but they may also occur at the point where the inferior turbinates meet the nasopharynx. Usually unilateral, they seem bilateral when blood runs from the bleeding side behind the nasal septum and out the opposite side. Epistaxis ranges from mild oozing to severe — possibly life-threatening — blood loss.

A rich supply of fragile blood vessels makes the nose particularly vulnerable to bleeding. Air moving through the nose can dry and irritate the mucous membranes, forming crusts that bleed when they're removed; dry mucous membranes are also more susceptible to infections, which can cause epistaxis as well. Trauma is another common cause of epistaxis. Additional causes include septal deviations; hematologic, coagulation, renal, and GI disorders; and certain drugs and treatments.

Emergency interventions

If your patient has severe epistaxis, quickly take his vital signs. Be alert for tachypnea, hypotension, and other signs of hypovolemic shock. Insert a large-gauge I.V. line for rapid fluid and blood replacement, and attempt to control bleeding by pinching the nares closed. (However, if you suspect a nasal fracture, *don't* pinch the nares. Instead, place gauze under the patient's nose to absorb the blood.)

Have a hypovolemic patient lie down and turn his head to the side to prevent blood from draining down the back of his throat, which could cause aspiration or vomiting of swallowed blood. If the patient isn't hypovolemic, have him sit upright and tilt his head forward. Constantly check airway patency. If the patient's condition is unstable, begin cardiac monitoring and give supplemental oxygen by mask.

History and physical examination

If your patient isn't in distress, take a history. Does he have a history of recent trauma? How often has he had nosebleeds in the past? On which side did the bleeding begin? How long has he been bleeding? Have the nosebleeds been long or unusually severe? Has the patient recently had surgery in the sinus area? Ask about a history of hypertension, bleeding or liver disorders, and other recent illnesses. Ask if the patient bruises easily. Find out what drugs he uses, especially anti-inflammatories such as aspirin and anticoagulants such as warfarin sodium.

Begin the physical examination by inspecting the patient's skin for other signs of bleeding, such as ecchymoses and petechiae, and noting jaundice, pallor, or other abnormalities. When examining a trauma patient, look for associated injuries, such as eye trauma or facial fractures.

Common medical causes

♦ ***Aplastic anemia.*** This disorder develops insidiously, eventually producing nosebleeds as well as ecchymoses, retinal hemorrhages, menorrhagia, petechiae, bleeding from the mouth, and signs of GI bleeding. Fatigue, dyspnea, headache, tachycardia, and pallor may also occur.

♦ ***Barotrauma.*** Commonly seen in airline passengers and scuba divers, barotrauma may cause severe, painful epistaxis in a patient with an upper respiratory infection.

♦ ***Chemical irritants.*** Some chemicals, including phosphorus, sulfuric acid, ammonia, printer's ink, and chromates, irritate the nasal mucosa, producing epistaxis.

♦ ***Coagulation disorders.*** Such disorders as hemophilia and thrombocytopenic purpura can cause epistaxis as well as with ecchymoses, petechiae, and bleeding from the gums, mouth, or I.V. puncture sites. Menorrhagia and signs of GI bleeding, such as melena and hematemesis, can also occur.

♦ ***Glomerulonephritis (chronic).*** This disorder causes nosebleeds as well as hypertension, proteinuria, hematuria, headache, edema, oliguria, hemoptysis, nausea, vomiting, pruritus, dyspnea, malaise, and fatigue.

♦ ***Hepatitis.*** When hepatitis interferes with the clotting mechanism, epistaxis and abnormal bleeding tendencies can result. Associated signs and symptoms typically include jaundice, clay-colored stools, pruritus, hepatomegaly, abdominal pain, fever, fatigue, weakness, dark amber urine, anorexia, nausea, and vomiting.

♦ ***Hypertension.*** Severe hypertension can cause extreme epistaxis, usually in the posterior nose, with pulsation above the middle turbinate. It may be accompanied by dizziness, a throbbing headache, anxiety, peripheral edema, nocturia, nausea, vomiting, drowsiness, and mental impairment.

♦ ***Leukemia.*** In *acute leukemia,* sudden epistaxis is accompanied by a high fever and other types of abnormal bleeding, such as bleeding gums, ecchymoses, petechiae, easy bruising, and prolonged menses. These may follow less noticeable signs, such as weakness, lassitude, pallor, chills, recurrent infections, and low-grade fever. Acute leukemia may also cause dyspnea, fatigue, malaise, tachycardia, palpitations, a systolic ejection murmur, or abdominal or bone pain.

In *chronic leukemia,* epistaxis is a late sign that may be accompanied by other types of abnormal bleeding, extreme fatigue, weight loss, hepatosplenomegaly, bone tenderness, edema, macular or nodular skin lesions, pallor, weakness, dyspnea, tachycardia, palpitations, or headache.

♦ ***Nasal fracture.*** Unilateral or bilateral epistaxis occurs with nasal swelling, periorbital ecchymoses and edema, pain, nasal deformity, and crepitation of the nasal bones.

♦ ***Polycythemia vera.*** A common sign of polycythemia vera, spontaneous epistaxis may be accompanied by bleeding gums; ecchymoses; ruddy cyanosis of the face, nose, ears, and lips; and congestion of the conjunctiva, retina, and oral mucous membranes. Other signs and symptoms vary according to the affected body system; they may include headache, dizziness, tinnitus, visual disturbances, hypertension, chest pain, intermittent claudication, early satiety and fullness, marked splenomegaly, epigastric pain, pruritus, or dyspnea.

♦ ***Sarcoidosis.*** Oozing epistaxis may occur with a nonproductive cough, substernal pain, malaise, and weight loss. Related findings include tachycardia, arrhythmias, parotid enlargement, cervical lymphadenopathy, skin lesions, hepatosplenomegaly, and arthritis in the ankles, knees, and wrists.

♦ ***Scleroma.*** Oozing epistaxis occurs with a watery nasal discharge that becomes foul-smelling and crusty. Progressive anosmia and turbinate atrophy may also occur.

♦ ***Sinusitis (acute).*** A bloody or blood-tinged nasal discharge may become purulent and copious after 24 to 48 hours. Associated signs and symptoms include

Controlling epistaxis with nasal packing

When direct pressure and cautery fail to control epistaxis, nasal packing may be required.

Anterior packing may be used if the patient has severe bleeding in the anterior nose. Horizontal layers of petroleum gauze strips are inserted into the nostrils near the turbinates.

Posterior packing may be needed if the patient has severe bleeding in the posterior nose or if blood from anterior bleeding starts flowing backward. This type of packing consists of a gauze pack secured by three strong silk sutures. After the nose is anesthetized, sutures are pulled through the nostrils with a soft catheter and the pack is positioned behind the soft palate. Two of the sutures are tied to a gauze roll under the patient's nose, which keeps the pack in place. The third suture is taped to his cheek. Instead of a gauze pack, an indwelling urinary or nasal epistaxis catheter may be inserted through the nose into the area behind the soft palate and inflated with 10 ml of water to compress the bleeding point.

PRECAUTIONS

If the patient has nasal packing, follow these guidelines:

◆ Watch for signs of respiratory distress, such as dyspnea, which may occur if the packing slips and obstructs the airway.

◆ Keep emergency equipment (flashlights, scissors, and hemostat) at the patient's bedside. Expect to cut the cheek suture (or deflate the catheter) and remove the pack at the first sign of airway obstruction.

◆ Avoid tension on the cheek suture, which could cause the posterior pack to slip out of place.

◆ Keep the call bell within easy reach.

◆ Monitor vital signs frequently. Watch for signs of hypoxia, such as tachycardia and restlessness.

◆ Elevate the head of the patient's bed, and remind him to breathe through his mouth.

◆ Administer humidified oxygen as needed.

◆ Instruct the patient *not* to blow his nose for 48 hours after the packing is removed.

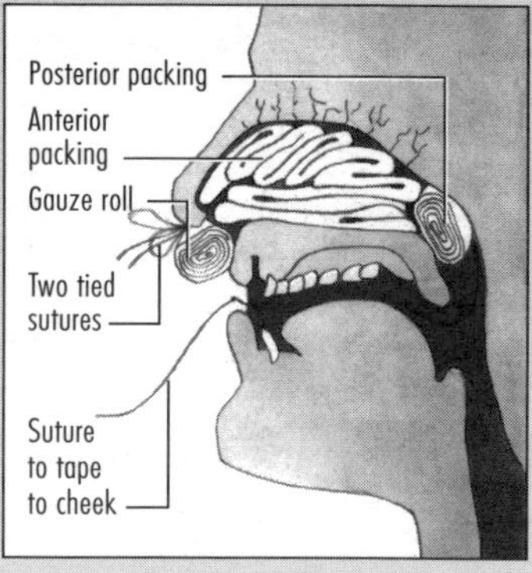

nasal congestion, pain, tenderness, malaise, headache, low-grade fever, and red, edematous nasal mucosa.

◆ ***Skull fracture.*** Depending on the type of fracture, epistaxis can be direct (when blood flows directly down the nares) or indirect (when blood drains through the eustachian tube and into the nose). Abrasions, contusions, lacerations, or avulsions are common. A severe skull fracture may cause severe headache, decreased level of consciousness, hemiparesis, dizziness, seizures, projectile vomiting, and decreased pulse and respiratory rates.

A *basilar fracture* may also cause bleeding from the pharynx, ears, and conjunctiva as well as raccoon eyes and Battle's sign. Cerebrospinal fluid or even brain tissue may leak from the nose or ears. A *sphenoid fracture* may also cause blindness, whereas a *temporal fracture* may also cause unilateral deafness or facial paralysis.

◆ ***Systemic lupus erythematosus (SLE).*** Usually affecting women under age 50, SLE causes oozing epistaxis. More characteristic signs and symptoms include butterfly rash, lymphadenopathy, joint pain and stiffness, anorexia, nausea, vomiting, myalgia, and weight loss.

Other causes

◆ ***Drugs.*** Anticoagulants such as Coumadin and anti-inflammatories, such as aspirin, can cause epistaxis.

◆ ***Surgery and procedures.*** Rarely, epistaxis results from facial and nasal surgery, including septoplasty, rhinoplasty, antrostomy, endoscopic sinus procedures, orbital decompression, and dental extraction.

Special considerations

Until the bleeding is completely under control, continue to monitor the patient for signs of hypovolemic shock, such as tachycardia and clammy skin. If external pressure doesn't control the bleeding, measures to control anterior bleeding include inserting a peldget soaked in vasoconstrictor and local anesthetic and pinching the patient's nostril for several minutes. This site can then be cauterized with silver nitrate for 30 seconds after removal of the pledget.

If bleeding persists, expect to insert anterior or posterior nasal packing. (See *Controlling epistaxis with nasal packing.*) Administer humidified oxygen by face mask to a patient with posterior packing.

A complete blood count may be ordered to evaluate blood loss and detect anemia. Clotting studies, such as prothrombin time and activated partial thromboplastin time, may be required to test coagulation time. Prepare the patient for X-rays if he has had a recent trauma.

Pediatric pointers

Children are more likely to experience anterior nosebleeds, usually the result of nose-picking or allergic rhinitis. Biliary atresia, cystic fibrosis, hereditary afibrinogenemia, and nasal trauma due to a foreign body can also cause epistaxis. Rubeola may cause an oozing nosebleed along with the characteristic maculopapular rash. Two rare childhood diseases — pertussis and diphtheria — can also cause oozing epistaxis.

Suspect a bleeding disorder if you see excess umbilical cord bleeding at birth or profuse bleeding during circumcision. Epistaxis frequently begins at puberty in a patient with hereditary hemorrhagic telangiectasia.

Geriatric pointers

Elderly patients are more likely to have posterior nosebleeds.

ERYTHEMA

[Erythroderma]

Dilated or congested blood vessels cause red skin, or erythema, the most common sign of skin inflammation or irritation. Erythema may be localized or generalized and may occur suddenly or gradually. Skin color can range from bright red in acute conditions to pale violet or brown in chronic problems. Erythema must be differentiated from purpura, which causes redness from bleeding into the skin. When pressure is applied directly to the skin, erythema blanches momentarily, but purpura doesn't

Erythema usually results from changes in the arteries, veins, and small vessels that lead to increased small-vessel perfusion. Drugs and neurogenic mechanisms can also allow extra blood to enter the small vessels. In addition, erythema can result from trauma and tissue damage as well as from changes in supporting tissues, which increase vessel visibility.

Emergency interventions

If your patient has sudden progressive erythema with rapid pulse, dyspnea, hoarseness, and agitation, quickly take his vital signs. These may be signs of anaphylactic shock. Provide emergency respiratory support and give epinephrine immediately.

History and physical examination

If erythema isn't associated with anaphylaxis, obtain a detailed health history. Find out how long the patient has had the erythema and where it first began. Has he had any associated pain or itching? Has he recently had a fever, upper respiratory infection, or joint pain? Does he have a history of skin disease or other illness? Does he or anyone in his family have allergies, asthma, or eczema? Has he been exposed to someone who has had a similar rash or who is now ill?

Obtain a complete drug history, including recent immunizations. Ask about food intake and exposure to chemicals.

Begin the physical examination by assessing the extent, distribution, and intensity of erythema. Look for edema and other skin lesions, such as hives, scales, papules, and purpura. Examine the affected area for warmth; gently palpate it to check for tenderness or crepitus.

Common medical causes

♦ ***Allergic reactions.*** Foods, drugs, chemicals, and other allergens can cause an allergic reaction and erythema. A *localized allergic reaction* also causes hive-like eruptions and edema.

Anaphylaxis, a life-threatening condition, causes relatively sudden erythema in the form of urticaria. It also causes flushing; facial edema; diaphoresis; weakness; sneezing; bronchospasm with dyspnea and tachypnea; shock with hypotension and cool, clammy skin; and possibly airway edema with hoarseness and stridor.

♦ ***Burns.*** In *thermal burns,* erythema and swelling appear first; deep or superficial blisters and other signs of damage that vary with the severity of the burn may follow. *Burns from ultraviolet rays* such as sunburn cause delayed erythema and tenderness on exposed areas of the skin.

♦ ***Dermatitis.*** Erythema commonly occurs in this family of inflammatory disorders. In *atopic dermatitis,* erythema and intense pruritus precede the development of small papules that may redden, weep, scale, and lichenify. These occur most commonly at skin folds of the extremities, neck, and eyelids.

Contact dermatitis occurs after exposure to an irritant. It quickly causes erythema and vesicles, blisters, or ulcerations on exposed skin.

In *seborrheic dermatitis,* dull red or yellow lesions accompany erythema. Sharply marginated, these lesions are sometimes ring-shaped and covered with greasy scales. They usually occur on the scalp, eyebrows, ears, and nasolabial folds, but they may form a butterfly rash on the face or spread to the chest or to skin folds on the trunk. This disorder is common in patients infected with the human immunodeficiency virus.

♦ ***Dermatomyositis.*** This disorder, most common in women over age 50, causes a dusky lilac rash on the face, neck, upper torso, and nail beds. Gottron's papules (violet, flat-topped lesions) may appear on finger joints.

♦ ***Erythema annulare centrifugum.*** Small, pink infiltrated papules appear on the trunk, buttocks, and inner thighs, slowly spreading at the margins and clearing in the center. Itching, scaling, and tissue hardening may occur.

♦ ***Erythema marginatum rheumaticum.*** Associated with rheumatic fever, this disorder causes erythematous lesions that are superficial, flat, and slightly hardened. They spread rapidly, and may last for hours or days, recurring after a time.

♦ ***Erythema multiforme.*** *Erythema multiforme major* (Stevens-Johnson syndrome) causes sudden hivelike erythema with blisters and pathognomic petechial or "iris" lesions that usually appear symmetrically and bilaterally on the face, hands, and feet. Erythema is characteristically preceded by blisters on the lips, tongue, and buccal mucosa; a thick, gray film over the mucous membranes; increased salivation; and an extremely sore throat.

Other early signs may include cough, vomiting, diarrhea, corneal ulcers, conjunctival injection with a copious purulent discharge, coryza, epistaxis, and severe inflammation of the urethra, vagina, and anus. Fever may range from 102° to 104° F (38.9° to 40° C). Tachypnea; a rapid, weak pulse; chest pain; malaise; and muscle and joint pain may also occur.

Erythematous macules and papules, purpura, and occasional blisters occur in *erythema multiforme minor.* Characteristic urticarial iris lesions may burn or itch slightly; they usually appear in groups and last for 2 to 3 weeks. After 1 week, individual lesions become flat or hyperpigmented. Early signs and symptoms may include a mild fever, cough, and sore throat.

Usually of unknown etiology, erythema multiforme can occur secondary to drug reactions or to infections, such as herpes simplex virus and mycoplasma.

♦ ***Erythema nodosum.*** Sudden bilateral eruption of tender erythematous nodules characterizes this disorder. The firm, round, protruding lesions usually appear in groups on the shins, knees, and ankles but may occur on the buttocks, arms, calves, and trunk as well. Other manifestations include mild fever, chills, malaise, muscle and joint pain and, possibly, swollen feet and ankles. Erythema nodosum is associated with various diseases, most notably inflammatory bowel disease, sarcoidosis, tuberculosis, and streptococcal or fungal infections.

♦ ***Lupus erythematosus.*** Both discoid and systemic lupus erythematosus (SLE) can cause a characteristic butterfly rash. This erythematous eruption may range from a blush with swelling to a scaly, sharply demarcated, macular rash with plaques that may spread to the forehead, chin, ears, chest, and other sun-exposed parts of the body.

In *discoid lupus erythematosus,* telangiectasia, hyperpigmentation, ear and nose deformity, and mouth, tongue, and eyelid lesions may occur.

In *SLE,* acute onset of erythema may also be accompanied by photosensitivity and mucous membrane ulcers, especially in the nose and mouth. Mottled erythema may occur on the hands, with edema around the nails and macular reddish purple lesions on the fingers. Telangiectasia occurs at the base of the nails or eyelids, along with purpura, petechiae, ecchymoses, and urticaria. Joint pain and stiffness are common. Other findings vary according to the body systems affected but typically include low-grade fever, malaise, weakness, headache, arthralgia, arthritis, depression, lymphadenopathy, fatigue, weight loss, anorexia, nausea, vomiting, diarrhea, and constipation.

♦ ***Psoriasis.*** Silvery white scales over a thickened erythematous base usually affect the elbows, knees, chest, scalp, and intergluteal folds. The fingernails may become thick and pitted.

♦ ***Raynaud's disease.*** Typically, the skin on hands and feet blanches and cools after exposure to cold and stress. Later, it becomes warm and purplish red.

♦ ***Rosacea.*** Scattered erythema initially develops across the center of the face, followed by superficial telangiectases, papules, pustules, and nodules. Rhinophyma may occur on the lower half of the nose.

♦ ***Rubella.*** Typically, flat solitary lesions join to form a blotchy pink erythematous rash that spreads rapidly to the trunk and extremities in this disorder. Occasionally, small red lesions (Forschheimer spots) occur on the soft palate. Lesions clear in 4 to 5 days. The rash usually follows fever (up to 102° F [38.9° C]), headache, malaise, sore throat, a gritty eye sensation, lymphadenopathy, pain in the joints, and coryza.

Drugs associated with erythema

Suspect drug-induced erythema in any patient who develops this sign within 1 week of starting a medication. Erythematous lesions can vary in size, shape, type, and amount, but they almost always appear suddenly and symmetrically on the trunk and inner arms. These drugs can produce erythematous lesions:

allopurinol	co-trimoxazole	isoniazid	phenytoin
anticoagulants	diazepam	lithium	quinidine
antimetabolites	erythromycin	nitrofurantoin	salicylates
barbiturates	gentamicin	oral contraceptives	sulfonamides
cephalosporins	gold	penicillin	sulfonylureas
chlordiazepoxide	griseofulvin	phenolphthalein	tetracyclines
codeine	indomethacin	phenothiazines	thiazides
corticosteroids	iodide bromides	phenylbutazone	

Some of these drugs — particularly barbiturates, oral contraceptives, phenolphthalein, phenylbutazone, salicylates, sulfonamides, and tetracycline — can cause a "fixed" drug eruption. In this type of reaction, lesions can appear in any body part and flake off after a few days, leaving a brownish purple pigmentation. Repeated drug administration causes the original lesions to recur and new ones to develop.

Other causes

◆ ***Drugs.*** Many drugs commonly cause erythema. (See *Drugs associated with erythema.*)

◆ **Herb alert** Ingestion of the fruit pulp of *Ginkgo biloba* can cause severe erythema and edema of the mouth and rapid formation of vesicles. St. John's wort can cause heightened sun sensitivity, resulting in erythema or sunburn.

◆ ***Radiation and other treatments.*** Radiation therapy may cause dull erythema and edema within 24 hours. As the erythema fades, the skin becomes light brown and mildly scaly. Any treatment that causes an allergic reaction can also cause erythema.

Special considerations

Because erythema can cause fluid loss, closely monitor and replace fluids and electrolytes, especially in patients with burns or widespread erythema. Be sure to withhold all medications until the cause of the erythema has been identified. Then expect to administer antibiotics and topical or systemic corticosteroids.

For the patient with itching skin, expect to give soothing baths or apply open wet dressings containing starch, bran, or sodium bicarbonate; also administer antihistamines and analgesics as needed. Advise a patient with leg erythema to keep his legs elevated above heart level. For a burn patient with erythema, immerse the affected area in cold water, or apply towels soaked in cold water to reduce pain, edema, and erythema.

Prepare the patient for diagnostic tests, such as skin biopsy to detect cancerous lesions, cultures to identify infectious organisms, and sensitivity studies to confirm allergies.

Pediatric pointers

Normally, newborn rash (erythema toxicum neonatorum), a pink papular rash, develops during the first 4 days after birth and spontaneously disappears by the 10th day. Newborns and infants can also develop erythema from infections and other disorders. For instance, candidiasis can cause thick white lesions over an erythematous base on the oral mucosa as well as diaper rash with beefy red erythema.

Roseola, rubeola, scarlet fever, granuloma annulare, and cutis marmorata also cause erythema in children.

Geriatric pointers

Elderly patients commonly have well-demarcated purple macules or patches, usually on the back of the hands and on the forearms. Known as actinic purpura, this condition results from blood leaking through fragile capillaries. The lesions disappear spontaneously.

Exophthalmos

[Proptosis]

Exophthalmos — the abnormal protrusion of one or both eyeballs — may result from hemorrhage, edema, or inflammation behind the eye; extraocular muscle relaxation; or space-occupying intraorbital lesions and metastatic tumors. It may also result from cavernous sinus thrombosis or from enlargement of the eyeball due to congenital glaucoma and unilateral high myopia. This sign may occur suddenly or gradually, causing mild to dramatic protrusion. Occasionally, the affected eye also pulsates. The most common cause of exophthalmos in adults is dysthyroid eye disease.

Exophthalmos is usually easily observed. However, lid retraction may mimic exophthalmos even when protrusion is absent. Similarly, ptosis in one eye may make the other eye appear exophthalmic by comparison. An exophthalmometer can differentiate these signs by measuring ocular protrusion.

History and physical examination

Begin by asking when the patient first noticed exophthalmos. Is it associated with pain in or around the eye? If so, how severe is it, and how long has he had it? Sudden unilateral onset is usually due to hemorrhage or inflammation of the orbit or paranasal sinuses. Then ask about recent sinus infection or vision problems. Take the patient's vital signs, noting fever, which may accompany eye infection. Next, evaluate the severity of exophthalmos with an exophthalmometer. (See *Detecting unilateral exophthalmos,* page 240.) If the eyes bulge severely, look for cloudiness on the cornea, which may indicate ulcer formation. Exposure of the globe of the eye may lead to corneal drying and infection as well as ulceration. Describe any eye discharge and observe for ptosis. Then check visual acuity, with and without correction, and evaluate extraocular movements. Visual acuity usually isn't affected unless the causative lesion arises from the optic nerve. If thyroid studies confirm normal thyroid function, a computed tomography scan or magnetic resonance imaging should be ordered to look for the cause.

On physical examination, small degrees of exophthalmos are most easily detected by standing behind the seated patient and looking down to compare the position of the two corneas.

EXAMINATION TIP

Detecting unilateral exophthalmos

If one of the patient's eyes seems more prominent than the other, examine both eyes from above the patient's head. Look down across his face, gently draw his lids up, and compare the relationship of the corneas to the lower lids. Abnormal protrusion of one eye suggests unilateral exophthalmos.

Remember: Do *not* perform this test if you suspect eye trauma.

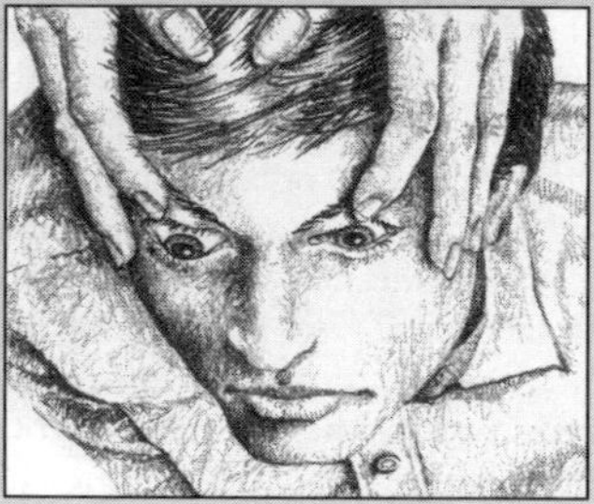

Common medical causes

◆ ***Cavernous sinus thrombosis.*** Usually, this disorder causes sudden onset of pulsating, unilateral exophthalmos. Accompanying it may be eyelid edema, decreased or absent pupillary reflexes, and impaired extraocular movement and visual acuity. Other features may include high fever with chills, papilledema, headache, nausea, vomiting, somnolence and, rarely, seizures.

◆ ***Dacryoadenitis.*** Unilateral, slowly progressive exophthalmos is the most common sign of dacryoadenitis. Assessment may also reveal limited extraocular movements (especially on elevation and abduction), ptosis, eyelid edema and erythema, conjunctival injection, eye pain, and diplopia.

◆ ***Foreign body in the eye.*** When a foreign body enters the eye, exophthalmos may accompany other signs and symptoms of ocular trauma, such as eye pain, redness, and tearing.

◆ ***Hemangioma.*** Most common in young adults, this orbital tumor causes progressive exophthalmos, which may be mild or severe and unilateral or bilateral. Other signs and symptoms may include ptosis, limited extraocular movements, and blurred vision.

◆ ***Lacrimal gland tumor.*** Exophthalmos usually develops slowly in one eye, causing its downward displacement toward the nose. The patient may also have ptosis and eye deviation and pain.

◆ ***Leiomyosarcoma.*** Most common in people older than age 45, this tumor is characterized by slowly developing, unilateral exophthalmos. Other effects include diplopia, impaired vision, and intermittent eye pain.

◆ ***Mucormycosis.*** This fungal infection of the orbit usually occurs in patients who have diabetes mellitus or are immunocompromised. It causes ischemic necrosis that manifests as pain and exophthalmos.

◆ ***Orbital choristoma.*** A common sign of this benign tumor, progressive exophthalmos may be associated with diplopia and blurred vision.

◆ ***Orbital emphysema.*** Air leaking from the sinus into the orbit usually causes unilateral exophthalmos. Palpation of the globe elicits crepitation.

◆ ***Parasite infestation.*** Usually, this disorder causes painless, progressive exophthalmos that begins in one eye and may spread to the other. Associated findings include limited extraocular movement, diplopia, eye pain, and impaired visual acuity.

◆ ***Scleritis (posterior).*** Gradual onset of mild to severe unilateral exophthalmos is common in patients with scleritis. Other signs and symptoms include severe eye pain, diplopia, papilledema, limited extraocular movement, and impaired visual acuity.

♦ ***Thyrotoxicosis.*** Although a classic sign of this disorder, exophthalmos is absent in many patients. It's usually bilateral, progressive, and severe. Associated ocular features include ptosis, increased tearing, lid lag and edema, photophobia, conjunctival injection, diplopia, and decreased visual acuity. Other findings include an enlarged thyroid, nervousness, heat intolerance, weight loss despite increased appetite, sweating, diarrhea, tremors, palpitations, and tachycardia.

Special considerations

Exophthalmos usually makes the patient self-conscious, so provide privacy and emotional support. Protect the affected eye from trauma, especially drying of the cornea. However, *never* place a gauze eye pad or other object over the affected eye; removal could damage the corneal epithelium. If a slit-lamp examination is indicated, explain the procedure to the patient. If necessary, refer him to an ophthalmologist for a complete examination. Etiology determines therapy.

Pediatric pointers

In children around age 5, a rare tumor—optic nerve glioma—may cause exophthalmos. Rhabdomyosarcoma, a more common tumor, usually affects children between ages 4 and 12 and causes rapid onset of exophthalmos. In Hand-Schüller-Christian syndrome, exophthalmos typically accompanies signs of diabetes insipidus and bone destruction. Most commonly, however, in children, orbital infection or tumor should be suspected.

EYE DISCHARGE

Usually associated with conjunctivitis, an eye discharge is the excretion of any substance other than tears. This common sign may occur in one or both eyes, producing scant to copious discharge. The discharge may be purulent, frothy, mucoid, cheesy, serous, or clear or stringy and white. Sometimes, the discharge can be expressed by applying pressure to the tear sac, punctum, meibomian glands, or canaliculus. (See *Sources of eye discharge,* page 242.)

An eye discharge commonly results from inflammatory or infectious eye disorders but may also occur in certain systemic disorders. Because this sign may accompany a disorder that threatens vision, it must be assessed and treated immediately.

History and physical examination

Begin your evaluation by finding out when the discharge began. Does it occur at certain times of day or in connection with certain activities? If the patient complains of pain, ask him to show you its exact location and to describe its character. Is the pain dull, continuous, sharp, or stabbing? Do his eyes itch or burn? Do they tear excessively? Are they sensitive to light? Does he feel like something is in them?

After taking vital signs, carefully inspect the eye; note the amount and consistency of the discharge. Then test visual acuity with and without correction. Examine external eye structures, beginning with the unaffected eye to prevent cross-contamination. Observe for eyelid edema, entropion, crusts, lesions, and trichiasis. Next, ask the patient to blink as you watch for impaired lid movement. If the eyes seem to bulge, measure them with an exophthalmometer. Test the six cardinal fields of gaze. Examine for conjunctival injection and follicles and for corneal cloudiness or white lesions.

Common medical causes

♦ ***Conjunctivitis.*** Five types of conjunctivitis may cause an eye discharge with redness, hyperemia, foreign-body sensation, periocular edema, and tearing.

EXAMINATION TIP

Sources of eye discharge

An eye discharge can come from the tear sac, punctum, meibomian glands, or canaliculi. If the patient reports a discharge that isn't immediately apparent, you can express a sample by pressing your fingertip lightly over these structures. Then characterize the discharge and note its source.

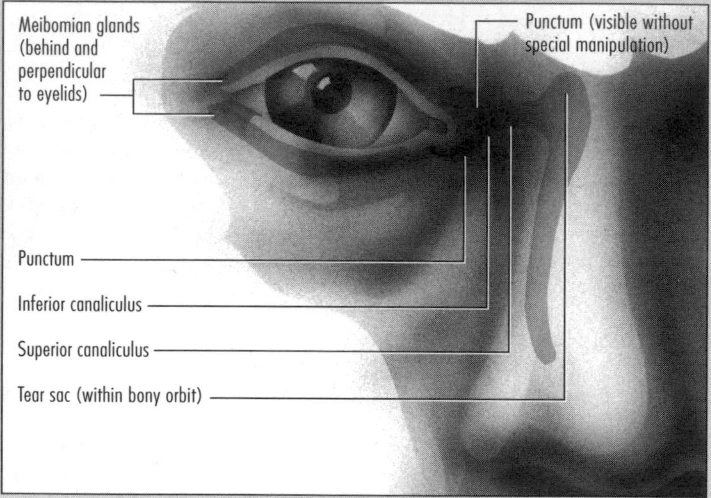

In *allergic conjunctivitis,* a bilateral stringy discharge is accompanied by itching and tearing.

Bacterial conjunctivitis causes a moderate purulent or mucopurulent discharge that may form sticky crusts on the eyelids during sleep. The discharge is commonly greenish white and usually occurs in one eye. The patient may also experience itching, burning, excessive tearing, and the sensation of a foreign body in the eye. Eye pain indicates corneal involvement. Preauricular adenopathy is uncommon.

Viral conjunctivitis is generally more common than the bacterial form. A serous, clear discharge and preauricular adenopathy are usually present. The history includes runny nose, upper respiratory infection, or recent contact with a person who had these symptoms. Onset is usually unilateral.

Fungal conjunctivitis causes a copious, thick, purulent discharge that makes the eyelids crusty and sticky. Patients may complain that their eyes are stuck together upon awakening from sleep. Also characteristic are eyelid edema, itching, burning, and tearing. Pain and photophobia occur only with corneal involvement.

Inclusion conjunctivitis causes scant mucoid discharge — especially in the morning — in both eyes, accompanied by pseudoptosis and conjunctival follicles.

♦ ***Corneal ulcers.*** Both bacterial and fungal ulcers cause a copious, purulent unilateral eye discharge. Related findings are crusty, sticky eyelids and, possibly, severe pain, photophobia, and impaired visual acuity. *Bacterial corneal ulcers* are also characterized by an irregular gray-white area on the cornea, blurred vision, unilateral pupil constriction, and conjunctival injection.

Fungal corneal ulcers are also characterized by conjunctival injection and eyelid edema and erythema. A painless, dense, whitish gray central ulcer develops slowly and may be surrounded by progressively clearer rings.

♦ ***Erythema multiforme major (Stevens-Johnson syndrome).*** A purulent discharge characterizes this disorder. Other ocular effects may include severe eye pain, entropion, trichiasis, photophobia, and decreased tear formation. Also typical are erythematous, urticarial, bullous lesions that suddenly erupt over the skin.

♦ ***Herpes zoster ophthalmicus.*** This disorder yields a moderate to copious serous eye discharge accompanied by excessive tearing. Examination reveals eyelid edema and erythema, conjunctival injection, and a white, cloudy cornea. The patient also complains of eye pain and severe unilateral facial pain that occurs several days before vesicles erupt.

♦ ***Keratoconjunctivitis sicca.*** Better known as dry eye syndrome, this disorder typically causes excessive, continuous mucoid discharge and insufficient tearing. Accompanying signs and symptoms may include eye pain, itching, burning, a foreign-body sensation, and dramatic conjunctival injection. The patient may also have difficulty closing his eyes.

♦ ***Meibomianitis.*** This disorder may cause a continuous frothy eye discharge. Applying pressure on the meibomian glands yields a soft, foul-smelling, cheesy yellow discharge. The eyes also appear chronically red, with inflamed lid margins.

♦ ***Orbital cellulitis.*** Although exophthalmos is the most obvious sign of this disorder, a unilateral purulent eye discharge may also be present. Related findings include eyelid edema, conjunctival injection, headache, orbital pain, impaired visual acuity, limited extraocular movement, and fever.

♦ ***Psoriasis vulgaris.*** Usually, psoriasis vulgaris causes a substantial mucus discharge in both eyes, accompanied by redness. Its characteristic lesions on the eyelids may extend into the conjunctiva, causing irritation, excessive tearing, and a foreign-body sensation.

♦ ***Trachoma.*** A bilateral eye discharge occurs in this disorder along with severe pain, excessive tearing, photophobia, eyelid edema, redness, and visible conjunctival follicles.

Special considerations

Apply warm soaks to soften crusts on eyelids and lashes, then gently wipe the eyes with a soft gauze pad. Carefully dispose of all used dressings, tissues, and cotton swabs to prevent the spread of infection. Teach the patient how to avoid contaminating the unaffected eye. Also, be sure to sterilize ophthalmic equipment after use.

Explain any ordered diagnostic tests, including culture and sensitivity studies to identify infectious organisms.

Hyperpurulent conjunctivitis with a copious purulent discharge suggests a gonococcal infection and warrants conjunctival cultures and an ophthalmic consultation. Gonococcal hyperpurulent conjunctivitis is a serious, potentially blinding disease.

Pediatric pointers

In infants, prophylactic eye medication (silver nitrate) frequently causes eye irritation and discharge. However, in children, discharges usually result from eye trauma, eye infection, or upper respiratory infection.

EYE PAIN
[Ophthalmalgia]

Eye pain may be described as a burning, throbbing, aching, or stabbing sensation in or around the eye. It may also be characterized as a foreign-body sensation. This sign varies from mild to severe; its duration and exact location provide clues to the causative disorder.

Eye pain usually results from corneal abrasion, but it may also be due to glaucoma or other eye disorders, trauma, and neurologic or systemic disorders. Any of these may stimulate nerve endings in the cornea or external eye, producing pain. Eye pain may result from a febrile illness, sinusitis, or endocrine eye lesions of thyrotoxicosis.

Emergency interventions

If the patient's eye pain results from a chemical burn, remove contact lenses, if present, and irrigate the eye with at least 1 L of normal saline solution over 10 minutes. Evert the lids and wipe the fornices with a cotton-tipped applicator to remove any particles or chemicals.

History and physical examination

If the patient's eye pain doesn't result from a chemical burn, take a complete history. Have the patient describe the pain fully. Is it an ache or a sharp pain? How long does it last? Is it accompanied by burning or itching? When did it begin? Is it worse in the morning or late in the evening? Ask about recent trauma or surgery, especially if the patient complains of sudden, severe pain. Does he have headaches? If so, find out how often and at what time of day they occur.

During the physical examination, *don't* manipulate the eye if you suspect trauma. Carefully assess the lids and conjunctiva for redness, inflammation, and swelling. Then examine the eyes for ptosis or exophthalmos. Finally, test visual acuity with and without correction, and assess extraocular movements. Characterize any discharge. (See *Examining the external eye.*)

Common medical causes

♦ ***Acute angle-closure glaucoma.*** Blurred vision and sudden, excruciating pain in and around the eye characterize this disorder; the pain may be so severe that it causes nausea, vomiting, and abdominal pain. Other findings are halo vision, rapidly decreasing visual acuity, and a fixed, nonreactive, moderately dilated pupil.

♦ ***Blepharitis.*** Burning pain in both eyelids is accompanied by itching, sticky discharge, and conjunctival injection. Related findings include foreign-body sensation, lid ulcerations, and loss of eyelashes.

♦ ***Chalazion.*** A chalazion causes localized tenderness and swelling on the upper or lower eyelid. Eversion of the lid reveals conjunctival injection and a small red lump.

♦ ***Conjunctivitis.*** Some degree of eye pain and excessive tearing occurs with five types of conjunctivitis. *Allergic conjunctivitis* causes mild, burning, bilateral pain accompanied by itching, conjunctival injection, and a characteristic stringy discharge. *Bacterial conjunctivitis* causes pain only when it affects the cornea. Otherwise, it causes burning and a foreign-body sensation. A purulent discharge and conjunctival injection are also typical.

If it affects the cornea, *fungal conjunctivitis* may cause pain and photophobia. Even without corneal involvement, it causes itching, burning eyes; a thick, purulent discharge; and conjunctival injection. *Viral conjunctivitis* causes itching, red eyes, foreign-body sensation, visible conjunctival follicles, and eyelid edema.

♦ ***Corneal abrasion.*** In this type of injury, eye pain is characterized by a foreign-body sensation. Excessive tearing, photo-

EXAMINATION TIP

Examining the external eye

For patients with eye pain or other ocular symptoms, examination of the external eye forms an important part of the ocular assessment.

First, inspect the eyelids for ptosis and incomplete closure. Also observe the lids for edema, erythema, cyanosis, hematoma, and masses. Evaluate skin lesions, growths, swelling, and tenderness by gross palpation. Are the lids everted or inverted? Do the eyelashes turn inward? Have some of them been lost? Do the lashes adhere to one another or contain a discharge? Next, examine the lid margins, noting especially any debris, scaling, lesions, or unusual secretions. Also watch for eyelid spasms.

Now gently retract the eyelid with your thumb and forefinger, and assess the conjunctiva for redness, cloudiness, follicles, and blisters or other lesions. Check for chemosis by pressing the lower lid against the eyeball and noting any bulging above this compression point. Observe the sclera,noting any change from its normal white color.

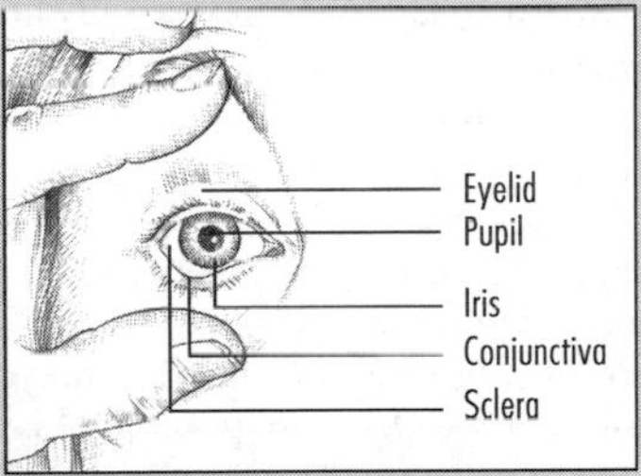

Next, shine a light across the cornea to detect scars, abrasions, or ulcers. Note any color changes, dots, or opaque or cloudy areas. Also assess the anterior eye chamber, which should be clean, deep, shadow-free, and filled with clear aqueous humor.

Inspect the color, shape, texture, and pattern of the iris. Then assess the pupils' size, shape, and equality. Finally evaluate their responses to light. Are they sluggish, fixed, or unresponsive? Does pupil dilation or constriction occur only on one side?

phobia, and conjunctival injection are also common.

◆ ***Corneal ulcers.*** Both bacterial and fungal corneal ulcers cause severe eye pain. They may also cause a purulent eye discharge, sticky eyelids, photophobia, and impaired visual acuity. In addition, *bacterial corneal ulcers* cause a grayish white, irregularly shaped ulcer on the cornea, unilateral pupil constriction, and conjunctival injection. *Fungal corneal ulcers* cause conjunctival injection, eyelid edema and erythema, and a dense, cloudy, central ulcer surrounded by progressively clearer rings.

◆ ***Dacryocystitis.*** Pain and tenderness near the tear sac characterize acute dacryocystitis. Additional signs include excessive tearing, a purulent discharge, eyelid erythema, and swelling in the lacrimal punctum area.

◆ ***Episcleritis.*** Deep eye pain occurs as tissues over sclera become inflamed. Related effects include photophobia, excessive tearing, conjunctival edema, and a red or purplish sclera.

◆ ***Erythema multiforme major.*** This disorder commonly causes severe eye pain, entropion, trichiasis, purulent conjunctivitis, photophobia, and decreased tear formation.

◆ ***Eye strain.*** Disorders of refraction or accommodation may cause pain in the orbits that radiates toward the occipital region, following the distribution of the ophthalmic nerve. The pain usually occurs when the eyes have been used intensively for some time, but the pain doesn't subside immediately with eye rest. The pain is attributed to sustained contraction of the intraocular and extraocular muscles.

♦ ***Foreign bodies in the cornea and conjunctiva.*** Sudden severe pain is common, but vision usually remains intact. Other findings include excessive tearing, photophobia, miosis, a foreign-body sensation, a dark speck on the cornea, and dramatic conjunctival injection.

♦ ***Iritis (acute).*** Moderate to severe eye pain occurs with severe photophobia, dramatic conjunctival injection, and blurred vision. The constricted pupil may respond poorly to light.

♦ ***Lacrimal gland tumor.*** This neoplastic lesion usually causes unilateral eye pain, impaired visual acuity, and some degree of exophthalmos.

♦ ***Ocular laceration and intraocular foreign bodies.*** Penetrating eye injuries usually cause mild to severe unilateral eye pain and impaired visual acuity. Eyelid edema, conjunctival injection, and an abnormal pupillary response may also occur.

♦ ***Optic neuritis.*** In this disorder, pain in and around the eye occurs with eye movement. Severe visual loss and tunnel vision develop but improve in 2 to 3 weeks. Pupils respond sluggishly to direct light but normally to consensual light.

♦ ***Orbital cellulitis.*** This disorder causes dull, aching pain in the affected eye, some degree of exophthalmos, eyelid edema and erythema, purulent discharge, impaired extraocular movement and, occasionally, decreased visual acuity and fever.

♦ ***Scleritis.*** This inflammation causes severe eye pain and tenderness, along with conjunctival injection, bluish purple sclera and, possibly, photophobia and excessive tearing.

♦ ***Sclerokeratitis.*** Inflammation of the sclera and cornea causes pain, burning, irritation, and photophobia.

♦ ***Subdural hematoma.*** Following head trauma, a subdural hematoma commonly causes severe eyeache and headache. Related neurologic signs depend on the hematoma's location and size.

♦ ***Trachoma.*** Along with pain in the affected eye, trachoma causes excessive tearing, photophobia, eye discharge, eyelid edema and redness, and visible conjunctival follicles.

♦ ***Uveitis.*** *Anterior uveitis* causes sudden onset of severe pain, dramatic conjunctival injection, photophobia, and a small, nonreactive pupil. *Posterior uveitis* causes insidious onset of similar features, plus gradual blurring of vision and distorted pupil shape. *Lens-induced uveitis* causes moderate eye pain, conjunctival injection, pupil constriction, and severely impaired visual acuity. In fact, the patient usually can perceive only light.

Other causes

♦ ***Treatments.*** Contact lenses may cause eye pain and a foreign-body sensation. Ocular surgery may also cause eye pain, ranging from a mild ache to a severe pounding or stabbing sensation.

Special considerations

To help ease eye pain, have the patient lie down in a darkened, quiet environment and close his eyes. Prepare him for diagnostic studies, including tonometry and orbital X-rays.

Pediatric pointers

Trauma and infection are the most common causes of eye pain in children. Be alert for nonverbal clues to pain, such as tightly shutting or frequently rubbing the eyes.

Geriatric pointers

Glaucoma, which can cause eye pain, is usually a disease of older patients, becoming clinically significant after age 40. It most commonly occurs bilaterally and leads to slowly progressive vision loss, especially in peripheral visual fields.

F

Fasciculations

Fasciculations are local muscle contractions representing the spontaneous discharge of a muscle fiber bundle innervated by a single motor nerve filament. These contractions cause visible dimpling or wavelike twitching of the skin, but they aren't strong enough to produce joint movement. They occur irregularly at frequencies ranging from once every several seconds to two or three times per second; infrequently, myokymia — continuous, rapid fasciculations that cause a rippling effect — may occur. Because fasciculations are brief and painless, they commonly go undetected or are ignored.

Benign, nonpathologic fasciculations are common and normal. They commonly occur in tense, anxious, or overtired people and typically affect the eyelid, thumb, or calf. However, fasciculations may also indicate a severe neurologic disorder, most notably a diffuse motor neuron disorder that causes loss of control over muscle fiber discharge. They're also an early sign of pesticide poisoning.

Emergency interventions

Begin by asking the patient about the nature, onset, and duration of the fasciculations. If the onset was sudden, ask about any precipitating events such as exposure to pesticides. Pesticide poisoning, although uncommon, is a medical emergency requiring prompt and vigorous intervention. You may need to maintain airway patency, monitor vital signs, give oxygen, and perform gastric lavage or induce vomiting.

History and physical examination

If the patient isn't in severe distress, find out if he has experienced sensory changes such as paresthesia or difficulty speaking, swallowing, breathing, or controlling bowel or bladder function. Ask him if he's in pain.

Explore the patient's medical history for neurologic disorders, cancer, and recent infections. Also ask about his lifestyle, especially stress at home, on the job, or at school.

Perform a physical examination, looking for fasciculations while the affected muscle is at rest. Compare each muscle group with its contralateral side while performing your assessment. Palpate muscle groups slowly from proximal to distal. Observe and test for motor and sensory abnormalities, particularly muscle atrophy and weakness, and decreased deep tendon reflexes. If you note these signs, suspect motor neuron disease, and perform a comprehensive neurologic examination.

Common medical causes

♦ ***Amyotrophic lateral sclerosis.*** Coarse fasciculations usually begin in the small muscles of the hands and feet, then spread to the forearms and legs. Widespread, symmetrical muscle atrophy and weakness may result in dysarthria; difficulty chewing, swallowing, or breathing; or, occasionally, choking and drooling.

♦ ***Bulbar palsy.*** Fasciculations of the face and tongue commonly appear early. Progressive signs include dysarthria, dysphagia, hoarseness, and drooling. Eventually, weakness spreads to the respiratory muscles.

♦ ***Pesticide poisoning.*** Ingestion of organophosphate or carbamate pesticides commonly causes acute onset of long, wavelike fasciculations and muscle weakness that rapidly progresses to flaccid paralysis. Other common effects include nausea, vomiting, diarrhea, loss of bowel and bladder control, hyperactive bowel sounds, and abdominal cramping. Cardiopulmonary findings may include bradycardia, dyspnea or bradypnea, and pallor or cyanosis. Seizures, visual disturbances (pupillary constriction or blurred vision), and increased secretions (tearing, salivation, pulmonary secretions, or diaphoresis) may also occur.

♦ ***Poliomyelitis (spinal paralytic).*** Coarse fasciculations, usually transient but occasionally persistent, accompany progressive muscle weakness, spasms, and atrophy. The patient may also exhibit decreased reflexes, paresthesia, coldness and cyanosis in the affected limbs, bladder paralysis, dyspnea, elevated blood pressure, or tachycardia.

♦ ***Spinal cord tumors.*** Fasciculations may develop along with muscle atrophy and cramps, asymmetrically at first and then bilaterally as cord compression progresses. Motor and sensory changes distal to the tumor include weakness or paralysis, areflexia, paresthesia, and a tightening band of pain. Bowel and bladder control may be lost.

Special considerations

Prepare the patient for diagnostic studies, such as spinal X-rays, myelography, computed tomography scan, magnetic resonance imaging, and electromyography with nerve conduction velocity tests. Help the patient with progressive neuromuscular degeneration to cope with activities of daily living, and provide appropriate assistive devices.

Pediatric pointers

Fasciculations, particularly of the tongue, are an important early sign of Werdnig-Hoffmann disease.

FATIGUE

Fatigue is a feeling of excessive tiredness, lack of energy, or exhaustion accompanied by a strong desire to rest or sleep. This common symptom is distinct from weakness, which involves the muscles, but they may occur together.

Fatigue is a normal and important response to physical overexertion, prolonged emotional stress, and sleep deprivation. However, it can also be a nonspecific symptom of a psychological or physiologic disorder — especially infection and endocrine, cardiovascular, or neurologic disease.

Fatigue reflects both hypermetabolic and hypometabolic states in which nutrients needed for cellular energy and growth are lacking because of overly rapid depletion, impaired replacement mechanisms, insufficient hormone production, or inadequate nutrient intake or metabolism.

History and physical examination

Obtain a careful history to identify the patient's fatigue pattern. Fatigue that worsens with activity and improves with rest usually indicates a physical disorder; the opposite pattern, commonly a psychological disorder. Fatigue lasting longer than 4 months, constant fatigue that's unrelieved by rest, and transient exhaustion that quickly gives way to bursts of energy are other findings associated with psychological disorders.

Ask about related symptoms and recent viral illness or stressful changes in lifestyle. Explore nutritional habits and appetite or weight changes. Carefully review the patient's medical and psychiatric history for any chronic disorders that commonly cause fatigue. Ask about a family history of such disorders.

Observe the patient's general appearance for overt signs of depression or organic illness. Is he unkempt or expressionless? Does he appear tired or sickly or have a slumped posture? If warranted, evaluate his mental status, noting especially mental clouding, attention deficits, agitation, or psychomotor retardation.

Common medical causes

◆ ***Acquired immunodeficiency syndrome.*** Besides fatigue, this syndrome may cause fever, night sweats, weight loss, diarrhea, or a cough, followed by any of several concurrent opportunistic infections.

◆ ***Adrenocortical insufficiency.*** Mild fatigue, the hallmark of this disorder, initially appears after exertion and stress but later becomes more severe and persistent. Weakness and weight loss typically accompany GI disturbances, such as nausea, vomiting, anorexia, abdominal pain, and chronic diarrhea; hyperpigmentation; orthostatic hypotension; and a weak, irregular pulse.

◆ ***Anemia.*** Fatigue following mild activity is commonly the first symptom of anemia. Associated findings vary but generally include pallor, tachycardia, and dyspnea.

◆ ***Anxiety.*** Chronic, unremitting anxiety invariably causes fatigue, commonly characterized as nervous exhaustion. Other persistent findings include apprehension, indecisiveness, restlessness, insomnia, trembling, and increased muscle tension.

◆ ***Cancer.*** Unexplained fatigue is commonly the earliest sign of cancer. Related findings reflect the type, location, and stage of the tumor and commonly include pain, nausea, vomiting, anorexia, weight loss, abnormal bleeding, or a palpable mass.

◆ ***Chronic fatigue syndrome.*** This syndrome, whose cause is unknown, is characterized by incapacitating fatigue. Other findings include sore throat, myalgia, and cognitive dysfunction.

◆ ***Chronic obstructive pulmonary disease.*** The earliest and most persistent symptoms of this disease are progressive fatigue and dyspnea. The patient may also experience a chronic and usually productive cough, weight loss, barrel chest, cyanosis, slight dependent edema, and poor exercise tolerance.

◆ ***Diabetes mellitus.*** Fatigue, the most common symptom in this disorder, may begin insidiously or abruptly. Related findings include weight loss, blurred vision, polyuria, polydipsia, and polyphagia.

◆ ***Heart failure.*** Persistent fatigue and lethargy characterize this disorder. Left-sided heart failure causes exertional and paroxysmal nocturnal dyspnea, orthopnea, and tachycardia. Right-sided heart failure causes distended neck veins and possibly a slight but persistent nonproductive cough. Right-sided heart failure may be caused by and accompanied by left-sided heart failure. In both types, slowed mental response accompanies later signs and symptoms, including nausea, anorexia, unexplained weight gain, and possibly oliguria. Cardiopulmonary findings include tachypnea, inspiratory crackles, palpitations and chest tightness, hypotension, narrowed pulse pressure, ventricular gallop, pallor, diaphoresis, clubbing, and dependent edema.

◆ ***Hypercortisolism.*** This disorder typically causes fatigue, related in part to accompanying sleep disturbances. Unmistakable signs include truncal obesity with slender extremities, buffalo hump, moon face, purple striae, acne, and hirsutism;

increased blood pressure and muscle weakness are other findings.

♦ ***Hypothyroidism.*** Fatigue occurs early in this disorder, along with forgetfulness, cold intolerance, weight gain, metrorrhagia, and constipation.

♦ ***Infection.*** In *chronic infection,* fatigue is commonly the most prominent symptom — and sometimes the only one. Low-grade fever and weight loss may accompany symptoms that reflect the type and location of infection, such as burning upon urination or swollen, painful gums. Subacute bacterial endocarditis is an example of a chronic infection that presents with fatigue or acute hemodynamic decompensation. In *acute infection,* brief fatigue typically accompanies headache, anorexia, arthralgia, chills, high fever, and such infection-specific signs as cough, vomiting, or diarrhea.

♦ ***Lyme disease.*** Besides fatigue and malaise, symptoms of this deer tickborne disease include intermittent headache, fever, chills, expanding red rash, and muscle and joint aches. In later stages, patients may manifest arthritis, fluctuating meningoencephalitis, and cardiac abnormalities such as a brief, fluctuating atrioventricular heart block.

♦ ***Malnutrition.*** Easy fatigability commonly occurs in protein-calorie malnutrition, along with lethargy and apathy. The patient may also exhibit weight loss, muscle wasting, sensations of coldness, pallor, edema, or dry, flaky skin.

♦ ***Myasthenia gravis.*** The cardinal symptoms of this disorder are easy fatigability and muscle weakness, which worsen as the day progresses. They also worsen with exertion and abate with rest. Related findings depend on the specific muscles affected.

♦ ***Renal failure.*** *Acute renal failure* commonly causes sudden fatigue, drowsiness, and lethargy. Oliguria, an early sign, is followed by severe systemic effects: ammonia breath odor, nausea, vomiting, diarrhea or constipation, and dry skin and mucous membranes. Neurologic findings include muscle twitching and changes in personality and level of consciousness, possibly progressing to seizures and coma.

In *chronic renal failure,* insidious fatigue and lethargy accompany marked changes in all body systems, including GI disturbances, ammonia breath odor, Kussmaul's respirations, bleeding tendencies, poor skin turgor, severe pruritus, paresthesia, visual disturbances, confusion, seizures, and coma.

♦ ***Systemic lupus erythematosus.*** Fatigue usually accompanies generalized aching, malaise, low-grade fever, headache, and irritability. Primary clinical features include joint pain and stiffness, butterfly rash, and photosensitivity. Also common are Raynaud's phenomenon, patchy alopecia, and mucous membrane ulcers.

♦ ***Valvular heart disease.*** All types of valvular heart disease commonly cause progressive fatigue and a cardiac murmur. Additional signs and symptoms vary but generally include exertional dyspnea, cough, and hemoptysis.

Other causes

♦ ***Drugs.*** Fatigue may result from various drugs, notably antihypertensives and sedatives. In patients receiving cardiac glycoside therapy, fatigue may indicate toxicity.

♦ ***Surgery.*** Most types of surgery cause temporary fatigue, probably due to the combined effects of hunger, anesthesia, and sleep deprivation.

Special considerations

If fatigue results from organic illness, help the patient determine which of his daily activities he may need help with and how to pace himself to ensure sufficient rest. You can help him reduce chronic fatigue by alleviating pain, which may interfere with rest, or nausea, which may lead to malnutrition. He may benefit from referral to a community health nurse or housekeeping service. If fatigue results from a psychogenic cause, refer him for psychological counseling.

Pediatric pointers

When evaluating a child for fatigue, ask his parents if they've noticed any change in his activity level. Fatigue without an organic cause occurs normally during accelerated growth phases in preschool-aged and prepubescent children. However, psychological causes of fatigue must be considered; for instance, a depressed child may try to escape problems at home or school by taking refuge in sleep. In the pubescent child, consider the possibility of drug abuse, particularly of hypnotics and tranquilizers.

Geriatric pointers

Always ask older patients about fatigue because this symptom may mask more serious underlying conditions in this age-group. Temporal arteritis, which is much more common in people over age 60, usually presents as fatigue, weight loss, jaw claudication, proximal muscle weakness, headache, visual disturbances, and associated anemia.

Fecal incontinence

Fecal incontinence, the involuntary passage of feces, follows any loss or impairment of external anal sphincter control. It can result from various GI, neurologic, and psychological disorders; the effects of drugs; and surgery. In some patients, it may even be a purposeful manipulative behavior.

Fecal incontinence may be temporary or permanent; its onset may be gradual, as in dementia, or sudden, as in spinal cord trauma. Although usually not a sign of severe illness, it can greatly affect the patient's physical and psychological well-being.

History and physical examination

Ask the patient with fecal incontinence about its onset, duration, and severity and about any discernible pattern — for instance, at night or with diarrhea. Note the frequency, consistency, and volume of stools passed within the last 24 hours, and obtain a stool sample. Focus your history taking on GI, neurologic, and psychological disorders.

Let the history guide your physical examination. If you suspect a brain or spinal cord lesion, perform a complete neurologic examination. (See *Neurologic control of defecation,* page 252.) If a GI disturbance seems likely, inspect the abdomen for distention, auscultate for bowel sounds, and percuss and palpate for a mass. Inspect the anal area for signs of excoriation or infection. If not contraindicated, check for fecal impaction, which may be associated with incontinence.

Common medical causes

♦ ***Dementias.*** Any of these chronic degenerative brain diseases can cause fecal as well as urinary incontinence. Associated signs and symptoms include impaired judgment and abstract thinking, amnesia, emotional lability, hyperactive deep tendon reflexes, aphasia or dysarthria and, possibly, diffuse choreoathetotic movements.

♦ ***Head trauma.*** Disruption of the neurologic pathways that control defecation can cause fecal incontinence. Additional findings depend on the location and severity of the injury and may include decreased level of consciousness, seizures, vomiting, and a wide range of motor and sensory impairments.

♦ ***Inflammatory bowel disease.*** Nocturnal fecal incontinence occurs occasionally with diarrhea. Related findings may include abdominal pain, anorexia, weight loss, blood in the stools, and hyperactive bowel sounds.

♦ ***Rectovaginal fistula.*** Fecal incontinence occurs in tandem with uninhibited passage of flatus.

♦ ***Spinal cord lesions.*** Any lesion that causes compression or transection of sensorimotor spinal tracts can lead to fecal

Neurologic control of defecation

Three neurologic mechanisms normally regulate defecation: the intrinsic defecation reflex in the colon, the parasympathetic defecation reflex involving sacral segments of the spinal cord, and voluntary control. Here's how they interact.

Fecal distention of the rectum activates the relatively weak intrinsic reflex, and afferent impulses spread through the mesenteric plexus, initiating peristalsis in the descending and sigmoid colon and in the rectum. Subsequent movement of feces toward the anus causes relaxation of the internal anal sphincter.

The parasympathetic reflex magnifies the intrinsic reflex. Stimulation of the afferent nerves in the rectal wall propels impulses through the spinal cord and back to the descending colon, rectum, and anus to intensify peristalsis (see illustration).

Fecal movement and internal sphincter relaxation, however, cause immediate contraction of the external anal sphincter and temporary fecal retention. At this point, conscious control of the external sphincter prevents or permits defecation. Except in infants or neurologically impaired patients, this voluntary mechanism further contracts the sphincter to prevent defecation at inappropriate times or relaxes it and allows defecation to occur.

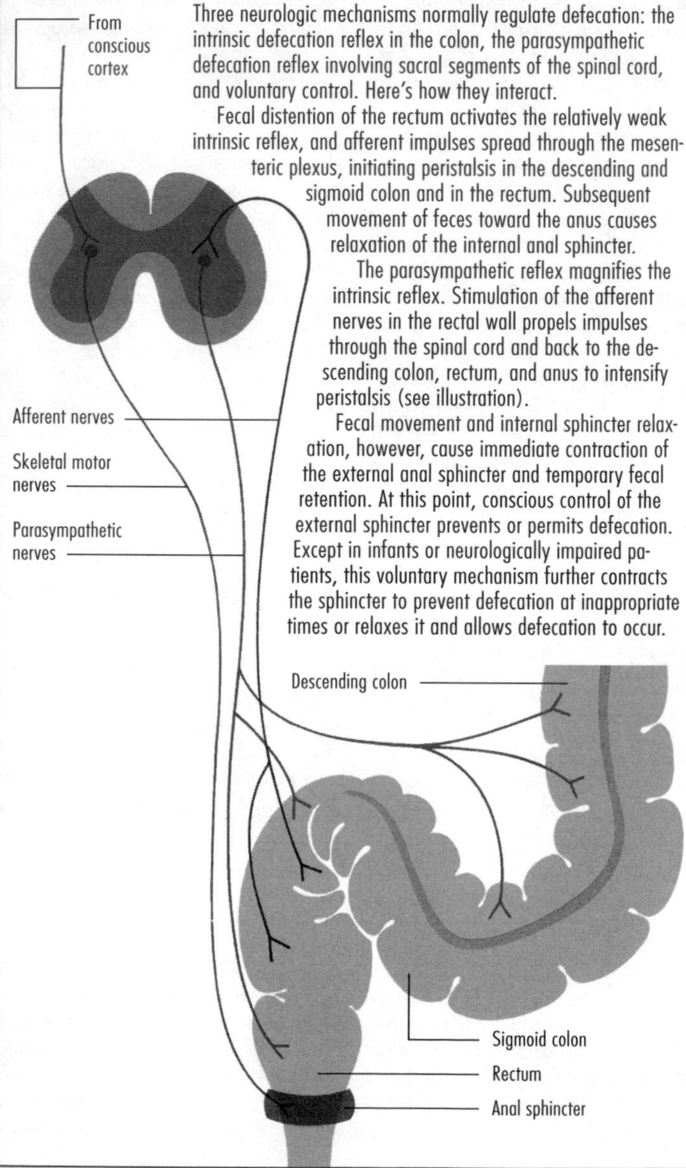

incontinence. Incontinence may be permanent, especially with severe lesions of the sacral segments. Other signs and symptoms reflect motor and sensory disturbances below the level of the lesion, such as urinary incontinence, weakness or paralysis, paresthesia, and analgesia and thermanesthesia.

Other causes

♦ ***Drugs.*** Chronic laxative abuse may cause insensitivity to the presence of a fecal mass or loss of the colonic defecation reflex.

♦ ***Surgery.*** Pelvic, prostate, or rectal surgery occasionally causes temporary fecal incontinence. Colostomy or ileostomy causes permanent or temporary fecal incontinence.

Special considerations

Maintain proper hygiene, including control of foul odors. Also, provide emotional support for the patient because he may feel deep embarrassment. For the patient with intermittent or temporary incontinence, encourage Kegel exercises to strengthen abdominal and perirectal muscles. For the neurologically capable patient with chronic incontinence, provide bowel retraining.

Pediatric pointers

Fecal incontinence is normal in infants and may occur temporarily in young children who experience stress-related psychological regression or a physical illness associated with diarrhea. Pediatric fecal incontinence can also result from myelomeningocele.

Geriatric pointers

Fecal incontinence is an important factor when long-term care is considered for an elderly patient. Leakage of liquid fecal material is especially common in males. Age-related changes affecting smooth muscle cells of the colon may change GI motility and lead to fecal incontinence. Before age is determined to be the cause, however, any pathology must be ruled out.

FETOR HEPATICUS

Fetor hepaticus — a distinctive musty, sweet breath odor — characterizes hepatic encephalopathy, a life-threatening complication of severe liver disease. The odor results from the damaged liver's inability to metabolize and detoxify mercaptans produced by bacterial degradation of methionine, a sulfur-containing amino acid. These substances circulate in the blood, are expelled by the lungs, and flavor the breath.

Emergency interventions

If you detect fetor hepaticus, quickly determine the patient's level of consciousness. If he's comatose, evaluate respiratory status. Prepare to intubate and provide ventilatory support, if necessary. Start a peripheral I.V. line for fluid administration, begin cardiac monitoring, and insert an indwelling urinary catheter to monitor output. Obtain arterial and venous samples for analysis of blood gases, ammonia, and electrolytes.

History and physical examination

If the patient is conscious, closely observe him for signs of impending coma. Evaluate deep tendon reflexes for asterixis, and test for Babinski's sign. Be alert for signs of GI bleeding and shock, common complications of end-stage liver failure. Also watch for increased anxiety, restlessness, tachycardia, tachypnea, hypotension, oliguria, hematemesis, melena, or cool, moist, pale skin. Place the patient in the supine position with his legs elevated 20 degrees, administer oxygen, and increase the infusion rate of I.V. fluids. Draw blood samples for a complete blood count, typing and crossmatching, a clotting profile, and ammonia level. Intubation, ventilation, or cardiopulmonary resuscitation may be necessary. Evaluate the degree of jaundice and abdominal distention and palpate the liver to assess the degree of enlargement.

Obtain a complete medical history, relying on the patient's family if necessary. Focus on any factors that may have precipitated hepatic disease or coma, such as recent severe infection; overuse of sedatives, analgesics, or diuretics; excessive protein intake; and recent blood transfusion, surgery, or GI bleeding.

Common medical causes

♦ ***Hepatic encephalopathy.*** Fetor hepaticus usually occurs in the final, comatose stage of this disorder but may occur earlier. Tremors progress to asterixis in the impending stage; lethargy, aberrant behavior, and apraxia also occur. Hyperventilation and stupor mark the stuporous stage, during which the patient acts agitated when aroused. Seizures and coma herald the final stage, along with decreased pulse and respiratory rates, positive Babinski's sign, hyperactive reflexes, decerebrate posture, and opisthotonos.

Special considerations

Effective treatment of hepatic encephalopathy reduces blood ammonia levels by eliminating ammonia from the GI tract. You may have to administer neomycin or lactulose to suppress bacterial production of ammonia, give sorbitol solution to induce osmotic diarrhea, give potassium supplements to correct alkalosis, provide continuous gastric aspiration of blood, or maintain the patient on a low-protein diet. If these methods aren't successful, hemodialysis or exchange transfusions may be performed.

During treatment, closely monitor the patient's level of consciousness, intake and output, and fluid and electrolyte balance.

Pediatric pointers

A child who's slipping into a hepatic coma may cry, be disobedient, or become preoccupied with an activity.

Geriatric pointers

In addition to fetor hepaticus, elderly patients with hepatic encephalopathy may exhibit disturbances of awareness and mentation, such as forgetfulness and confusion.

FEVER

[Pyrexia]

Fever is a common sign that can arise from disorders affecting virtually any body system. As a result, fever in the absence of other signs usually has little diagnostic significance. A persistent high fever, though, represents an emergency.

Fever can be classified as low (oral reading of 99° to 100.4° F [37.2° to 38° C]), moderate (100.5° to 104° F [38° to 40° C]), or high (above 104° F). Fever over 106° F (41.1° C) causes unconsciousness and, if sustained, leads to permanent brain damage.

Fever may also be classified as remittent, intermittent, sustained, relapsing, or undulant. *Remittent fever,* the most common type, is characterized by daily temperature fluctuations above the normal range. *Intermittent fever* is marked by a daily temperature drop into the normal range, then a rise back to above normal. An intermittent fever that fluctuates widely, typically producing chills and sweating, is called *hectic* or *septic fever. Sustained fever* is a persistent temperature elevation with little fluctuation. *Relapsing fever* consists of alternating feverish and afebrile periods. *Undulant fever* refers to a gradual increase in temperature that stays high for a few days and then decreases gradually.

Further classification involves duration — either brief (less than 3 weeks) or prolonged. Prolonged fevers include fever of unknown origin, a classification used when careful examination fails to detect an underlying cause.

Emergency interventions

If you detect a fever higher than 106° F (41.1° C), take the patient's other vital signs and determine his level of consciousness. Administer antipyretic drugs and begin rapid cooling measures: Apply ice packs to the axillae and groin, give tepid sponge baths, or apply a hypothermia blanket. These methods may evoke a hypothermic response; to prevent this, constantly monitor the patient's rectal temperature.

History and physical examination

If the patient's fever is only mild to moderate, ask him when it began and how high his temperature reached. Did the fever disappear, only to reappear later? Did he experience any other symptoms, such as chills, fatigue, or pain?

Obtain a complete medical history, noting especially immunosuppressive treatments or disorders, infection, trauma, surgery, diagnostic testing, and use of anesthesia or other medications. Ask about recent travel because certain diseases are endemic to specific areas.

Let the history findings direct your physical examination. Because fever can accompany diverse disorders, the examination may range from a brief evaluation of one body system to a comprehensive review of all systems. (See *How fever develops,* page 256.)

Common medical causes

◆ ***Immune complex disease.*** When present, fever usually remains low, although moderate elevations may accompany erythema multiforme. Fever may be remittent or intermittent, as in acquired immunodeficiency syndrome (AIDS) or systemic lupus erythematosus, or sustained, as in polyarteritis. As one of several vague prodromal complaints (such as fatigue, anorexia, and weight loss), fever causes nocturnal diaphoresis and accompanies such associated signs as diarrhea and a persistent cough (in AIDS) or morning stiffness (in rheumatoid arthritis). Other disease-specific findings include headache and possible vision loss (temporal arteritis); pain and stiffness in the neck, shoulders, back, or pelvis (ankylosing spondylitis and polymyalgia rheumatica); skin and mucous membrane lesions (erythema multiforme); and urethritis with urethral discharge and conjunctivitis (Reiter's syndrome).

◆ ***Infectious and inflammatory disorders.*** Fever ranges from low (in Crohn's disease and ulcerative colitis) to extremely high (in bacterial pneumonia, necrotizing fasciitis, and Ebola and Hanta virus infections). It may be remittent, as in infectious mononucleosis and otitis media; hectic (recurring daily with sweating, chills, and flushing), as in lung abscess, influenza, and endocarditis; sustained, as in meningitis; or relapsing, as in malaria. Fever may arise abruptly, as in toxic shock syndrome and Rocky Mountain spotted fever, or insidiously, as in mycoplasmal pneumonia. In hepatitis, fever may represent a disease prodrome; in appendicitis, it follows the acute stage. Its sudden late appearance with tachycardia, tachypnea, and confusion heralds life-threatening septic shock in peritonitis and gram-negative bacteremia.

Associated signs and symptoms involve every system. The cyclic variations of hectic fever typically cause alternating chills and diaphoresis. General systemic complaints include weakness, anorexia, and malaise.

◆ ***Neoplasms.*** Primary neoplasms and metastases can cause prolonged fever of varying elevations. For instance, acute leukemia may present insidiously with low fever, pallor, and bleeding tendencies or abruptly with high fever, frank bleeding, and prostration. Occasionally, Hodgkin's disease causes undulant fever or Pel-Ebstein fever, an irregularly relapsing fever.

How fever develops

Body temperature is regulated by the hypothalamic thermostat, which has a specific set point under normal conditions. Fever can result from a resetting of the set point or from an abnormality in the thermoregulatory system itself.

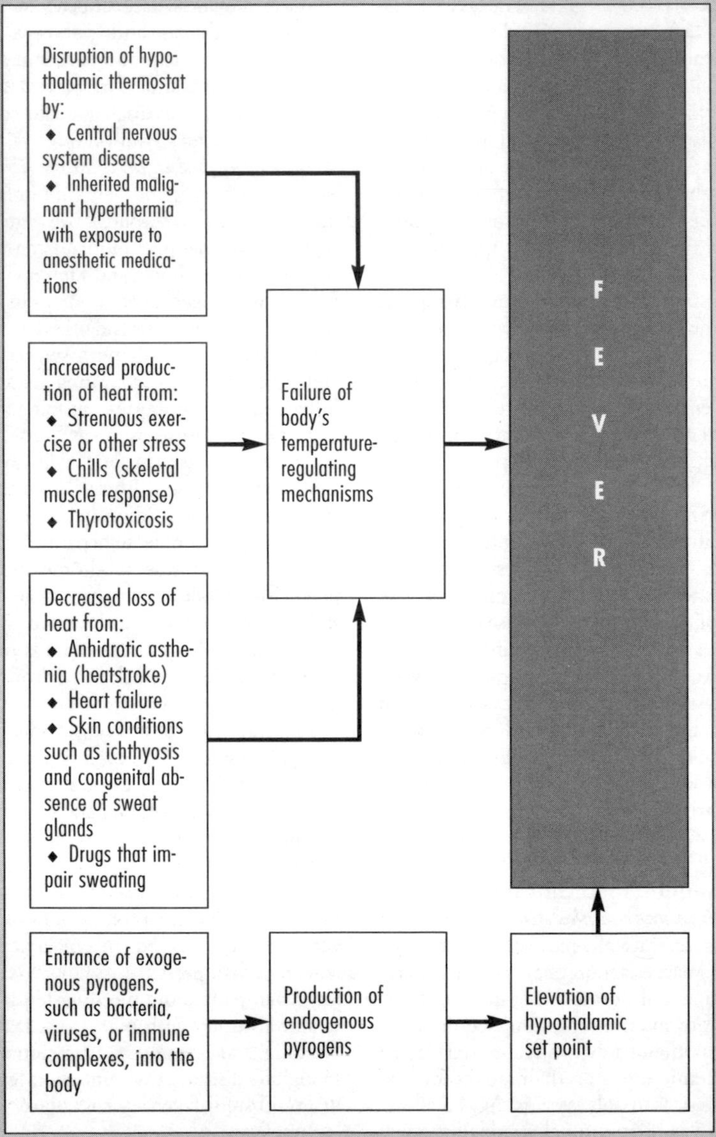

Besides fever and nocturnal diaphoresis, neoplastic disease commonly causes anorexia, fatigue, malaise, and weight loss. Examination may reveal lesions, lymphadenopathy, palpable masses, or hepatosplenomegaly.

◆ ***Thermoregulatory dysfunction.*** Sudden onset of fever that rises rapidly and remains as high as 107° F (41.7° C) occurs in life-threatening disorders, such as heatstroke, thyroid storm, neuroleptic malignant syndrome, and malignant hyperthermia, and in lesions of the central nervous system (CNS). Low or moderate fever appears in dehydration.

Prolonged high fever commonly causes vomiting, anhidrosis, decreased level of consciousness (LOC), and hot, flushed skin. Related cardiovascular effects may include tachycardia, tachypnea, and hypotension. Other disease-specific findings may include skin changes: dry skin and mucous membranes and poor skin turgor in dehydration; mottled cyanosis in malignant hyperthermia; diarrhea in thyroid storm; oliguria in dehydration; and ominous signs of increased intracranial pressure (decreased LOC with bradycardia, widened pulse pressure, and increased systolic pressure) in CNS tumor, trauma, or hemorrhage.

◆ ***West Nile encephalitis.*** This brain infection is caused by West Nile virus, a mosquito-borne flavivirus commonly found in Africa, West Asia, and the Middle East, and becoming more common in North America. Mild infection is common; signs and symptoms include fever, headache, and body aches, commonly with skin rash and swollen lymph glands. More severe infection is marked by high fever, headache, neck stiffness, stupor, disorientation, coma, tremors, occasional seizures, paralysis and, rarely, death.

Other causes

◆ ***Diagnostic tests.*** Immediate or delayed fever infrequently follows radiographic tests that use contrast medium.

◆ ***Drugs.*** Fever and rash commonly result from hypersensitivity to antifungals, sulfonamides, penicillins, cephalosporins, tetracyclines, barbiturates, phenytoin, quinidine, iodides, phenolphthalein, methyldopa, procainamide, and some antitoxins. Fever can accompany chemotherapy, especially with bleomycin, vincristine, or asparaginase. It can result from drugs that impair sweating, such as anticholinergics, phenothiazines, or monoamine oxidase inhibitors. A drug-induced fever typically disappears after the involved drug is discontinued. Fever can also stem from toxic doses of salicylates, amphetamines, and tricyclic antidepressants. Inhalant anesthetics and muscle relaxants can trigger malignant hyperthermia in patients with this inherited trait.

◆ ***Treatments.*** Remittent or intermittent low fever may occur for several days after surgery. Transfusion reactions characteristically cause abrupt onset of fever and chills.

Special considerations

Regularly monitor the patient's temperature, and record it on a chart for easy follow-up of the temperature curve. Provide increased fluid and nutritional intake. When administering prescribed antipyretic drugs, minimize resultant chills and diaphoresis by following a regular dosage schedule. Promote patient comfort by maintaining a stable room temperature and providing frequent changes of bedding and clothing.

Pediatric pointers

Infants and young children experience higher and more prolonged fevers, more rapid temperature increases, and greater temperature fluctuations than older children and adults.

Keep in mind that seizures commonly accompany extremely high fever, so take appropriate precautions. Also, instruct parents not to give aspirin to a child with varicella or flulike symptoms because of the risk of precipitating Reye's syndrome.

Common pediatric causes of fever include varicella, croup syndrome, dehydration, meningitis, mumps, otitis media, pertussis, roseola infantum, rubella, rubeola, and tonsillitis. Fever can also occur as a reaction to immunizations or antibiotics.

Geriatric pointers

Elderly people may have an altered sweating mechanism that predisposes them to heatstroke when exposed to high temperatures; they may also have an impaired thermoregulatory mechanism, making temperature change a less reliable measure of disease severity.

FLANK PAIN

Pain in the flank, the area extending from the ribs to the ilium, is a leading indicator of renal and upper urinary tract disease or trauma. Depending on the cause, this symptom may vary from a dull ache to severe stabbing or throbbing pain and may be unilateral or bilateral, constant or intermittent. It's aggravated by costovertebral angle (CVA) percussion and, in patients with renal or urinary tract obstruction, by increased fluid intake or ingestion of alcohol, caffeine, or diuretic drugs. Unaffected by position changes, flank pain typically responds only to analgesics or, of course, to treatment of the underlying disorder.

Emergency interventions

If the patient has suffered trauma, quickly look for a visible or palpable flank mass, associated injuries, CVA pain, hematuria, Turner's sign, and signs of shock (such as tachycardia and cool, clammy skin). If any of these is present, insert an I.V. line to allow fluid or drug infusion. Insert an indwelling urinary catheter to monitor urine output and evaluate hematuria. Obtain blood samples for typing and crossmatching, complete blood count, and electrolyte levels.

History and physical examination

If the patient's condition isn't critical, take a thorough history. Ask about the pain's onset and apparent precipitating events. Have him describe the pain's location, intensity, pattern, and duration. Find out if anything aggravates or alleviates it.

Ask the patient about changes in his normal pattern of fluid intake and urine output. Explore his history for urinary tract infection (UTI) or obstruction, renal disease, or recent streptococcal infection.

During the physical examination, palpate the patient's flank area and percuss the CVA to determine the extent of pain. (See *Flank pain: Common causes and associated findings,* pages 260 and 261.)

Common medical causes

◆ ***Calculi.*** Renal and ureteral calculi cause intense unilateral, colicky flank pain. Typically, initial CVA pain radiates to the flank, suprapubic region, and perhaps the genitalia; abdominal and lower back pains are also possible. Nausea and vomiting commonly accompany severe pain. Associated findings include CVA tenderness, hematuria, hypoactive bowel sounds and, possibly, signs of UTI (urinary frequency and urgency, dysuria, nocturia, fatigue, low-grade fever, and tenesmus).

◆ ***Cortical necrosis (acute).*** Unilateral flank pain is usually severe. Accompanying findings include gross hematuria, anuria, leukocytosis, and fever.

◆ ***Obstructive uropathy.*** In acute obstruction, flank pain may be excruciating; in gradual obstruction, it's typically a dull ache. In both, the pain may also localize in the upper abdomen and may radiate to the groin. Nausea and vomiting, abdominal distention, anuria alternating with periods of oliguria and polyuria, and hypoactive bowel sounds may also occur. Additional findings — a palpable abdominal mass, CVA tenderness, and bladder distention — vary with the site and cause of the obstruction.

♦ ***Papillary necrosis (acute).*** Intense bilateral flank pain is accompanied by renal colic, CVA tenderness, and abdominal pain and rigidity. Possible urinary signs include oliguria or anuria, hematuria, and pyuria, with associated high fever, chills, vomiting, and hypoactive bowel sounds.

♦ ***Perirenal abscess.*** Intense unilateral flank pain and CVA tenderness accompany dysuria, persistent high fever, chills and, in some patients, a palpable abdominal mass.

♦ ***Polycystic kidney disease.*** Dull, aching, bilateral flank pain is commonly the earliest symptom of this renal disorder. The pain can become severe and colicky if cysts rupture and clots migrate or cause obstruction. Nonspecific early findings may include polyuria, increased blood pressure, and signs of UTI. Later findings include hematuria and perineal, lower back, and suprapubic pain.

♦ ***Pyelonephritis (acute).*** Intense, constant, unilateral or bilateral flank pain develops over a few hours or days along with typical urinary features: dysuria, nocturia, hematuria, urgency, frequency, and tenesmus. Other common findings include persistent high fever, chills, anorexia, weakness, fatigue, generalized myalgia, abdominal pain, and marked CVA tenderness.

♦ ***Renal infarction.*** Unilateral, constant, severe flank pain and tenderness typically accompany persistent, severe upper abdominal pain. The patient may also develop CVA tenderness, anorexia, nausea and vomiting, fever, hypoactive bowel sounds, hematuria, and oliguria or anuria.

♦ ***Renal neoplasm.*** Unilateral flank pain, gross hematuria, and a palpable flank mass form the classic clinical triad. Flank pain is usually dull and vague, although severe colicky pain can occur during bleeding or passage of clots. Possible associated signs and symptoms include fever, increased blood pressure, and urine retention. Weight loss, leg edema, nausea, and vomiting point to advanced disease.

♦ ***Renal trauma.*** Variable bilateral or unilateral flank pain is a common symptom. A visible or palpable flank mass may also exist, along with CVA or abdominal pain — possibly severe and radiating to the groin. Other findings may include hematuria, oliguria, abdominal distention, Turner's sign, hypoactive bowel sounds, and nausea or vomiting. Severe injury may cause signs of shock, such as tachycardia and cool, clammy skin.

♦ ***Renal vein thrombosis.*** Severe unilateral flank and lower back pain with CVA and epigastric tenderness typify the rapid onset of venous obstruction. Other features may include fever, hematuria, and leg edema. Bilateral flank pain, oliguria, and other uremic signs (nausea, vomiting, and uremic fetor) typify bilateral obstruction.

Special considerations

Administer pain medication. Continue to monitor the patient's vital signs, and maintain precise intake and output records.

Diagnostic evaluation may involve serial urine and serum analysis, excretory urography, flank ultrasonography, computed tomography scan, voiding cystourethrography, cystoscopy, and retrograde ureteropyelography, urethrography, and cystography.

Pediatric pointers

Assessment of flank pain can be difficult if a child can't describe the pain. In such cases, transillumination of the abdomen and flanks may facilitate assessment of bladder distention and identification of masses. Common causes of flank pain in children include obstructive uropathy, acute poststreptococcal glomerulonephritis, infantile polycystic kidney disease, and nephroblastoma.

Flank pain: Common causes and associated findings

CAUSES	MAJOR ASSOCIATED SIGNS AND SYMPTOMS									
	Abdominal distention	Abdominal mass	Abdominal pain	Anuria	Back pain	Bladder distention	Blood pressure, increased	Bowel sounds, hypoactive	Chills	Costovertebral angle tenderness
Calculi			◆					◆		◆
Cortical necrosis (acute)				◆						
Obstructive uropathy	◆	◆	◆	◆		◆		◆		◆
Papillary necrosis (acute)			◆	◆				◆	◆	◆
Perirenal abscess		◆							◆	◆
Polycystic kidney disease					◆		◆			
Pyelonephritis (acute)			◆						◆	◆
Renal infarction			◆	◆				◆		◆
Renal neoplasm							◆			
Renal trauma	◆		◆					◆		◆
Renal vein thrombosis					◆					◆

FONTANEL BULGING

In a normal infant, the anterior fontanel, or "soft spot," is flat, soft yet firm, and well demarcated against surrounding skull bones. The posterior fontanel, if not fused at birth, usually closes by age 2 months. (See *Locating fontanels,* page 262.) Subtle pulsations may be visible, reflecting the arterial pulse.

A bulging fontanel (widened, tense, and with marked pulsations) is a cardinal sign of meningitis associated with increased intracranial pressure (ICP), a medical emergency. It can also reflect encephalitis or fluid overload. Because prolonged coughing, crying, or lying down can cause transient, physiologic bulging, the infant's head should be observed and palpated while the infant is upright and relaxed.

Emergency interventions

If you detect a bulging fontanel, measure fontanel size and head circumference, and note overall head shape. Take vital signs, and check

Dysuria	Fatigue	Fever	Flank mass	Groin pain	Hematuria	Nausea	Nocturia	Oliguria	Perineal pain	Polyuria	Pyuria	Suprapubic pain	Tenesmus	Urinary frequency	Urinary urgency	Urine retention	Vomiting
◆	◆	◆		◆	◆	◆	◆					◆	◆	◆	◆		◆
		◆			◆												
				◆		◆		◆		◆							◆
		◆			◆			◆			◆						◆
◆		◆															
					◆				◆	◆		◆	◆	◆	◆		
◆	◆	◆			◆		◆						◆	◆	◆		
		◆				◆		◆									◆
		◆	◆		◆	◆										◆	◆
			◆	◆	◆	◆		◆									◆
		◆			◆	◆		◆									◆

level of consciousness (LOC) by observing spontaneous postural reflex activity and sensory responses. Note whether the infant assumes a normal, flexed posture or one of extreme extension, opisthotonos, or hypotonia. Observe limb movements; excessive tremulousness or frequent twitching may herald the onset of a seizure. Look for other signs of increased ICP: abnormal respiratory patterns and a distinctive, high-pitched cry. Ensure airway patency, and have size-appropriate emergency equipment on hand. Provide oxygen, establish I.V. access and, if the infant is having a seizure, stay with him to prevent injury and administer anticonvulsants. Administer antibiotics, antipyretics, and osmotic diuretics to help reduce cerebral edema and ICP, and dexamethasone for edema secondary to head trauma. If these measures fail to reduce ICP, neuromuscular blockade, intubation, mechanical ventilation and, in rare cases, barbiturate coma and total body hypothermia may be necessary.

EXAMINATION TIP

Locating fontanels

The anterior fontanel lies at the junction of the sagittal, coronal, and frontal sutures. It normally measures about 2.5 cm by 4 to 5 cm at birth and usually closes by age 12 to 20 months.

The posterior fontanel lies at the junction of the sagittal and lambdoidal sutures. If it hasn't already fused by the time of birth, it measures 1 to 2 cm and normally closes by age 2 months.

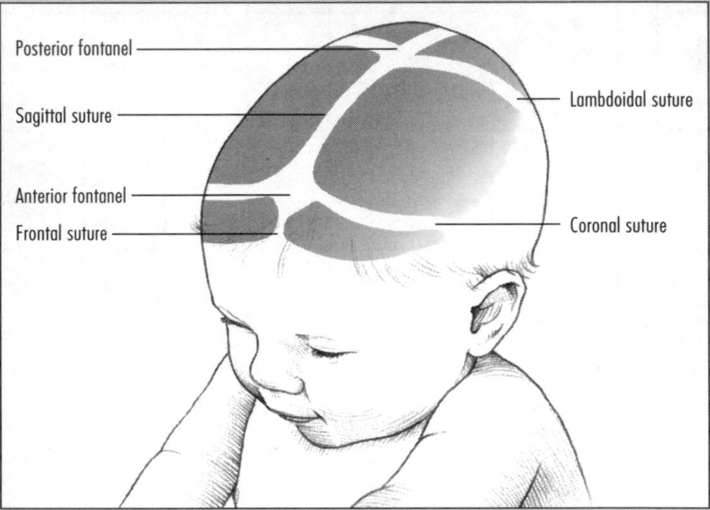

History

Once the infant's condition is stabilized, you can begin investigating the underlying cause of increased ICP. Obtain the child's medical history from a parent or caretaker, paying particular attention to recent infection or trauma, including birth trauma. Has the infant or a family member had a recent rash or fever? Ask about changes in the infant's behavior, such as frequent vomiting, lethargy, or disinterest in feeding.

Common medical causes

♦ ***Increased ICP.*** Besides a bulging fontanel and increased head circumference, other early signs and symptoms are commonly subtle and difficult to discern. They may include behavioral changes, irritability, fatigue, and vomiting. As ICP rises, the infant's pupils may dilate and his LOC may decrease to drowsiness and eventual coma. Seizures commonly occur.

Special considerations

Closely monitor the infant, including urine output (via indwelling urinary catheter, if necessary); continue to observe for seizures. Restrict fluid. Keep the infant in a supine position, with his body tilted 30 degrees and his head up, to enhance cerebral venous drainage and reduce intracranial blood volume.

Explain the purpose and procedure of diagnostic tests to the infant's parents or caretaker. Such tests may include intracranial computed tomography scan or skull X-ray, cerebral angiography, and a full sepsis workup, including blood studies and urine cultures.

FONTANEL DEPRESSION

Depression of the anterior fontanel below the surrounding bony ridges of the skull is a sign of dehydration. A common disorder of infancy and early childhood, dehydration can result from insufficient fluid intake, but it typically reflects excessive fluid loss from severe vomiting or diarrhea. It may also reflect insensible water loss, pyloric stenosis, or tracheoesophageal fistula. It's best to assess the fontanel when the infant is in an upright position and isn't crying.

Emergency interventions

If you detect a markedly depressed fontanel, take vital signs, weigh the infant, and check for signs of shock — tachycardia, tachypnea, and cool, clammy skin. If these signs are present, insert an I.V. line and administer fluids. Have size-appropriate emergency equipment on hand. Anticipate oxygen administration. Monitor urine output by weighing the wet diapers.

History

Obtain a thorough patient history from a parent or caretaker, focusing on recent fever, vomiting, diarrhea, and behavioral changes. Monitor the infant's fluid intake and urine output over the last 24 hours, including the number of wet diapers during that time. Ask about the child's pre-illness weight, and compare it with current weight; weight loss in an infant reflects water loss.

Common medical causes

♦ ***Dehydration.*** In *mild dehydration* (5% weight loss), the anterior fontanel appears slightly depressed. The infant has pale, dry skin and mucous membranes, decreased urine output, a normal or slightly elevated pulse rate and, possibly, irritability and a decreased level of activity.

Moderate dehydration (10% weight loss) causes slightly more pronounced fontanel depression, along with gray skin with poor turgor, dry mucous membranes, and decreased urine output. The infant has normal or decreased blood pressure, an increased pulse rate and, possibly, lethargy and seizures.

Severe dehydration (15% or greater weight loss) may result in a markedly depressed fontanel, extremely poor skin turgor, parched mucous membranes, marked oliguria, lethargy, and signs of shock, such as rapid, thready pulse and very low blood pressure.

Special considerations

Continue to monitor the infant's vital signs and intake and output, and watch for signs of worsening dehydration. Obtain serum electrolyte values to check for increased or decreased sodium, chloride, or potassium. In mild dehydration, frequently provide small amounts of clear fluids. If the infant can't ingest sufficient fluid, begin I.V. parenteral nutrition.

In patients with moderate to severe dehydration, your first priority is rapid restoration of extracellular fluid volume to treat or prevent shock. Continue to administer I.V. solution with sodium bicarbonate added to combat acidosis. As renal function improves, administer I.V. potassium replacements. Once the infant's fluid status stabilizes, begin to replace depleted fat and protein stores through diet.

Tests to evaluate dehydration include urinalysis for specific gravity and possibly blood tests to determine blood urea nitrogen and serum creatinine levels, osmolality, and acid-base status.

G

GAG REFLEX ABNORMALITIES

[Pharyngeal reflex abnormalities]

The gag reflex — a protective mechanism that prevents aspiration of food, fluid, and vomitus — normally can be elicited by touching the posterior wall of the oropharynx with a tongue blade or by suctioning the throat. Prompt elevation of the palate, constriction of the pharyngeal musculature, and a sensation of gagging indicate a normal gag reflex. An abnormal gag reflex — either decreased or absent — interferes with the ability to swallow and, more important, increases susceptibility to life-threatening aspiration.

An impaired gag reflex can result from any lesion that affects its mediators — cranial nerves IX (glossopharyngeal) and X (vagus) or the pons or medulla. It can also occur during a coma, in muscle diseases such as severe myasthenia gravis, or as a temporary result of anesthesia.

Emergency interventions

If you detect an abnormal gag reflex, immediately stop the patient's oral intake to prevent aspiration. Prepare the patient for a swallowing test. Quickly evaluate level of consciousness (LOC). If it's decreased, place him in a side-lying position to prevent aspiration; if not, place him in Fowler's position. Have suction equipment at hand.

History and physical examination

Ask the patient (or a family member if the patient can't communicate) about the onset and duration of swallowing difficulties. Are liquids more difficult to swallow than solids? Is swallowing more difficult at certain times of the day (as occurs in the bulbar palsy associated with myasthenia gravis)? If the patient also has trouble chewing, suspect more widespread neurologic involvement because chewing involves different cranial nerves.

Explore the patient's medical history for vascular and degenerative disorders. Then assess his respiratory status for evidence of aspiration, and perform a neurologic examination.

Common medical causes

♦ ***Basilar artery occlusion.*** This disorder may suddenly diminish or obliterate the gag reflex. It also causes diffuse sensory loss, dysarthria, facial weakness, extraocular muscle palsies, quadriplegia, and decreased LOC.

♦ ***Brain stem glioma.*** This lesion causes gradual loss of the gag reflex. Related symptoms reflect bilateral brain stem involvement and include diplopia and facial weakness. Common involvement of the corticospinal pathways causes spasticity and paresis of the arms and legs as well as gait disturbances.

◆ ***Bulbar palsy.*** Loss of the gag reflex reflects temporary or permanent paralysis of muscles supplied by cranial nerves IX and X. Other indicators of this paralysis include jaw and facial muscle weakness, dysphagia, loss of sensation at the base of the tongue, increased salivation, possible difficulty articulating and breathing, and fasciculations.

◆ ***Wallenberg's syndrome.*** Paresis of the palate and an impaired gag reflex usually develop within hours to days of thrombosis. The patient may experience analgesia and thermanesthesia (ipsilaterally on the face and contralaterally on the body) and vertigo. He may also display nystagmus, ipsilateral ataxia of the arm and leg, and signs of Horner's syndrome (unilateral ptosis and miosis, hemifacial anhidrosis).

Other causes

◆ ***Anesthesia.*** General and local (throat) anesthesia can produce temporary loss of the gag reflex.

Special considerations

Continually assess the patient's ability to swallow. If his gag reflex is absent, provide tube feedings; if it's merely diminished, try pureed foods. Advise the patient to take small amounts and eat slowly while sitting or in high Fowler's position. Stay with him while he eats, and observe for choking. Remember to keep suction equipment handy in case of aspiration. Keep accurate intake and output records, and assess the patient's nutritional status daily.

Prepare the patient for diagnostic studies, such as computed tomography scan, magnetic resonance imaging, electroencephalography, lumbar puncture, or arteriography.

Pediatric pointers

Brain stem glioma is an important cause of abnormal gag reflex in children.

GAIT, BIZARRE

[Hysterical gait]

A bizarre gait has no obvious organic basis; rather, it's produced unconsciously by a person with a somatoform disorder (hysterical neurosis) or consciously by a malingerer. The gait has no consistent pattern. It may mimic an organic impairment but characteristically has a more theatrical or bizarre quality with key elements missing, such as a spastic gait without hip circumduction, or leg "paralysis" with normal reflexes and motor strength. Its manifestations may include wild gyrations, exaggerated stepping, leg dragging, or mimicking unusual walks such as that of a tightrope walker.

History and physical examination

If you suspect that the patient's gait impairment has no organic cause, begin to investigate other possibilities. Ask the patient when he first developed the impairment and whether it coincided with a stressful period or event, such as the death of a loved one or loss of a job. Ask about associated symptoms, and explore reports of frequent unexplained illnesses and multiple doctor's visits. Subtly try to determine if he'll gain anything from malingering; for instance, added attention or an insurance settlement.

Begin the physical examination by testing the patient's reflexes and sensorimotor function, noting abnormal response patterns. To quickly check his reports of leg weakness or paralysis, perform Hoover's test: Place the patient in the supine position and stand at his feet. Cradle a heel in each of your palms, and rest your hands on the table. Ask the patient to raise the affected leg against resistance. In true motor weakness, the heel of the other leg will press downward; in hysteria, this movement will be absent. As a further check, observe the patient for normal movements when he's unaware of being watched.

Common medical causes

♦ ***Conversion disorder.*** In this rare somatoform disorder, a bizarre gait or paralysis may develop after severe stress and isn't accompanied by other symptoms. The patient typically shows indifference toward his impairment (la belle indifference.)

♦ ***Malingering.*** In this rare cause of bizarre gait, the patient may also complain of headache as well as chest and back pain.

♦ ***Somatization disorder.*** Bizarre gait is one of many possible somatic complaints. The patient may exhibit a combination of pseudoneurologic signs and symptoms — fainting, weakness, memory loss, dysphagia, visual problems (diplopia, vision loss, blurred vision), loss of voice, seizures, or bladder dysfunction. He may also report pain in the back, joints, and extremities (most commonly the legs) and complaints in almost any body system. For example, characteristic GI complaints include pain, bloating, nausea, and vomiting.

The patient's reflexes and motor strength remain normal, but peculiar contractures and arm or leg rigidity may occur. His reputed sensory loss doesn't conform to a known sensory dermatome. In some cases, he won't stand or walk (astasia-abasia), remaining bedridden although still able to move his legs in bed.

Special considerations

A full neurologic workup may be necessary to completely rule out an organic cause of the patient's abnormal gait. Remember, even though bizarre gait has no organic basis, it's real to the patient (unless, of course, he's malingering). Avoid expressing judgment on the patient's actions or motives; you'll need to be supportive and reinforce positive progress. Because muscle atrophy and bone demineralization can develop in bedridden patients, encourage ambulation and resumption of normal activities. Consider a referral for psychiatric counseling as appropriate.

Pediatric pointers

Bizarre gait is rare before age 8. More common in prepubescence, it usually results from conversion disorder.

GAIT, PROPULSIVE

[Festinating gait]

Propulsive gait is characterized by a stooped, rigid posture — the patient's head and neck are bent forward; his flexed, stiffened arms are held away from the body; his fingers are extended; and his knees and hips are stiffly bent. During ambulation, this posture results in a forward shifting of the body's center of gravity and consequent impairment of balance, causing increasingly rapid, short, shuffling steps with involuntary acceleration (festination) and lack of control over forward motion (propulsion) or backward motion (retropulsion). (See *Identifying gait abnormalities,* pages 268 and 269.)

Propulsive gait is a cardinal sign of advanced Parkinson's disease; it results from progressive degeneration of the ganglia, which are primarily responsible for smooth muscle movement. Because this sign develops gradually and its accompanying effects are commonly wrongly attributed to aging; propulsive gait commonly goes unnoticed or unreported until severe disability results.

History and physical examination

Ask the patient when his gait impairment first developed and whether it has recently worsened. Because he may have difficulty remembering, having attributed the gait to "old age," you may be able to gain information from family members or friends, especially those who see the patient only sporadically.

Also, obtain a thorough drug history, including both medication type and dosage. Ask the patient if he has been taking tranquilizers, especially phenothiazines. If he knows he has Parkinson's disease and has been taking levodopa, pay particular attention to the dosage because an overdose can cause acute exacerbation of signs and symptoms. If Parkinson's disease isn't a known or suspected diagnosis, ask the patient if he has been acutely or routinely exposed to carbon monoxide or manganese.

Begin the physical examination by testing the patient's reflexes and sensorimotor function, noting abnormal response patterns.

Common medical causes

♦ ***Carbon monoxide poisoning.*** Propulsive gait commonly appears several weeks after acute carbon monoxide intoxication. Earlier effects include muscle rigidity, choreoathetotic movements, generalized seizures, myoclonic jerks, masklike facies, and dementia.

♦ ***Manganese poisoning.*** Chronic overexposure to manganese can cause an insidious, usually permanent, propulsive gait. Typical early findings include fatigue, muscle weakness and rigidity, dystonia, resting tremor, choreoathetotic movements, masklike facies, and personality changes.

♦ ***Parkinson's disease.*** The characteristic and permanent propulsive gait begins early as a shuffle. As the disease progresses, the gait slows. Cardinal signs of the disease are progressive muscle rigidity, which may be uniform (lead-pipe rigidity) or jerky (cogwheel rigidity); akinesia; and an insidious tremor that begins in the fingers, increases during stress or anxiety, and decreases with purposeful movement and sleep. Besides the gait, akinesia also typically produces a monotone voice, drooling, masklike facies, stooped posture, and dysarthria or dysphagia. Occasionally, it also causes oculogyric crises or blepharospasm.

Other causes

♦ ***Drugs.*** Propulsive gait and possibly other extrapyramidal effects can result from the use of phenothiazines, other antipsychotics (notably haloperidol, thiothixene, and loxapine) or, infrequently, metoclopramide or metyrosine. Such effects are usually temporary, disappearing within a few weeks after therapy is discontinued.

Special considerations

Because of his gait and associated motor impairment, the patient may have problems performing activities of daily living. Assist him as appropriate, at the same time encouraging his independence and self-reliance. Advise the patient and his family to allow plenty of time for these activities, especially walking, because he's particularly susceptible to falls due to festination and poor balance. Encourage the patient to maintain ambulation; for safety reasons, remember to stay with him while he's walking, especially if he's on unfamiliar or uneven ground. You may need to refer him to a physical therapist for exercise therapy and gait retraining.

Pediatric pointers

Propulsive gait, usually with severe tremors, typically occurs in juvenile parkinsonism, a rare form. Other possible but rare causes include Hallervorden-Spatz disease and kernicterus.

GAIT, SCISSORS

Resulting from bilateral spastic paresis (diplegia), scissors gait affects both legs and has little or no effect on the arms. The patient's legs flex slightly at the hips and knees, so he looks as if he's crouching. With each step, his thighs adduct

EXAMINATION TIP

Identifying gait abnormalities

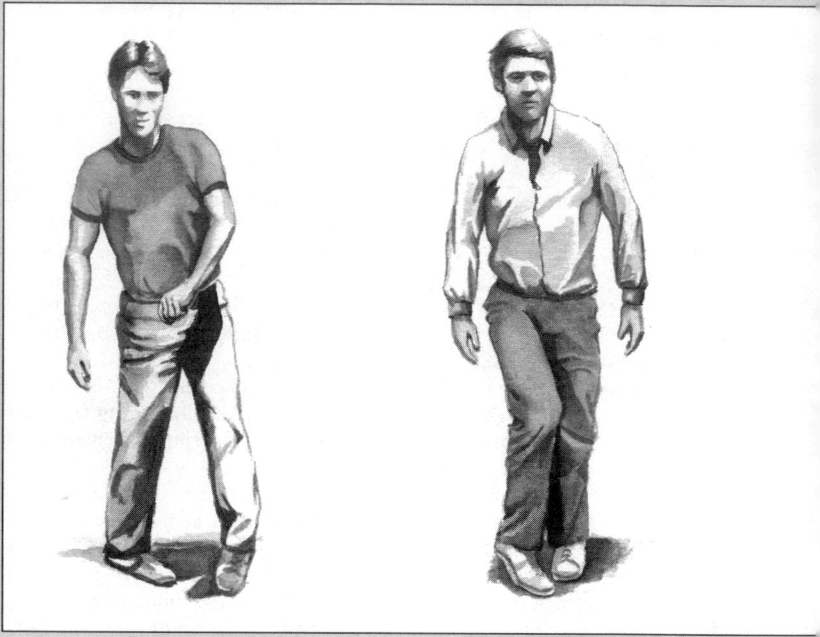

and his knees hit or cross in a scissors-like movement. (See *Identifying gait abnormalities.*) His steps are short, regular, and laborious, as if he were wading through waist-deep water. His feet may be plantarflexed and turned inward, with a shortened Achilles tendon; as a result, he walks on his toes or on the balls of his feet and may scrape his toes on the ground.

History and physical examination

Ask the patient (or a family member, if the patient can't answer) about the onset and duration of the gait. Has it progressively worsened or remained constant? Ask about a history of trauma, including birth trauma, and neurologic disorders. Thoroughly evaluate motor and sensory function and deep tendon reflexes in the legs.

Common medical causes

◆ ***Cerebral palsy.*** In the spastic form of this disorder, patients walk on their toes with a scissors gait. Other features include hyperactive deep tendon reflexes, increased stretch reflexes, rapid alternating muscle contraction and relaxation, muscle weakness, underdevelopment of affected limbs, and a tendency toward contractures.

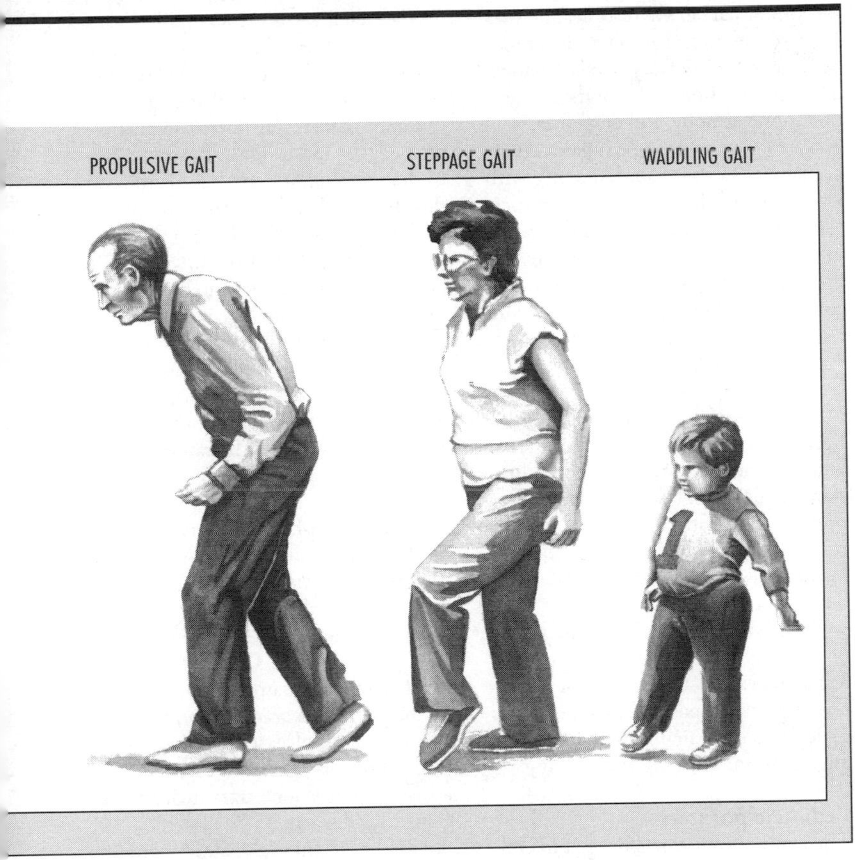
PROPULSIVE GAIT
STEPPAGE GAIT
WADDLING GAIT

♦ ***Cervical spondylosis with myelopathy.*** Scissors gait develops in the late stages of this degenerative disease and steadily worsens. Related findings mimic those of a herniated disk: severe lower back pain, which may radiate to the buttocks, legs, and feet; muscle spasms; sensorimotor loss; and muscle weakness and atrophy.

♦ ***Multiple sclerosis.*** Progressive scissors gait usually develops gradually, with infrequent remissions. Characteristic muscle weakness, usually in the legs, ranges from minor fatigability to paraparesis with urinary urgency and constipation. Related findings include facial pain, visual disturbances, paresthesia, incoordination, and loss of proprioception and vibration sensation in the ankle and toes.

♦ ***Spinal cord tumor.*** Scissors gait can develop gradually from a thoracic or lumbar tumor. Other findings reflect the location of the tumor and may include radicular, subscapular, shoulder, groin, leg, or flank pain; muscle spasms or fasciculations; muscle atrophy; sensory deficits, such as paresthesia and a girdle sensation of the abdomen and chest; hyperactive deep tendon reflexes; bilateral Babinski's reflex; spastic neurogenic bladder; and sexual dysfunction.

♦ ***Syphilitic meningomyelitis.*** Scissors gait appears late in this disorder and may improve with treatment. The patient may also experience sensory ataxia, changes in proprioception and vibration sensation, optic atrophy, and dementia.

♦ ***Syringomyelia.*** Scissors gait usually occurs late in this disorder, along with analgesia and thermanesthesia, muscle atrophy and weakness, and Charcot's joints. Other effects may include loss of fingernails, fingers, or toes; Dupuytren's contracture of the palms; scoliosis; and clubfoot. Skin in the affected areas is commonly dry, scaly, and grooved.

Special considerations

Because of the sensory loss associated with scissors gait, provide meticulous skin care to prevent skin breakdown and pressure ulcer formation. Also, give the patient and his family complete skin care instructions. If appropriate, provide bladder and bowel retraining.

Provide daily active and passive range-of-motion exercises. Referral to a physical therapist may be required for gait retraining and for possible in-shoe splints or leg braces to maintain proper foot alignment for standing and walking.

Pediatric pointers

The major causes of scissors gait in children are cerebral palsy, hereditary spastic paraplegia, and spinal injury at birth. If spastic paraplegia is present at birth, scissors gait becomes apparent when the child begins to walk, which is usually later than normal.

GAIT, SPASTIC
[Hemiplegic gait]

Spastic gait — sometimes referred to as paretic or weak gait — is a stiff, foot-dragging walk caused by unilateral leg muscle hypertonicity. This gait reflects focal damage to the corticospinal tract. The affected leg becomes rigid, with a marked decrease in flexion at the hip and knee and possibly plantar flexion and equinovarus deformity of the foot. Because the patient's leg doesn't swing normally at the hip or knee, his foot tends to drag or shuffle, scraping his toes on the ground. (See *Identifying gait abnormalities,* pages 268 and 269.) To compensate, the pelvis of the affected side tilts upward in an attempt to lift the toes, causing the patient's leg to abduct and circumduct. Also, arm swing is hindered on the same side as the affected leg.

Spastic gait usually develops after a period of flaccidity (hypotonicity) in the affected leg. Whatever the cause, the gait is usually permanent once it develops.

History and physical examination

Find out when the patient first noticed the gait impairment and whether it developed suddenly or gradually. Ask him if it waxes and wanes or if it has worsened progressively. Does fatigue, hot weather, or warm baths or showers worsen the gait? Such exacerbation typically occurs in multiple sclerosis. Focus your medical history questions on neurologic disorders, recent head trauma, and degenerative diseases.

During the physical examination, test and compare strength, range of motion, and sensory function in all limbs. Also, observe and palpate for muscle flaccidity or atrophy.

Common medical causes

♦ ***Brain abscess.*** In this disorder, spastic gait generally develops slowly after a period of muscle flaccidity and fever. Early signs and symptoms of abscess reflect increased intracranial pressure (ICP): headache, nausea, vomiting, and focal or generalized seizures. Later, site-specific features may include hemiparesis, tremors, vision disturbances, nystagmus, and pupillary inequality. The patient's level of consciousness may range from drowsiness to stupor.

◆ ***Brain tumor.*** Depending on the site and type of tumor, spastic gait usually develops gradually and worsens over time. Accompanying effects may include signs of increased ICP (headache, nausea, vomiting, and focal or generalized seizures), papilledema, sensory loss on the affected side, dysarthria, ocular palsies, aphasia, and personality changes.

◆ ***Cerebrovascular accident.*** Spastic gait usually appears after a period of muscle weakness and hypotonicity on the affected side. Associated effects may include unilateral muscle atrophy, sensory loss, and footdrop; aphasia; dysarthria; dysphagia; visual field deficits; diplopia; and ocular palsies.

◆ ***Head trauma.*** Spastic gait typically follows the acute stage of head trauma. The patient may also experience focal or generalized seizures, personality changes, headache, and focal neurologic signs, such as aphasia and visual field deficits.

◆ ***Multiple sclerosis.*** Spastic gait begins insidiously and follows this disorder's characteristic cycle of remission and exacerbation. The gait, as well as other signs and symptoms, commonly worsens in warm weather or after a warm bath or shower. Characteristic weakness, usually affecting the legs, ranges from minor fatigability to paraparesis with urinary urgency and constipation. Other effects include facial pain, paresthesia, incoordination, loss of proprioception and vibration sensation in the ankle and toes, and vision disturbances.

Special considerations

Because leg muscle contractures are commonly associated with spastic gait, promote daily exercise — active and passive. The patient may have poor balance and a tendency to fall to the paralyzed side, so stay with him while he's walking. Provide a cane or a walker, as indicated. As appropriate, refer the patient to a physical therapist for gait retraining and possible in-shoe splints or leg braces to maintain proper foot alignment for standing and walking.

Pediatric pointers

Causes of spastic gait in children include sickle cell crisis, cerebral palsy, porencephalic cysts, and arteriovenous malformation that causes hemorrhage or ischemia.

GAIT, STEPPAGE

[Equine gait, paretic gait, prancing gait, weak gait]

Steppage gait typically results from footdrop caused by weakness or paralysis of pretibial and peroneal muscles, usually from lower motor neuron lesions. Footdrop causes the foot to hang with the toes pointing down, causing the toes to scrape the ground during ambulation. To compensate, the hip rotates outward and the hip and knee flex in an exaggerated fashion to lift the advancing leg off the ground. The foot is thrown forward and the toes hit the ground first, producing an audible slap. (See *Identifying gait abnormalities,* pages 268 and 269.) The rhythm of the gait is usually regular, with even steps and normal upper body posture and arm swing. Steppage gait can be unilateral or bilateral and permanent or transient, depending on the site and type of neural damage.

History and physical examination

Begin by asking the patient about the onset of the gait and recent changes in its character. Does a family member have a similar gait? Find out if the patient has had a traumatic injury to the buttocks, hips, legs, or knees. Ask about a history of chronic disorders that may be associated with polyneuropathy, such as diabetes mellitus, polyarteritis nodosa, and alcoholism. While you're taking the history, observe whether the patient crosses his legs while sitting because this may put pressure on the peroneal nerve.

Inspect and palpate the patient's calves and feet for muscle atrophy and wasting. Using a pin, test for sensory deficits along the entire length of both legs.

Common medical causes

♦ ***Guillain-Barré syndrome.*** Typically occurring after recovery from the acute stage of this disorder, steppage gait can be mild or severe and unilateral or bilateral; it's invariably permanent. Muscle weakness usually begins in the legs, extends to the arms and face within 72 hours, and can progress to total motor paralysis and respiratory failure. Other effects include footdrop, transient paresthesia, hypernasality, dysphagia, diaphoresis, tachycardia, orthostatic hypotension, and incontinence.

♦ ***Herniated lumbar disk.*** Unilateral steppage gait and footdrop commonly occur with late-stage weakness and atrophy of leg muscles. However, the most pronounced symptom is severe lower back pain, which may radiate to the buttocks, legs, and feet, usually unilaterally. Sciatic pain follows, commonly accompanied by muscle spasms and sensorimotor loss. Paresthesia and fasciculations may occur.

♦ ***Multiple sclerosis.*** Steppage gait and footdrop typically fluctuate in severity with this disorder's characteristic cycle of periodic exacerbation and remission. Muscle weakness, usually affecting the legs, can range from minor fatigability to paraparesis with urinary urgency and constipation. Related findings include facial pain, vision disturbances, paresthesia, incoordination, and sensory loss in the ankle and toes.

♦ ***Peroneal muscle atrophy.*** Bilateral steppage gait and footdrop begin insidiously in this disorder. Foot, peroneal, and ankle dorsiflexor muscles are affected first. Other early signs and symptoms include paresthesia, aching, and cramping in the feet and legs along with coldness, swelling, and cyanosis. As the disorder progresses, all leg muscles become weak and atrophic, with hypoactive or absent deep tendon reflexes. Later, atrophy and sensory losses spread to the hands and arms.

♦ ***Peroneal nerve trauma.*** Temporary ipsilateral steppage gait occurs suddenly but resolves with the release of peroneal nerve pressure. The gait is associated with footdrop and muscle weakness and sensory loss over the lateral surface of the calf and foot.

Special considerations

The patient with steppage gait may tire rapidly when walking because of the extra effort he must expend to lift his feet off the ground. When he tires, he may stub his toes, causing a fall. To prevent this, help the patient recognize his exercise limits, and encourage him to get adequate rest. Refer him to a physical therapist, if appropriate, for gait retraining and possible application of in-shoe splints or leg braces to maintain correct foot alignment.

GAIT, WADDLING

Waddling gait, a distinctive ducklike walk, is an important sign of muscular dystrophy, spinal muscle atrophy or, rarely, congenital hip displacement. It may be present when the child begins to walk or may appear only later in life. The gait results from deterioration of the pelvic girdle muscles — primarily the gluteus medius, hip flexors, and hip extensors. Weakness in these muscles hinders stabilization of the weight-bearing hip during walking, causing the opposite hip to drop and the trunk to lean toward that side in an attempt to maintain balance. (See *Identifying gait abnormalities,* pages 268 and 269.)

Typically, the legs assume a wide stance, and the trunk is thrown back to further improve stability, exaggerating lordosis and abdominal protrusion. In severe cases, leg and foot muscle contractures may cause equinovarus deformity of the foot combined with circumduction or bowing of the legs.

History and physical examination

Ask the patient (or a family member, if the patient is a young child) when the gait first appeared and if it has recently worsened. To determine the extent of pelvic girdle and leg muscle weakness, ask if the patient falls frequently or has difficulty climbing stairs, rising from a chair, or walking. Also, find out if he was late in learning to walk or holding his head upright. Obtain a family history, focusing on problems of muscle weakness and gait and on congenital motor disorders.

Inspect and palpate leg muscles, especially in the calves, for size and tone. Check for a positive Gowers' sign, which reflects pelvic muscle weakness. Next, assess motor strength and function in the shoulders, arms, and hands, looking for weakness or asymmetrical movements.

Common medical causes

◆ ***Congenital hip dysplasia.*** Bilateral hip dislocation produces a waddling gait with lordosis and pain.

◆ ***Muscular dystrophy.*** In *Duchenne's muscular dystrophy,* waddling gait becomes clinically evident by age 3 to 5. The gait worsens as the disease progresses, until the child loses the ability to walk and becomes wheelchair-bound, usually between ages 10 and 12. Early signs are usually subtle: delay in learning to walk, frequent falls, gait or posture abnormalities, and intermittent calf pain. Common later findings include lordosis with abdominal protrusion, a positive Gowers' sign, and equinovarus foot position. As the disease progresses, its effects become more prominent; they commonly include rapid muscle wasting beginning in the legs and spreading to the arms (although calf and upper arm muscles may become hypertrophied, firm, and rubbery), muscle contractures, limited dorsiflexion of the feet and extension of the knees and elbows, obesity and, possibly, mild mental retardation. Serious complications result when kyphoscoliosis develops, leading to respiratory dysfunction and, eventually, death from cardiac or respiratory failure.

In *Becker's muscular dystrophy,* waddling gait typically becomes apparent in late adolescence, slowly worsens during the third decade, and culminates in total loss of ambulation. Muscle weakness first appears in the pelvic and upper arm muscles. Progressive wasting with selected muscle hypertrophy produces lordosis with abdominal protrusion, poor balance, a positive Gowers' sign and, possibly, mental retardation.

In *facioscapulohumeral muscular dystrophy,* which usually occurs late in childhood and during adolescence, waddling gait appears after muscle wasting has spread downward from the face and shoulder girdle to the pelvic girdle and legs. Earlier effects include progressive weakness and atrophy of facial, shoulder, and arm muscles; slight lordosis; and pelvic instability.

◆ ***Spinal muscle atrophy.*** In *Kugelberg-Welander syndrome,* waddling gait occurs early (usually after age 2) and typically progresses slowly, culminating in total loss of ambulation up to 20 years later. Related findings may include muscle atrophy in the legs and pelvis that progresses to the shoulders, a positive Gowers' sign, ophthalmoplegia, or tongue fasciculations.

In *Werdnig-Hoffmann disease,* waddling gait typically begins when the child learns to walk. Reflexes may be absent. The gait progressively worsens, culminating in complete loss of ambulation by adolescence. Associated findings include lordosis with abdominal protrusion and muscle weakness in the hips and thighs.

Special considerations

Although there's no cure for this gait, daily passive and active muscle-stretching exercises should be performed for both arms and legs. If possible, have the patient walk at least 3 hours each day (with leg braces, if necessary) to maintain muscle strength, reduce contractures, and delay further gait deterioration. Stay near the patient during the walk, especially if he's on unfamiliar or uneven ground. Provide a balanced diet to maintain energy levels and prevent obesity. Because of the grim prognosis associated with muscular dystrophy and spinal muscle atrophy, provide emotional support for the patient and his family.

Patient counseling

Caution the patient against long, unbroken periods of bed rest, which accelerate muscle deterioration. As indicated, refer him to a local Muscular Dystrophy Association chapter. Suggest genetic testing and counseling for the parents, if they're considering having another child.

GALLOP, ATRIAL

[S_4]

An atrial or presystolic gallop is an extra heart sound (known as S_4) that's heard or commonly palpated immediately before the first heart sound. This low-pitched sound is heard best with the bell of the stethoscope pressed lightly against the cardiac apex. Some clinicians say that an S_4 has the cadence of the "Ten" in Tennessee (Ten = S_4; nes = S_1; see = S_2).

This gallop typically results from hypertension, conduction defects, valvular disorders, or other problems such as ischemia. Occasionally, it helps differentiate angina from other causes of chest pain. Atrial gallop results from abnormal forceful atrial contraction caused by elevated ventricular filling pressures or by decreased left ventricular compliance. It usually originates from left atrial contraction, is heard at the apex, and doesn't vary with inspiration. The gallop may also originate from right atrial contraction. If so, it's heard best at the lower left sternal border and intensifies with inspiration.

An atrial gallop seldom occurs in normal hearts; however, it may occur in athletes with physiologic hypertrophy of the left ventricle.

Emergency interventions

Suspect myocardial ischemia if you auscultate an atrial gallop in a patient with chest pain. (See *Locating heart sounds.* See also *Interpreting heart sounds,* pages 276 and 277.) Take the patient's vital signs, and quickly look for signs of heart failure, such as dyspnea, crackles, and distended neck veins. If you detect these signs, connect the patient to a cardiac monitor and obtain an electrocardiogram. Administer antianginal drugs. If the patient has dyspnea, elevate the head of the bed and then auscultate for abnormal breath sounds. If you detect coarse crackles, start an I.V. line and give oxygen and diuretics as needed. If the patient has bradycardia, he may require atropine and a pacemaker.

History

When the patient's condition permits, ask about a history of hypertension, angina, valvular stenosis, or cardiomyopathy. If appropriate, have him describe the frequency and severity of anginal attacks.

Common medical causes

♦ ***Angina.*** An intermittent atrial gallop characteristically occurs during an anginal attack and disappears when angina subsides. This gallop may be accompanied by a paradoxical S_2 or a new mur-

EXAMINATION TIP

Locating heart sounds

When auscultating heart sounds, remember that certain sounds are heard best in specific areas. Use the auscultatory points shown here to locate heart sounds quickly and accurately. Then expand your auscultation to nearby areas. Note that the numbers indicate pertinent intercostal spaces.

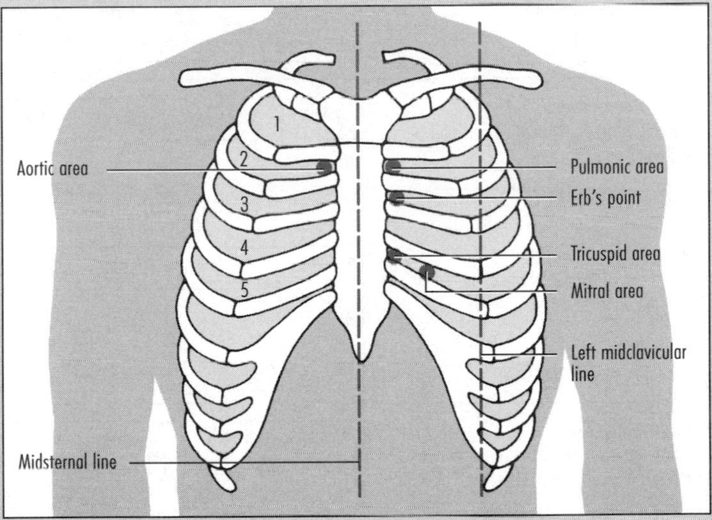

mur. Typically, the patient complains of anginal chest pain — a feeling of tightness, pressure, achiness, or burning that usually radiates from the retrosternal area to the neck, jaws, left shoulder, and arm. He may also exhibit dyspnea, tachycardia, palpitations, increased blood pressure, dizziness, diaphoresis, belching, nausea, and vomiting.

♦ ***Aortic insufficiency (acute).*** This disorder causes an atrial gallop accompanied by a soft, short diastolic murmur along the left sternal border. S_2 may be soft or absent. Sometimes, a soft, short midsystolic murmur may be heard over the second right intercostal space. Related cardiopulmonary findings may include tachycardia, S_3, dyspnea, neck vein distention, and crackles. The patient may also be fatigued and have cool extremities.

♦ ***Aortic stenosis.*** This disorder usually causes an atrial gallop, especially when valvular obstruction is severe. Auscultation reveals a harsh, crescendo-decrescendo, systolic ejection murmur that's loudest at the right sternal border near the second intercostal space. Dyspnea, anginal chest pain, and syncope are cardinal associated findings. The patient may also display crackles, palpitations, fatigue, and diminished carotid pulses.

♦ ***Atrioventricular (AV) block.*** *First-degree AV block* may cause an atrial gal-

Interpreting heart sounds

Detecting subtle variations in heart sounds requires both concentration and practice. Once you recognize normal heart sounds, the abnormal sounds become more obvious.

HEART SOUNDS AND CAUSES | **TIMING AND CADENCE**

First heart sound (S_1)
Vibrations associated with mitral and tricuspid valve closure

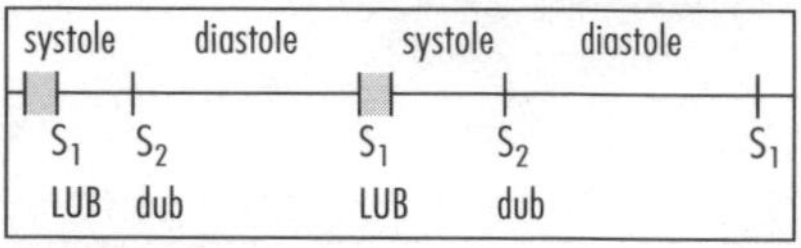

Second heart sound (S_2)
Vibrations associated with aortic and pulmonic valve closure

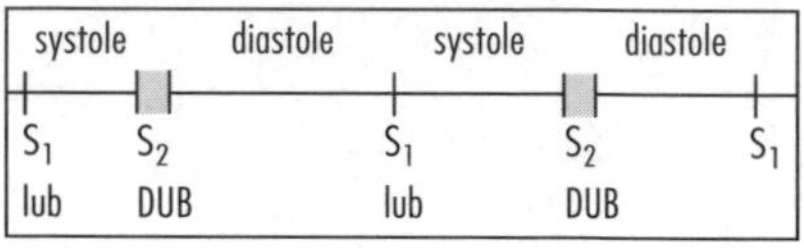

Ventricular gallop (S_3)
Vibrations produced by rapid blood flow into the ventricles

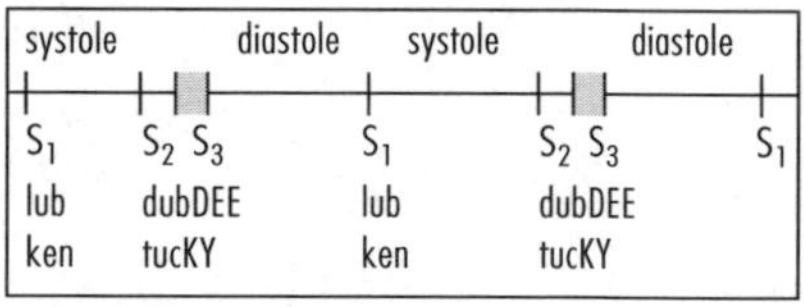

Atrial gallop (S_4)
Vibrations produced by an increased resistance to sudden, forceful ejection of atrial blood

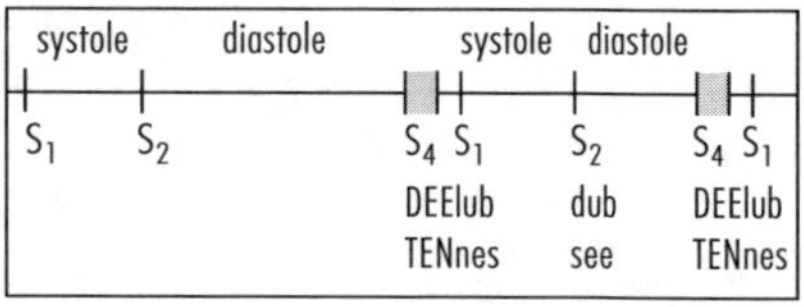

Summation gallop
Vibrations produced in middiastole by simultaneous ventricular and atrial gallops, caused by tachycardia

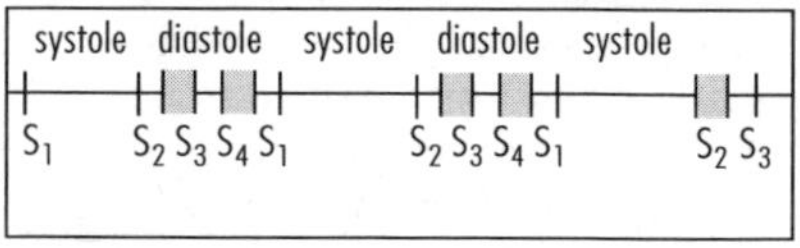

lop accompanied by a faint first heart sound (S_1). Although the patient may have bradycardia, he's usually asymptomatic. In *second-degree AV block,* an atrial gallop is easily heard. If bradycardia develops, the patient may also experience hypotension, light-headedness, dizziness, and fatigue. An atrial gallop is also common in *third-degree AV block.* It varies in intensity with S_1 and is loudest when atrial systole coincides with early, rapid ventricular filling during diastole. The

AUSCULTATION TIPS

Best heard with the diaphragm of the stethoscope at the apex (mitral area).

Best heard with the diaphragm of the stethoscope in the second or third right and left parasternal intercostal spaces with the patient sitting or supine.

Best heard though the bell of the stethoscope at the apex with the patient in the left lateral position. May be visible and palpable during early diastole at the midclavicular line between the fourth and fifth intercostal spaces.

Best heard through the bell of the stethoscope at the apex with the patient in the left semilateral position. May be visible in the diastole at the midclavicular line between the fourth and fifth intercostal spaces. May also be palpable in the midclavicular area with the patient in the left lateral decubitus position.

Best heard through the bell of the stethoscope at the apex with the patient in the left lateral position. May be louder than S_1 or S_2. May be visible and palpable during diastole.

patient may be asymptomatic or have hypotension, light-headedness, dizziness, or syncope, depending on the ventricular rate. Bradycardia may also aggravate or provoke angina or symptoms of heart failure such as dyspnea.

♦ ***Cardiomyopathy.*** An atrial gallop is a sign associated with cardiomyopathy, regardless of the type — dilated (most common), hypertrophic, or restrictive (least common). Additional findings may include dyspnea, orthopnea, crackles, fatigue, syncope, chest pain, palpitations, edema, neck vein distention, S_3, and transient or sustained bradycardia usually associated with tachycardia.

♦ ***Hypertension.*** One of the earliest findings in systemic arterial hypertension is an atrial gallop. The patient may be asymptomatic, or he may experience headache, weakness, epistaxis, tinnitus, dizziness, or fatigue.

♦ ***Myocardial infarction (MI).*** An atrial gallop is a classic sign of life-threatening MI; in fact, it may persist even after the infarction heals. Typically, the patient reports crushing substernal chest pain that may radiate to the back, neck, jaw, shoulder, and left arm. Associated signs and symptoms include dyspnea, restlessness, anxiety, a feeling of impending doom, diaphoresis, pallor, clammy skin, nausea, vomiting, and increased or decreased blood pressure.

♦ ***Pulmonary embolism.*** This life-threatening disorder causes a right-sided atrial gallop that's usually heard along the lower left sternal border with a loud pulmonic closure sound. Other features include tachycardia, tachypnea, fever, chest pain, dyspnea, decreased breath sounds, crackles, a pleural chest rub, apprehension, diaphoresis, syncope, and cyanosis. The patient may have a productive cough with blood-tinged sputum or a nonproductive cough.

♦ ***Thyrotoxicosis.*** An atrial gallop and an S_3 may both be auscultated in thyroid hormone overproduction. Other cardinal features include tachycardia, palpitations, weight loss despite increased appetite, diarrhea, tremors, an enlarged thyroid, dyspnea, nervousness, diaphoresis, heat intolerance, and exophthalmos.

Special considerations

Prepare the patient for diagnostic tests, such as electrocardiography, echocardiography, cardiac catheterization and, possibly, a lung scan.

Pediatric pointers

An atrial gallop may occur normally in children, especially after exercise. However, it may also result from congenital heart diseases, such as atrial septal defect, ventricular septal defect, patent ductus arteriosus, and severe pulmonary valvular stenosis.

Geriatric pointers

Because the absolute intensity of an atrial gallop doesn't decrease with age, as it does with an S_1, the relative intensity of S_4 increases compared with S_1. This explains the increased frequency of an audible S_4 in elderly patients.

GALLOP, VENTRICULAR

[S_3]

A ventricular gallop is a heart sound (known as S_3) associated with rapid ventricular filling in early diastole. Usually palpable, this low-frequency sound occurs about 0.15 second after the second heart sound (S_2). It may originate in either the left or right ventricle. A right-sided gallop usually sounds louder on inspiration and is heard best along the lower left sternal border or over the xiphoid region. A left-sided gallop usually sounds louder on expiration and is heard best at the apex.

Ventricular gallops are easily overlooked because they're usually faint. Fortunately, certain techniques make their detection more likely. These include auscultating in a quiet environment; examining the patient in the supine, left lateral, and semi-Fowler's positions; and having the patient cough or raise his legs to augment the sound.

A physiologic ventricular gallop normally occurs in children and young adults; however, most people lose this third heart sound by age 40. This gallop may also occur during the third trimester of pregnancy. Although the physiologic S_3 has the same timing as the pathologic S_3, its intensity waxes and wanes with respiration. It's also heard more faintly if the patient is sitting or standing.

A pathologic ventricular gallop may be one of the earliest signs of ventricular failure. It may result from one of two mechanisms: rapid deceleration of blood entering a stiff, noncompliant ventricle or rapid acceleration of blood associated with increased flow into the ventricle. A gallop that persists despite therapy indicates a poor prognosis.

Patients with cardiomyopathy or heart failure may develop a ventricular gallop and an atrial gallop—a condition known as a summation gallop. (See *Summation gallop: Two gallops in one.*)

History and physical examination

After auscultating a ventricular gallop, focus your history and examination on the cardiovascular system. Begin the history by asking the patient if he has had chest pain. If so, have him describe its character, location, frequency, duration, and any alleviating or aggravating factors. Also, ask about palpitations, dizziness, or syncope. Does the patient have difficulty breathing after exertion? While lying down? At rest? Does he have a cough? Ask about a history of cardiac disorders. Is the patient currently receiving treatment for heart failure? If so, which medications is he taking?

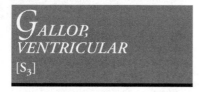

During the physical examination, carefully auscultate for murmurs or abnormalities in the first and second heart sounds. Then listen for pulmonary crackles. Next, assess peripheral pulses, noting pulsus alternans, an alternating strong and weak pulse. Finally, palpate the liver to detect enlargement or tenderness, and assess for neck vein distention and peripheral edema.

Common medical causes

◆ ***Aortic insufficiency.*** This occurs secondary to reduced ejection fraction and elevated end-systolic volume. Acute and chronic aortic insufficiency may produce an S_3. Typically, acute aortic insufficiency also causes an atrial gallop and a soft, short diastolic murmur over the left sternal border. S_2 may be soft or absent. At times, a soft, short midsystolic murmur may be heard over the second right intercostal space. Related findings include tachycardia, dyspnea, neck vein distention, and crackles.

Chronic aortic insufficiency produces a ventricular gallop and a high-pitched, blowing, decrescendo diastolic murmur that's best heard over the second or third right intercostal space or the left sternal border. An Austin Flint murmur — an apical, rumbling, mid- to late-diastolic murmur — may also occur. Typical related findings include palpitations, tachycardia, anginal chest pain, fatigue, dyspnea, orthopnea, and crackles.

◆ ***Cardiomyopathy.*** A ventricular gallop is characteristic of this disorder. When accompanied by pulsus alternans and altered first and second heart sounds, this gallop usually signals advanced heart disease. Other effects may include fatigue, dyspnea, orthopnea, chest pain, palpitations, syncope, crackles, peripheral edema, neck vein distention, or an atrial gallop.

◆ ***Heart failure.*** A cardinal sign of heart failure is a ventricular gallop. When it's loud and accompanied by sinus tachycardia, this gallop may indicate severe heart failure. The patient with left-sided heart failure also exhibits fatigue, exertional dyspnea, paroxysmal nocturnal dyspnea, orthopnea and, possibly, a dry cough; with right-sided heart failure, neck vein distention occurs. Other late features include tachypnea, chest tightness, palpitations, anorexia, nausea, dependent edema, weight gain, slowed mental response, diaphoresis, pallor, hypotension, narrowed pulse pressure and, possibly, oliguria. In some patients, inspiratory crackles, clubbing, and a tender, palpable liver may be present. As heart failure progresses, hemoptysis, cyanosis, severe pitting edema, and marked hepatomegaly may develop.

Summation gallop: Two gallops in one

When atrial and ventricular gallops occur simultaneously, they produce a short, low-pitched sound known as *summation gallop*. This relatively uncommon sound occurs during middiastole (between S_2 and S_1) and is best heard with the bell of the stethoscope pressed lightly against the cardiac apex. It may be louder than either S_1 or S_2 and may cause visible apical movement during diastole.

A summation gallop may result from tachycardia or from delayed or blocked atrioventricular (AV) conduction. Tachycardia shortens ventricular filing time during diastole, causing it to coincide with atrial contraction. When the heart rate slows, the summation gallop is replaced by a quadruple rhythm much like the canter of a horse. Delayed AV conduction also brings atrial contraction closer to ventricular filing, creating a summation gallop.

A summation gallop usually results from heart failure or dilated congestive cardiomyopathy, but it may accompany other cardiac disorders. Occasionally, it signals further cardiac deterioration. For example, consider the hypertensive patient with a chronic atrial gallop who develops tachycardia and a superimposed ventricular gallop. If this patient abruptly displays a summation gallop, heart failure is the likely cause.

◆ ***Mitral insufficiency.*** Both acute and chronic mitral insufficiency may produce a ventricular gallop. In *acute mitral insufficiency,* auscultation may also reveal an early or holosystolic decrescendo murmur at the apex, an atrial gallop, and a widely split second heart sound. Typically, the patient displays sinus tachycardia, tachypnea, orthopnea, dyspnea, crackles, distended neck veins, and fatigue.

In *chronic mitral insufficiency,* a progressively severe ventricular gallop is typical. Auscultation also reveals a holosystolic, blowing, high-pitched apical murmur. The patient may report fatigue, exertional dyspnea, and palpitations, or he may be asymptomatic.

◆ ***Thyrotoxicosis.*** This disorder may produce ventricular and atrial gallops, but its cardinal features are an enlarged thyroid gland, weight loss despite increased appetite, heat intolerance, diaphoresis, nervousness, tremors, tachycardia, palpitations, diarrhea, and dyspnea.

Special considerations

Monitor the patient for and report tachycardia, dyspnea, crackles, and neck vein distention. Give oxygen, diuretics, and other drugs, such as digoxin and angiotensin-converting enzyme inhibitors, to prevent pulmonary edema. Prepare the patient for echocardiography, gated blood pool imaging, and cardiac catheterization.

Pediatric pointers

A ventricular gallop is normally heard in children. However, it may accompany congenital abnormalities associated with heart failure, such as large ventricular septal defect and patent ductus arteriosus. It may also result from sickle cell anemia. Clearly, this gallop must be correlated with the patient's associated signs and symptoms to be of diagnostic value.

GENITAL LESIONS IN THE MALE

Among the diverse lesions that may affect the male genitalia are warts, papules, ulcers, scales, and pustules. These common lesions may be painful or painless, singular or multiple. They may be limited to the genitalia or may also occur elsewhere on the body. (See *Recognizing common male genital lesions.*)

Genital lesions may result from infection, neoplasms, parasites, allergy, or the effects of drugs. These lesions can profoundly affect the patient's self-image. In fact, the patient may hesitate to seek medical attention because he fears cancer or sexually transmitted disease (STD).

Genital lesions that arise from an STD could mean that the patient is at risk for infection with human immunodeficiency virus (HIV). Genital ulcers make HIV transmission between sexual partners more likely. Unfortunately, if the patient is treating himself, he may alter the lesions, making differential diagnosis especially difficult.

History and physical examination

Begin by asking the patient when he first noticed the lesion. Did it erupt after he began taking a new drug or after a trip out of the country? Has he had similar lesions before? If so, did he get medical treatment for them? Find out if he has been treating the lesion himself. If so, how? Does the lesion itch? If so, is the itching constant, or does it bother him only at night? Note whether the lesion is painful. Next, take a complete sexual history, noting the frequency of relations and the number of sexual partners.

Before you examine the patient, observe his clothing. Do his pants fit properly? Tight pants or underwear, especially those made of nonabsorbent fabrics, can promote the growth of bacteria and fun-

Recognizing common male genital lesions

A variety of lesions may affect the male genitalia. Some of the more common ones and their causes are shown here.

PENILE CANCER

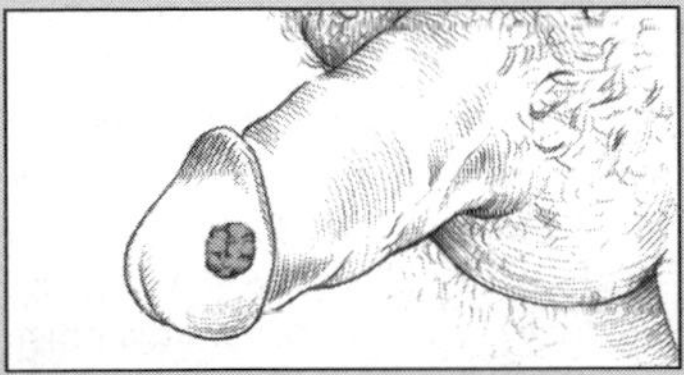

Penile cancer causes a painless ulcerative lesion on the glans or foreskin, possibly accompanied by a foul-smelling discharge.

FIXED DRUG ERUPTION

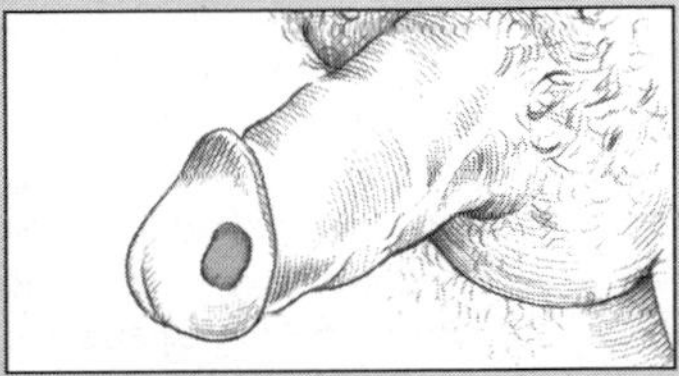

A *fixed drug eruption* causes a bright red to purplish lesion on the glans penis.

GENITAL WARTS

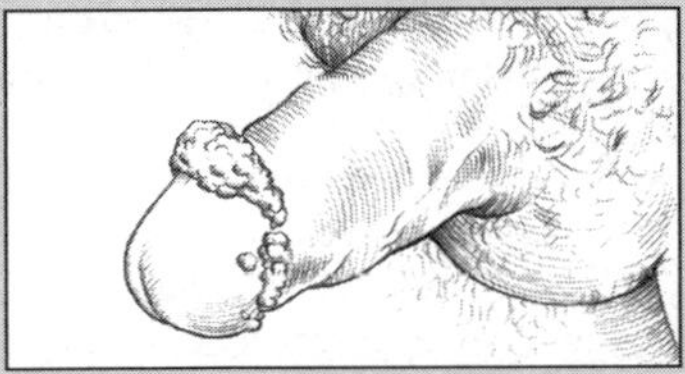

Genital warts are marked by clusters of flesh-colored papillary growths that may be barely visible or several inches in diameter.

GENITAL HERPES

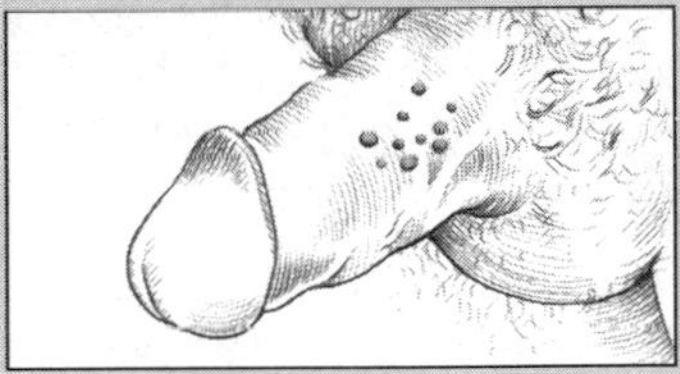

Genital herpes begins as a swollen, slightly pruritic wheal and later becomes a group of small vesicles or blisters on the foreskin, glans, or penile shaft.

TINEA CRURIS

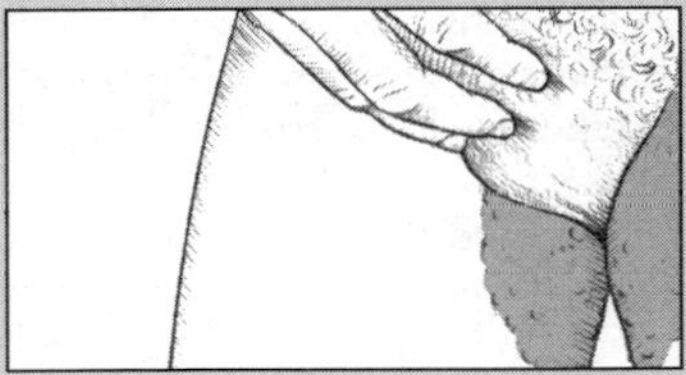

Tinea cruris (commonly known as "jock itch") produces itchy patches of well-defined, slightly raised, scaly lesions that usually affect the inner thighs and groin.

CHANCROID

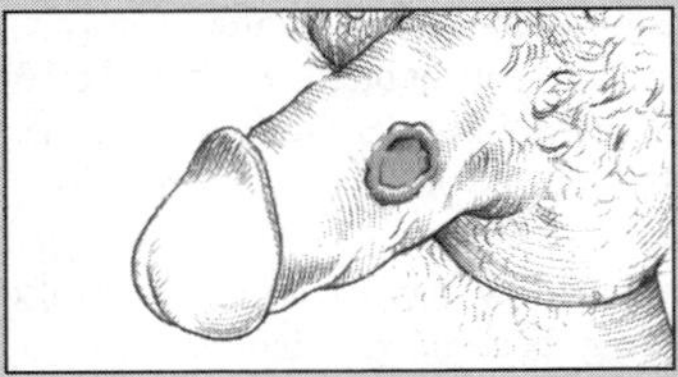

Chancroid causes a painful ulcer that's usually less than 2 cm in diameter and bleeds easily. The lesion may be deep and covered by gray or yellow exudates at its base.

gi. Examine the entire skin surface, noting the location, size, color, and pattern of the lesions. Do genital lesions resemble those on other parts of the body? Palpate for nodules, masses, and tenderness. Also, look for bleeding, edema, or signs of infection such as erythema. Finally, take the patient's vital signs.

Common medical causes

♦ ***Balanitis and balanoposthitis.*** Typically, balanitis (glans infection) and posthitis (prepuce infection) occur together (balanoposthitis), causing painful ulceration on the glans, foreskin, or penile shaft. Ulceration is usually preceded by 2 to 3 days of prepuce irritation and soreness, followed by a foul discharge and edema. The patient may then develop features of acute infection, such as fever with chills, malaise, and dysuria. Without treatment, the ulcers may deepen and multiply. Eventually, the entire penis and scrotum may become gangrenous, resulting in life-threatening sepsis.

♦ ***Bowen's disease.*** This painless, premalignant lesion commonly occurs on the penis or scrotum but may also appear elsewhere. It appears as a brownish red, raised, scaly, indurated plaque with well-defined borders, which may ulcerate at its center.

♦ ***Chancroid.*** This STD is characterized by the eruption of one or more lesions, usually on the groin, inner thigh, or penis. Within 24 hours, the lesion changes from a reddened area to a small papule. (A similar papule may erupt on the tongue, lip, breast, or umbilicus.) It then becomes an inflamed pustule that rapidly ulcerates. This painful — and usually deep — ulcer bleeds easily and commonly has a purulent gray or yellow exudate covering its base. Rarely more than 2 cm in diameter, it's typically irregular in shape. The inguinal lymph nodes also enlarge, become very tender, and may drain pus.

♦ ***Folliculitis and furunculosis.*** Hair follicle infection may cause red, sharply pointed lesions that are tender and swollen with central pustules. If folliculitis progresses to furunculosis, these lesions become hard, painful nodules that may gradually enlarge and rupture, discharging pus and necrotic material. Rupture relieves the pain, but erythema and edema may persist for days or weeks.

♦ ***Genital herpes.*** Caused by herpesvirus Type 1 or Type 2, this STD produces fluid-filled vesicles on the glans penis, foreskin, or penile shaft and, occasionally, on the mouth or anus. Usually painless at first, these vesicles may rupture and become extensive, shallow, painful ulcers accompanied by redness, marked edema, and tender, inguinal lymph nodes. Other findings may include fever, malaise, and dysuria. If the vesicles recur in the same area, the patient usually feels localized numbness and tingling before they erupt. Associated inflammation is typically less marked.

♦ ***Genital warts.*** Most common in sexually active males, genital warts initially develop on the subpreputial sac or urethral meatus and less commonly on the penile shaft; they then spread to the perineum and the perianal area. These painless warts start as tiny red or pink swellings that may grow to 4″ (10.2 cm) and become pedunculated. Multiple swellings are common, giving the warts a cauliflower appearance. Infected warts are malodorous.

♦ ***Leukoplakia.*** This precancerous disorder is characterized by white, scaly patches on the glans and prepuce accompanied by skin thickening and occasionally fissures.

♦ ***Pediculosis pubis.*** This parasitic infestation is characterized by erythematous, itching papules in the pubic area and around the anus, abdomen, and thigh. Inspection may detect grayish white specks (lice eggs) attached to hair shafts. Skin irritation from scratching in these areas is common.

♦ ***Penile cancer.*** This cancer usually produces a painless, enlarging wartlike lesion on the glans or foreskin. The patient may experience localized pain, however, if the foreskin becomes unretractable. Examination may reveal a foul-smelling discharge from the prepuce, a firm lump in the glans, and enlarged lymph nodes. Late signs and symptoms may include dysuria, pain, bleeding from the lesion, and urine retention and bladder distention associated with obstruction of the urinary tract.

♦ ***Scabies.*** Mites that burrow under the skin in this disorder may cause crusted lesions or large papules on the glans and shaft of the penis and on the scrotum. Lesions may also occur on the wrists, elbows, axillae, and waist. They're usually threadlike and 1 to 10 cm long and have a swollen nodule or red papule that contains the mite. Nocturnal itching is typical and commonly causes excoriation.

♦ ***Syphilis.*** Two to 4 weeks after exposure to *Treponema pallidum,* one or more primary lesions, or chancres, may erupt on the genitalia; occasionally, they also erupt elsewhere on the body, typically on the mouth or perianal area. The chancre usually starts as a small, red, fluid-filled papule and then erodes to form a painless, firm, indurated, shallow ulcer with a clear base and a scant, yellow serous discharge or, less commonly, a hard papule. This lesion gradually involutes and disappears. Painless, unilateral regional lymphadenopathy is also typical.

♦ ***Tinea cruris.*** Also called "jock itch," this fungal infection usually causes sharply defined, slightly raised, scaling patches on the inner thigh or groin (commonly bilaterally) and, less commonly, on the scrotum and penis. Pruritus may be severe.

♦ ***Urticaria.*** This common allergic reaction is characterized by intensely pruritic hives, which may appear on the genitalia, especially on the foreskin or shaft of the penis. These distinct, raised, evanescent wheals are surrounded by an erythematous flare.

Other causes

♦ ***Drugs.*** Phenolphthalein, barbiturates, and certain broad-spectrum antibiotics, such as tetracycline and sulfonamides, may cause a fixed drug eruption and a genital lesion.

Special considerations

Many disorders produce penile lesions that resemble those of syphilis. Expect to screen every patient with penile lesions for STDs, using the dark-field examination and the Venereal Disease Research Laboratory test. In addition, you may need to prepare the patient for a biopsy to confirm or rule out penile cancer. Provide emotional support, especially if cancer is suspected.

To prevent cross-contamination, wash your hands before and after every patient contact. Wear gloves when handling urine or performing catheter care. Dispose of all needles carefully, and double-bag all material contaminated by secretions.

Pediatric pointers

In infants, contact dermatitis ("diaper rash") may produce minor irritation or bright-red, weepy, excoriated lesions. Use of disposable diapers and careful cleaning of the penis and scrotum can help reduce diaper rash.

In children, impetigo may cause pustules with thick, yellow, weepy crusts. Like adults, children may develop genital warts, but they'll need more reassurance that the treatment (excision) won't hurt or castrate them. Children with an STD must be evaluated for signs of sexual abuse.

Adolescents ages 15 to 19 have a high incidence of STDs and related genital lesions. Syphilis, however, may also be congenital.

Geriatric pointers

Elderly adults who are sexually active with multiple partners have as high a risk of developing STDs as do younger adults. However, because of decreased immunity, poor hygiene, poor symptom reporting and, possibly, several concurrent conditions, they may present with different symptoms.

GUM BLEEDING
[Gingival bleeding]

Bleeding gums usually result from dental disorders; less commonly, they may stem from blood dyscrasias or the effects of certain drugs. Physiologic causes of this common sign include pregnancy, which can produce gum swelling in the first or second trimester (pregnancy epulis); atmospheric pressure changes, which usually affect divers and aviators; and oral trauma. Bleeding ranges from slight oozing to life-threatening hemorrhage. It may be spontaneous or may follow trauma. Occasionally, direct pressure can control it.

Emergency interventions

If you detect profuse, spontaneous bleeding in the oral cavity, quickly check the patient's airway and look for signs of cardiovascular collapse, such as tachycardia and hypotension. Suction the patient. Apply direct pressure to the bleeding site. Expect to insert an airway, administer I.V. fluids, and collect serum samples for diagnostic evaluation.

History and physical examination

If gum bleeding isn't an emergency, obtain a history. Find out when the bleeding began. Has it been continuous or intermittent? Does it occur spontaneously or when the patient brushes his teeth? Have the patient show you the site of the bleeding, if possible.

Find out if the patient or a family member has bleeding tendencies; for example, ask about easy bruising and frequent nosebleeds. How much does the patient bleed after a tooth extraction? Does he have a history of liver or spleen disease? Next, check the patient's dental history. Find out how often he brushes his teeth and goes to the dentist. Has he seen a dentist recently? To evaluate nutritional status, have the patient describe his normal diet and intake of alcohol. Finally, note any prescription and over-the-counter drugs he takes.

Next, perform a complete oral examination. If the patient wears dentures, have him remove them. Examine the gums to determine the site and amount of bleeding. Gums normally appear pink and rippled with their margins snugly against the teeth. Check for inflammation, pockets around the teeth, swelling, retraction, hypertrophy, discoloration, and gum hyperplasia. Note obvious decay, discoloration, foreign material such as food, and absence of any teeth.

Common medical causes

- ***Agranulocytosis.*** Spontaneous gum bleeding and other systemic hemorrhages may occur in this hematologic disorder, which typically causes progressive fatigue and weakness, followed by signs of infection, such as fever and chills. Inspection may reveal oral and perianal lesions, which are usually rough-edged with a gray or black membrane.
- ***Aplastic anemia.*** In this disorder, profuse or scant gum bleeding may follow trauma. Other signs of bleeding, such as epistaxis or ecchymoses, are also characteristic. The patient exhibits progressive weakness and fatigue, shortness of breath, headache, pallor and, possibly, fever. Eventually, tachycardia and signs of heart failure, such as neck vein distention and dyspnea, also develop.
- ***Ehlers-Danlos syndrome.*** In this congenital syndrome, gums bleed easily after toothbrushing. Easy bruising and other signs of abnormal bleeding are also typical. Skin is fragile and hyperelastic; joints are hyperextendible.
- ***Gingivitis.*** Reddened and edematous gums are characteristic of this disorder. The gingivae between the teeth become bulbous and bleed easily with slight trauma. However, in *acute necrotizing ulcerative gingivitis,* bleeding is spontaneous, and the gums become so painful that the

patient may be unable to eat. A characteristic grayish yellow pseudomembrane develops over punched-out gum erosions. Offensive halitosis is typical and may be accompanied by headache, malaise, fever, and cervical adenopathy.

♦ ***Hemophilia.*** Hemorrhage occurs from many sites in the oral cavity, especially the gums. *Mild hemophilia* causes easy bruising, hematomas, epistaxis, bleeding gums, and prolonged bleeding during even minor surgery and up to 8 days afterward. *Moderate hemophilia* produces more frequent episodes of abnormal bleeding and occasional bleeding into the joints, which may cause swelling and pain. *Severe hemophilia* causes spontaneous or severe bleeding after minor trauma, possibly resulting in large subcutaneous and intramuscular hematomas. Bleeding into joints and muscles causes pain, swelling, extreme tenderness and, possibly, permanent deformity. Bleeding near peripheral nerves causes peripheral neuropathies, pain, paresthesia, and muscle atrophy. Signs of anemia and fever may follow bleeding. Severe blood loss may lead to shock and death.

♦ ***Hereditary hemorrhagic telangiectasia.*** This disorder is characterized by red to violet spiderlike hemorrhagic areas on the gums, which blanch on pressure and bleed spontaneously. These telangiectases may also occur on the lips, buccal mucosa, and palate; on the face, ears, scalp, hands, arms, and feet; and under the nails. Epistaxis commonly occurs early and is difficult to control. Hemoptysis and signs of GI bleeding may develop.

♦ ***Leukemia.*** Easy gum bleeding, which is an early sign of acute monocytic, lymphocytic, or myelocytic leukemia, is accompanied by gum swelling, necrosis, and petechiae. The soft, tender gums appear glossy and bluish. *Acute leukemia* causes severe prostration marked by high fever and bleeding tendencies, such as epistaxis and prolonged menses. It may also cause dyspnea, tachycardia, palpitations, and abdominal or bone pain. Later effects may include confusion, headaches, vomiting, seizures, papilledema, and nuchal rigidity.

Chronic leukemia usually develops insidiously, producing less-severe bleeding tendencies. Other effects may include anorexia, weight loss, low-grade fever, chills, skin eruptions, and enlarged spleen, tonsils, and lymph nodes. Signs of anemia, such as fatigue and pallor, may occur.

♦ ***Pemphigoid (benign mucosal).*** Most common in women between ages 40 and 50, this uncommon autoimmune disorder typically causes thick-walled gum lesions that rupture, desquamate, and then bleed easily. Extensive scars form with healing, and the gums remain red for months. Lesions may also develop on other parts of the oral mucosa, conjunctiva and, less commonly, the skin. Secondary fibrous bands may lead to dysphagia, hoarseness, or blindness.

♦ ***Periodontal disease.*** Gum bleeding typically occurs after chewing, toothbrushing, or gum probing but may also occur spontaneously. As gingivae separate from the bone, pus-filled pockets develop around the teeth; occasionally, pus can be expressed. Other findings include unpleasant taste with halitosis, facial pain, loose teeth, and dental calculi and plaque.

♦ ***Polycythemia vera.*** In this disorder, engorged gums ooze blood after even a slight trauma. Polycythemia vera usually turns the oral mucosa — especially the gums and tongue — a deep red-violet. Among associated findings are headache, dyspnea, dizziness, fatigue, paresthesia, tinnitus, double or blurred vision, aquagenic pruritus, epigastric distress, weight loss, increased blood pressure, ruddy cyanosis, ecchymosis, and hepatosplenomegaly.

♦ ***Thrombocytopenia.*** Blood usually oozes between the teeth and gums; however, severe bleeding may follow minor trauma. Associated signs of hemorrhage include large blood-filled bullae in the mouth, petechiae, ecchymosis, epistaxis, and hematuria. Malaise, fatigue, weakness, and lethargy eventually develop.

♦ ***Thrombocytopenic purpura (idiopathic).*** Profuse gum bleeding occurs in this disorder. Its classic feature, however, is spontaneous hemorrhagic skin lesions that range from pinpoint petechiae to massive hemorrhages. The patient has a tendency to bruise easily, develops petechiae on the oral mucosa, and may exhibit melena, epistaxis, or hematuria.

♦ ***Vitamin K deficiency.*** The first sign of this deficiency usually is gum bleeding after toothbrushing. Other signs of abnormal bleeding, such as ecchymosis, epistaxis, or hematuria, may also occur. GI bleeding may produce hematemesis and melena; intracranial bleeding may cause decreased level of consciousness and focal neurologic deficits.

Other causes

♦ ***Drugs.*** Coumadin and heparin interfere with blood clotting and may cause prolonged gum bleeding. Abuse of aspirin and nonsteroidal anti-inflammatory drugs may alter platelets, producing bleeding gums. Localized gum bleeding may also occur with mucosal "aspirin burn" caused by dissolving aspirin near an aching tooth.

Special considerations

Prepare the patient for diagnostic tests, such as blood studies or facial X-rays. When providing mouth care, avoid using lemon-glycerin swabs, which may burn or dry the gums.

Pediatric pointers

In newborns, bleeding gums may result from vitamin K deficiency associated with a lack of normal intestinal flora or poor maternal nutrition. In infants who primarily drink cow's milk and don't receive vitamin supplements, bleeding gums can result from vitamin C deficiency.

Encourage parents to teach proper oral hygiene early. Daily toothbrushing in the morning and before bedtime should begin with eruption of the first tooth. When the child has all of his baby teeth, he should begin receiving regular dental checkups.

Geriatric pointers

In patients who have no teeth, constant gum trauma and bleeding may result from using a dental prosthesis.

GYNECOMASTIA

Occurring only in males, gynecomastia refers to benign increased breast size due to excessive mammary gland development. This change in breast size may be barely palpable or immediately obvious. Usually bilateral, gynecomastia may be associated with breast tenderness and milk secretion. It may also be asssociated with breast cancer, which is unilateral and usually an eccentric hard mass.

Normally, several hormones regulate breast development. Estrogens, growth hormone, and corticosteroids stimulate ductal growth, whereas progesterone and prolactin stimulate growth of the alveolar lobules. Although the pathophysiology of gynecomastia isn't fully understood, a hormonal imbalance — particularly a change in the estrogen-androgen ratio and an increase in prolactin — is a likely contributing factor. This explains why gynecomastia commonly results from the effects of estrogens and other drugs. It may also result from hormone-secreting tumors and from endocrine, genetic, hepatic, or adrenal disorders. Physiologic gynecomastia may occur in neonatal, pubertal, and geriatric males because of normal fluctuations in hormone levels.

History and physical examination

Begin the history by asking the patient when he first noticed his breast enlargement. How old was he at the time? Since then, have his breasts gotten progressively larger, smaller, or stayed the same? Does he also have breast tenderness or discharge? Next, take a thorough drug history, including prescription, over-the-counter, herbal, and street drugs, as well as alcohol ingestion. Then explore associated signs and symptoms, such as testicular mass or pain; loss of libido; decreased potency; loss of chest, axillary, or facial hair; and symptoms of hyperthyroidism.

Focus the physical examination on the breasts, testicles, and penis. As you examine the breasts, note asymmetry, dimpling, abnormal pigmentation, or ulceration. Observe the testicles for size and symmetry. Then palpate them to detect nodules, tenderness, or unusual consistency. Look for normal penile development after puberty, and note hypospadias. Also examine the liver; look for signs of cirrhosis and portal hypertension.

Common medical causes

◆ ***Adrenal carcinoma.*** Estrogen production by an adrenal tumor may produce a feminizing syndrome in males characterized by bilateral gynecomastia, loss of libido, impotence, testicular atrophy, and reduced facial hair growth. Cushingoid signs, such as moon face and purple striae, may also occur.

◆ ***Breast cancer.*** Painful unilateral gynecomastia develops rapidly in males with breast cancer. Palpation may reveal a hard or stony breast lump suggesting a malignant tumor. Breast examination may also detect changes in breast symmetry; skin changes, such as thickening, dimpling, peau d'orange, or ulceration; a warm, reddened area; and nipple changes, such as itching, burning, erosion, deviation, flattening, retraction, and a watery, bloody, or purulent discharge.

◆ ***Hepatic cancer.*** This type of cancer may produce bilateral gynecomastia and other characteristics of feminization, such as testicular atrophy, impotence, and reduced facial hair growth. The patient may complain of severe epigastric or right-upper-quadrant pain associated with a right-upper-quadrant mass. A large tumor may also produce a bruit on auscultation. Related findings may include anorexia, weight loss, dependent edema, fever, cachexia and, possibly, jaundice or ascites.

◆ ***Hypothyroidism.*** Typically, this disorder produces bilateral gynecomastia and bradycardia, cold intolerance, weight gain despite anorexia, or mental dullness. The patient may display periorbital edema and puffiness in the face, hands, and feet. His hair appears brittle and sparse, and his skin is dry, pale, cool, and doughy.

◆ ***Klinefelter's syndrome.*** Painless bilateral gynecomastia first appears during adolescence in this genetic disorder. Before puberty, symptoms also include abnormally small testicles and slight mental deficiency; after puberty, sparse facial hair, a small penis, decreased libido, and impotence.

◆ ***Pituitary tumor.*** Prolactin-secreting tumors cause bilateral gynecomastia accompanied by galactorrhea, impotence, and decreased libido. Other hormonal effects may include enlarged hands and feet, coarse facial features with prognathism, voice deepening, weight gain, increased blood pressure, diaphoresis, heat intolerance, hyperpigmentation, and thickened, oily skin. Paresthesia or sensory loss and muscle weakness commonly affect the limbs. If the tumor expands, it may cause blurred vision, diplopia, headache, or partial bitemporal hemianopsia that may progress to blindness.

◆ ***Reifenstein's syndrome.*** This genetic disorder produces painless bilateral gynecomastia at puberty. Associated signs may include hypospadias, testicular atrophy, and an underdeveloped penis.

Other causes

◆ ***Drugs.*** When gynecomastia is an effect of drugs, it's typically painful and bilateral. Estrogens used to treat prostate cancer, including diethylstilbestrol and estramustine, directly affect the estrogen-androgen ratio. Drugs that have an estrogen-like effect, such as cardiac glycosides and human chorionic gonadotropin, may do the same. Regular use of alcohol, marijuana, or heroin reduces plasma testosterone levels, causing gynecomastia. Other drugs—such as flutamide, cyproterone, spironolactone, cimetidine, and ketoconazole—produce this sign by interfering with androgen production or action. Some common drugs—including phenothiazines, tricyclic antidepressants, antihypertensives (including calcium channel blockers and angiotensin-converting enzyme inhibitors), sulindac, ranitidine, and omeprazole—produce gynecomastia in an unknown way.

♦ ***Treatments.*** Gynecomastia may develop within weeks of starting hemodialysis for chronic renal failure. It may also follow major surgery or testicular irradiation.

Special considerations

To make the patient as comfortable as possible, apply cold compresses to his breasts and administer analgesics. Prepare him for diagnostic tests, including chest and skull X-rays and blood hormone levels.

Because gynecomastia may alter the patient's body image, provide emotional support. Reassure the patient that treatment can reduce gynecomastia. Some patients are helped by tamoxifen, an antiestrogen, or by testolactone, an inhibitor of testosterone-to-estrogen conversion. Surgical removal of breast tissue may be an option if drug treatment fails.

Pediatric pointers

In newborns, gynecomastia may be associated with galactorrhea ("witch's milk"). This sign usually disappears within a few weeks but may persist until age 2.

Most males have physiologic gynecomastia at some time during adolescence, usually around age 14. This gynecomastia is usually asymmetrical and tender; it commonly resolves within 2 years and rarely persists beyond age 20.

H

Halo vision

Halo vision refers to seeing rainbowlike, colored rings around lights or bright objects. The rainbowlike effect can be explained by this physical principle: As light passes through water (in the eye, through tears or the cells of various anteretinal media), it breaks up into spectral colors.

Halo vision usually develops suddenly; its duration depends on the causative disorder. This symptom may occur in disorders associated with excessive tearing and corneal epithelial edema. Among these causes, the most common and significant is acute angle-closure glaucoma, which can lead to blindness. In fact, rainbowlike fringes or colored halos seen around a point of light are usually a symptom of corneal edema, commonly resulting from an abrupt rise in intraocular pressure (IOP). Thus, colored halos are a danger symptom suggesting acute glaucoma. In this disorder, increased IOP forces fluid into corneal tissues anterior to Bowman's membrane, causing edema. Halo vision is also an early symptom of cataracts, resulting from dispersion of light by abnormal opacities on the lens.

Nonpathologic causes of excessive tearing associated with halo vision include poorly fitted or overworn contact lenses, emotional extremes, and exposure to intense light, as in snow blindness.

History and physical examination

First, ask the patient how long he has been seeing halos around lights and when he usually sees them. Patients with glaucoma typically see halos most frequently in the morning, when IOP is most elevated. Ask the patient if light bothers his eyes. Does he have eye pain? If so, have him describe it. Remember that halos associated with excruciating eye pain or a severe headache may point to acute angle-closure glaucoma, an ocular emergency. Note a history of glaucoma or cataracts.

Next, examine the patient's eyes, noting conjunctival injection, excessive tearing, and lens changes. Examine pupil size, shape, and response to light. Then test visual acuity by performing an ophthalmoscopic examination.

Common medical causes

- ***Cataract.*** Halo vision may be an early symptom of painless, progressive cataract formation. The glare of headlights may blind the patient, making nighttime driving impossible. Other features include blurred vision, impaired visual acuity, and lens opacity, all of which develop gradually.
- ***Corneal endothelial dystrophy.*** Typically, halo vision is a late symptom. Impaired visual acuity may also occur.
- ***Glaucoma.*** Halo vision characterizes all types of glaucoma. *Acute angle-closure glaucoma*—an ophthalmic emergency—also causes blurred vision, followed by a

Safety considerations for poor vision

Halo vision poses a particular safety hazard for elderly people, who have a high incidence of cataracts and glaucoma. Encourage your older patients to have annual eye examinations and to comply with medical therapies, such as wearing eyeglasses and instilling eye drops. Make sure the patient's room and stairwells are well lit. Place brightly colored tape on the edges of steps.

If the patient drives, discuss his safety with family members. If he needs to take medications, assist him with his daily routine. For instance, draw up a week's worth of insulin in syringes, and label and store them in the refrigerator. Encourage the patient to use a weekly pill container to display the week's supply of pills. Magnifiers and reading aids are also available.

severe headache or excruciating pain in and around the affected eye. Examination reveals a moderately dilated fixed pupil that doesn't respond to light, conjunctival injection, a cloudy cornea, impaired visual acuity and, possibly, nausea and vomiting. *Chronic angle-closure glaucoma* is usually asymptomatic until pain and blindness occur in advanced disease. Sometimes, halos and blurred vision develop slowly. In *chronic open-angle glaucoma,* halo vision is a late symptom that's accompanied by mild eye ache, peripheral vision loss, and impaired visual acuity.

Other causes

♦ ***Drugs.*** Intoxication with digoxin, a widely used cardiovascular drug, may cause halos.

Special considerations

To help minimize halo vision, remind the patient not to look directly at bright lights. White halos may be perceived on dark objects, or objects may seem frosted in appearance. Unusual fatigue and weakness also occur, but the visual disturbances commonly dominate the patient's complaints. (See *Safety considerations for poor vision.*)

Pediatric pointers

Halo vision in a child usually results from congenital cataracts or glaucoma. In a young child, limited verbal ability may make halo vision difficult to assess.

Geriatric pointers

Primary glaucoma, the most common cause of halo vision, occurs more frequently in older patients.

HEADACHE

The most common neurologic symptom, headaches may be localized or generalized, producing mild to severe pain. About 90% of all headaches are benign and can be described as vascular, muscle-contraction, or a combination. (See *Comparing benign headaches.*) Occasionally, however, headaches indicate a severe neurologic disorder associated with intracranial inflammation, increased intracranial pressure (ICP), or meningeal irritation. They may also result from ocular or sinus disorders and the effects of drugs, tests, or treatments.

Other causes of headache include fever, eyestrain, dehydration, and systemic febrile illnesses. Headaches may occur in certain metabolic disturbances — such as hypoxemia, hypercapnia, hyperglycemia, and hypoglycemia — but they aren't a diagnostic or prominent symptom. Some individuals get headaches after seizures or from coughing, sneezing, heavy lifting, or stooping.

Comparing benign headaches

Of the many patients who report headaches, only about 10% have an underlying medical disorder. The other 90% suffer from benign headaches, which may be classified as muscle-contraction (tension), vascular (migraine and cluster), or a combination of both. This chart describes the two major types — muscle-contraction and vascular headache or late-stage migraine. Treatment of a combined headache includes analgesics and sedatives.

CHARACTERISTICS	MUSCLE-CONTRACTION HEADACHES	VASCULAR HEADACHES
Incidence	◆ Most common type, accounting for 80% of all headaches	◆ More common in women and people with a family history of migraines ◆ Onset after puberty
Precipitating factors	◆ Stress, anxiety, tension, improper posture and body alignment ◆ Prolonged muscle contraction without structural damage ◆ Eye, ear, and paranasal sinus disorders that produce reflex muscle contractions	◆ Hormone fluctuation ◆ Alcohol ◆ Emotional upset ◆ Too little or too much sleep ◆ Foods such as chocolate, cheese, monosodium glutamate, cured meats; caffeine withdrawal ◆ Weather changes, such as shifts in barometric pressure
Intensity and duration	◆ Produce an aching tightness or a band of pain around the head, especially in the neck and occipital and temporal areas ◆ Occur frequently and usually last for several hours	◆ May begin with an awareness of an impending migraine or a 5- to 15-minute prodrome of neurologic deficits, such as vision disturbances, dizziness, unsteady gait, or tingling of the face, lips, or hands ◆ Produce severe, constant, throbbing pain that's typically unilateral and may be incapacitating ◆ Lasts for 4 to 6 hours
Associated signs and symptoms	◆ Tense neck and facial muscles	◆ Anorexia, nausea, and vomiting ◆ Occasionally, photophobia, sensitivity to loud noises, weakness, fatigue ◆ Depending on the type (cluster headache or classic, common or hemiplegic migraine), possibly chills, depression, eye pain, ptosis, tearing, rhinorrhea, diaphoresis, facial flushing
Alleviating factors	◆ Mild analgesics, muscle relaxants, or other drugs during an attack ◆ Biofeedback, relaxation techniques, and counseling; posture correction	◆ Methysergide and propranolol to prevent vascular headache ◆ Ergot alkaloids or serotonin-receptor drugs at first sign of a migraine ◆ Rest in a quiet, darkened room ◆ Elimination of irritating foods from diet

History and physical examination

If the patient reports a headache, ask him to describe its characteristics and location. How often does he get a headache? How long does a typical headache last? Does the patient notice any pattern to the headaches? If the patient is female, does she notice any relationship to the headaches and the onset of her menstrual cycle? Try to identify precipitating factors, such as certain foods and exposure to bright lights. Is the patient under stress? Does he have trouble sleeping?

Take a drug history and ask about head trauma within the past 4 weeks. Has the patient recently experienced nausea, vomiting, photophobia, or vision changes? Does he feel drowsy, confused, or dizzy? Has he recently developed seizures, or does he have a history of seizures?

Begin the physical examination by evaluating the patient's level of consciousness (LOC). Then check his vital signs. Be alert for signs of increased ICP — widened pulse pressure, bradycardia, altered respiratory pattern, and increased blood pressure. Check pupil size and response to light, and note any neck stiffness.

Common medical causes

♦ ***Arteriovenous malformations.*** Less common than cerebral aneurysms, vascular malformations usually result from developmental defects of the cerebral veins and arteries. Although many are present from birth, they manifest in adulthood with a triad of symptoms: headache, hemorrhage, and seizures.

♦ ***Brain abscess.*** In this disorder, headache is localized to the abscess site. Usually, it intensifies over a few days and is aggravated by straining. Accompanying the headache may be nausea, vomiting, and focal or generalized seizures. The patient's LOC varies from drowsiness to deep stupor. Depending on the abscess site, associated signs and symptoms may include aphasia, impaired visual acuity, hemiparesis, ataxia, tremors, and personality changes. Signs of infection, such as fever and pallor, usually develop late; however, if the abscess remains encapsulated, these signs may not appear.

♦ ***Brain tumor.*** Initially, a tumor causes a localized headache near the tumor site; as the tumor grows, the headache eventually becomes generalized. The pain is usually intermittent, deep-seated, dull, and most intense in the morning. It's aggravated by coughing, stooping, Valsalva's maneuver, and changes in head position and is relieved by sitting and rest. Associated signs and symptoms may include personality changes, altered LOC, motor or sensory dysfunction, and eventually signs of increased ICP, such as vomiting, increased systolic blood pressure, and widened pulse pressure.

♦ ***Cerebral aneurysm (ruptured).*** This life-threatening disorder is characterized by a sudden, excruciating headache, which may be unilateral and usually peaks within minutes of the rupture. The patient may lose consciousness immediately or display a variably altered LOC. Depending on the severity and location of the bleeding, he may also exhibit nausea and vomiting as well as signs of meningeal irritation, such as nuchal rigidity, blurred vision, or hemiparesis.

♦ ***Ebola virus infection.*** Headache is usually abrupt in onset, commonly occurring on the 5th day of illness. Additionally, the patient has a history of malaise, myalgia, high fever, diarrhea, abdominal pain, dehydration, and lethargy. A maculopapular skin rash develops between the 5th and 7th days of the illness. Other possible findings include pleuritic chest pain; a dry, hacking cough; pronounced pharyngitis; hematemesis; melena; and bleeding from the nose, gums, and vagina. Death usually occurs in the 2nd week of the illness, following severe blood loss and shock.

♦ ***Encephalitis.*** A severe, generalized headache is characteristic in this disorder. Within 48 hours, the patient's LOC typically deteriorates — perhaps from lethargy to coma. Associated signs and symptoms include fever, nuchal rigidity, irritability, seizures, nausea and vomiting, photophobia, cranial nerve palsies such as ptosis, and focal neurologic deficits, such as hemiparesis and hemiplegia.

♦ ***Epidural hemorrhage (acute).*** Head trauma and a sudden, brief loss of consciousness usually precede this hemorrhage, which causes a progressively severe headache that's accompanied by nausea and vomiting, bladder distention, confusion, and then a rapid decrease in LOC. Other signs and symptoms may include unilateral seizures, hemiparesis, hemiplegia, high fever, decreased pulse rate and bounding pulse, widened pulse pressure, increased blood pressure, a positive Babinski's reflex, and decerebrate posture.

If the patient slips into a coma, his respirations deepen and become stertorous, then become shallow and irregular, and eventually cease. Pupil dilation may occur on the same side as the hemorrhage.

♦ ***Glaucoma (acute angle-closure).*** This ophthalmic emergency may cause an excruciating headache as well as acute eye pain, blurred vision, halo vision, nausea, and vomiting. Assessment reveals conjunctival injection, a cloudy cornea, and a moderately dilated, fixed pupil.

♦ ***Hantavirus pulmonary syndrome.*** Noncardiogenic pulmonary edema distinguishes this viral disease, which was first reported in the United States in 1993. Common chief complaints include flulike symptoms — headache, myalgia, fever, nausea, vomiting, and a cough — followed by respiratory distress. Fever, hypoxia, and serious hypotension typify the hospital course. Other signs and symptoms include a rising respiratory rate (28 breaths/minute or more) and an increased heart rate (120 beats/minute or more).

♦ ***Hypertension.*** This disorder may cause a slightly throbbing occipital headache on awakening that decreases in severity during the day. However, if the patient's diastolic blood pressure exceeds 120 mm Hg, the headache remains constant. Associated signs and symptoms may include an atrial gallop, restlessness, confusion, nausea and vomiting, blurred vision, seizures, or altered LOC.

♦ ***Influenza.*** A severe generalized or frontal headache usually begins suddenly with the flu. Accompanying signs and symptoms may last for 3 to 5 days and include stabbing retro-orbital pain, weakness, diffuse myalgia, fever, chills, coughing, rhinorrhea, and occasionally hoarseness.

♦ ***Meningitis.*** This disorder is marked by the sudden onset of a severe, constant, generalized headache that worsens with movement. Associated signs include nuchal rigidity, positive Kernig's and Brudzinski's signs, hyperreflexia and, possibly, opisthotonos. Fever occurs early in meningitis and may be accompanied by chills. As ICP increases, vomiting and, occasionally, papilledema develop. Other features may include altered LOC, seizures, ocular palsies, facial weakness, and hearing loss.

♦ ***Postconcussion syndrome.*** A generalized or localized headache may develop 1 to 30 days after head trauma and last for 2 to 3 weeks. This characteristic symptom may be described as an aching, pounding, pressing, stabbing, or throbbing pain. The patient's neurologic examination is normal, but he may experience dizziness, blurred vision, fatigue, insomnia, inability to concentrate, and noise and alcohol intolerance.

♦ ***Subarachnoid hemorrhage.*** This hemorrhage commonly causes a sudden, violent headache with nuchal rigidity, nausea and vomiting, seizures, dizziness, ipsilateral pupil dilation, and altered LOC, which may rapidly progress to coma. The patient also exhibits positive Kernig's and Brudzinski's signs, photophobia, blurred vision and, possibly, fever. Focal signs and symptoms (such as hemiparesis, hemiplegia, sensory or vision disturbances, and aphasia) and signs of elevated ICP (such as bradycardia and increased blood pressure) may also occur.

ALTERNATIVE THERAPY

Relieving headache with reflexotherapy

Also known as reflexology, this bodywork technique is used to treat tension and migraine headaches, among other conditions. It's similar to acupressure in which hand pressure is applied to specific points on the feet or, less commonly, on the hands or ears.

Reflexotherapy is based on the theory that sensitive nerve endings at reference points on the feet, hands, or ears correspond to all major organs and other parts of the body. Practitioners maintain that applying pressure to these points facilitates movement of the energy along channels in the body to the corresponding body organ or area.

◆ ***Subdural hematoma.*** Typically associated with head trauma, both acute and chronic subdural hematomas may cause headache and decreased LOC. In the patient with *acute subdural hematoma,* drowsiness, confusion, and agitation may progress to coma; later findings may include signs of increased ICP and focal neurologic deficits, such as hemiparesis.

Chronic subdural hematoma causes a dull, pounding headache that fluctuates in severity and is located over the hematoma. Weeks or months after the initial head trauma, the patient may experience dizziness, personality changes, confusion, seizures, and progressively worsening LOC. Late signs may include unilateral pupil dilation, sluggish pupil reaction to light, or ptosis.

◆ ***West Nile encephalitis.*** This brain infection is caused by West Nile virus, a mosquito-borne flavivirus commonly found in Africa, West Asia, and the Middle East. Mild infection is common; signs and symptoms include fever, headache, and body aches, commonly with skin rash and swollen lymph glands. More severe infection is marked by high fever, headache, neck stiffness, stupor, disorientation, coma, tremors, occasional seizures, paralysis and, rarely, death.

Other causes

◆ ***Diagnostic tests.*** A lumbar puncture or myelogram may cause a throbbing frontal headache that worsens on standing.

◆ ***Drugs.*** A variety of drugs may cause headaches. For example, indomethacin causes morning headaches in many patients. Vasodilators and drugs with a vasodilating effect, such as nitrates, typically cause a throbbing headache. Headaches may also follow withdrawal from vasopressors, such as caffeine, ergotamine, and sympathomimetics.

◆ **Herb alert** Herbal medicines, such as St. John's wort, ginseng, or ephedra (ma huang), may cause adverse effects, including headaches.

◆ ***Traction.*** Cervical traction with pins commonly causes headache, which may be generalized or localized to pin insertion sites.

Special considerations

Continue to monitor the patient's vital signs and LOC. Watch for a change in the headache's severity or location. To help ease the headache, administer analgesics, darken the patient's room, and minimize other stimuli. (See *Relieving headache with reflexotherapy.*)

Prepare the patient for diagnostic tests, such as skull X-rays, computed tomography scan, lumbar puncture, or cerebral arteriography.

Pediatric pointers

If a child is too young to describe his symptom, suspect a headache if you see him banging or holding his head. In an infant, a shrill cry or bulging fontanels may reflect increased ICP and headache. Ask the parents about the school-aged child's recent scholastic performance and about problems at home that may cause a tension headache. Twice as many young boys have migraine headaches as girls. In children over age 3, headache is the most common symptom of a brain tumor.

Hearing loss

Affecting nearly 16 million Americans, hearing loss may be temporary or permanent, partial or complete. This common symptom may involve reception of low-, middle-, or high-frequency tones. If the hearing loss doesn't affect speech frequencies, the patient may be unaware of it.

Normally, sound waves enter the external auditory canal, then travel to the middle ear's tympanic membrane and ossicles (incus, malleus, and stapes) and into the inner ear's cochlea. The cochlear division of the eighth cranial (auditory) nerve (CN VIII) carries the sound impulse to the brain. This type of sound transmission, called *air conduction,* is normally better than *bone conduction*—sound transmission through bone to the inner ear.

Hearing loss can be classified as conductive, sensorineural, mixed, or functional. *Conductive hearing loss* results from external or middle ear disorders that block sound transmission. This type of hearing loss usually responds to medical or surgical intervention (or, in some cases, both). *Sensorineural hearing loss* results from disorders of the inner ear or of CN VIII. *Mixed hearing loss* combines aspects of conductive and sensorineural hearing loss. *Functional hearing loss* results from psychological factors rather than identifiable organic damage.

Hearing loss may also result from trauma, infection, allergy, tumors, systemic disorders, hereditary conditions, or the effects of ototoxic drugs and treatments. In most cases, however, it results from presbycusis, a type of sensorineural hearing loss that usually affects people over age 50. Other physiologic causes of hearing loss include cerumen (earwax) impaction; barotitis media (unequal pressure on the eardrum) associated with descent in an airplane or elevator, diving, or proximity to an explosion; and chronic exposure to noise over 90 decibels, which can occur on the job, with certain hobbies, or from listening to live or recorded music.

History and physical examination

If the patient reports hearing loss, ask him to describe it fully. Is it unilateral or bilateral? Continuous or intermittent? Ask about a family history of hearing loss. Then obtain the patient's medical history, noting chronic ear infections, ear surgery, and ear or head trauma. Has the patient recently had an upper respiratory infection? After taking a drug history, have the patient describe his occupation and work environment.

Next, explore associated signs and symptoms. Does the patient have ear pain? If so, is it unilateral or bilateral? Continuous or intermittent? Ask the patient if he has noticed a discharge from one or both ears. If so, have him describe its color and consistency and note when it began. Does he hear ringing, buzzing, hissing, or other noises in one or both ears? If so, are the noises constant or intermittent? Does he experience dizziness? If so, when did he first notice it?

Begin the physical examination by inspecting the external ear for inflammation, boils, foreign bodies, and discharge. Then apply pressure to the tragus and mastoid to elicit tenderness. (See *Using an otoscope correctly,* page 221.) During the otoscopic examination, note a color change, perforation, bulging, or retraction of the tympanic membrane, which normally looks like a shiny, pearl gray cone.

Next, evaluate the patient's hearing acuity, using the ticking watch and whispered voice tests. Then perform the Weber and Rinne tests to obtain a preliminary evaluation of the type and degree of hearing loss.

Common medical causes

◆ ***Acoustic neuroma.*** This tumor of CN VIII causes unilateral, progressive, sensorineural hearing loss. The patient may also develop tinnitus, vertigo, and—with cranial nerve compression—facial paralysis.

◆ ***Adenoid hypertrophy.*** This condition blocks the eustachian tubes, preventing free air flow to the middle ear. The consequent retraction of the tympanic membrane reduces its mobility and promotes accumulation of an effusion, which thickens with time and may eventually erode the ossicles. These changes result in a conductive hearing loss and may be reflected in delayed speech in children. The patient also tends to breathe through his mouth and may complain of a sensation of ear fullness.

◆ ***Aural polyps.*** If a polyp occludes the external auditory canal, partial hearing loss may occur. The polyp typically bleeds easily and is covered by a purulent discharge. Aural polyps should be considered cholesteatoma until proven otherwise.

◆ ***Cholesteatoma.*** Gradual hearing loss is characteristic; possibly accompanied by vertigo and, at times, facial paralysis. Examination reveals pearly white masses in the ear canal and possible discharge. Most patients present with purulent otorrhea, which is commonly malodorous, and a history of chronic otitis. It may be congenital (without perforation of the ear drum) or acquired (with perforation). Cholesteatoma may present as an aural polyp.

◆ ***Cyst.*** Ear canal obstruction by a sebaceous or dermoid cyst causes progressive conductive hearing loss. On inspection, the cyst looks like a soft mass.

◆ ***External ear canal tumor (malignant).*** Progressive conductive hearing loss is characteristic and is accompanied by deep, boring ear pain, purulent discharge, and eventually facial paralysis. Examination may detect the granular, bleeding tumor.

◆ ***Glomus jugulare tumor.*** Initially, this benign tumor causes mild, unilateral conductive hearing loss that becomes progressively more severe. The patient may report tinnitus that sounds like his heartbeat. Associated signs and symptoms include gradual congestion in the affected ear, throbbing or pulsating discomfort, bloody otorrhea, facial nerve paralysis, and vertigo. Although the tympanic membrane is normal, a reddened mass appears behind it.

◆ ***Head trauma.*** Sudden conductive or sensorineural hearing loss may result from ossicle disruption, ear canal fracture, tympanic membrane perforation, or cochlear fracture associated with head trauma. Typically, the patient reports a headache and exhibits bleeding from his ear. Neurologic features vary and may include impaired vision and altered level of consciousness.

◆ ***Ménière's disease.*** Initially, this inner ear disorder causes intermittent, unilateral sensorineural hearing loss that involves only low tones. Later, hearing loss becomes constant and affects other tones. Associated signs and symptoms include intermittent severe vertigo, nausea and vomiting, a feeling of fullness in the ear, a roaring or hollow-seashell tinnitus, diaphoresis, and nystagmus.

◆ ***Nasopharyngeal cancer.*** This type of cancer causes mild unilateral conductive hearing loss when it compresses the eustachian tube. Bone conduction is normal, and inspection reveals a retracted tympanic membrane backed by fluid. When the tumor obstructs the nasal airway, the patient may exhibit nasal speech and a bloody nasal and postnasal discharge. Cranial nerve involvement causes other findings, such as diplopia and rectus muscle paralysis.

◆ ***Otitis externa.*** Conductive hearing loss resulting from debris in the ear canal characterizes both acute and malignant otitis externa. In *acute otitis externa,* ear canal inflammation causes pain, itching, and a foul-smelling, sticky yellow discharge. Severe tenderness is typically elicited by chewing, opening the mouth, and pressing on the tragus or mastoid. The patient may also develop a low-grade fever, regional lymphadenopathy, headache on the affected side, or mild to moderate pain around the ear that may later intensify. Examination may reveal greenish white debris or edema in the canal.

Malignant otitis externa is a life-threatening disorder, which most commonly occurs in diabetics; it causes sensorineural hearing loss, pruritus, tinnitus, and severe ear pain.

◆ ***Otitis media.*** This middle ear inflammation typically causes unilateral conductive hearing loss. In *acute suppurative otitis media,* the hearing loss develops gradually over a few hours and is usually accompanied by an upper respiratory infection with sore throat, cough, nasal discharge, and headache. Related signs and symptoms may include dizziness, a sensation of fullness in the ear, intermittent or constant ear pain, fever, nausea, and vomiting. Rupture of the bulging, swollen tympanic membrane relieves the pain and causes a brief, bloody, purulent discharge. Hearing returns after the infection subsides.

Hearing loss also develops gradually in *chronic otitis media.* Examination may reveal a perforated tympanic membrane, purulent ear drainage, earache, nausea, and vertigo.

Commonly associated with an upper respiratory infection or nasopharyngeal cancer, *serous otitis media* commonly causes a stuffy feeling in the ear and pain that worsens at night. Examination reveals a retracted, perhaps discolored tympanic membrane and, possibly, air bubbles behind the membrane.

◆ ***Otosclerosis.*** In this hereditary disorder, which is the leading cause of hearing loss in adults, unilateral conductive hearing loss usually begins when the patient is in his early twenties and may gradually progress to bilateral mixed loss. The patient may report tinnitus and an ability to hear better in a noisy environment. Associated signs may include a dip in bone conduction threshold at 2,000 Hz on audiometric testing and a reddish hue on the promontory on otoscopic examination (Schwartze's sign).

◆ ***Skull fracture.*** Auditory nerve injury causes sudden unilateral sensorineural hearing loss. Accompanying signs and symptoms may include ringing tinnitus, blood behind the tympanic membrane, or scalp wounds.

◆ ***Temporal bone fracture.*** This fracture can cause sudden unilateral sensorineural hearing loss accompanied by hissing tinnitus. The tympanic membrane may be perforated, depending on the fracture's location. Loss of consciousness, Battle's sign, and facial paralysis may also occur.

◆ ***Tympanic membrane perforation.*** Commonly caused by trauma from sharp objects or rapid pressure changes, perforation of the tympanic membrane causes abrupt hearing loss with ear pain, tinnitus, vertigo, and a sensation of fullness in the ear.

Other causes

◆ ***Drugs.*** Ototoxic drugs typically cause ringing or buzzing tinnitus and a feeling of fullness in the ear. Chloroquine, cisplatin, vancomycin, and aminoglycosides (especially neomycin, kanamycin, and amikacin) may cause irreversible hearing loss. Loop diuretics, such as furosemide, ethacrynic acid, and bumetanide, usually cause a brief, reversible hearing loss. Quinine, quinidine, and high doses of erythromycin or salicylates (such as aspirin) may also cause reversible hearing loss.

◆ ***Radiation therapy.*** Irradiation of the middle ear, thyroid, face, skull, or nasopharynx may cause eustachian tube dysfunction, resulting in hearing loss.

◆ ***Surgery.*** Myringotomy, myringoplasty, simple or radical mastoidectomy, or fenestrations may cause scarring that interferes with hearing.

Compensating for hearing loss

Hearing loss isn't only a safety hazard but also a major impediment to social interaction. Make sure your patient's regular medical checkups include hearing tests. If he uses a hearing aid, encourage him to use it. Inform him and his family about devices that can make his life easier, such as amplifiers or light signals for the phone or doorbell, smoke detectors with strobe light or vibrating pod attachments, and communication systems activated by voice or button that can alert the person by a pulse sensation.

When speaking to an elderly person whose behavior suggests hearing impairment, address him in a louder tone. Don't cover your mouth because he may be trying to read your lips. Ask him to repeat what you said, if appropriate, to ensure that he heard you correctly.

Special considerations

When talking with the patient, remember to face him and speak slowly. Don't shout, smoke, eat, or chew gum when talking. (See *Compensating for hearing loss.*)

Prepare the patient for audiometry and auditory evoked-response testing. After testing, the patient may require a hearing aid or cochlear implant to improve his hearing.

Pediatric pointers

About 3,000 profoundly deaf infants are born in the United States each year. In about one-half of these infants, hereditary disorders (such as Paget's disease and Alport's, Hurler's, and Klippel-Feil syndromes) cause the typically sensorineural hearing loss. Nonhereditary disorders associated with congenital sensorineural hearing loss include albinism, onychodystrophy, cochlear dysplasias, and Pendred's, Waardenburg's, Usher's, and Jervell and Lange-Nielsen syndromes. This type of hearing loss may also result from maternal use of ototoxic drugs, birth trauma, and anoxia during or after birth.

Mumps is the most common pediatric cause of unilateral sensorineural hearing loss. Other causes are meningitis, measles, influenza, and acute febrile illness.

Disorders that may cause congenital *conductive* hearing loss include atresia, ossicle malformation, and other abnormalities. Serous otitis media commonly causes *bilateral* conductive hearing loss in children. Conductive hearing loss may also occur in children who put objects in their ears.

Hearing disorders in children may lead to speech, language, and learning problems. Early identification and treatment of hearing loss is thus crucial to avoid incorrectly labeling the child as mentally retarded, brain damaged, or a slow learner.

When assessing an infant or a young child for hearing loss, remember that you can't use a tuning fork. Instead, test the startle reflex in infants under age 6 months, or have an audiologist test brain stem evoked response in neonates, infants, and young children. Also, obtain a gestational, perinatal, and family history from the parents.

Geriatric pointers

In older patients, presbycusis may be aggravated by exposure to noise as well as other factors.

HEAT INTOLERANCE

Heat intolerance refers to the inability to withstand high temperatures or to maintain a comfortable body temperature. This symptom causes a continuous feeling of being overheated and, at times, profuse diaphoresis. It usually develops gradually and is chronic.

Most cases of heat intolerance result from thyrotoxicosis. In this disorder, excess thyroid hormone stimulates peripheral tissues, increasing basal metabolism and producing excess heat. Although rare, hypothalamic disease may also cause intolerance to heat and cold.

History and physical examination

Ask the patient when he first noticed his heat intolerance. Did he gradually use fewer blankets at night? Does he have to turn up the air conditioning to keep cool? Is it hard for him to adjust to warm weather? Does he sweat in a hot environment? Find out if his appetite or weight has changed. Also, ask about unusual nervousness or other personality changes. Then take a drug history, especially noting use of amphetamines or amphetamine-like drugs. Ask the patient if he takes prescribed thyroid drugs. If so, what's the daily dose? When did he last take it?

As you begin the examination, notice how much clothing the patient is wearing. After taking vital signs, inspect the patient's skin for flushing and diaphoresis. Also note tremors and lid lag.

Common medical causes

♦ ***Hypothalamic disease.*** In this rare disease, body temperature fluctuates dramatically, causing alternating heat and cold intolerance. Related features include amenorrhea, disturbed sleep patterns, increased thirst and urination, increased appetite with weight gain, impaired visual acuity, headache, and personality changes, such as bursts of rage or laughter. Common causes of hypothalamic disease are pituitary adenoma and hypothalamic and pineal tumors.

♦ ***Thyrotoxicosis.*** A classic symptom of thyrotoxicosis, heat intolerance may be accompanied by an enlarged thyroid, nervousness, weight loss despite increased appetite, diaphoresis, diarrhea, tremor, and palpitations. Although exophthalmos is characteristic, many patients don't display this sign. Associated findings may affect virtually every body system. Some common findings include irritability, difficulty concentrating, mood swings, insomnia, muscle weakness, fatigue, lid lag, tachycardia, full and bounding pulse, widened pulse pressure, dyspnea, amenorrhea, and gynecomastia. Typically, the patient's skin is warm and flushed; premature graying and alopecia occur in both sexes.

Other causes

♦ ***Drugs.*** Amphetamines, amphetamine-like appetite suppressants, and excessive doses of thyroid hormone may cause heat intolerance. Anticholinergics and phenothiazines may block sweating and temperature regulation, especially in elderly patients.

Special considerations

Adjust room temperature to make the patient comfortable. If the patient is diaphoretic, change his clothing and bed linens as necessary, and encourage him to drink fluids.

Pediatric pointers

Rarely, maternal thyrotoxicosis may be passed to the neonate, resulting in heat intolerance. More commonly, acquired thyrotoxicosis appears between ages 12 and 14, although this, too, is infrequent. Dehydration may also make a child sensitive to heat.

HEMATEMESIS

Hematemesis, the vomiting of blood, usually indicates GI bleeding above the ligament of Treitz, which suspends the duodenum at its junction with the jejunum. Bright red or blood-streaked vomitus indicates fresh or recent bleeding. Dark red, brown, or black vomitus (the color and consistency of coffee grounds) indicates that blood has been retained in the stomach and partially digested.

Although hematemesis usually results from GI disorders, it may stem from coagulation disorders or from treatments that irritate the GI tract. Swallowed blood from epistaxis or oropharyngeal erosion may also cause bloody vomitus.

Hematemesis is always an important sign, but its severity depends on the amount, source, and rapidity of the bleeding. Massive hematemesis (vomiting of 500 to 1,000 ml of blood) may rapidly be life-threatening. Hematemesis may be precipitated by straining, emotional stress, or the use of anti-inflammatory drugs or alcohol.

Emergency interventions

If the patient has massive hematemesis, quickly check his vital signs. If you detect signs of shock, such as tachypnea, hypotension, and tachycardia, place the patient in a supine position and elevate his feet 20 to 30 degrees. Start a large-bore I.V. line for emergency fluid replacement. Also, send a blood sample for typing and crossmatching, and begin oxygen administration. Emergency endoscopy may be necessary to locate the source of bleeding. Prepare to insert a nasogastric tube for suction or iced lavage. A Sengstaken-Blakemore tube may be used to compress esophageal varices. (See *Managing hematemesis with intubation.*)

History and physical examination

If the patient's hematemesis isn't immediately life-threatening, begin with a thorough history. First, have the patient describe the amount, color, and consistency of the vomitus. When did he first notice this sign? Has he ever had hematemesis before? Find out if he also has bloody or black tarry stools. Note whether hematemesis is usually preceded by nausea, flatulence, diarrhea, or weakness. Has he recently had bouts of retching with or without vomiting?

Next, ask about a history of ulcers or of liver or coagulation disorders. Find out how much alcohol the patient drinks, if any. Does he regularly take aspirin or another nonsteroidal anti-inflammatory drug (NSAID), such as phenylbutazone or indomethacin? These drugs may cause erosive gastritis or ulcers.

Begin the physical examination by checking for orthostatic hypotension, an early warning sign of hypovolemia. Take blood pressure and pulse with the patient supine, sitting, then standing. A decrease of 10 mm Hg or more in systolic pressure or an increase of 10 beats/minute or more in pulse rate indicates volume depletion. After obtaining other vital signs, inspect the mucous membranes, nasopharynx, and skin for signs of bleeding or other abnormalities. Finally, palpate the abdomen for tenderness, pain, or masses. Note lymphadenopathy.

Common medical causes

♦ ***Coagulation disorders.*** Any disorder that disrupts normal clotting may result in GI bleeding and moderate to severe hematemesis. Bleeding may occur in other body systems as well, resulting in such signs as epistaxis, ecchymosis, and gum bleeding. Other associated effects vary, depending on the specific coagulation disorder, such as thrombocytopenia or hemophilia.

♦ ***Esophageal cancer.*** A late sign of this cancer, hematemesis may be accompanied by steady chest pain that radiates to the back. Other features include substernal fullness, severe dysphagia, nausea, vomiting with nocturnal regurgitation and aspiration, hemoptysis, fever, hiccups, sore throat, melena, and halitosis.

♦ ***Esophageal rupture.*** The severity of hematemesis depends on the cause of the rupture. When an instrument damages the esophagus, hematemesis is usually slight. However, rupture due to Boerhaave's syndrome (increased esophageal pressure from vomiting or retching) or other esophageal disorders typically causes more severe hematemesis. This life-threatening disorder may also cause se-

Managing hematemesis with intubation

A patient with hematemesis will need to have a gastrointestinal (GI) tube inserted to allow blood drainage, to aspirate gastric contents, or in case gastric lavage must be performed. Here are the most common tubes and their uses.

NASOGASTRIC TUBES

The Salem-Sump tube, a double-lumen nasogastric (NG) tube, is used to remove stomach fluid and gas or to aspirate gastric contents. It may also be used for gastric lavage, drug administration, or feeding. Its main advantage over the Levin tube — a single-lumen NG device — is that it allows atmospheric air to enter the patient's stomach so that the tube can float freely instead of risking adhesion and damage to the gastric mucosa.

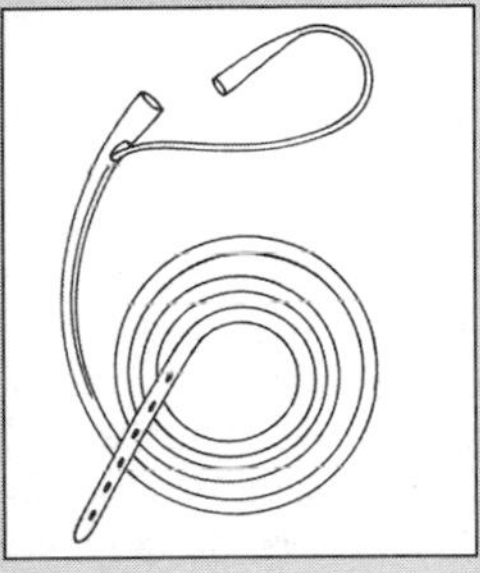

WIDE-BORE GASTRIC TUBES

The Edlich tube has one wide-bore lumen with four openings near the closed distal tip. A funnel or syringe can be connected at the proximal end. Like the other tubes, the Edlich can aspirate a large volume of gastric contents quickly.

The Ewald tube, a wide-bore tube that allows quick passage of a large volume of fluid and clots, is especially useful for gastric lavage in patients with profuse GI bleeding and in those who have ingested poison. Another wide-bore tube, the double-lumen Levacuator, has a large lumen for evacuation of gastric contents and a small one for lavage.

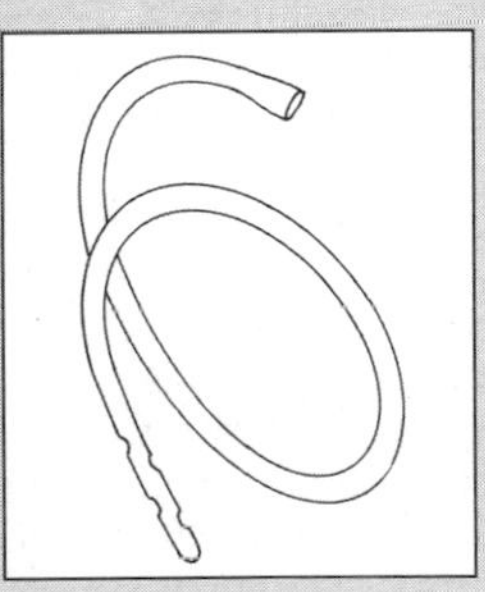

ESOPHAGEAL TUBES

The Sengstaken-Blakemore tube, a triple-lumen double-balloon esophageal tube, provides a gastric aspiration port that allows drainage from below the gastric balloon. It can also be used for instilling medication. A similar tube, the Linton, can aspirate esophageal and gastric contents without risking necrosis because it has no esophageal balloon. The Minnesota esophagogastric tamponade tube, which has four lumina and two balloons, provides pressure-monitoring ports for both balloons without the need for Y-connectors.

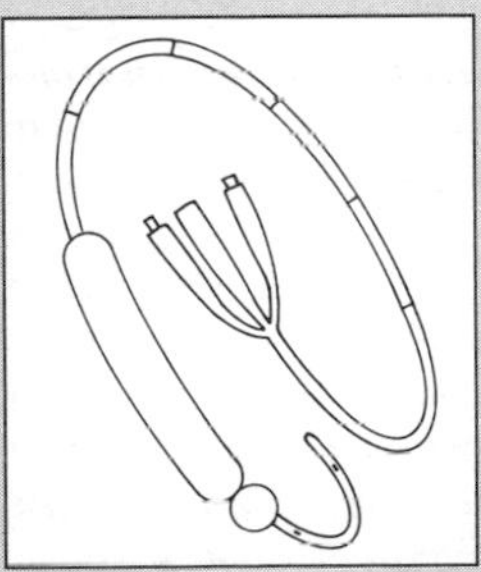

vere retrosternal, epigastric, neck, or scapular pain accompanied by chest and neck edema. Examination reveals subcutaneous crepitation in the chest wall, supraclavicular fossa, and neck. The patient may also show signs of respiratory distress, such as dyspnea and cyanosis.

◆ ***Esophageal varices (ruptured).*** Life-threatening rupture of esophageal varices may cause "coffee-ground" or massive, bright red vomitus. Signs of shock, such as hypotension or tachycardia, may follow or even precede hematemesis if the stomach fills with blood before vomiting occurs. Other symptoms may include abdominal distention and melena or painless hematochezia, ranging from slight oozing to massive rectal hemorrhage.

♦ ***Gastric carcinoma.*** Painless bright red or dark brown vomitus is a late sign of this uncommon cancer, which usually begins insidiously with upper abdominal discomfort. The patient then develops anorexia, mild nausea, and chronic dyspepsia unrelieved by antacids and exacerbated by food. Later symptoms may include fatigue, weakness, weight loss, feelings of fullness, melena, altered bowel habits, and signs of malnutrition, such as muscle wasting and dry skin.

♦ ***Gastritis (acute).*** Hematemesis and melena are the most common signs of acute gastritis. They may even be the only signs, although mild epigastric discomfort, nausea, fever, and malaise may also occur. Massive blood loss triggers signs of shock. Typically, the patient has a history of alcohol abuse or has used aspirin or some other NSAID. Gastritis may also occur secondary to *Helicobacter pylori* infection.

♦ ***Mallory-Weiss syndrome.*** Characterized by a mucosal tear of the cardia or lower esophagus, this syndrome may cause hematemesis and melena. It's commonly triggered by severe vomiting, retching, or straining (as from coughing). Severe bleeding may precipitate signs of shock, such as tachycardia, hypotension, dyspnea, and cool, clammy skin.

♦ ***Peptic ulcer.*** Hematemesis may occur when a peptic ulcer penetrates an artery, vein, or highly vascular tissue. Massive—and possibly life-threatening—hematemesis is typical when an artery is penetrated. Other features include melena or hematochezia, chills, fever, and signs of shock and dehydration, such as tachycardia, hypotension, poor skin turgor, or thirst. Most patients have a history of nausea, vomiting, epigastric tenderness, and epigastric pain that's relieved by foods or antacids. The patient may also have a history of habitual use of tobacco, alcohol, or NSAIDs.

Other causes

♦ ***Treatments.*** Traumatic nasogastric or endotracheal intubation may cause hematemesis associated with swallowed blood. Nose or throat surgery may also cause this sign in the same way.

Special considerations

Closely monitor the patient's vital signs every 15 minutes, and watch for signs of shock. Check the patient's stools regularly for occult blood, and keep accurate intake and output records. Place the patient on bed rest in a low or semi-Fowler's position to prevent aspiration of vomitus. Keep suctioning equipment nearby and use it as needed. Provide frequent oral hygiene and emotional support—the sight of bloody vomitus can be very frightening. Administer I.V. histamine-2 blockers; vasopressin may be required for variceal hemorrhage. As the bleeding tapers off, give hourly doses of antacids by nasogastric tube.

Pediatric pointers

Hematemesis is much less common in children than in adults and may be related to foreign-body ingestion. Occasionally, neonates develop hematemesis after swallowing maternal blood during delivery or breast-feeding from a cracked nipple. Hemorrhagic disease of the newborn and esophageal erosion may also cause hematemesis in infants; such cases require immediate fluid replacement.

Geriatric pointers

In elderly patients, hematemesis may be caused by vascular anomalies, aortoenteric fistulas, and upper GI cancers. In addition, chronic obstructive pulmonary disease, chronic liver or renal failure, and chronic NSAID use all predispose elderly people to hemorrhage secondary to coexisting ulcerative disorders.

HEMATOCHEZIA
[Rectal bleeding]

The passage of bloody stools, hematochezia usually indicates — and may be the first sign of — GI bleeding below the ligament of Treitz. However, this sign — usually preceded by hematemesis — may also accompany rapid hemorrhage of 1 L or more from the upper GI tract.

Hematochezia ranges from formed, blood-streaked stools to liquid, bloody stools that may be bright red, dark mahogany, or maroon in color. This sign usually develops abruptly and is heralded by abdominal pain.

Although hematochezia commonly is associated with GI disorders, it may also result from coagulation disorders, the effects of toxins, medications, and certain diagnostic tests. Always a significant sign, hematochezia may precipitate life-threatening hypovolemia.

Emergency interventions

If the patient has severe hematochezia, quickly check his vital signs. If you detect signs of shock, such as hypotension and tachycardia, place the patient in a supine position and elevate his feet 20 to 30 degrees. Prepare to administer oxygen, and start a large-bore I.V. line for emergency fluid replacement. Next, obtain a blood sample for typing and crossmatching. Insert a nasogastric tube. Iced lavage may be indicated to control bleeding. Endoscopy may be necessary to detect the source of the bleeding.

History and physical examination

If the hematochezia isn't immediately life-threatening, ask the patient to fully describe the amount, color, and consistency of his bloody stools. (If possible, also inspect and characterize the stools yourself.) How long have the stools been bloody? Do they always look the same, or does the amount of blood seem to vary? Ask about associated signs and symptoms.

Next, explore the patient's medical history, focusing on GI and coagulation disorders. Ask about use of GI irritants, such as alcohol, aspirin, and other nonsteroidal anti-inflammatory drugs.

Begin the physical examination by checking for orthostatic hypotension, an early sign of shock. Take the patient's blood pressure and pulse while he's lying down, sitting, and standing. If systolic pressure decreases by 10 mm Hg or more, or pulse rate increases by 10 beats/minute or more when he changes position, suspect volume depletion and impending shock.

Examine the skin for petechiae or spider angiomas. Palpate the abdomen for tenderness, pain, or masses. Also, note lymphadenopathy. Finally, a digital rectal examination must be done to rule out any rectal masses.

Common medical causes

◆ ***Anal fissure.*** Slight hematochezia characterizes this disorder; blood may streak the stools or appear on toilet tissue. Accompanying hematochezia is severe rectal pain that may make the patient reluctant to defecate, thereby causing constipation.

◆ ***Angiodysplastic lesions.*** Most common in the elderly, usually those with aortic stenosis, these arteriovenous lesions of the ascending colon typically cause chronic, bright red rectal bleeding. Occasionally, this painless hematochezia may cause life-threatening blood loss and signs of shock, such as tachycardia and hypotension.

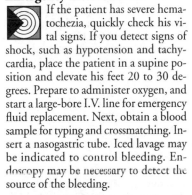

◆ ***Coagulation disorders.*** Patients with a coagulation disorder (such as thrombocytopenia or disseminated intravascular coagulation) may experience GI bleeding with moderate to severe hematochezia. Bleeding in other body systems may cause such signs as epistaxis or purpura. Associated findings vary with the specific coagulation disorder.

◆ ***Colitis.*** *Ischemic colitis* commonly causes bloody diarrhea, especially in the elderly. The hematochezia may be slight or massive and is usually accompanied by severe, cramping lower abdominal pain and hypotension. Other effects include abdominal tenderness, distention, and absent bowel sounds. Severe colitis may cause life-threatening hypovolemic shock and peritonitis.

Ulcerative colitis typically causes bloody diarrhea that may contain mucus. The hematochezia is preceded by mild to severe abdominal cramps and may cause slight to massive blood loss. Associated signs and symptoms include fever, tenesmus, anorexia, nausea, vomiting, hyperactive bowel sounds and, occasionally, tachycardia. Weight loss and weakness occur late.

◆ ***Colon cancer.*** Bright red rectal bleeding with or without pain is a telling sign, especially in cancer of the left colon.

Usually, a left colon tumor causes early signs of obstruction, such as rectal pressure, bleeding, and intermittent fullness or cramping. As the disease progresses, the patient also develops obstipation, diarrhea, or ribbon-shaped stools and pain, which typically is relieved by passage of stools or flatus. Stools are grossly bloody.

Early tumor growth in the right colon may cause melena, abdominal aching, pressure, and dull cramps. As the disease progresses, the patient develops weakness and fatigue. Later, he may also experience diarrhea, anorexia, weight loss, anemia, vomiting, abdominal mass, and signs of obstruction, such as abdominal distention or abnormal bowel sounds.

◆ ***Colorectal polyps.*** These polyps are the most common cause of intermittent hematochezia in adults under age 60; however, such polyps may cause no symptoms. Polyps high in the colon may cause blood-streaked stools. The stools yield a positive response when tested with guaiac If the polyps are closer to the rectum, they may bleed freely.

◆ ***Diverticulitis.*** Most common in the elderly, this disorder can suddenly cause mild to moderate rectal bleeding after the patient feels the urge to defecate. The bleeding may end abruptly or may progress to life-threatening blood loss with signs of shock. Associated signs and symptoms may include left-lower-quadrant pain that's relieved by defecation, alternating episodes of constipation and diarrhea, anorexia, nausea and vomiting, rebound tenderness, and a distended tympanic abdomen.

◆ ***Esophageal varices (ruptured).*** In this life-threatening disorder, hematochezia may range from slight rectal oozing to grossly bloody stools and may be accompanied by mild to severe hematemesis or melena. This painless but massive hemorrhage may precipitate signs of shock, such as tachycardia or hypotension. In fact, signs of shock occasionally precede overt signs of bleeding. Typically, the patient has a history of chronic liver disease.

◆ ***Food poisoning (staphylococcal).*** The patient may have bloody diarrhea 1 to 6 hours after ingesting contaminated food. Accompanying signs and symptoms include severe, cramping abdominal pain, nausea and vomiting, and prostration, all of which last a few hours.

◆ ***Hemorrhoids.*** Hematochezia may accompany external hemorrhoids, which typically cause painful defecation, resulting in constipation. Less painful internal hemorrhoids usually cause more chronic bleeding with bowel movements, which may eventually lead to signs of anemia, such as weakness and fatigue.

◆ ***Leptospirosis.*** The severe form of this infection — Weil's syndrome — causes hematochezia or melena and other signs of bleeding, such as epistaxis and hemoptysis. The bleeding is typically preceded by a sudden frontal headache and severe thigh and lumbar myalgia that may be accompanied by cutaneous hyperesthesia. Conjunctival suffusion is indicative. Bleeding is followed by chills, a rapidly rising fever and, perhaps, nausea and vomiting. Fever, headache, and myalgia usually intensify and persist for weeks. Other findings may include right-upper-quadrant tenderness, hepatomegaly, and jaundice.

♦ ***Peptic ulcer.*** Upper GI bleeding is a frequent complication in this disorder. The patient may display hematochezia, hematemesis, or melena, depending on the rapidity and amount of bleeding. If the peptic ulcer penetrates an artery or vein, massive bleeding may precipitate signs of shock, such as hypotension and tachycardia. Other findings may include chills, fever, nausea and vomiting, and signs of dehydration, such as dry mucous membranes, poor skin turgor, and thirst. The patient typically has a history of epigastric pain that's relieved by foods or antacids; he may also have a history of habitual use of tobacco, alcohol, or nonsteroidal anti-inflammatory drugs.

♦ ***Ulcerative proctitis.*** This disorder typically causes an intense urge to defecate, but the patient passes only bright red blood, pus, or mucus. Other common signs and symptoms include acute constipation and tenesmus.

Other causes

♦ ***Tests.*** Certain procedures, especially colonoscopy, polypectomy, and proctosigmoidoscopy, may cause rectal bleeding. Bowel perforation is rare.

Special considerations

Place the patient on bed rest and check his vital signs every 15 minutes, watching for signs of shock, such as hypotension and tachycardia. Monitor the patient's intake and output hourly. Remember to provide emotional support because hematochezia may frighten the patient.

Prepare the patient for blood tests and GI procedures, such as endoscopy and X-rays. Visually examine the patient's stools and test them for occult blood. If necessary, send a stool sample to the laboratory to check for parasites.

Pediatric pointers

Hematochezia is much less common in children than in adults. It may result from structural disorders, such as intussusception or Meckel's diverticulum, or from inflammatory disorders, such as peptic ulcer disease or ulcerative colitis.

In children, ulcerative colitis typically causes chronic, rather than acute, signs and symptoms; it may also cause slow growth and maturation related to malnutrition. Suspect sexual abuse in all cases of rectal bleeding in children.

Geriatric pointers

Because older people have an increased risk of colon cancer, hematochezia should be evaluated with colonoscopy after perirectal lesions have been ruled out as the cause of bleeding.

HEMATURIA

A cardinal sign of renal and urinary tract disorders, hematuria is the presence of blood in the urine. Strictly defined, it means three or more red blood cells per high-power microscopic field in the urine. Microscopic hematuria is confirmed by an occult blood test, whereas macroscopic hematuria is immediately visible. Macroscopic hematuria may be continuous or intermittent, is commonly accompanied by pain, and may be aggravated by prolonged standing or walking.

Hematuria may be classified by the stage of urination it predominantly affects. *Initial hematuria* (at the start of urination) usually indicates urethral pathology; *total hematuria* (throughout urination), pathology above the bladder neck; and *terminal hematuria* (at the end of urination), pathology of the bladder neck, posterior urethra, or prostate.

Hematuria may result from one of two mechanisms: rupture or perforation of vessels in the renal system or urinary tract or impaired glomerular filtration, which allows red blood cells to seep into the urine. The color of the bloody urine provides a clue to the source of the bleeding: *dark or brownish,* renal or upper urinary tract bleeding; *bright red,* lower urinary tract.

Although hematuria usually results from renal and urinary tract disorders, it may also result from certain GI, prostate, vaginal, or coagulation disorders or from the effects of certain drugs. Invasive therapy and diagnostic tests that involve manipulative instrumentation of the renal and urologic systems may also cause hematuria. Nonpathologic hematuria may result from fever and hypercatabolic states. Transient hematuria may follow strenuous exercise.

History and physical examination

After detecting hematuria, take a pertinent health history. If hematuria is macroscopic, ask the patient when he first noticed blood in his urine. Does it vary in severity between voidings? Is it worse at the beginning, middle, or end of urination? Has it occurred before? Is the patient passing any clots? To rule out artifactitious hematuria, ask about bleeding hemorrhoids or the onset of menses, if appropriate.

Ask about recent abdominal or flank trauma. Has the patient been exercising strenuously? Note a history of renal, urinary, prostatic, or coagulation disorders. Then obtain a drug history.

Begin the physical examination by palpating and percussing the abdomen and flanks. Next, percuss the costovertebral angle (CVA) to elicit tenderness. Check the urinary meatus for bleeding or other abnormalities. Using a chemical reagent strip, test a urine specimen for protein. A vaginal or digital rectal examination may be necessary. (See *Hematuria: Common causes and associated findings,* pages 308 to 311.)

Common medical causes

♦ ***Bladder cancer.*** A primary cause of gross hematuria in men, this disorder may also cause pain in the bladder, rectum, pelvis, flank, back, or leg. Other common features are nocturia, dysuria, urinary frequency and urgency, vomiting, diarrhea, and insomnia.

♦ ***Bladder trauma.*** Gross hematuria is characteristic in traumatic rupture or perforation of the bladder. Typically, the hematuria is accompanied by lower abdominal pain and, occasionally, anuria despite a strong urge to void. The patient may also develop swelling of the scrotum, buttocks, or perineum and signs of shock, such as tachycardia and hypotension.

♦ ***Calculi.*** Bladder and renal calculi cause hematuria, which may be associated with signs of urinary tract infection, such as dysuria or urinary frequency and urgency. *Bladder calculi* usually cause gross hematuria, referred pain to the lower back or penile or vulvar area and, in some patients, bladder distention.

Renal calculi may cause microscopic or gross hematuria. The cardinal symptom, though, is colicky pain that travels from the CVA to the flank, suprapubic region, and external genitalia when a calculus is passed. The pain may be excruciating at its peak. Other signs and symptoms may include nausea and vomiting, restlessness, fever, chills, abdominal distention, or decreased bowel sounds.

♦ ***Coagulation disorders.*** Macroscopic hematuria is commonly the first sign of hemorrhage in coagulation disorders, such as thrombocytopenia or disseminated intravascular coagulation. Among other features are epistaxis, purpura (petechiae, ecchymoses), and signs of GI bleeding.

♦ ***Cortical necrosis (acute).*** Accompanying gross hematuria in this renal disorder are intense flank pain, anuria, leukocytosis, and fever.

♦ ***Cystitis.*** Hematuria is a telling sign in all types of cystitis. *Bacterial cystitis* usually causes macroscopic hematuria with urinary urgency and frequency, dysuria, nocturia, and tenesmus. The patient complains of perineal and lumbar pain, suprapubic discomfort, and fatigue and occasionally has a low-grade fever.

More common in women, *chronic interstitial cystitis* occasionally causes grossly bloody hematuria. Associated features include urinary frequency, dysuria, nocturia, and tenesmus. Both microscopic and macroscopic hematuria may occur in *tubercular cystitis*, which may also cause urinary urgency and frequency, dysuria, tenesmus, flank pain, fatigue, or anorexia. *Viral cystitis* usually causes hematuria, urinary urgency and frequency, dysuria, nocturia, tenesmus, and fever.

♦ ***Diverticulitis.*** When this disorder involves the bladder, it usually causes microscopic hematuria, urinary frequency and urgency, dysuria, and nocturia. Characteristic findings include left-lower-quadrant pain, abdominal tenderness, constipation or diarrhea and, at times, a palpable, firm, fixed, tender abdominal mass. The patient may also develop mild nausea, flatulence, and a low-grade fever.

♦ ***Glomerulonephritis.*** *Acute glomerulonephritis* usually begins with gross hematuria that tapers off to microscopic hematuria and red cell casts, which may persist for months. It may also cause oliguria or anuria, proteinuria, mild fever, fatigue, flank and abdominal pain, generalized edema, increased blood pressure, nausea, vomiting, and signs of lung congestion, such as crackles and a productive cough.

Chronic glomerulonephritis usually causes microscopic hematuria accompanied by proteinuria, generalized edema, and increased blood pressure. Signs and symptoms of uremia may also occur in advanced disease.

♦ ***Nephritis (interstitial).*** Typically, this infection causes microscopic hematuria. However, some patients with *acute interstitial nephritis* may develop gross hematuria. Other findings are fever, maculopapular rash, and oliguria or anuria. In *chronic interstitial nephritis,* the patient has dilute — almost colorless — urine, which may be accompanied by polyuria and increased blood pressure.

♦ ***Nephropathy (obstructive).*** This disorder may cause microscopic or macroscopic hematuria, but urine is seldom grossly bloody. The patient may report colicky flank and abdominal pain, CVA tenderness, or anuria or oliguria alternating with polyuria.

♦ ***Polycystic kidney disease.*** This hereditary disorder may cause recurrent microscopic or gross hematuria. Although commonly asymptomatic before age 40, it may cause increased blood pressure, polyuria, dull flank pain, or signs of urinary tract infection, such as dysuria and urinary frequency and urgency. Later, the patient develops a swollen, tender abdomen and lumbar pain that's aggravated by exertion and relieved by lying down. He may also have proteinuria and colicky abdominal pain from the ureteral passage of clots or stones.

♦ ***Prostatitis.*** Whether acute or chronic, prostatitis may cause macroscopic hematuria, usually at the end of urination. It may also cause urinary frequency and urgency and dysuria followed by visible bladder distention. *Acute prostatitis* also causes fatigue, malaise, myalgia, polyarthralgia, fever with chills, nausea, vomiting, perineal and lower back pain, and decreased libido. Rectal palpation reveals a tender, swollen, boggy prostate. *Chronic prostatitis* commonly follows an acute attack. It may cause persistent urethral discharge, dull perineal pain, ejaculatory pain, and decreased libido.

♦ ***Pyelonephritis (acute).*** This infection typically causes microscopic or macroscopic hematuria that progresses to grossly bloody hematuria. After the infection resolves, microscopic hematuria may persist for a few months. Related signs and symptoms include persistent high fever, unilateral or bilateral flank pain, CVA tenderness, shaking chills, weakness, fatigue, dysuria, urinary frequency and urgency, nocturia, and tenes-

(Text continues on page 310.)

Hematuria: Common causes and associated findings

CAUSES	MAJOR ASSOCIATED SIGNS AND SYMPTOMS											
	Abdominal distention	Abdominal pain	Anuria	Bladder distention	Blood pressure increase	Bowel sounds, hypoactive	Colicky pain	Costovertebral angle tenderness	Dysuria	Edema, generalized	Edema of the legs	Fever
Bladder cancer									◆			
Bladder trauma		◆	◆									
Calculi (bladder)				◆					◆			
Calculi (renal)	◆	◆				◆	◆	◆	◆			◆
Coagulation disorders												
Cortical necrosis (acute)			◆									◆
Cystitis (bacterial)									◆			◆
Cystitis (chronic interstitial)									◆			
Cystitis (tubercular)									◆			
Cystitis (viral)									◆			◆
Glomerulonephritis (chronic)		◆	◆		◆					◆		◆
Nephritis (acute interstitial)			◆									◆
Nephropathy (obstructive)		◆	◆				◆	◆				
Polycystic kidney disease		◆			◆		◆		◆			
Prostatitis (acute)				◆					◆			◆
Prostatitis (chronic)				◆					◆			
Pyelonephritis (acute)	◆					◆		◆	◆			◆
Renal cancer					◆		◆	◆			◆	◆

	Flank mass	Flank pain	Lumbar pain	Murmers	Nausea	Nocturia	Oligurea	Perineal pain	Polyarthralgia	Polyuria	Proteinurea	Purpura	Rash	Urethral discharge	Urinary frequency	Urinary hesitancy	Urinary urgency	Vomiting
		◆				◆		◆							◆		◆	◆
								◆							◆		◆	
		◆			◆										◆		◆	◆
												◆						
		◆																
			◆			◆		◆							◆		◆	
						◆									◆			
		◆													◆		◆	
						◆									◆		◆	
		◆			◆		◆				◆							◆
							◆						◆					
		◆					◆			◆								
			◆							◆	◆				◆		◆	
			◆		◆			◆	◆						◆		◆	◆
								◆						◆	◆		◆	
		◆			◆	◆									◆	◆	◆	◆
	◆	◆			◆													◆

(continued)

Hematuria: Common causes and associated findings *(continued)*

CAUSES	Abdominal distention	Abdominal pain	Anuria	Bladder distention	Blood pressure increase	Bowel sounds, hypoactive	Colicky pain	Costovertebral angle tenderness	Dysuria	Edema, generalized	Edema of the legs	Fever
Renal infarction		◆	◆		◆	◆		◆				◆
Renal papillary necrosis (acute)		◆	◆			◆	◆	◆				◆
Renal trauma						◆						
Renal tuberculosis		◆					◆		◆			
Renal vein thrombosis			◆					◆			◆	◆
Schistosomiasis							◆		◆			
Sickle cell anemia												
Vasculitis			◆		◆							◆

mus. The patient may also exhibit nausea, anorexia, vomiting, and signs of paralytic ileus, such as hypoactive or absent bowel sounds and abdominal distention.

♦ ***Renal cancer.*** The classic triad of signs and symptoms includes grossly bloody hematuria; dull, aching flank pain; and a smooth, firm, palpable flank mass. Colicky pain may accompany the passage of clots. Other findings include fever, CVA tenderness, and increased blood pressure. In advanced disease, the patient may develop weight loss, nausea and vomiting, and leg edema with varicoceles.

♦ ***Renal infarction.*** Typically, this disorder causes gross hematuria. The patient may complain of constant, severe flank and upper abdominal pain accompanied by CVA tenderness, anorexia, and nausea and vomiting. Other findings include oliguria or anuria, proteinuria, hypoactive bowel sounds and, a day or two after infarction, fever and increased blood pressure.

♦ ***Renal papillary necrosis (acute).*** This disorder usually causes grossly bloody hematuria, which may be accompanied by intense flank pain, CVA tenderness, abdominal rigidity and colicky pain, oliguria or anuria, pyuria, fever, chills, vomiting, and hypoactive bowel sounds. Arthralgia and hypertension are common.

♦ ***Renal trauma.*** About 80% of patients with renal trauma have microscopic or gross hematuria. Accompanying signs and symptoms may include flank pain, a palpable flank mass, oliguria, hematoma or ecchymoses over the upper abdomen or flank, nausea and vomiting, and hy-

Flank mass	Flank pain	Lumbar pain	Murmers	Nausea	Nocturia	Oligurea	Perineal pain	Polyarthralgia	Polyuria	Proteinurea	Purpura	Rash	Urethral discharge	Urinary frequency	Urinary hesitancy	Urinary urgency	Vomiting
	◆			◆		◆				◆							◆
	◆					◆											◆
◆	◆			◆		◆					◆						◆
		◆								◆				◆			
	◆	◆				◆				◆							
			◆					◆									
								◆			◆	◆					

poactive bowel sounds. Severe trauma may precipitate signs of shock, such as tachycardia and hypotension.

◆ ***Renal tuberculosis.*** Gross hematuria is commonly the first sign of this disorder. It may be accompanied by urinary frequency, dysuria, pyuria, tenesmus, colicky abdominal pain, lumbar pain, and proteinuria.

◆ ***Renal vein thrombosis.*** Grossly bloody hematuria usually occurs in this type of thrombosis. In abrupt venous obstruction, the patient experiences severe flank and lumbar pain as well as epigastric and CVA tenderness. Other features include fever, pallor, proteinuria, peripheral edema and, when the obstruction is bilateral, oliguria or anuria and other uremic signs. The kidneys are easily palpable. Gradual venous obstruction causes signs of nephrotic syndrome, proteinuria and, occasionally, peripheral edema.

◆ ***Schistosomiasis.*** This infection usually causes intermittent hematuria at the end of urination. It may be accompanied by dysuria, colicky renal and bladder pain, and palpable lower abdominal masses.

◆ ***Sickle cell anemia.*** In this hereditary disorder, gross hematuria may result from congestion of the renal papillae. Associated signs and symptoms may include pallor, dehydration, chronic fatigue, polyarthralgia, leg ulcers, dyspnea, chest pain, impaired growth and development, hepatomegaly, or jaundice. Auscultation reveals tachycardia and systolic and diastolic murmurs.

◆ ***Systemic lupus erythematosus.*** Gross hematuria and proteinuria may occur when this disorder involves the kidneys. Cardinal associated features include nondeforming joint pain and stiffness, a butterfly rash, photosensitivity, Raynaud's phenomenon, seizures or psychoses, recurrent fever, lymphadenopathy, oral or nasopharyngeal ulcers, anorexia, and weight loss.

♦ ***Urethral trauma.*** Initial hematuria may occur, possibly with blood at the urinary meatus, local pain, and penile or vulvar ecchymoses.

♦ ***Vasculitis.*** Hematuria is usually microscopic in this disorder. Associated signs and symptoms include malaise, myalgia, polyarthralgia, fever, increased blood pressure, pallor and, occasionally, anuria. Other features, such as urticaria and purpura, may reflect the etiology of vasculitis.

Other causes

♦ ***Diagnostic tests.*** Renal biopsy is the diagnostic test most commonly associated with hematuria. This sign may also result from biopsy or manipulative instrumentation of the urinary tract, as in cystoscopy.

♦ ***Drugs.*** Drugs that commonly cause hematuria are anticoagulants, analgesics, cyclophosphamide (Cytoxan), metyrosine, phenylbutazone, penicillin, rifampin, and thiabendazole.

♦ **Herb alert** Herbal medicines, such as garlic and ginkgo biloba, may cause adverse effects, including excessive bleeding and hematuria, when taken with anticoagulants.

♦ ***Treatments.*** Any therapy that involves manipulative instrumentation of the urinary tract, such as transurethral prostatectomy, may cause microscopic or macroscopic hematuria.

Special considerations

Because hematuria may frighten and upset the patient, be sure to provide emotional support. Check his vital signs at least every 4 hours and monitor intake and output, including the amount and pattern of hematuria. Administer prescribed analgesics, and enforce bed rest as indicated. Prepare the patient for diagnostic tests, such as blood and urine studies, cystoscopy, and renal X-rays or biopsy.

Pediatric pointers

Many of the causes described above also cause hematuria in children. However, cyclophosphamide is more likely to cause hematuria in children than in adults.

Common causes of hematuria that chiefly affect children include congenital anomalies, such as obstructive uropathy and renal dysplasia; birth trauma; hematologic disorders, such as vitamin K deficiency, hemophilia, and hemolytic-uremic syndrome; certain neoplasms, such as Wilms' tumor, bladder cancer, and rhabdomyosarcoma; allergies; and foreign bodies in the urinary tract. Artifactual hematuria may follow circumcision.

Geriatric pointers

Evaluation of hematuria in elderly patients should include a urine culture, excretory urography or sonography, and consultation with a urologist.

HEMIANOPSIA

Hemianopsia is loss of vision in half the visual field (usually the right or left half) of one or both eyes. However, if the visual field defects are identical in both eyes but affect less than half the field of vision in each eye (incomplete homonymous hemianopsia), the lesion may be in the occipital lobe; otherwise, it probably involves the parietal or temporal lobe. (See *Recognizing types of hemianopsia.*)

Hemianopsia is caused by a lesion affecting the optic chiasm, tract, or radiation. Defects in visual perception due to

Recognizing types of hemianopsia

Lesions of the optic pathways cause visual field defects. The lesion's site determines the type of defect. For example, a lesion of the optic chiasm involving only fibers that cross over to the opposite side causes bitemporal hemianopsia — visual loss in the temporal half of each field. However, a lesion of the optic tract or a complete lesion of the optic radiation produces visual loss in the same half of each field— either left or right homonymous hemianopsia.

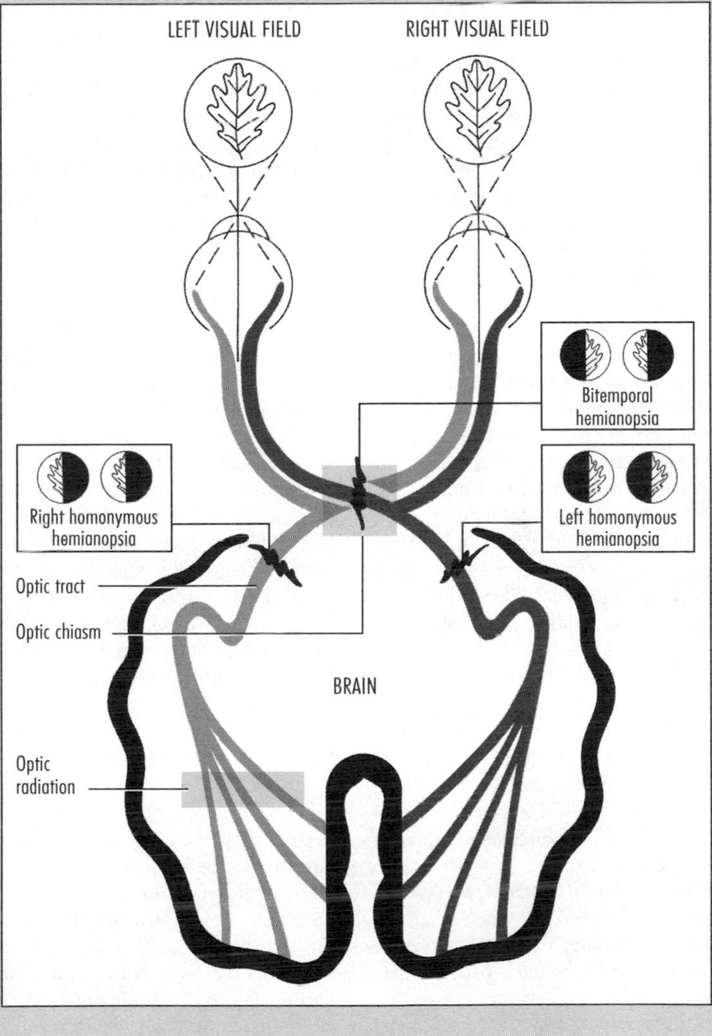

cerebral lesions are usually associated with impaired color vision.

History and physical examination

Suspect a visual field defect if the patient seems startled when you approach him from one side or if he fails to see objects placed directly in front of him. To help determine the type of defect, compare the patient's visual fields with your own — if yours are normal. First, ask the patient to cover his right eye while you cover your left eye. Then move a pen or similarly shaped object from the periphery of his (and your) uncovered eye into his field of vision. Ask the patient to indicate when he first sees the object. Does he see it at the same time you do? After you do? Repeat this test in each quadrant of both eyes. Then, for each eye, plot the defect by shading the area of a circle that corresponds to the area of vision loss.

Next, evaluate the patient's level of consciousness (LOC), take his vital signs, and check his pupillary reaction and motor response. Ask if he has recently experienced headache, dysarthria, or seizures. Does he have ptosis or facial or extremity weakness? Hallucinations or loss of color vision? When did neurologic symptoms start? Obtain a medical history, noting especially eye disorders, hypertension, and diabetes mellitus.

Common medical causes

♦ ***Carotid artery aneurysm.*** An aneurysm in the internal carotid artery can cause contralateral or bilateral defects in the visual fields. It can also cause hemiplegia, decreased LOC, headache, aphasia, behavior disturbances, and unilateral hypoesthesia.

♦ ***Cerebrovascular accident (CVA).*** Hemianopsia can result when a hemorrhagic, thrombotic, or embolic CVA affects any part of the optic pathway. Associated signs and symptoms vary according to the location and size of the CVA but may include decreased LOC, intellectual deficits (such as memory loss or poor judgment), personality changes, emotional lability, headache, or seizures. Other possible manifestations include contralateral hemiplegia, dysarthria, dysphagia, ataxia, a unilateral sensory loss, apraxia, agnosia, aphasia, blurred vision, decreased visual acuity, diplopia, urine retention or incontinence, constipation, and vomiting.

♦ ***Occipital lobe lesion.*** The most common symptoms arising from a lesion of one occipital lobe are incomplete homonymous hemianopsia, scotomas, and impaired color vision. The patient may also experience visual hallucinations: flashes of light or color or visions of objects, people, animals, or geometric forms. These may appear in the defective field or may move toward it from the intact field.

♦ ***Parietal lobe lesion.*** This disorder causes homonymous hemianopsia and sensory deficits, such as an inability to perceive body position or passive movement or to localize tactile, thermal, or vibratory stimuli. It may also cause apraxia and visual or tactile agnosia.

♦ ***Pituitary tumor.*** A tumor that compresses nerve fibers supplying the nasal half of both retinas causes complete or partial bitemporal hemianopsia that first occurs in the upper visual fields but later can progress to blindness. Related findings include blurred vision, diplopia, headache, and (rarely) somnolence, hypothermia, and seizures.

Special considerations

If the patient's visual field defect is significant, further visual field testing, such as perimetry or a tangent screen examination, may be indicated.

To avoid startling the patient, approach him from the unaffected side and position his bed so that his unaffected side faces the door. If he's ambulatory, remove objects that could cause falls, and alert him to other possible hazards. Place his clock and other personal objects within his field of vision, and avoid putting dangerous objects (such as hot dishes) where he can't see them.

Pediatric pointers

In children, a brain tumor is the most common cause of hemianopsia. To help detect this sign, look for nonverbal clues, such as the child reaching for a toy but missing it. To help the child compensate for hemianopsia, place objects within his visual field; teach his parents to do this as well.

Hemoptysis

Frightening to the patient and commonly ominous, hemoptysis is the expectoration of blood or bloody sputum from the lungs or tracheobronchial tree. It's sometimes confused with bleeding from the mouth, throat, nasopharynx, or GI tract. (See *Identifying hemoptysis,* page 316.)

Expectoration of 300 ml in 24 hours is considered *massive* and signals a life-threatening crisis. *Mild to moderate* hemoptysis is most common in acute and chronic bronchitis (30%), bronchiectasis (25%), and bronchogenic carcinoma (20%). *Moderate to severe* hemoptysis occurs most commonly in tuberculosis (30%), bronchiectasis (30%), and bronchiogenic carcinoma (15%). However, hemoptysis may also result from other inflammatory infections or cardiovascular or coagulation disorders. A number of pathophysiologic processes can cause hemoptysis. (See *What happens in hemoptysis,* page 317.)

Emergency interventions

If the patient coughs up copious amounts of blood, endotracheal intubation may be required. Suction frequently to remove blood. Massive hemoptysis can cause airway obstruction and asphyxiation. Insert an I.V. line to allow fluid replacement, drug administration, and blood transfusions, if needed. An emergency bronchoscopy should be performed to identify the bleeding site. Monitor blood pressure and pulse to detect hypotension and tachycardia, and draw an arterial blood sample for laboratory analysis to monitor respiratory status.

History and physical examination

If the hemoptysis is mild, ask the patient when it began. Has he ever coughed up blood before? About how much blood is he coughing up now? And how often? Ask about coughing up sputum and other signs of infection. Ask about a history of cardiac, pulmonary, or bleeding disorders. If he's receiving anticoagulant therapy, find out the drug, its dosage and schedule, and the duration of therapy. Is he taking other prescription drugs? Does he smoke?

Take the patient's vital signs and examine his nose, mouth, and pharynx for sources of bleeding. Inspect the configuration of his chest and look for abnormal movement during breathing, use of accessory muscles, and retractions. Observe his respiratory rate, depth, and rhythm. Finally, examine his skin for lesions.

Next, palpate the patient's chest for diaphragm level and for tenderness, respiratory excursion, fremitus, and abnormal pulsations; then percuss for flatness, dullness, resonance, hyperresonance, and tympany. Finally, auscultate the lungs, noting especially the quality and intensity of breath sounds. Also auscultate for heart murmurs, bruits, and pleural friction rubs. Obtain a sputum sample and examine it for overall quantity, for the amount of blood it contains, and for its color, odor, and consistency.

Common medical causes

♦ ***Bronchial adenoma.*** This insidious disorder causes recurring hemoptysis in up to 30% of patients, along with a chronic cough and local wheezing.

EXAMINATION TIP

Identifying hemoptysis

These guidelines will help you distinguish hemoptysis from epistaxis, hematemesis, and brown, red, or pink sputum.

HEMOPTYSIS
Often frothy because it is mixed with air, hemoptysis is typically bright red with an alkaline pH (tested with nitrazine paper). It's strongly suggested by the presence of respiratory signs and symptoms, including a cough, a tickling sensation in the throat, and blood produced from repeated coughing episodes. You can rule out epistaxis because the patient's nasal passages and posterior pharynx are usually clear.

HEMATEMESIS
The usual site of hematemesis is the GI tract; the patient vomits or regurgitates coffee-ground material that contains food particles, tests positive for occult blood, and has an acid pH. But he may vomit bright red blood or swallowed blood from the oral cavity and nasopharynx. After an episode of hematemesis, the patient's stools may have traces of blood. Many patients with hematemesis also complain of dyspepsia.

BROWN, RED, OR PINK SPUTUM
Brown, red, or pink sputum can result from oxidation of inhaled bronchodilators. Sputum that looks like old blood may result from rupture of an amoebic abscess into the bronchus. Red or brown sputum may occur in a patient with pneumonia caused by the enterobactum *Serratia marcescens.* "Current-jelly" sputum suggests *Klebsiella* infections.

◆ ***Bronchiectasis.*** Inflamed bronchial surfaces and eroded bronchial blood vessels cause hemoptysis, which can vary from blood-tinged sputum to blood (in about 20% of patients). The patient's sputum may also be copious, foul-smelling, and purulent. He may exhibit a chronic cough, coarse crackles, clubbing (a late sign), fever, weight loss, fatigue, weakness, malaise, or dyspnea on exertion.

◆ ***Bronchitis (chronic).*** The first sign of this disorder is typically a productive cough that lasts at least 3 months. Eventually this leads to production of blood-streaked sputum; massive hemorrhage is unusual. Other respiratory effects include dyspnea, prolonged expirations, wheezing, scattered rhonchi, accessory muscle use, barrel chest, tachypnea, and clubbing (a late sign).

◆ ***Bronchogenic carcinoma.*** Ulceration of the bronchus commonly causes recurring hemoptysis (an early sign), which can vary from blood-streaked sputum to blood. Related findings include a productive cough, dyspnea, fever, anorexia, weight loss, wheezing, and chest pain (a late symptom).

◆ ***Coagulation disorders.*** Such disorders as thrombocytopenia and disseminated intravascular coagulation can cause hemoptysis. Besides their specific related findings, these disorders may share such general signs as multisystem hemorrhaging (for example, GI bleeding or epistaxis) and purpuric lesions.

◆ ***Lung abscess.*** In about 50% of patients, this disorder causes blood-streaked sputum resulting from bronchial ulceration, necrosis, and granulation tissue. Common associated findings include a cough with large amounts of purulent, foul-smelling sputum; fever with chills; diaphoresis; anorexia; weight loss; headache; weakness; dyspnea; pleuritic or dull chest pain; and clubbing. Auscultation reveals tubular or cavernous breath sounds and crackles. Percussion reveals dullness on the affected side.

◆ ***Pneumonia.*** In up to 50% of patients with *Klebsiella* pneumonia, dark brown or red ("currant-jelly") sputum is so tenacious that the patient has difficulty expelling it from his mouth. This type of pneumonia begins abruptly with chills, fever, dyspnea, a productive cough, and severe pleuritic chest pain. Associated findings may include cyanosis, prostration, tachycardia, decreased breath sounds, and crackles.

Pneumococcal pneumonia causes pinkish or rusty mucoid sputum. It begins with sudden shaking chills, a rapidly rising temperature and, in over 80% of patients, tachycardia and tachypnea. Within a few hours, the patient typically experiences a productive cough along with severe, stabbing, pleuritic pain. The agonizing chest pain leads to rapid, shallow, grunting respirations with splinting. Examination reveals respiratory distress with dyspnea and accessory muscle use, crackles, and dullness on percussion over the affected lung. Malaise, weakness, myalgia, and prostration accompany high fever.

◆ ***Pulmonary edema.*** Severe cardiogenic or noncardiogenic pulmonary edema commonly causes frothy, blood-tinged pink sputum, which accompanies severe dyspnea, orthopnea, gasping, anxiety, cyanosis, diffuse crackles, a ventricular gallop, and cold, clammy skin. This life-threatening condition may also cause tachycardia, lethargy, cardiac arrhythmias, tachypnea, hypotension, and a thready pulse.

◆ ***Pulmonary embolism with infarction.*** Hemoptysis is a common finding in this life-threatening disorder, although massive hemoptysis is infrequent. Typical initial symptoms are dyspnea and anginal or pleuritic chest pain. Other common clinical features include tachycardia, tachypnea, low-grade fever, and diaphoresis. Less common signs are splinting of the chest, leg edema, and—with a large embolus—cyanosis, syncope, and distended neck veins. Examination reveals decreased breath sounds, pleural friction rub, crackles, diffuse wheezing, dullness on percussion, and signs of circulatory collapse (weak, rapid pulse, hypotension), cerebral ischemia (transient loss of consciousness, seizures), or hypoxemia (restlessness and, particularly in the elderly, hemiplegia and other focal neurologic deficits).

◆ ***Pulmonary hypertension (primary).*** Features generally develop late. He-

What happens in hemoptysis

Hemoptysis results from bleeding into the respiratory tract by bronchial or pulmonary vessels. Bleeding reflects alterations in the vascular walls and in blood-clotting mechanisms. It can result from these pathophysiologic processes:

◆ hemorrhage and diapedesis of red blood cells from the pulmonary microvasculature into the alveoli
◆ necrosis of lung tissue that causes inflammation and rupture of blood vessels or hemorrhage into the alveolar spaces
◆ rupture of an aortic aneurysm into the tracheobronchial tree
◆ rupture of distended endobronchial blood vessels from pulmonary hypertension due to mitral stenosis
◆ rupture of a pulmonary arteriovenous fistula or of bronchial or pulmonary artery or pulmonary venous collateral channels
◆ sloughing of a caseous lesion into the tracheobronchial tree
◆ ulceration and erosion of the bronchial epithelium.

moptysis, exertional dyspnea, and fatigue are common. Angina-like pain usually occurs with exertion and may radiate to the neck but not to the arms. Other findings include arrhythmias, syncope, cough, and hoarseness.

♦ ***Pulmonary tuberculosis.*** Blood-streaked or -tinged sputum is common in this disorder; massive hemoptysis may occur in advanced cavitary tuberculosis. Accompanying respiratory findings include a chronic productive cough, fine crackles after coughing, dyspnea, dullness to percussion, increased tactile fremitus, and possible amphoric breath sounds. The patient may also develop night sweats, malaise, fatigue, fever, anorexia, weight loss, or pleuritic chest pain.

♦ ***Systemic lupus erythematosus.*** In 50% of patients with this disorder, pleuritis and pneumonitis cause hemoptysis, cough, dyspnea, pleuritic chest pain, and crackles. Related findings are a butterfly rash in the acute phase, nondeforming joint pain and stiffness, photosensitivity, Raynaud's phenomenon, seizures or psychoses, anorexia with weight loss, and lymphadenopathy.

♦ ***Tracheal trauma.*** Torn tracheal mucosa may cause hemoptysis, hoarseness, dysphagia, neck pain, airway occlusion, and respiratory distress.

Other causes

♦ ***Diagnostic tests.*** Lung or airway injury from bronchoscopy, laryngoscopy, mediastinoscopy, or lung biopsy can cause bleeding and hemoptysis.

Special considerations

Comfort and reassure the patient, who may react to this alarming sign with anxiety and apprehension. Place him in a slight Trendelenburg position to promote drainage of blood from the lung. If necessary to protect the nonbleeding lung, place him in the lateral decubitus position, with the suspected bleeding lung facing down. Perform this maneuver with caution, however, because hypoxemia may worsen with the healthy lung facing up.

Prepare the patient for diagnostic tests to determine the cause of bleeding. These may include a complete blood count, a sputum culture and smear, chest X-rays, coagulation studies, bronchoscopy, lung biopsy, pulmonary arteriography, lung scan, or a high-resolution computed tomography scan.

Pediatric pointers

Hemoptysis in children may stem from Goodpasture's syndrome, cystic fibrosis, or (rarely) idiopathic primary pulmonary hemosiderosis. Sometimes no cause can be found for pulmonary hemorrhage occurring in the first 2 weeks of life; in such cases, the prognosis is poor.

Geriatric pointers

If the patient is receiving anticoagulants, evaluate his diet and medications (including over-the-counter and natural supplements) for ingredients that may affect clotting.

HEPATOMEGALY

Hepatomegaly, an enlarged liver, indicates potentially reversible primary or secondary liver disease. This sign may stem from diverse pathophysiologic mechanisms, including dilated hepatic sinusoids (in heart failure), persistently high venous pressure leading to liver congestion (in chronic constrictive pericarditis), dysfunction and engorgement of hepatocytes (in hepatitis), fatty infiltration of parenchymal cells causing fibrous tissue (in cirrhosis), distention of liver cells with glycogen (in diabetes), and infiltration of amyloid (in amyloidosis).

Hepatomegaly may be confirmed by palpation, percussion, or radiologic tests. It may be mistaken for displacement of the liver by the diaphragm, in a respiratory disorder; by an abdominal tumor; by a spinal deformity such as kyphosis; by the gallbladder; or by fecal material or a tumor in the colon.

History and physical examination

Hepatomegaly is seldom a patient's chief complaint. It usually comes to light during palpation and percussion of the abdomen.

If you suspect hepatomegaly, ask the patient about his use of alcohol and exposure to hepatitis. Also ask if he's currently ill or taking prescribed drugs. If he complains of abdominal pain, ask him to locate and describe it.

Inspect the patient's skin and sclera for jaundice, dilated veins (suggesting generalized congestion), scars from previous surgery, and spider angiomas (commonly occurring in cirrhosis). Next, inspect the contour of his abdomen. Is it protuberant over the liver or distended (possibly from ascites)? Measure his abdominal girth.

Percuss the liver, but be careful to identify structures and conditions that can obscure dull percussion notes, such as the sternum, ribs, breast tissue, pleural effusions, and gas in the colon. (See *Percussing for liver size and position.*) Next, during deep inspiration, palpate the liver's edge; it's tender and rounded in hepatitis and cardiac decompensation, rocklike in carcinoma, and firm in cirrhosis.

Take the patient's baseline vital signs, and assess his nutritional status. An enlarged liver that's functioning poorly causes muscle wasting, exaggerated skeletal prominences, weight loss, thin hair, and edema.

Evaluate the patient's level of consciousness. When an enlarged liver loses its ability to detoxify waste products, the result is accumulation of metabolic substances toxic to brain cells. As a result, watch for personality changes, irritability, agitation, memory loss, inability to concentrate, and — in a severely ill patient — coma.

Percussing for liver size and position

With your patient supine, begin at the right iliac crest to percuss up the right midclavicular line (MCL), as shown here. The percussion note becomes dull when you reach the liver's inferior border — usually at the costal margin but sometimes at a lower point in a patient with liver disease. Mark this point and then percuss down from the right clavicle, again along the right MCL. The liver's superior border usually lies between the fifth and seventh intercostal spaces. Mark the superior border. The distance between the two marked points represents the approximate span of the liver's right lobe, which normally ranges from 2⅜″ to 4¾″ (6 to 12 cm).

Next, assess the liver's left lobe similarly, percussing along the sternal midline. Again, mark the points where you hear dull percussion notes. Also, measure the span of the left lobe, which normally ranges from 1½″ to 3⅛″ (3.5 to 8 cm). Record your findings for use as a baseline.

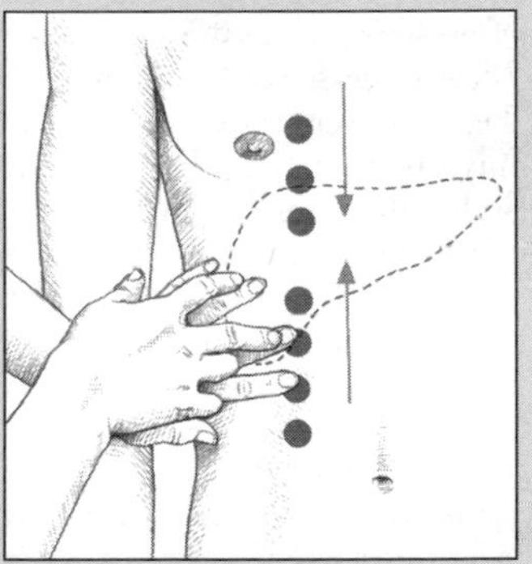

Common medical causes

♦ ***Amyloidosis.*** This rare disorder can cause hepatomegaly and mild jaundice as well as renal, cardiac, and other GI effects.

♦ ***Cirrhosis.*** Late in this disorder, the liver becomes enlarged, nodular, and hard. Other late signs and symptoms affect all body systems. *Respiratory* findings include limited thoracic expansion due to abdominal ascites, leading to hypoxia. *Central nervous system* findings include signs and symptoms of hepatic encephalopathy, such as lethargy, slurred speech, asterixis, peripheral neuritis, paranoia, hallucinations, extreme obtundation, and coma. *Hematologic* signs include epistaxis, easy bruising, and bleeding gums. *Endocrine* findings include testicular atrophy, gynecomastia, loss of chest and axillary hair, or menstrual irregularities. *Integumentary* effects include abnormal pigmentation, severe pruritus, extreme dryness, poor tissue turgor, spider angiomas, and palmar erythema.

The patient may also develop fetor hepaticus, enlarged superficial abdominal veins, muscle atrophy, right-upper-quadrant pain that worsens when he sits up or leans forward, and a palpable spleen. Portal hypertension — elevated pressure in the portal vein — causes bleeding from esophageal varices.

♦ ***Diabetes mellitus.*** Poorly controlled diabetes in overweight patients commonly causes fatty infiltration of the liver, hepatomegaly, and right-upper-quadrant tenderness along with polydipsia, polyphagia, and polyuria. These features are more common in type 2 than in type 1 diabetes. A chronically enlarged fatty liver typically causes no symptoms except for slight tenderness.

♦ ***Granulomatous disorders.*** Sarcoidosis, histoplasmosis, and other such disorders commonly cause a slightly enlarged, firm liver.

♦ ***Hepatic abscess.*** Hepatomegaly may accompany fever (a primary sign), nausea, vomiting, chills, weakness, diarrhea, anorexia, elevated right hemidiaphragm, and right-upper-quadrant pain and tenderness.

♦ ***Hepatic neoplasms.*** Primary tumors commonly cause irregular, nodular, firm hepatomegaly, with pain or tenderness in the right upper quadrant and a friction rub or bruit over the liver. Common related findings are weight loss, anorexia, nausea, and vomiting. Peripheral edema, ascites, jaundice, and a palpable right-upper-quadrant mass may also develop. When metastatic liver tumors cause hepatomegaly, accompanying signs and symptoms reflect the patient's primary cancer.

♦ ***Hepatitis.*** In viral hepatitis, early signs and symptoms include nausea, anorexia, vomiting, fatigue, malaise, photophobia, sore throat, cough, and headache. Hepatomegaly occurs in the icteric phase and continues during the recovery phase. Also, during the icteric phase, the early signs and symptoms diminish and others appear: liver tenderness, slight weight loss, dark urine, clay-colored stools, jaundice, pruritus, right-upper-quadrant pain, and splenomegaly.

♦ ***Infectious mononucleosis.*** Occasionally, this disorder causes hepatomegaly. Prodromal symptoms include headache, malaise, and fatigue. After 3 to 5 days, the patient typically develops sore throat, cervical lymphadenopathy, and temperature fluctuations. He may also develop stomatitis, palatal petechiae, periorbital edema, splenomegaly, exudative tonsillitis, pharyngitis and, possibly, a maculopapular rash.

♦ ***Leukemia and lymphomas.*** These proliferative blood cell disorders frequently cause moderate to massive hepatomegaly and splenomegaly as well as abdominal discomfort. General signs and symptoms include malaise, low-grade fever, fatigue, weakness, tachycardia, weight loss, bleeding disorders, and anorexia.

♦ ***Obesity.*** Hepatomegaly can result from fatty infiltration of the liver. Weight loss reduces the liver's size.

♦ ***Pancreatic cancer.*** In this disease, hepatomegaly accompanies such classic signs and symptoms as anorexia, weight loss, abdominal or back pain, and jaundice. Other findings include nausea, vomiting, fever, fatigue, weakness, pruritus, and skin lesions (usually on the legs).

♦ ***Pericarditis.*** In chronic constrictive pericarditis, an increase in systemic venous pressure causes marked congestive hepatomegaly. Distended neck veins (more prominent on inspiration) are a common finding. The usual signs of cardiac disease typically are absent; other features include peripheral edema, ascites, fatigue, and decreased muscle mass.

Special considerations

Prepare the patient for hepatic enzyme, alkaline phosphatase, bilirubin, albumin, and globulin studies to evaluate liver function and for X-rays, liver scan, celiac arteriography, computed tomography scan, and ultrasonography to confirm hepatomegaly.

Bed rest, relief from stress, and adequate nutrition are important for the patient with hepatomegaly to help protect liver cells from further damage and to allow the liver to regenerate functioning cells. Hepatotoxic drugs or drugs metabolized by the liver should be given in very small doses, if at all.

Pediatric pointers

Assess hepatomegaly in children the same way you do in adults. Childhood hepatomegaly may stem from Reye's syndrome; biliary atresia; rare disorders such as Wilson's, Gaucher's, or Niemann-Pick disease; or poorly controlled type 1 diabetes mellitus.

Hoarseness

Hoarseness — a rough or harsh sound to the voice — can result from infections or inflammatory lesions or exudates of the larynx, laryngeal edema, or compression or disruption of the vocal cords or recurrent laryngeal nerve. This common sign can also result from a thoracic aortic aneurysm, vocal cord paralysis, or a systemic disorder, such as Sjögren's syndrome or rheumatoid arthritis. It's characteristically worsened by excessive alcohol intake, smoking, inhalation of noxious fumes, excessive talking, and shouting.

Hoarseness can be acute or chronic. For example, chronic hoarseness and laryngitis result when irritating polyps or nodules develop on the vocal cords. Gastroesophageal reflux into the larynx should also be considered as a possible cause of chronic hoarseness. Hoarseness may also result from progressive atrophy of the laryngeal muscles and mucosa due to aging, which leads to diminished control of the vocal cords.

History and physical examination

Obtain a patient history. First, consider his age and sex; laryngeal cancer is most common in men between the ages of 50 and 70. Be sure to ask about the onset of hoarseness. Has the patient been overusing his voice? Has he experienced shortness of breath, a sore throat, dry mouth, a cough, or difficulty swallowing dry food? In addition, ask if he has been in or near a fire within the past 48 hours. Be aware that inhalation injury can cause sudden airway obstruction.

Next, explore associated symptoms. Does the patient have a history of cancer, rheumatoid arthritis, or aortic aneurysm? Does he regularly drink alcohol or smoke? Has he had any recent neck trauma? Has he had any recent surgery requiring endotracheal intubation placement?

Inspect the oral cavity and pharynx for redness or exudate, possibly indicating an upper respiratory infection. Palpate the neck for masses and the cervical lymph nodes and the thyroid for enlargement. Palpate the trachea — is it midline? Ask the patient to stick out his tongue; if he can't, he may have paralysis from cranial nerve involvement. Examine the eyes for corneal ulcers and enlarged lacrimal ducts (signs of Sjögren's syndrome). Dilated neck and chest veins may indicate compression by an aortic aneurysm.

Take the patient's vital signs, noting especially fever and bradycardia. Inspect for asymmetrical chest expansion or signs of respiratory distress — nasal flaring, stridor, and intercostal retractions. Then auscultate for crackles, rhonchi, wheezing, and tubular sounds, and percuss for dullness.

Common medical causes

♦ ***Gastroesophageal reflux.*** In this disorder, gastric juices flow retrograde into the esophagus and may then spill into the hypopharynx. The resulting laryngeal irritation manifests as hoarseness, possibly with sore throat, cough, throat clearing, and a sensation of a lump in the throat. The adenoids and the vocal cords may appear red and swollen.

♦ ***Hypothyroidism.*** Gradually progressive hoarseness may be an early sign of this disorder. Others include fatigue, cold intolerance, weight gain despite anorexia, and menorrhagia.

♦ ***Laryngeal cancer.*** Hoarseness is an early sign of vocal cord cancer but may not occur until later in cancer of other laryngeal areas. Alcohol consumption has a synergistic effect with smoking in increasing the risk of laryngeal cancer. Other common findings include a mild, dry cough; minor throat discomfort; otalgia; and, sometimes, hemoptysis.

♦ ***Laryngeal leukoplakia.*** Leukoplakia is a common cause of hoarseness, especially in smokers. Histologic examination from direct laryngoscopy usually reveals mild, moderate, or severe dysphasia.

♦ ***Laryngitis.*** Persistent hoarseness may be the only sign of *chronic laryngitis.* In *acute laryngitis,* hoarseness or a complete loss of voice develops suddenly. Related findings include pain (especially during swallowing or speaking), cough, fever, profuse diaphoresis, sore throat, and rhinorrhea.

♦ ***Rheumatoid arthritis.*** Hoarseness may signal laryngeal involvement. Other common findings include pain, dysphagia, a sensation of fullness or tension in the throat, dyspnea on exertion, and stridor.

♦ ***Thoracic aortic aneurysm.*** This type of aneurysm typically causes no symptoms but may cause hoarseness. Its most common symptom is penetrating pain that's especially severe when the patient is supine. Other clinical features include a brassy cough; dyspnea; wheezing; a substernal aching in the shoulders, lower back, or abdomen; a tracheal tug; facial and neck edema; jugular vein distention; dysphagia; prominent chest veins; stridor; and possibly paresthesia or neuralgia.

♦ ***Tracheal trauma.*** A blow to the neck may fracture the larynx, resulting in mucosal bleeding and edema. Symptoms may include hoarseness, hemoptysis, dysphagia, neck pain, and airway obstruction.

♦ ***Vocal cord paralysis.*** Paralysis of the laryngeal nerve can be the result of inflammatory, metabolic, neoplastic, compressive, traumatic, or idiopathic causes. These causes include diabetes, lupus, rheumatid arthritis, polyarteritis nodosa, drug toxicity, chronic alcoholism, sarcoidosis, myasthenia gravis, Eaton-Lambert syndrome, polymyositis, dermatomyositis, muscular dystrophy, and tuberculosis. Skull base lesions cause vocal cord paralysis, pharyngeal paralysis, and sensory loss causing aspiration.

♦ ***Vocal cord polyps or nodules.*** Raspy hoarseness, the chief complaint, accompanies a chronic cough and a crackling voice.

Other causes

♦ ***Inhalation injury.*** Inhalation injury from a fire or explosion causes hoarseness and coughing, singed nasal hairs, orofacial burns, and soot-stained sputum. Subsequent signs and symptoms include crackles, rhonchi, and wheezing, which rapidly deteriorate to respiratory distress.

◆ ***Treatments.*** Occasionally, surgical trauma to the recurrent laryngeal nerve results in temporary or permanent unilateral vocal cord paralysis, leading to hoarseness. Prolonged intubation may cause temporary hoarseness.

Special considerations

Carefully observe the patient for stridor, which may indicate bilateral vocal cord paralysis. When hoarseness lasts for longer than 2 weeks, indirect or fiberoptic laryngoscopy is indicated to observe the larynx at rest and during speech.

Pediatric pointers

In children, hoarseness may result from congenital anomalies, such as laryngocele or dysphonia plicae ventricularis. In prepubescent boys, it can reflect juvenile papillomatosis of the upper respiratory tract.

In infants and young children, hoarseness commonly stems from acute laryngotracheobronchitis (croup). Temporary hoarseness frequently results from laryngeal irritation due to aspiration of liquids, foreign bodies, or stomach contents. Hoarseness may also be a symptom of diphtheria, although immunization has made this disease rare.

Help the child with hoarseness rest his voice. Comfort an infant to minimize crying, play quiet games with him, and humidify his environment.

HOMANS' SIGN

Homans' sign is positive when deep calf pain results from dorsiflexion of the ankle. This pain results from venous thrombosis or inflammation of the calf muscles. However, because a positive Homans' sign appears in only 35% of patients with these conditions, it's an unreliable indicator. (See *Eliciting Homans' sign,* page 324.) Even when accurate, a positive Homans' sign doesn't indicate the extent of the venous disorder.

This elicited sign may be confused with continuous calf pain, which can result from strains, contusions, cellulitis, or arterial occlusion, or with pain in the posterior ankle or Achilles tendon (for example, in a woman with Achilles tendons shortened from wearing high heels).

History and physical examination

When you detect a positive Homans' sign, focus your patient history on signs and symptoms that can accompany deep vein thrombosis or thrombophlebitis. These include throbbing, aching, heavy, or tight sensations in the calf and leg pain during or after exercise or routine activity. Also, ask about shortness of breath, cough, hemoptysis, or chest pain, which may indicate pulmonary embolism. Be sure to ask about predisposing events, such as leg injury, recent surgery, childbirth, use of contraceptive pills, associated diseases (cancer, nephrosis, hypercoagulable states), and prolonged inactivity.

Next, inspect and palpate the patient's calf for warmth, tenderness, redness, swelling, and the presence of a palpable vein. If you strongly suspect deep vein thrombosis, elicit Homans' sign very carefully to avoid detaching the clot, which could cause pulmonary embolism, a life-threatening condition.

In addition, measure the circumferences of both the patient's calves. The calf with the positive Homans' sign may be larger because of edema and swelling.

Common medical causes

◆ ***Deep vein thrombophlebitis.*** A positive Homans' sign and calf tenderness may be the only clinical features of this disorder. But the patient may also have

EXAMINATION TIP

Eliciting Homans' sign

To elicit Homans' sign, first support the patient's thigh with one hand and his foot with the other. Bend the leg slightly at the knee; then firmly dorsiflex the ankle. The resulting deep calf pain indicates a positive Homans' sign. The patient may also resist ankle dorsiflexion or flex the knee involuntarily if Homans' sign is positive.

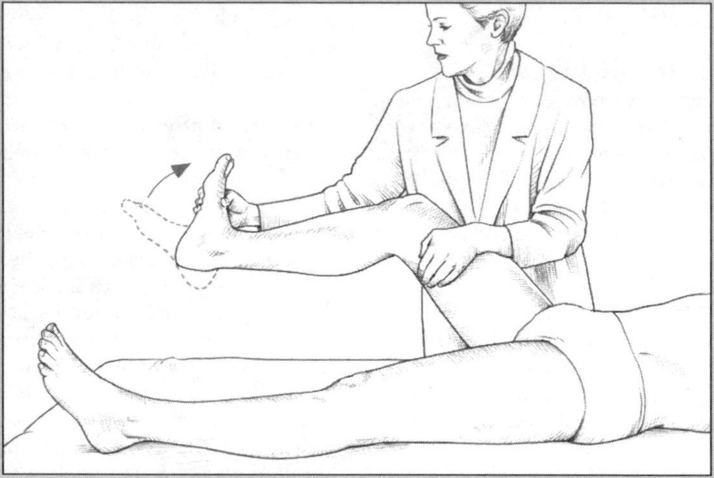

severe pain, heaviness, warmth, and swelling of the affected leg; visible, engorged superficial veins or palpable, cordlike veins; and fever, chills, and malaise.

◆ ***Deep vein thrombosis (DVT).*** DVT causes a positive Homans' sign along with tenderness over the deep calf veins, slight edema of the calves and thighs, a low-grade fever, and tachycardia. If DVT affects the femoral and iliac veins, you'll notice marked local swelling and tenderness. If DVT causes venous obstruction, you'll notice cyanosis and possibly cool skin in the affected leg.

◆ ***Popliteal cyst (ruptured).*** Rupture of this synovial cyst may cause a positive Homans' sign as well as sudden onset of calf tenderness, swelling, and redness.

◆ ***Cellulitis (superficial).*** This disorder typically affects the legs but can also affect the arms, producing pain, redness, tenderness, and edema. Some patients also experience fever, chills, tachycardia, headache, and hypotension.

Special considerations

Be sure to place the patient on bed rest, with the affected leg elevated above the heart level. Apply warm, moist compresses to the affected area, and administer mild oral analgesics. In addition, prepare the patient for further diagnostic tests, such as Doppler studies and venograms.

Once the patient is ambulatory, advise him to wear elastic support stockings after his discomfort decreases (usually in 5 to 10 days) and to continue wearing them for at least 3 months. In addition, instruct the patient to keep the affected leg elevated while sitting and to avoid crossing his legs at the knees. Why? Because this may impair circulation to the popliteal area. (Crossing at the ankles is acceptable.)

Pediatric pointers

Homans' sign is seldom assessed in children, who rarely have DVT or thrombophlebitis.

Hyperpnea

Hyperpnea reflects increased respiratory effort — a normal rate (at least 12 breaths/ minute) with increased depth (tidal volume greater than 7.5 ml/ kg), or increased rate and depth — for a sustained period. This sign differs from sighing (intermittent deep inspirations) and may or may not be associated with tachypnea (increased respiratory frequency).

The typical patient with hyperpnea breathes at a normal or increased rate and inhales deeply, displaying marked chest expansion. He may complain of shortness of breath if a respiratory disorder is causing hypoxemia, or he may not be aware of his breathing if a metabolic or neurologic disorder is causing involuntary hyperpnea. Other causes of hyperpnea include profuse diarrhea or dehydration, loss of pancreatic juice or bile from GI drainage, and ureterosigmoidostomy. All these conditions and procedures cause a loss of bicarbonate ions, resulting in metabolic acidosis. Of course, hyperpnea may also accompany strenuous exercise, and voluntary hyperpnea can promote relaxation in patients experiencing stress or pain — for example, women in labor.

Hyperventilation, a consequence of hyperpnea, is characterized by respiratory alkalosis (arterial pH above 7.45 and partial pressure of carbon dioxide below 35 mm Hg). In central neurogenic hyperventilation, brain stem dysfunction (such as that which results from a severe cranial injury) increases the rate and depth of respirations. In acute intermittent hyperventilation, the respiratory pattern may be a response to hypoxemia, anxiety, fear, pain, or excitement. Hyperpnea may also be a compensatory mechanism to metabolic acidosis. Under these conditions, it's known as *Kussmaul's respirations.* (See *Kussmaul's respirations,* page 326.)

History and physical examination

If you observe hyperpnea in a patient whose other signs and symptoms signal a life-threatening emergency, you must intervene quickly and effectively. (See *Managing hyperpnea,* page 327.) However, if the patient's condition isn't grave, first determine his level of consciousness (LOC). If he's alert (and if his hyperpnea isn't interfering with speaking), ask about recent illnesses or infections and about ingestion of aspirin or other drugs or chemicals. Find out if the patient has diabetes mellitus or renal disease. Is he excessively thirsty or hungry? Has he recently had severe diarrhea or an upper respiratory infection?

Next, observe the patient for clues to his abnormal breathing pattern. Is he unable to speak, or does he speak only in brief, choppy phrases? Is his breathing abnormally rapid? Examine the patient for cyanosis (especially of the mouth, lips, mucous membranes, and earlobes), restlessness, and anxiety — all signs of decreased tissue oxygenation, as occurs in shock. In addition, observe for intercostal and abdominal retractions, use of accessory muscles, and diaphoresis, all of which may indicate deep breathing related to an insufficient supply of oxygen. Next, inspect for draining wounds or signs of infection, and ask about nausea and vomiting. Take the patient's vital signs, noting fever, and examine his

Kussmaul's respirations

Kussmaul's respirations — fast, deep breathing without pauses — characteristically sound labored, with deep breaths that resemble sighs. This breathing pattern develops when respiratory centers in the medulla detect decreased blood pH, thereby triggering compensatory fast and deep breathing to remove carbon dioxide and restore pH balance.

Disorders (such as diabetes mellitus and renal failure), drug effects, and other conditions causing metabolic acidosis (loss of bicarbonate ions and retention of acid).

↓

Blood pH decreases.

↓

Kussmaul's respirations develop to blow off carbon dioxide to match loss of bicarbonate.

↓

Blood pH rises.

↓

Respiratory rate and depth decreases (corrected pH) in effective compensation.

skin and mucous membranes for turgor, possibly indicating dehydration.

Common medical causes

♦ ***Head injury.*** Hyperpnea that results from a severe head injury is called *central neurogenic hyperventilation.* Whether its onset is acute or gradual, this type of hyperpnea indicates damage to the lower midbrain or upper pons. Accompanying signs reflect the site and extent of injury and can include loss of consciousness; soft-tissue injury or bony deformity of the face, head, or neck; facial edema; clear or bloody drainage from the mouth, nose, or ears; raccoon eyes; Battle's sign; an absent doll's eye reflex; and motor and sensory disturbances.

Signs of increased intracranial pressure include decreased response to painful stimulation, loss of pupillary reaction, bradycardia, increased systolic pressure, and widening pulse pressure.

♦ ***Hyperventilation syndrome.*** Acute anxiety triggers episodic hyperpnea, resulting in respiratory alkalosis. Other findings may include agitation, vertigo, syncope, pallor, circumoral and peripheral paresthesia, muscle twitching, carpopedal spasm, weakness, and arrhythmias.

♦ ***Hypoxemia.*** Many pulmonary disorders that cause hypoxemia — for example, pneumonia, pulmonary edema, chronic obstructive pulmonary disease, and pneumothorax — may cause hyperpnea and episodes of hyperventilation with chest pain, dizziness, and paresthesia. Other effects include dyspnea, cough, crackles, rhonchi, wheezing, and decreased breath sounds.

♦ ***Ketoacidosis.*** *Alcoholic ketoacidosis* (occurring most commonly in females with a history of alcohol abuse) typically follows cessation of drinking after a marked increase in alcohol consumption has caused severe vomiting. Kussmaul's respirations begin abruptly and are accompanied by vomiting for several days, fruity breath odor, slight dehydration, abdominal pain and distention, and absent bowel sounds. The patient is alert and has a normal blood glucose level, unlike the patient with diabetic ketoacidosis.

Diabetic ketoacidosis is potentially life-threatening and typically causes Kussmaul's respirations. The patient usually

EMERGENCY INTERVENTIONS

Managing hyperpnea

Carefully examine the patient with hyperpnea or related signs of life-threatening conditions, such as increased intracranial pressure (ICP), metabolic acidosis, diabetic ketoacidosis, and uremia. Be prepared for rapid intervention.

INCREASED ICP

If you observe hyperpnea in a patient who has signs of head trauma (soft-tissue injury, edema, or ecchymoses on the face or head) from a recent accident and has lost consciousness, act quickly to prevent further brain stem injury and irreversible deterioration. Then take the patient's vital signs, noting bradycardia, increased systolic blood pressure, and widening pulse pressure — signs of increased ICP.

Examine his pupillary reaction. Elevate the head of the bed 30 degrees (unless you suspect spinal cord injury); if the patient is unconscious, insert an artificial airway. Connect him to a cardiac monitor, and continuously observe his respiratory pattern. (Irregular respirations signal deterioration.) Start an I.V. line at a slow infusion rate and prepare to administer an osmotic diuretic, such as mannitol, to decrease cerebral edema. Catheterize the patient to measure urine output, give supplemental oxygen, and keep emergency resuscitation equipment close by.

METABOLIC ACIDOSIS

If the patient doesn't have a head injury, his increased respiratory rate suggests metabolic acidosis. If his level of consciousness is decreased, check his chart for history data to help you determine the cause of his metabolic acidosis and intervene appropriately. Suspect shock if the patient has cold, clammy skin. Palpate for a rapid, thready pulse and take his blood pressure, noting hypotension. Elevate the patient's legs 30 degrees, apply pressure dressings to any obvious hemorrhage, start several large-bore I.V. lines, and prepare to administer fluids, vasopressors, and blood transfusions.

A patient with hyperpnea who has a history of alcohol abuse, is vomiting profusely, has diarrhea or profuse abdominal drainage, has ingested an overdose of aspirin, or is cachectic and has a history of starvation may also have metabolic acidosis. Inspect his skin for dryness and poor turgor, indicating dehydration. Take his vital signs, looking for low-grade fever and hypotension. Start an I.V. line for fluid replacement. Draw blood for electrolyte studies, and prepare to administer sodium bicarbonate.

DIABETIC KETOACIDOSIS

If the patient has a history of diabetes mellitus, is vomiting, and has a fruity breath odor (acetone breath), suspect diabetic ketoacidosis. Catheterize him to monitor increased urine output, and infuse saline solution. Perform a finger stick to estimate blood glucose levels with a reagent strip. Obtain a urine specimen to test for glucose and acetone and draw blood for glucose and ketone tests. Also, administer fluids, insulin, potassium, and sodium bicarbonate I.V.

UREMIA

If the patient has a history of renal disease, an ammonia breath odor (uremic fetor), and a fine, white powder on his skin (uremic frost), suspect uremia. Start and I.V. line at a slow rate, and prepare to administer sodium bicarbonate. Monitor his electrocardiogram for arrhythmias due to hyperkalemia. Monitor his serum electrolyte, blood urea nitrogen, and creatinine levels until hemodialysis or peritoneal dialysis begins.

experiences polydipsia, polyphagia, and polyuria before the onset of acidosis; he may or may not have a history of diabetes mellitus. Other clinical features include fruity breath odor; orthostatic hypotension; rapid, thready pulse; generalized weakness; decreased LOC (lethargy to coma); nausea; vomiting; anorexia; and abdominal pain.

Starvation ketoacidosis is also potentially life-threatening and can cause Kussmaul's respirations. Its onset is gradual; typical findings include signs of cachexia and dehydration, decreased LOC, bradycardia, and a history of severely limited food intake.

◆ ***Renal failure.*** Acute or chronic renal failure can cause life-threatening acidosis with Kussmaul's respirations. Signs and symptoms of severe renal failure include oliguria or anuria, uremic fetor, and yellow, dry, scaly skin. Other cutaneous signs include severe pruritus, uremic frost, purpura, and ecchymoses. The patient may complain of nausea and vomiting, weakness, burning pain in the legs and feet, and diarrhea or constipation.

As acidosis progresses, corresponding clinical features include frothy sputum, pleuritic chest pain, and signs of heart failure and pleural or pericardial effusion. Neurologic signs include altered LOC (lethargy to coma), twitching, and seizures. Hyperkalemia and hypertension, if present, require rapid intervention to prevent cardiovascular collapse.

◆ ***Sepsis.*** A severe infection may cause lactic acidosis, resulting in Kussmaul's respirations. Other possible findings include tachycardia, fever, chills, headache, lethargy, profuse diaphoresis, anorexia, cough, wound drainage, burning on urination, and other signs of local infection.

◆ ***Shock.*** Potentially life-threatening metabolic acidosis causes Kussmaul's respirations, hypotension, tachycardia, narrowed pulse pressure, weak pulse, dyspnea, oliguria, anxiety, restlessness, stupor that can progress to coma, and cool, clammy skin. Other clinical features may include external or internal bleeding (in hypovolemic shock); chest pain or arrhythmias and signs of heart failure (in cardiogenic shock); high fever, chills and, rarely, hypothermia (in septic shock); or stridor due to laryngeal edema (in anaphylactic shock). Onset is usually acute in hypovolemic, cardiogenic, or anaphylactic shock, but it may be gradual in septic shock.

Other causes

◆ ***Drugs.*** Toxic levels of salicylates, ammonium chloride, acetazolamide, and other carbonic anhydrase inhibitors can cause Kussmaul's respirations. So can ingestion of methanol and ethylene glycol, found in antifreeze solutions.

Special considerations

Monitor vital signs in all patients with hyperpnea, and observe for increasing respiratory distress or an irregular respiratory pattern signaling deterioration. Prepare for immediate intervention to prevent cardiovascular collapse: Start an I.V. line for administration of fluids, blood transfusions, and vasopressor drugs for hemodynamic stabilization, as ordered, and prepare to give ventilatory support. Prepare the patient for arterial blood gas analysis and blood chemistry studies.

Pediatric pointers

Hyperpnea in children indicates the same metabolic or neurologic causes as in adults and requires the same prompt intervention. The most common cause of metabolic acidosis in children is diarrhea, which can cause a life-threatening crisis. In infants, Kussmaul's respirations may accompany acidosis due to inborn errors of metabolism.

I

IMPOTENCE

Impotence is the inability to achieve and maintain penile erection sufficient to complete satisfactory intercourse; ejaculation may or may not be affected. Impotence varies from occasional and minimal to permanent and complete. Occasional impotence occurs in about half of adult American men, whereas chronic impotence affects about 10 million American men.

Impotence can be classified as primary or secondary. A man with *primary impotence* has never been potent with a sexual partner but may achieve normal erections in other situations. This uncommon condition is difficult to treat. *Secondary impotence* carries a more favorable prognosis because, despite present erectile dysfunction, the patient has succeeded in completing intercourse in the past.

Penile erection involves increased arterial blood flow secondary to psychological, tactile, and other sensory stimulation. Trapping of blood within the penis produces increased length, circumference, and rigidity. Impotence results when any component of this process — psychological, vascular, neurologic, or hormonal — malfunctions.

Organic causes of impotence include vascular disease, diabetes mellitus, hypogonadism, a spinal cord lesion, alcohol and drug abuse, and surgical complications. (The incidence of organic impotence associated with other medical problems increases after age 50.) Psychogenic causes range from performance anxiety and marital discord to moral or religious conflicts.

History and physical examination

If the patient complains of impotence or of a condition that may be causing it, let him describe his problem without interruption. Then begin your examination in a systematic way, moving from less sensitive to more sensitive matters. Begin with a psychosocial history. Is the patient married, single, or widowed? How long has he been married or had a sexual relationship? What's the age and health status of his sexual partner? Find out about past marriages, if any, and ask him why he thinks they ended. If you can do so discreetly, ask about sexual activity outside marriage or his primary sexual relationship. Also ask about his job history, his typical daily activities, and his living situation. How well does he get along with others in his household?

Focus your medical history on the causes of erectile dysfunction. Does the patient have type 2 diabetes mellitus, hypertension, or heart disease? If so, ask about its onset and treatment. Also ask about neurologic diseases, such as multiple sclerosis. Obtain a surgical history, emphasizing neurologic, vascular, and urologic surgery. If trauma may be causing the patient's impotence, find out the

Drugs that may cause impotence

Many commonly used drugs — especially antihypertensives — can cause impotence, which may be reversible if the drug is discontinued or the dosage reduced. Here are some examples.

- Amitriptyline
- Atenolol
- Cimetidine
- Clonidine
- Desipramine
- Digoxin
- Hydralazine
- Imipramine
- Methantheline bromide
- Methyldopa
- Naproxen
- Nortriptyline
- Perphenazine
- Prazosin
- Propranolol
- Thiazide diuretics
- Thioridazine
- Tranylcypromine

date of the injury as well as its severity, associated effects, and treatment. Ask about intake of alcohol, drug use or abuse, smoking, diet, and exercise. Obtain a urologic history, including voiding problems and past injury.

Next, ask the patient when his impotence began. How did it progress? What's its current status? Make your questions specific, but remember that many patients have difficulty discussing sexual problems, and many don't understand the physiology involved. The following sample questions may yield helpful data:

When was the first time you remember not being able to initiate or maintain an erection? How often do you wake in the morning or at night with an erection? Do you have wet dreams? Has your sexual drive changed? How often do you try to have intercourse with your partner? How often would you *like* to? Can you ejaculate with or without an erection? Do you experience orgasm with ejaculation?

Ask the patient to rate the quality of a typical erection on a scale of 0 to 10, with 0 being completely flaccid and 10 being completely erect. Using the same scale, also ask him to rate his ability to ejaculate during sexual activity, with 0 being never and 10 being always.

Next, perform a brief physical examination. Inspect and palpate the genitalia and prostate for structural abnormalities. Assess the patient's sensory function, concentrating on the perineal area. Next, test motor strength and deep tendon reflexes in all extremities, and note other neurologic deficits. Take the patient's vital signs and palpate his pulses for quality. Note any signs of peripheral vascular disease, such as cyanosis and cool extremities. Auscultate for abdominal aortic, femoral, carotid, or iliac bruits, and palpate for thyroid gland enlargement.

Common medical causes

◆ ***Endocrine disorders.*** Hypogonadism from pituitary dysfunction may lead to impotence from deficient secretion of androgens (primarily testosterone). Adrenocortical and thyroid dysfunction and chronic hepatic disease may also cause impotence because these organs play a role (although minor) in sex hormone regulation.

◆ ***Nervous system disorders.*** Spinal cord lesions from trauma produce sudden impotence. A complete lesion above the second sacral vertebra (upper-motor-neuron lesion) disrupts descending motor tracts to the genital area, causing loss of voluntary erectile control but not of reflex erection and reflex ejaculation. However, a complete lesion in the lumbosacral spinal cord (lower-motor-neuron lesion) causes loss of reflex ejaculation and reflex erection. Spinal cord tumors and degenerative diseases of the brain and spinal cord (such as multiple sclerosis and amyotrophic lateral sclerosis) cause progressive impotence.

♦ ***Penile disorders.*** In Peyronie's disease, the penis is bent, making erection painful and penetration difficult and eventually impossible. Phimosis prevents erection until circumcision releases the constricted foreskin. Other inflammatory, infectious, or destructive diseases of the penis may also cause impotence.

♦ ***Psychological distress.*** Impotence can result from diverse psychological causes, including depression, performance anxiety, memories of previous traumatic sexual experiences, moral or religious conflicts, and troubled emotional or sexual relationships.

Other causes

♦ ***Alcohol and drugs.*** Alcoholism and drug abuse are associated with impotence, as are many prescription drugs, especially antihypertensives. (See *Drugs that may cause impotence.*)

♦ ***Surgery.*** Surgical injury to the penis, bladder neck, urinary sphincter, rectum, or perineum can cause impotence, as can injury to local nerves or blood vessels.

Special considerations

Care begins by establishing a rapport with the patient. Probably no other medical condition affecting males is as potentially frustrating, humiliating, even devastating to self-esteem and significant relationships. Help the patient feel comfortable about discussing his sexuality. This begins with feeling comfortable about your own sexuality and adopting an accepting attitude about the sexual experiences and preferences of others.

Prepare the patient for screening tests for hormonal irregularities and for Doppler studies of penile blood pressure to rule out vascular insufficiency. Other possible tests include voiding studies, nerve conduction tests, evaluation of nocturnal penile tumescence, and psychological screening.

Treatment for psychogenic impotence may include counseling of both the patient and his sexual partner; treatment for organic impotence focuses on reversing the cause, if possible. Other forms of treatment include surgical revascularization, drug-induced erection, surgical repair of a venous leak, and penile prostheses. Encourage the patient to maintain follow-up appointments and treatment for underlying medical disorders.

Geriatric pointers

Most people believe that sexual performance normally declines with age. Many also believe (erroneously) that elderly people are incapable of or aren't interested in sex or that they can't find elderly partners who are interested in sex. In elderly people who suffer from sexual dysfunction, organic disease must be ruled out before counseling to improve sexual performance can start.

INSOMNIA

Insomnia is the inability to fall asleep, remain asleep, or feel refreshed by sleep. The sleep-wake cycle is governed by circadian rhythms, which generally run on 25-hour cycles. These cycles include two natural daily peak times for sleeping; at night and at mid-day. Acute and transient during periods of stress, insomnia may become chronic, causing constant fatigue, extreme anxiety as bedtime approaches, and even psychiatric disorders. This common complaint is experienced occasionally by about 25% of Americans, chronically by another 10%.

Physiologic causes of insomnia include jet lag, emotional conflict, and lack of exercise. Pathophysiologic causes range from medical and psychiatric disorders to pain, drug adverse effects, and idiopathic factors. Complaints of insomnia are subjective and require close investigation; the patient may mistakenly attribute to insomnia his fatigue from an organic cause such as anemia. (See *Tips for relieving insomnia.*)

History

Take a thorough sleep and health history. Find out when the patient's insomnia began and the attending circumstances. Is the patient trying to stop using sedatives? Does he use central nervous system (CNS) stimulants, such as amphetamines, pseudoephedrine, theophylline derivatives, phenylpropanolamine, cocaine, or caffeine-containing drugs and beverages?

Find out if the patient has any chronic or acute conditions whose effects may be disturbing his sleep, particularly cardiac or respiratory disease, or painful or pruritic conditions. What about endocrine or neurologic disorders or a history of drug or alcohol abuse? Is he a frequent traveler who suffers from jet lag? Does he use his legs a lot during the day, then feel restless at night? Ask about daytime fatigue and regular exercise. Also ask if he experiences periods of gasping for air or apnea and frequent body repositioning. If possible, consult the patient's spouse or sleep partner because the patient may not be aware of his own behavior.

Assess the patient's emotional status, and try to estimate his level of self-esteem. Ask about personal and professional problems and psychological stress. Also ask if he has had hallucinations, and note behavior that may indicate alcohol withdrawal. After reviewing complaints that suggest an undiagnosed disorder, perform a physical examination.

Common medical causes

◆ ***Alcohol withdrawal syndrome.*** Abrupt cessation of alcohol after long-term use causes insomnia that may persist for up to 2 years. Other early effects of this acute syndrome include excessive diaphoresis, tachycardia, hypertension, tremors, restlessness, irritability, headache, nausea, flushing, and nightmares. Progression to delirium tremens produces confusion, disorientation, paranoia, delusions, hallucinations, and seizures.

◆ ***Generalized anxiety disorder.*** Anxiety can cause chronic insomnia as well as signs of tension, such as fatigue and restlessness; signs of autonomic hyperactivity, such as diaphoresis, dyspepsia, and high resting pulse and respiratory rates; or signs of apprehension.

◆ ***Hormonal fluctuation in women.*** Fluctuating levels of female hormones play a role in insomnia. Progesterone promotes sleep. When progesterone levels drop during menstruation, insomnia may result. During pregnancy, progesterone levels in the first and third trimesters can disrupt sleep. Insomnia is also a major problem in perimenopause when hormone levels are fluctuating.

◆ ***Mood (affective) disorders.*** At least 70% of people with depression complain of insomnia. Depression commonly causes chronic insomnia with difficulty falling asleep, waking and inability to fall back to sleep, or waking early in the morning. Related findings include dysphoria (a primary symptom), decreased appetite with weight loss or increased appetite with weight gain, and psychomotor agitation or retardation. The patient experiences loss of interest in his usual activities, feelings of worthlessness and guilt, fatigue, difficulty concentrating, indecisiveness, or recurrent thoughts of death.

Episodes of *mania* produce a decreased need for sleep, elevated mood, and irritability. Related findings include increased energy and activity, fast speech, speeding thoughts, inflated self-esteem, easy distractibility, and involvement in high-risk activities such as reckless driving.

◆ ***Nocturnal myoclonus.*** In this seizure disorder, involuntary and fleeting muscle jerks of the legs occur every 20 to 40 seconds, disturbing sleep.

Tips for relieving insomnia

COMMON PROBLEMS	CAUSES	INTERVENTIONS
Acroparesthesia	Improper position may compress superficial (ulnar, radial, and peroneal) nerves, disrupting circulation to the compressed nerve. This causes numbness and tingling in an arm or leg.	Teach the patient to assume a comfortable position in bed, with limbs unrestricted. If he tends to awaken with a numb leg or arm, tell him to massage and move it until sensation returns completely, then to assume an unrestricted position.
Anxiety	Physical or emotional stress produces anxiety, which causes autonomic stimulation.	Encourage the patient to discuss his fears and concerns, and teach him relaxation techniques, such as guided imagery and deep breathing. If ordered, administer a mild sedative, such as diazepam, before bedtime.
Dyspnea	In many cardiac and pulmonary disorders, a recumbent position and inactivity cause restricted chest expansion, secretion pooling, and pulmonary vascular congestion, leading to coughing and shortness of breath.	Elevate the head of the bed, or provide at least two pillows or a reclining chair to help the patient sleep. Suction him when he awakens, and encourage deep breathing every 2 to 4 hours. Also, provide supplementary oxygen by nasal cannula.
Pain	Chronic or acute pain from any cause can prevent or disrupt sleep.	Administer pain medication, as ordered, 20 minutes before bedtime, and teach deep, even, slow breathing to promote relaxation. Help the patient with back pain lie on his side with his legs flexed. Encourage the patient with epigastric pain to take an antacid before bedtime and elevate the head of the bed.
Pruritus	A localized skin infection or a systemic disorder, such as liver failure, may cause intensely annoying itching.	Wash the patient's skin with a mild soap and water, and dry the skin thoroughly. Apply moisturizing lotion on dry, unbroken skin and an antipruritic, such as calamine lotion, on pruritic areas.
Restless leg	Excessive exercise during the day may cause tired, aching legs at night, requiring movement for relief.	Help the patient exercise his legs gently by slowly walking with him around the room and down the hall. If ordered, administer a muscle relaxant such as diazepam.

♦ ***Sleep apnea syndrome.*** Apneic periods begin with the onset of sleep, continue for 10 to 90 seconds, and end with a series of gasps and arousal. In *central sleep apnea,* respiratory movement ceases during the apneic period; in *obstructive sleep apnea,* upper airway obstruction blocks incoming air, although breathing movements continue. Some patients display both types of apnea. Repeated possibly hundreds of times during the night, this cycle alternates with bradycardia and tachycardia. Associated findings include morning headache, daytime fatigue, hypertension, ankle edema, and personality changes, such as hostility, paranoia, or agitated depression.
♦ ***Thyrotoxicosis.*** Difficulty falling asleep and then sleeping for only a brief period is one of the characteristic symptoms of this disorder. Cardiopulmonary features include dyspnea, tachycardia, palpitations, and atrial or ventricular gallop. Other findings include weight loss despite increased appetite, diarrhea, tremors, nervousness, diaphoresis, hypersensitivity to heat, an enlarged thyroid, and exophthalmos.

Other causes

♦ ***Drugs.*** Use of, abuse of, or withdrawal from sedatives or hypnotics may produce insomnia. CNS stimulants — including amphetamines, theophylline derivatives, pseudoephedrine, phenylpropanolamine, cocaine, and caffeine-containing beverages — may also produce insomnia.
♦ **Herb alert** Herbal medicines, such as ginseng and green tea, can cause adverse effects including insomnia.
♦ ***Other.*** People who work night shifts or alternating schedules of two and three shifts tend to suffer more from insomnia than those on day shifts. It has also been found that excessive computer work is associated with insomnia.

Special considerations

Prepare the patient for tests to evaluate his insomnia, such as blood and urine studies for 17-hydroxycorticosteroids and catecholamines; polysomnography (including an EEG, electrooculography, and electrocardiography); and sleep EEG.

Pediatric pointers

Insomnia in early childhood may develop along with separation anxiety at age 2 or 3, after a stressful or tiring day, or during illness or teething. In children ages 6 to 11, insomnia usually reflects residual excitement from the day's activities; a few children continue to have bedtime fears. Foster children commonly display sleep problems.

INTERMITTENT CLAUDICATION

Most common in the legs, intermittent claudication is cramping limb pain brought on by exercise and relieved by 1 or 2 minutes of rest. This pain may be acute or chronic; when acute, it may signal acute arterial occlusion. Intermittent claudication occurs most commonly in men ages 50 to 60 with a history of diabetes mellitus, hyperlipidemia, hypertension, or tobacco use. Without treatment, it may progress to pain at rest. In chronic arterial occlusion, limb loss is uncommon because collateral circulation usually develops.

In occlusive artery disease, intermittent claudication results from an inadequate blood supply. Pain in the calf (the most common area) or foot indicates disease of the femoral or popliteal arteries; pain in the buttocks and upper thigh, disease of the aortoiliac arteries. During exercise, the pain typically results from the release of lactic acid due to anaerobic metabolism in the ischemic segment, secondary to obstruction. When exercise stops, the lactic acid clears and the pain subsides.

Intermittent claudication may also have a neurologic cause: narrowing of the vertebral column at the level of the cauda equina. This condition creates pressure on the nerve roots to the lower extremities. Walking stimulates circulation to the cauda equina, causing increased pressure on those nerves and resultant pain.

Emergency interventions

If the patient has *sudden* intermittent claudication with severe or aching leg pain at rest, check the leg's temperature and color and palpate pulses. Ask about numbness and tingling. Suspect acute arterial occlusion if pulses are absent; the leg feels cold and looks pale, cyanotic, or mottled; and paresthesia and pain are present.

Don't elevate the leg. Protect it and let nothing press on it. Prepare the patient for preoperative blood tests, urinalysis, electrocardiography, and chest X-rays. Start an I.V. line, and administer an anticoagulant and pain medication.

History and physical examination

If the patient has *chronic intermittent claudication,* gather history data first. Ask how far he can walk before pain occurs and how long he must rest before it subsides. Can he walk less far now than before, or does he need to rest longer? Does the pain-rest pattern vary? Has this symptom affected his lifestyle?

Get a history of risk factors for atherosclerosis, such as smoking, diabetes, hypertension, and hyperlipidemia. Next, ask about associated signs and symptoms, such as paresthesia in the affected limb and visible changes in the color of the fingers (white to blue to pink) when he's smoking, exposed to cold, or under stress. If the patient is male, does he experience impotence?

Focus the physical examination on the cardiovascular system. Palpate for femoral, popliteal, dorsalis pedis, and posterior tibial pulses. Note character, amplitude, and bilateral equality. Diminished or absent popliteal and pedal pulses with the femoral pulse present may indicate atherosclerotic disease of the femoral artery. Diminished femoral and distal pulses may indicate disease of the terminal aorta or iliac branches. Absent pedal pulses with normal femoral and popliteal pulses may indicate Buerger's disease.

Listen for bruits over the major arteries. Note color and temperature differences between the legs or compared with the arms; also note the leg level where changes in temperature and color occur. Elevate the affected leg for 2 minutes; if it becomes pale or white, blood flow is severely decreased. When the leg hangs down, how long does it take for color to return? (Thirty seconds or longer indicates severe disease.) Check the patient's deep tendon reflexes after exercise; note if they're diminished in his lower extremities.

Examine the feet, toes, and fingers for ulceration, and inspect the hands and lower legs for small, tender nodules and erythema along blood vessels.

In the patient with arm pain, inspect the arms for a change in color (to white) on elevation. Next, palpate for changes in temperature, for muscle wasting, and for a pulsating mass in the subclavian area. Palpate and compare the radial, ulnar, brachial, axillary, and subclavian pulses to identify obstructed areas.

Common medical causes

- ***Arterial occlusion (acute).*** This disorder produces intense intermittent claudication — sudden severe or aching leg pain aggravated by exercise. A saddle embolus may affect both legs. Associated findings include paresthesia, paresis, and a sensation of cold in the affected limb. The limb is cool, pale, and cyanotic (mottled) with absent pulses below the occlusion. Capillary refill time is prolonged.
- ***Arteriosclerosis obliterans.*** This disorder usually affects the femoral and

Improving circulation in the legs

To help circulation in the legs, have your patient perform these exercises (called Berger's exercises) as part of her regular exercise program. Advise doing them four times each day or as often as the doctor specifies. Instruct the patient as follows:

Begin by lying flat on your back; then raise your legs straight up and hold this position for 2 minutes.

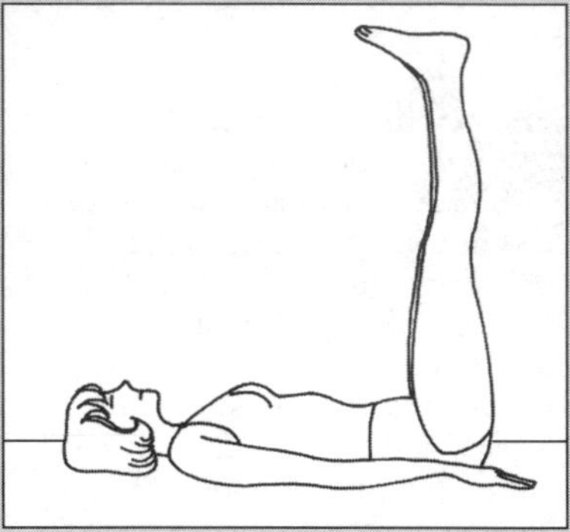

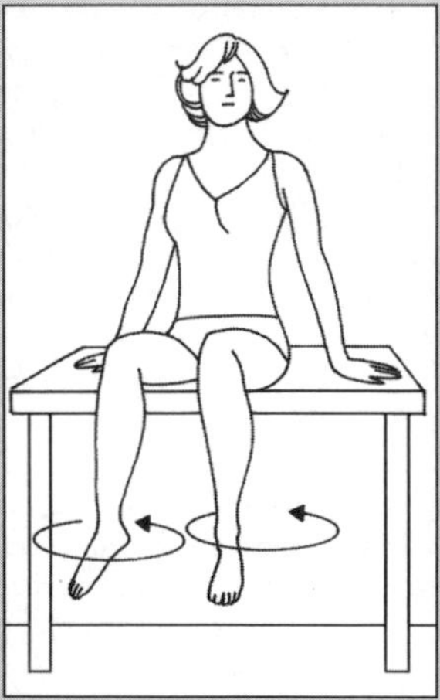

Now sit on the edge of a table or any flat surface that's high enough so that your legs don't touch the floor. Dangle your legs and swirl them in circles for 2 minutes.

Finally, lie flat for 2 minutes; then repeat the sequence twice.

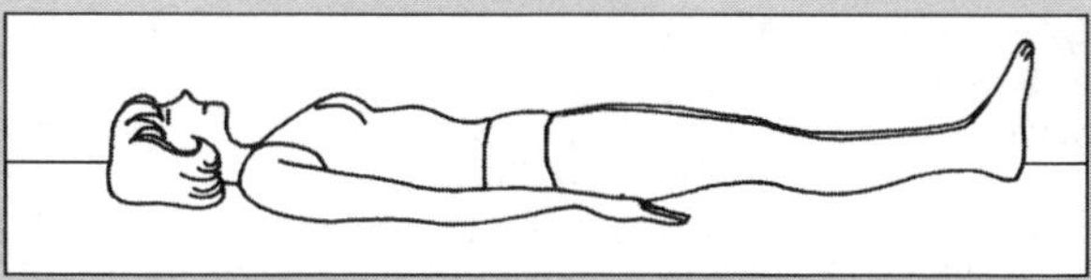

popliteal arteries, causing intermittent claudication (the most common symptom) in the calf. Typical associated findings include diminished or absent popliteal and pedal pulses, coolness in the affected limb, pallor on elevation, and profound limb weakness with continuing exercise. Other possible findings include numbness, paresthesia, and — in severe disease — pain at rest in the toes or foot, ulceration, and gangrene.

♦ ***Buerger's disease.*** This disorder typically produces intermittent claudication of the instep. Early signs include migratory superficial nodules and erythema along extremity blood vessels (nodular phlebitis) as well as migratory venous phlebitis. With exposure to cold, the feet initially become cold, cyanotic, and numb; later, they redden, become hot, and tingle. Occasionally, Buerger's disease also affects the hands and can cause painful fingertip ulcerations. Other characteristic findings include impaired peripheral pulses, paresthesia of the hands and feet, and migratory superficial thrombophlebitis.

♦ ***Neurogenic claudication.*** Neurospinal disease causes pain from neurogenic intermittent claudication that requires a longer rest time than the 2 to 3 minutes needed in vascular claudication. Associated findings include paresthesia, weakness and clumsiness when walking, and hypoactive deep tendon reflexes after walking. Pulses aren't affected in this disorder.

Special considerations

Encourage the patient to exercise to improve collateral circulation and increase venous return, and advise him to avoid prolonged sitting or standing as well as crossing his legs at the knees. (See *Improving circulation in the legs.*) If intermittent claudication interferes with the patient's lifestyle, he may require diagnostic tests (Doppler flow studies, arteriography, and digital subtraction angiography) to determine the location and degree of occlusion.

Pediatric pointers

Intermittent claudication rarely occurs in children. Although it sometimes develops in coarctation of the aorta, extensive compensatory collateral circulation typically prevents manifestation of this sign. Muscle cramps from exercise and growing pains may be mistaken for intermittent claudication in children.

J

JAUNDICE
[Icterus]

Jaundice, a yellow discoloration of the skin or mucous membranes, indicates excessive levels of conjugated or unconjugated bilirubin in the blood. In fair-skinned patients, it's most noticeable on the face, trunk, and sclera; in dark-skinned patients, on the hard palate, sclera, and conjunctiva.

Jaundice is most apparent in natural sunlight. In fact, it may be undetectable in artificial or poor light. It's commonly accompanied by pruritus (because bile pigment damages sensory nerves), dark urine, and clay-colored stools.

Jaundice may result from any of three pathophysiologic processes. (See *Jaundice: Impaired bilirubin metabolism.*) It may be the only warning sign of certain disorders such as pancreatic cancer.

History and physical examination

Documenting a history of the patient's jaundice is critical in determining its cause. Begin by asking the patient when he first noted the jaundice. Does he also have pruritus, clay-colored stools, or dark urine? Ask about past episodes or a family history of jaundice. Does he have any nonspecific signs or symptoms, such as fatigue, fever, or chills; GI signs or symptoms, such as anorexia, abdominal pain, nausea, or vomiting; or cardiopulmonary symptoms, such as shortness of breath or palpitations? Ask about alcohol use and a history of cancer or liver or gallbladder disease. Has the patient lost weight recently? Also, obtain a drug history.

Perform the physical examination in a room with natural light. Inspect the skin for texture and dryness and for hyperpigmentation and xanthomas. Look for spider angiomas or petechiae, clubbed fingers, and gynecomastia. If the patient has heart failure, auscultate for arrhythmias, murmurs, and gallops. For all patients, auscultate for crackles and abnormal bowel sounds. Palpate the lymph nodes for swelling and the abdomen for tenderness, pain, and swelling. Palpate and percuss the liver and spleen for enlargement, and test for ascites with the shifting dullness and fluid-wave techniques. Obtain baseline data on the patient's mental status: Slight changes in sensorium may be an early sign of deteriorating hepatic function.

Common medical causes

♦ ***Carcinoma.*** *Cancer of the ampulla of Vater* initially produces fluctuating jaundice, mild abdominal pain, recurrent fever, and chills. Occult bleeding may be its first sign. Other findings include weight loss, pruritus, and back pain.

Hepatic cancer (primary liver cancer or another cancer that has metastasized to the liver) may cause jaundice by causing obstruction of the bile duct. Even

Jaundice: Impaired bilirubin metabolism

Jaundice occurs in three forms: prehepatic, hepatic, and posthepatic. In all three, bilirubin levels in the blood increase due to impaired metabolism.

PREHEPATIC JAUNDICE

In *prehepatic jaundice,* certain conditions and disorders, such as transfusion reactions and sickle cell anemia, cause massive hemolysis. Red blood cells rupture faster than the liver can conjugate bilirubin, so large amounts of unconjugated bilirubin pass into the blood, causing increased intestinal conversion of this bilirubin to water-soluble urobilinogen for excretion in urine and stools. (Unconjugated bilirubin is insoluble in water, so it can't be directly excreted in urine.)

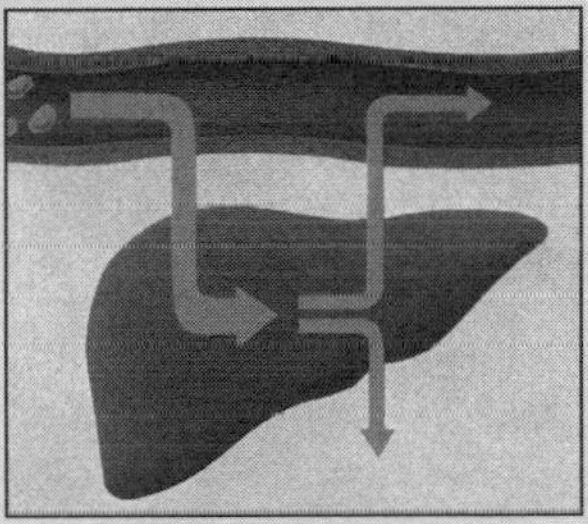

HEPATIC JAUNDICE

Hepatic jaundice results from the liver's inability to conjugate or excrete bilirubin, leading to increased blood levels of conjugated and unconjugated bilirubin. This occurs in such disorders as hepatitis, cirrhosis, and metastatic cancer and during prolonged use of drugs metabolized by the liver.

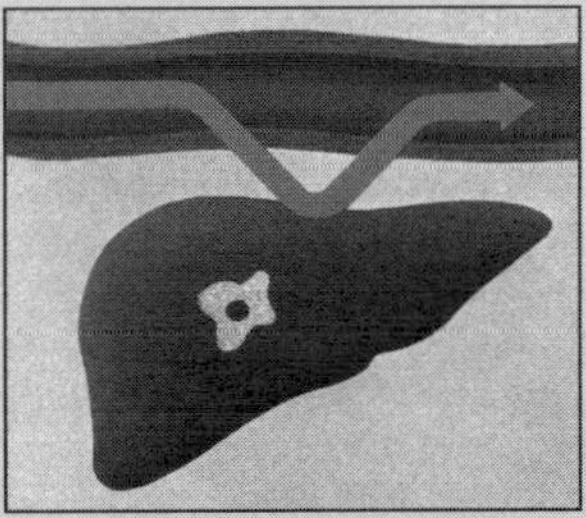

POSTHEPATIC JAUNDICE

In *posthepatic jaundice,* which occurs in biliary and pancreatic disorders, bilirubin forms at its normal rate, but inflammation, scar tissue, a tumor, or gallstones block the flow of bile into the intestine. This causes an accumulation of conjugated bilirubin in the blood. Water-soluble, conjugated bilirubin is excreted in the urine.

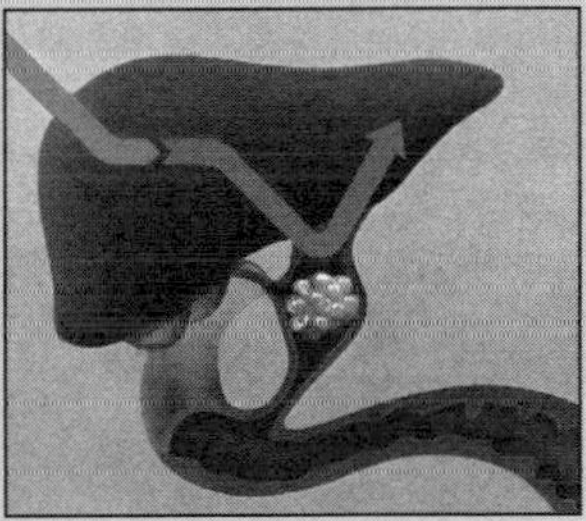

advanced cancer causes nonspecific signs and symptoms, such as right-upper-quadrant discomfort and tenderness, nausea, and slight fever. Examination may reveal irregular, nodular, firm hepatomegaly; ascites; peripheral edema; a bruit heard over the liver; and a right-upper-quadrant mass.

In *pancreatic cancer,* progressive jaundice — possibly with pruritus — may be the only sign. Related early findings are nonspecific, such as weight loss and back or abdominal pain. Other clinical features include anorexia, nausea and vomiting, fever, steatorrhea, fatigue, weakness, diarrhea, pruritus, and skin lesions (usually on the legs).

◆ ***Cholecystitis.*** This disorder produces nonobstructive jaundice in about 25% of patients. Biliary colic typically peaks abruptly and persists at that level for 2 to 4 hours. The pain then localizes to the right upper quadrant and becomes constant. Local inflammation or passage of stones to the common bile duct causes jaundice. Other findings include nausea, vomiting (usually indicating the presence of a stone), fever, profuse diaphoresis, chills, tenderness on palpation, a positive Murphy's sign and, possibly, abdominal distention and rigidity.

◆ ***Cholelithiasis.*** This disorder commonly causes jaundice and biliary colic. It's characterized by severe, steady pain in the right upper quadrant or epigastrium that radiates to the right scapula or shoulder and intensifies over several hours. Accompanying signs and symptoms include nausea and vomiting, tachycardia, and restlessness. Occlusion of the common bile duct causes fever, chills, jaundice, clay-colored stools, and abdominal tenderness. After consuming a fatty meal, the patient may experience vague epigastric fullness and dyspepsia.

◆ ***Cirrhosis.*** In *Laënnec's cirrhosis,* mild to moderate jaundice with pruritus usually signals hepatocellular necrosis or progressive hepatic insufficiency. Common early findings include ascites, weakness, leg edema, nausea and vomiting, diarrhea or constipation, anorexia, weight loss, and right-upper-quadrant pain. Massive hematemesis and other bleeding tendencies may also occur. Other findings may include enlarged liver and parotid gland, clubbed fingers, Dupuytren's contracture, mental changes, asterixis, fetor hepaticus, spider angiomas, and palmar erythema. Males may exhibit gynecomastia, scanty chest and axillary hair, and testicular atrophy; females may experience menstrual irregularities.

In *primary biliary cirrhosis,* fluctuating jaundice may appear years after the onset of other signs and symptoms, such as pruritus that worsens at bedtime (commonly the first sign), weakness, fatigue, weight loss, and vague abdominal pain. Itching frequently leads to skin excoriation. Associated findings include hyperpigmentation; indications of malabsorption, such as nocturnal diarrhea, steatorrhea, purpura, and osteomalacia; hematemesis from esophageal varices; ascites; edema; xanthelasmas; xanthomas on the palms, soles, and elbows; and hepatomegaly.

◆ ***Dubin-Johnson syndrome.*** In this inherited syndrome, fluctuating jaundice that increases with stress is the major sign, appearing as late as age 40. Related findings include slight hepatic enlargement and tenderness, upper abdominal pain, nausea, and vomiting.

◆ ***Heart failure.*** Jaundice due to liver dysfunction occurs in severe right-sided heart failure. Other effects may include jugular vein distention, cyanosis, dependent edema of the legs and sacrum, steady weight gain, confusion, hepatomegaly, nausea and vomiting, abdominal discomfort, and anorexia due to visceral edema. Ascites is a late sign. Oliguria and marked weakness and anxiety may also occur. If left-sided heart failure develops first, other findings may include fatigue, dyspnea, orthopnea, paroxysmal nocturnal dyspnea, tachypnea, arrhythmias, and tachycardia.

◆ ***Hepatic abscess.*** Multiple abscesses may cause jaundice, but the primary effects are persistent fever with chills and sweating. Other, possibly misleading, findings include steady, severe pain in the right upper quadrant or midepigastrium that may be referred to the shoulder; nausea and vomiting; anorexia; hepatomegaly; elevated right hemidiaphragm; and ascites.

◆ ***Hepatitis.*** Dark urine and clay-colored stools usually develop before jaundice in the late stages of acute viral hepatitis. Early systemic signs and symptoms vary and include fatigue, nausea, vomiting, malaise, arthralgias, myalgias, headache, anorexia, photophobia, pharyngitis, cough, diarrhea or constipation, and a low-grade fever associated with liver and lymph node enlargement. During the icteric phase (which subsides within 2 or 3 weeks unless complications occur), systemic signs subside, but an enlarged, palpable liver may be present along with weight loss, anorexia, and right-upper-quadrant pain and tenderness.

♦ ***Pancreatitis (acute).*** Edema of the head of the pancreas and obstruction of the common bile duct can cause jaundice; however, this disorder's primary symptom is usually severe epigastric pain that commonly radiates to the back. Lying with the knees flexed on the chest or sitting up and leaning forward brings relief. Early associated signs and symptoms include nausea, persistent vomiting, abdominal distention, and Turner's or Cullen's sign. Other findings include fever, tachycardia, abdominal rigidity and tenderness, hypoactive bowel sounds, and crackles.

Severe pancreatitis produces extreme restlessness; mottled skin; cold, diaphoretic extremities; paresthesia, and tetany — the last two being signs of hypocalcemia. Fulminant pancreatitis causes massive hemorrhage.

♦ ***Sickle cell anemia.*** Hemolysis produces jaundice in this disorder. Other findings include impaired growth and development, increased susceptibility to infection, life-threatening thrombotic complications and, commonly, leg ulcers and painful, swollen joints with fever and chills. Bone aches and chest pain may also occur. Severe hemolysis may cause hematuria and pallor, chronic fatigue, dyspnea (or dyspnea on exertion), and tachycardia. During a sickle cell crisis, the patient may have severe bone, abdominal, thoracic, and muscular pain; low-grade fever; and increased weakness, jaundice, and dyspnea.

Other causes

♦ ***Drugs.*** Many drugs may cause hepatic injury and resultant jaundice. Some examples include phenylbutazone, I.V. tetracycline, isoniazid, oral contraceptives, sulfonamides, mercaptopurine, erythromycin estolate, niacin, troleandomycin, androgenic steroids, HMG-CoA reductase inhibitors, and phenothiazines.

♦ ***Treatments.*** Upper abdominal surgery may cause postoperative jaundice, which occurs secondary to hepatocellular damage from manipulation of organs, leading to edema and obstructed bile flow; from administration of halothane; or from prolonged surgery resulting in shock, blood loss, or blood transfusion.

A surgical shunt used to reduce portal hypertension (such as a portacaval shunt) may also produce jaundice.

Special considerations

To help decrease pruritus, bathe the patient frequently, and apply an antipruritic lotion such as calamine. Prepare the patient for diagnostic tests to evaluate biliary and hepatic function. Laboratory studies may include urine and fecal urobilinogen, serum bilirubin, hepatic enzymes and cholesterol, prothrombin time, and a complete blood count. Other tests may include ultrasonography, cholangiography, liver biopsy, and exploratory laparotomy.

Pediatric pointers

Physiologic jaundice is common in neonates, developing 3 to 5 days after birth. In infants, obstructive jaundice usually results from congenital biliary atresia. A choledochal cyst — a congenital cystic dilation of the common bile duct — may also cause jaundice in children, particularly those of Japanese descent.

Other causes of jaundice include Crigler-Najjar syndrome, Gilbert's syndrome, Rotor's syndrome, thalassemia major, hereditary spherocytosis, erythroblastosis fetalis, Hodgkin's disease, and infectious mononucleosis.

Geriatric pointers

In patients older than age 60, jaundice is usually caused by cholestasis resulting from extrahepatic obstruction.

JAW PAIN

Jaw pain may arise from either or both of the bones that hold the teeth in the jaw — the maxilla (upper jaw) and the mandible (lower jaw). Jaw pain also includes pain in the temporomandibular joint (TMJ), where the mandible meets the temporal bone.

Jaw pain may develop gradually or abruptly and may range from barely noticeable to excruciating, depending on its cause. Jaw pain is seldom a primary indicator of any one disorder; however, some of its causes are medical emergencies. It usually results from disorders of the teeth, soft tissue, or glands of the mouth or throat or from local trauma or infection. Systemic causes include musculoskeletal, neurologic, cardiovascular, endocrine, immunologic, metabolic, or infectious disorders. Life-threatening disorders, such as myocardial infarction (MI) and tetany, also produce jaw pain, as do drugs (especially phenothiazines) and dental or surgical procedures. Jaw pain may result from dental abscess and gingivitis.

Emergency interventions

Ask the patient when his jaw pain began. Did it arise suddenly or gradually? Is it more severe or frequent now than when it first occurred? Sudden severe jaw pain, especially when associated with chest pain, shortness of breath, or arm pain, requires prompt evaluation because it may herald a life-threatening disorder.

History and physical examination

Begin the patient history by asking the patient to describe the pain's character, intensity, and frequency. When did he first notice the jaw pain? Where on the jaw does he feel pain? Does the pain radiate to other areas? Sharp or burning pain arises from the skin or subcutaneous tissues. Causalgia, an intense burning sensation, usually results from damage to the fifth cranial or trigeminal nerve. This type of superficial pain is easily localized, unlike dull, aching, boring, or throbbing pain, which originates in muscle, bone, or joints. Also, ask about aggravating or alleviating factors.

Ask about associated signs and symptoms, such as joint or chest pain, fatigue, headache, malaise, anorexia, weight loss, intermittent claudication, diplopia, and hearing loss. (Keep in mind that jaw pain may accompany more characteristic signs and symptoms of life-threatening disorders such as chest pain in MI.)

Focus your physical examination on the jaw. Inspect the painful area for redness, and palpate for edema or warmth. Facing the patient directly, look for facial asymmetry indicating swelling. Check the TMJs by placing your fingertips just anterior to the external auditory meatus and asking the patient to open and close and to thrust out and retract his jaw. Note the presence of crepitus, an abnormal scraping or grinding sensation in the joint. (Clicks heard when the jaw is widely spread apart are normal.) How wide can the patient open his mouth? Less than 3 cm or more than 6 cm between upper and lower teeth is abnormal. Next, palpate the parotid area for pain and swelling, and inspect and palpate the oral cavity for lesions, elevation of the tongue, or masses.

Common medical causes

♦ ***Angina pectoris.*** Angina may produce jaw pain (usually radiating from the substernal area) and left arm pain. Anginal pain is less severe than that of MI. It's commonly triggered by exertion, emotional stress, or ingestion of a heavy meal and usually subsides with rest and administration of nitroglycerin. Other signs and symptoms may include shortness of breath, nausea and vomiting, tachycardia, dizziness, diaphoresis, belching, and palpitations.

♦ ***Arthritis.*** In *osteoarthritis,* which usually affects the small hand joints, aching jaw pain increases with activity (talking, eating) and subsides with rest. Other features are crepitus heard and felt over the TMJ, enlarged joints with a restricted range of motion, and stiffness on awakening that improves with a few minutes of activity. Redness and warmth are usually absent.

Rheumatoid arthritis causes symmetrical pain in all the joints (frequently affecting proximal finger joints first), including the jaw. The joints display limited range of motion and are tender, warm, swollen, and stiff after inactivity, especially in the morning. Myalgia is common. Systemic signs and symptoms include fatigue, weight loss, malaise, anorexia, lymphadenopathy, and mild fever. Painless, movable rheumatoid nodules may appear on the elbows, knees, and knuckles. Progressive disease causes deformities, crepitation with joint rotation, muscle weakness and atrophy around the involved joint, and multiple systemic complications.

◆ ***Head and neck cancer.*** Many types of head and neck cancer, especially of the oral cavity and nasopharynx, produce aching jaw pain of insidious onset. Other findings include a history of leukoplakia ulcers of the mucous membranes; palpable masses in the jaw, mouth, and neck; dysphagia; bloody discharges; drooling; lymphadenopathy; and trismus.

◆ ***Hypocalcemic tetany.*** Besides painful muscle contractions of the jaw and mouth, this life-threatening disorder produces paresthesia and carpopedal spasms. The patient may complain of weakness, fatigue, and palpitations. Examination reveals hyperreflexia and positive Chvostek's and Trousseau's signs. Muscle twitching, choreiform movements, and muscle cramps may also occur. In severe hypocalcemia, laryngeal spasm may occur with stridor, cyanosis, seizures, and cardiac arrhythmias.

◆ ***Myocardial infarction.*** Initially, this life-threatening disorder causes intense, crushing substernal pain that's unrelieved by rest or nitroglycerin. The pain may radiate to the lower jaw, left arm, neck, back, or shoulder blades. (Rarely, jaw pain occurs without chest pain.) Other findings may include pallor, clammy skin, dyspnea, excessive diaphoresis, nausea and vomiting, anxiety, restlessness, a feeling of impending doom, low-grade fever, decreased or increased blood pressure, arrhythmias, an atrial gallop, new murmurs (frequently from mitral insufficiency), and crackles.

◆ ***Sinusitis.*** Maxillary sinusitis produces intense boring pain in the maxilla and cheek that may radiate to the eye. This type of sinusitis also causes a feeling of fullness, increased pain on percussion of the first and second molars, and — in nasal obstruction — loss of the sense of smell. Sphenoid sinusitis causes a scanty nasal discharge and chronic pain at the mandibular ramus and vertex of the head and in the temporal area. Other signs and symptoms of both types of sinusitis include fever, halitosis, headache, malaise, cough, sore throat, and fever.

◆ ***Suppurative parotitis.*** Bacterial infection of the parotid gland by *Staphylococcus aureus* tends to develop in debilitated patients with dry mouth or poor oral hygiene. Besides abrupt onset of jaw pain, high fever, and chills, findings include redness and edema of the overlying skin; a tender, swollen gland; and pus at the second top molar (Stensen's ducts). Infection commonly leads to disorientation; shock and death are common.

◆ ***Temporal arteritis.*** Common in patients over age 60, this disorder produces sharp jaw pain after chewing or talking. Nonspecific signs and symptoms include low-grade fever, generalized muscle pain, malaise, fatigue, anorexia, and weight loss. Vascular lesions produce jaw pain; throbbing, unilateral headache in the frontotemporal region; swollen, nodular, tender temporal arteries; and, at times, erythema of the overlying skin.

◆ ***TMJ syndrome.*** This common syndrome produces jaw pain at the TMJ; spasm and pain of the masticating muscle; clicking, popping, or crepitus of the TMJ; and restricted jaw movement. Unilateral, localized pain may radiate to other head and neck areas. The patient typically reports teeth clenching, bruxism, and emotional stress. He may also experience ear pain, headache, deviation of the jaw to the affected side upon opening the mouth, and jaw subluxation or dislocation, especially after yawning.

♦ ***Tetanus.*** A rare life-threatening disorder caused by a bacterial toxin, tetanus produces stiffness and pain in the jaw and difficulty opening the mouth. Early nonspecific signs and symptoms (commonly unnoticed or mistaken for influenza) include headache, irritability, restlessness, low-grade fever, and chills. Examination reveals tachycardia, profuse diaphoresis, and hyperreflexia. Progressive disease leads to painful, involuntary muscle spasms that spread to the abdomen, back, or face. The slightest stimulus may produce reflex spasms of any muscle group. Ultimately, laryngospasm, respiratory distress, and seizures may occur.

♦ ***Trigeminal neuralgia.*** This disorder is marked by paroxysmal attacks of intense unilateral jaw pain (stopping at the facial midline) or rapid-fire shooting sensations in one of the divisions of the trigeminal nerve (usually the mandibular or maxillary division). This superficial pain, felt mainly over the lips and chin and in the teeth, lasts from 1 to 15 minutes. Mouth and nose areas may be hypersensitive. Involvement of the ophthalmic branch of the trigeminal nerve causes a diminished or absent corneal reflex on the same side. Attacks can be triggered by even mild stimulation of the nerve (for example, lightly touching the cheeks), exposure to heat or cold, or consuming hot or cold foods or beverages.

Other causes

♦ ***Drugs.*** Some drugs, such as phenothiazines, affect the extrapyramidal tract, causing dyskinesias; others cause tetany of the jaw secondary to hypocalcemia.

Special considerations

If the patient is in severe pain, withhold food, liquids, and normally taken drugs until the diagnosis is confirmed. Administer pain medications. Prepare the patient for diagnostic tests such as jaw X-rays. Apply an ice pack if the jaw is swollen, and discourage the patient from talking or moving his jaws.

Pediatric pointers

Be alert for nonverbal signs of jaw pain, such as rubbing the affected area or wincing while talking or swallowing. In infants, initial signs of tetany from hypocalcemia may include episodes of apnea and generalized jitteriness progressing to facial grimaces and generalized rigidity. Finally, seizures may occur.

Jaw pain in children sometimes stems from disorders not common in adults. Mumps, for example, causes unilateral or bilateral swelling from the lower mandible to the zygomatic arch. Parotitis due to cystic fibrosis also causes jaw pain. When trauma causes jaw pain in children, always consider the possibility of abuse.

JUGULAR VEIN DISTENTION

Jugular vein distention is abnormal fullness and height of the pulse waves in the internal or external jugular veins. When a supine patient's head is elevated 45 degrees, a pulse wave height greater than 3 cm above the angle of Louis indicates distention. Engorged, distended veins reflect increased venous pressure in the right side of the heart. This common sign characteristically occurs in heart failure and other cardiovascular disorders.

Emergency interventions

Evaluating jugular vein distention involves visualizing and assessing venous pulsations. (See

EXAMINATION TIP

Evaluating jugular vein distention

First, position the patient so that you can visualize pulsations reflected from the right atrium. Elevate the head of the bed 45 to 90 degrees. (In the normal patient, veins distend only when the patient lies flat.) Next, locate the angle of Louis (sternal notch) — the reference point for measuring venous pressure. To do so, palpate the clavicles where they join the sternum (the suprasternal notch). Place your first two fingers on the suprasternal notch. Then, without lifting them from the skin, slide them down the sternum until you feel a bony protuberance — this is the angle of Louis.

Find the right internal jugular vein (which indicates venous pressure more reliably than the external jugular vein). Shine a flashlight across the patient's neck to create shadows that highlight his venous pulse. Be sure to distinguish jugular venous pulsations from carotid arterial pulsations. One way to do this is to palpate the vessel: Arterial pulsations continue, whereas venous pulsations disappear with light finger pressure. Also, venous pulsations increase or decrease with changes in body position, but arterial pulsations remain constant.

Next, locate the highest point along the vein, where you can see the pulsations. Using a centimeter ruler, measure the vertical distance between that high point and the sternal notch. Record this finding as well as the angle at which the patient was lying. A finding greater than 1¼" (3 cm) above the sternal notch, with the head of the bed at a 45-degree angle, indicates jugular vein distention.

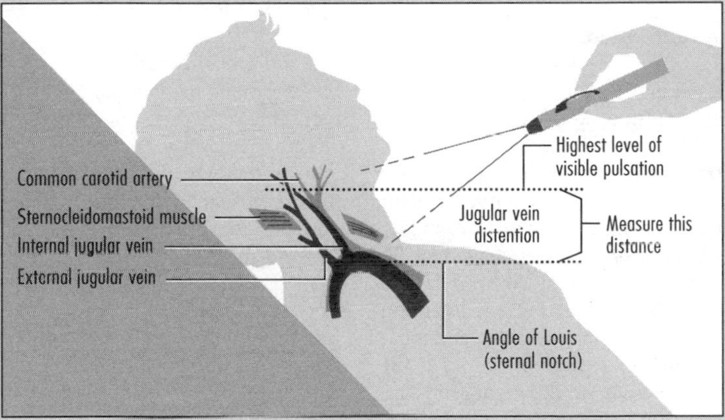

Evaluating jugular vein distention.) If you detect jugular vein distention in a patient with pale, clammy skin who suddenly appears anxious and dyspneic, take his blood pressure. If you note hypotension and pulsus paradoxus, suspect cardiac tamponade. Elevate the foot of the bed 20 to 30 degrees, give supplemental oxygen, and monitor cardiac status. Start an I.V. line for fluid administration, and keep cardiopulmonary resuscitation equipment close by. Assemble the needed equipment for emergency pericardiocentesis (to relieve pressure on the heart.) Throughout the procedure, monitor the patient's blood pressure, heart rhythm, and respirations.

History and physical examination

If the patient isn't in severe distress, obtain a history. Has he gained weight recently? Does he have difficulty putting on shoes? Are his ankles swollen? Ask about chest pain, shortness of breath, paroxysmal nocturnal dyspnea, anorexia, nausea or vomiting, and a history of cancer or heart, pulmonary, or renal disease.

Next, perform a physical examination, beginning with vital signs. Tachycardia, tachypnea, and increased blood pressure indicate fluid overload that's stressing the heart. Inspect and palpate the extremities and face for edema. Then weigh the patient.

Auscultate the lungs for crackles and the heart for gallops and a pericardial friction rub. Inspect the abdomen for distention, and palpate and percuss for an enlarged liver. Finally monitor urine output and note any decrease.

Common medical causes

♦ ***Cardiac tamponade.*** This life-threatening condition produces jugular vein distention along with anxiety, restlessness, cyanosis, chest pain, dyspnea, hypotension, and clammy skin. It also causes tachycardia, tachypnea, pulsus paradoxus, and muffled heart sounds.

♦ ***Heart failure.*** Sudden or gradual development of right-sided heart failure commonly causes jugular vein distention along with possible weakness and anxiety, cyanosis, dependent edema of the legs and sacrum, steady weight gain, confusion, and hepatomegaly. Other findings may include nausea and vomiting, abdominal discomfort, and anorexia due to visceral edema. Ascites is a late sign. Massive right-sided heart failure may produce anasarca and oliguria.

If left-sided heart failure precedes right-sided heart failure, jugular vein distention is a late sign. Other clinical features include fatigue, dyspnea, orthopnea, paroxysmal nocturnal dyspnea, tachypnea, tachycardia, and arrhythmias. Auscultation reveals crackles and a ventricular gallop.

♦ ***Hypervolemia.*** Markedly increased intravascular fluid volume causes jugular vein distention along with rapid weight gain, elevated blood pressure, bounding pulse, peripheral edema, dyspnea, and crackles.

♦ ***Pericarditis (chronic constrictive).*** Progressive signs and symptoms of restricted heart filling cause jugular vein distention that's more prominent on inspiration (Kussmaul's sign). The patient usually complains of chest pain. Other features typically include fluid retention with dependent edema, hepatomegaly, ascites, and pericardial friction rub.

♦ ***Superior vena cava obstruction.*** A tumor or, rarely, thrombosis may gradually lead to jugular vein distention when the veins of the head, neck, and arms fail to empty effectively, causing facial, neck, and upper arm edema. Metastasis to the mediastinum may cause dyspnea, cough, substernal chest pain, and hoarseness.

Special considerations

If the patient has cardiac tamponade, prepare him for pericardiocentesis. If he doesn't have cardiac tamponade, restrict fluids and monitor intake and output. If the patient has heart failure, administer diuretics. Routinely change his position to avoid skin breakdown.

Pediatric pointers

Jugular vein distention is difficult (sometimes impossible) to evaluate in most infants and toddlers because of their short, thick necks. Even in school-age children, measurement can be unreliable because the sternal angle may not be the same distance (5 to 7 cm) above the right atrium as it is in adults.

K

KEHR'S SIGN

A cardinal sign of hemorrhage within the peritoneal cavity, Kehr's sign is referred left shoulder pain that arises when intraperitoneal blood irritates the diaphragm. The pain usually begins when the patient lies supine or lowers his head. Such positioning increases the contact of free blood or clots with the left diaphragm, irritating the phrenic nerve.

Kehr's sign usually develops immediately after the hemorrhage, although onset is sometimes delayed up to 48 hours. A classic symptom of a ruptured spleen, Kehr's sign also occurs in ruptured ectopic pregnancy.

Emergency interventions

After you detect Kehr's sign, quickly take the patient's vital signs. If the patient shows signs of hypovolemia, elevate his feet 30 degrees. In addition, insert a large-bore I.V. line for fluid and blood replacement and an indwelling urinary catheter. Begin monitoring intake and output. Draw blood to determine hematocrit level, and provide supplemental oxygen.

Inspect the patient's abdomen for bruises and distention, and palpate for tenderness. Percuss for Ballance's sign — an indicator of massive perisplenic clotting and free blood in the peritoneal cavity from a ruptured spleen.

Common medical causes

♦ ***Intra-abdominal hemorrhage.*** Kehr's sign usually accompanies intense abdominal pain, abdominal rigidity, and muscle spasm. Other findings vary with the cause of bleeding, such as blunt or penetrating abdominal injuries.

Special considerations

In anticipation of surgery, withhold oral intake and prepare the patient for abdominal X-rays, computed tomography and ultrasound scans and, possibly, paracentesis, peritoneal lavage, and culdocentesis. Give analgesics as needed.

Pediatric pointers

Because a child may have difficulty describing pain, watch for nonverbal clues such as rubbing the shoulder.

KERNIG'S SIGN

A reliable early indicator of meningeal irritation, Kernig's sign elicits resistance and hamstring muscle pain when the examiner attempts to extend the knee while hip and knee are flexed 90 degrees. (See *Eliciting Kernig's sign,* page 348.) This sign is usually elicited in meningitis or subarachnoid hemorrhage. In these potentially life-threatening disorders, stretching blood- or exudate-irritated meninges surrounding spinal nerve roots causes hamstring muscle resistance.

EXAMINATION TIP

Eliciting Kernig's sign

To elicit Kernig's sign, place the patient in a supine position. Flex the leg at the hip and knee, as shown here. Then try to extend the leg while you keep the hip flexed. If the patient experiences pain and possibly spasm in the hamstring muscle and resists further extension, you can assume that meningeal irritation has occurred.

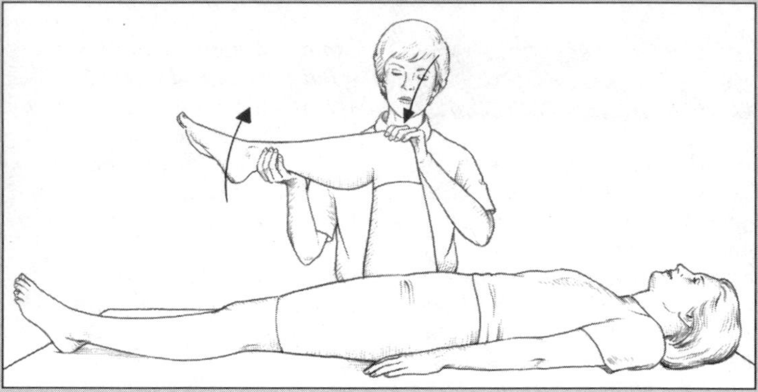

Kernig's sign can also suggest herniated disk and spinal tumor. In these disorders, sciatic pain results from disk or tumor pressure on spinal nerve roots.

History and physical examination

If you elicit a positive Kernig's sign and suspect meningitis or subarachnoid hemorrhage, immediately prepare for emergency intervention. (See *When Kernig's sign signals CNS crisis.*)

If you don't suspect meningeal irritation, ask the patient if he feels back pain that radiates down one or both legs. Does he also feel leg numbness, tingling, or weakness? Ask about other signs and symptoms, and find out if he has a history of cancer or back injury. Then perform a physical examination, concentrating on motor and sensory function.

Common medical causes

♦ ***Lumbosacral herniated disk.*** A positive Kernig's sign may be elicited in this disorder, but the cardinal and earliest feature is sciatic pain on the affected side or on both sides. Associated findings include postural deformity (lumbar lordosis or scoliosis), paresthesia, hypoactive deep tendon reflexes in the involved leg, and dorsiflexor muscle weakness.

♦ ***Meningitis.*** A positive Kernig's sign usually occurs early in meningitis along with fever and possibly chills. Other signs and symptoms of meningeal irritation may include nuchal rigidity, hyperreflexia, Brudzinski's sign, and opisthotonos. As intracranial pressure (ICP) increases, headache and vomiting may occur. In severe meningitis, the patient may experience stupor, coma, and seizures. Cranial nerve involvement may produce ocular palsies, facial weakness, deafness, and photophobia. An erythematous maculopapular rash may occur in viral meningitis; a purpuric rash may be seen in meningococcal meningitis.

EMERGENCY INTERVENTIONS

When Kernig's sign signals CNS crisis

Because Kernig's sign may signal meningitis or subarachnoid hemorrhage — both life-threatening central nervous system (CNS) disorders — take the patient's vital signs at once to obtain baseline information. Then test for Brudzinski's sign to obtain further evidence of meningeal irritation. (See *Testing for Brudzinski's' sign*, page 108.) Next, ask the patient or his family to describe the onset of illness. Typically, progressive onset of headache, fever, nuchal rigidity, and confusion suggests meningitis. Conversely, sudden onset of a severe headache, nuchal rigidity, photophobia, and possible loss of consciousness usually indicates subarachnoid hemorrhage.

MENINGITIS

If you suspect meningitis, ask about recent infections, especially tooth abscesses. Ask about exposure to infected persons or places where meningitis is endemic. Meningitis is usually a complication of another bacterial infection, so you'll need to draw blood for culture studies to determine the causative organism. Prepare the patient for lumbar puncture (if tumor or abscess can be ruled out). Also, find out if the patient has a history of I.V. drug abuse, an open head injury, or endocarditis. Insert an I.V line and administer antibiotics immediately.

SUBARACHNOID HEMORRHAGE

If you suspect subarachnoid hemorrhage, ask about a history of hypertension, cerebral aneurysm, head trauma, or arteriovenous malformation. Also ask about sudden withdrawal of antihypertensive drugs.

Check the patient's pupils for dilation, and assess for signs of increasing intracranial pressure, such as bradycardia, increased systolic blood pressure, and a widened pulse pressure. Insert an I.V. line and administer supplemental oxygen.

♦ ***Spinal cord tumor.*** Kernig's sign can be elicited occasionally, but the earliest symptom is commonly pain felt locally or along the spinal nerve, usually in the leg. Other findings may include weakness or paralysis distal to the tumor, paresthesia, urine retention, urinary or fecal incontinence, and sexual dysfunction.

♦ ***Subarachnoid hemorrhage.*** Kernig's sign and Brudzinski's sign can be elicited within minutes after the initial hemorrhage. The patient experiences sudden onset of severe headache, nuchal rigidity, and decreased level of consciousness. Photophobia, fever, nausea and vomiting, dizziness, and seizures are possible. Focal signs may include hemiparesis or hemiplegia, aphasia, and sensory or vision disturbances. Increasing ICP may produce bradycardia, increased blood pressure, respiratory pattern change, and rapid progression to coma.

Special considerations

Prepare the patient for diagnostic tests, such as computed tomography scan, magnetic resonance imaging, spinal X-ray, and myelography. Closely monitor his vital signs, ICP, and cardiopulmonary and neurologic status. Ensure bed rest, quiet, and minimal stress.

If the patient has a subarachnoid hemorrhage, darken the room and raise the head of the bed at least 30 degrees to lower ICP. If he has a herniated disk or spinal tumor, he may need pelvic traction.

Pediatric pointers

Kernig's sign is considered ominous in children because of their greater potential for rapid deterioration.

L

Leg pain

Although leg pain commonly signifies a musculoskeletal disorder, it can also result from more serious vascular or neurologic disorders. The pain may arise suddenly or gradually and may be localized or affect the entire leg. Constant or intermittent, it may feel dull, burning, sharp, shooting, or tingling. Leg pain commonly affects locomotion, limiting weight bearing. Severe leg pain that follows cast application for a fracture may signal limb-threatening compartment syndrome. Sudden onset of severe leg pain in a patient with underlying vascular insufficiency may signal acute deterioration, possibly requiring an arterial graft or amputation. (See *Causes of local leg pain.*)

Emergency interventions

If the patient has acute leg pain and a history of trauma, quickly take his vital signs and determine the leg's neurovascular status. Observe the patient's leg position and check for swelling, gross deformities, or abnormal rotation. Also, be sure to check distal pulses and note skin color and temperature. A pale, cool, and pulseless leg may indicate impaired circulation, which may require emergency surgery.

History and physical examination

If the patient's condition permits, ask him when the pain began and have him describe its intensity, character, and pattern. Is the pain worse in the morning, at night, or with movement? If it doesn't prevent him from walking, must he rely on a crutch or other assistive device? Also, ask him about the presence of other signs and symptoms.

Find out if the patient has a history of leg injury or surgery and if he or a family member has a history of joint, vascular, or back problems. Also, ask what medications he's taking and whether they've helped to relieve his leg pain.

Begin the physical examination by watching the patient walk, if his condition permits. Observe how he holds his leg while standing and sitting. Palpate the legs, buttocks, and lower back to determine the extent of pain and tenderness. If fracture has been ruled out, test range of motion in the hip and knee. Also, check reflexes with the patient's leg straightened and raised, noting any action that causes pain. Then compare both legs for symmetry, movement, and active range of motion. Also, assess sensation and strength. If the patient wears a leg cast, splint, or restrictive dressing, carefully check distal circulation, sensation, and mobility, and stretch his toes to elicit associated pain.

Causes of local leg pain

Various disorders cause hip, knee, ankle, or foot pain, which may radiate to surrounding tissues and be reported as leg pain. Local pain is commonly accompanied by tenderness, swelling, and deformity in the affected area.

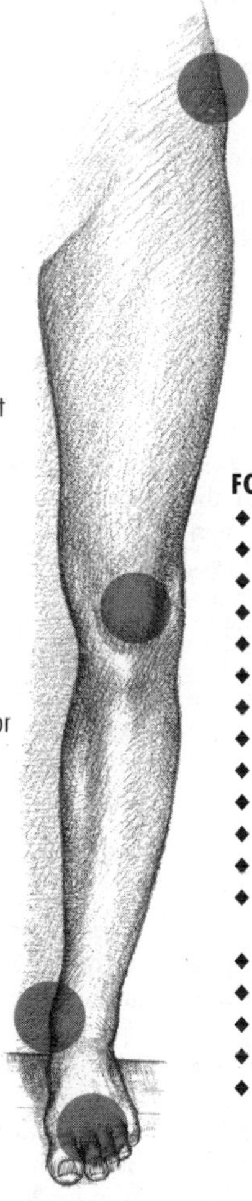

HIP PAIN
- Arthritis
- Avascular necrosis
- Bursitis
- Dislocation
- Fracture
- Sepsis
- Tumor

KNEE PAIN
- Arthritis
- Bursitis
- Chondromalacia
- Contusion
- Cruciate ligament injury
- Dislocation
- Fracture
- Meniscal injury
- Osteochondritis dissecans
- Phlebitis
- Popliteal cyst
- Radiculopathy
- Ruptured extensor mechanism
- Sprain

FOOT PAIN
- Arthritis
- Bunion
- Callus or corn
- Dislocation
- Flatfoot
- Fracture
- Gout
- Hallux rigidus
- Hammer toe
- Ingrown toenail
- Köhler's disease
- Morton's neuroma
- Occlusive vascular disease
- Plantar fascitis
- Plantar wart
- Radiculopathy
- Tabes dorsalis
- Tarsal tunnel syndrome

ANKLE PAIN
- Achilles tendon fracture
- Arthritis
- Dislocation
- Fracture
- Sprain
- Tenosynovitis

Common medical causes

♦ ***Bone neoplasm.*** Continuous deep or boring pain, commonly worse at night, may be the first symptom. Later, skin breakdown and impaired circulation may occur, along with cachexia, fever, and impaired mobility.

♦ ***Compartment syndrome.*** Progressive, intense lower leg pain that increases with passive muscle stretching is a cardinal sign of this limb-threatening disorder. Restrictive dressings or traction may aggravate the pain, which typically worsens despite analgesic administration. Other findings may include muscle weakness and paresthesia but apparently normal distal circulation. With irreversible muscle ischemia, paralysis and absent pulse also occur.

♦ ***Fracture.*** Severe, acute pain accompanies swelling and ecchymosis in the affected leg. Movement produces extreme pain, and the leg may be unable to bear weight. Neurovascular status distal to the fracture may be impaired, causing paresthesia, absent pulse, mottled cyanosis, and cool skin. Deformity, muscle spasms, and bony crepitation may also occur.

♦ ***Infection.*** Local leg pain, erythema, swelling, and warmth characterize both soft-tissue and bone infections. Fever and tachycardia may be present with other systemic signs.

♦ ***Occlusive vascular disease.*** Continuous cramping pain in the legs and feet may worsen with walking, inducing claudication. The patient may report increased pain at night and complain of cold feet and cold intolerance. Examination may reveal ankle and lower leg edema, decreased or absent pulses, and decreased capillary refill time.

♦ ***Sciatica.*** Pain, described as shooting, aching, or tingling, radiates down the back of the leg along the sciatic nerve. Typically, activity exacerbates the pain and rest relieves it. The patient may limp to avoid exacerbating the pain and may have difficulty moving from a sitting to a standing position.

♦ ***Strain or sprain.*** Acute strain causes sharp, transient pain and rapid swelling, followed by leg tenderness and ecchymosis. Chronic strain produces stiffness, soreness, and generalized leg tenderness several hours after the injury; active and passive motion may be painful or impossible. A sprain causes local pain, especially during joint movement; ecchymosis and possibly local swelling and loss of mobility develop.

♦ ***Thrombophlebitis.*** Discomfort may range from calf tenderness to severe pain accompanied by swelling, warmth, and a feeling of heaviness in the affected leg. The patient may also develop fever, chills, malaise, muscle cramps, and a positive Homans' sign. Assessment may reveal visibly engorged, palpable superficial veins.

♦ ***Varicose veins.*** Mild to severe leg symptoms may develop, including nocturnal cramping; a feeling of heaviness; diffuse, dull aching after prolonged standing or walking; and aching during menses. Assessment may reveal palpable nodules, orthostatic edema, and stasis pigmentation of the calves and ankles.

♦ ***Venous stasis ulcers.*** Localized pain and bleeding arise from infected ulcerations on the calves. Mottled, bluish pigmentation is characteristic, and local edema may also occur.

Special considerations

If the patient has acute leg pain, closely monitor his neurovascular status by frequently checking distal pulses and evaluating the temperature and color of both legs. Also monitor thigh and calf circumference to evaluate bleeding into tissues from a possible fracture site. Prepare him for X-rays. Use sandbags to immobilize the leg; apply ice and possibly skeletal traction. If a fracture isn't suspected, prepare the patient for laboratory tests to detect an infectious agent or for venography, Doppler ultrasonography, or plethysmography to determine vascular competency. Withhold food and fluids until the need for surgery has been ruled out, and withhold analgesics until a preliminary diagnosis is made.

Pediatric pointers

Common pediatric causes of leg pain include fracture, osteomyelitis, and bone cancer. If parents fail to give an adequate explanation for a leg fracture, consider the possibility of child abuse.

LEVEL OF CONSCIOUSNESS, DECREASED

A decrease in level of consciousness (LOC), from lethargy to stupor to coma, usually results from neurologic disorders and commonly signals life-threatening complications of hemorrhage, trauma, or cerebral edema. However, this sign can also result from metabolic, GI, musculoskeletal, urologic, and cardiopulmonary disorders; severe nutritional deficiency; the effects of toxins; or drug use. LOC can deteriorate suddenly or gradually and can remain altered temporarily or permanently.

Consciousness is affected by the reticular activating system (RAS), an intricate network of neurons whose axons extend from the brain stem, thalamus, and hypothalamus to the cerebral cortex. A disturbance in any part of this integrated system prevents the intercommunication that makes consciousness possible. Loss of consciousness can result from a bilateral cerebral disturbance, an RAS disturbance, or both. Cerebral dysfunction characteristically produces the least dramatic decrease in a patient's LOC. In contrast, dysfunction of the RAS produces the most dramatic decrease in LOC—coma.

The most sensitive indicator of decreased LOC is a change in the patient's mental status. The Glasgow Coma Scale, which measures ability to respond to verbal, sensory, and motor stimulation, can be used to quickly evaluate a patient's LOC.

Emergency interventions

After evaluating the patient's airway, breathing, and circulation, use the Glasgow Coma Scale to quickly determine LOC and to obtain baseline data. (See *Glasgow Coma Scale,* page 354.) If the patient's score is 13 or less, emergency surgery may be necessary. Insert an artificial airway, elevate the head of the bed 30 degrees and, if spinal cord injury has been ruled out, turn the patient's head to the side. Prepare to suction the patient if necessary. Remember to hyperventilate him first to reduce carbon dioxide levels. Then determine the rate, rhythm, and depth of spontaneous respirations. Support his breathing with a handheld resuscitation bag, if necessary. If the patient's Glasgow Coma Scale score is 7 or less, intubation and resuscitation may be necessary.

Continue to monitor the patient's vital signs, being alert for signs of increasing intracranial pressure (ICP), such as bradycardia and widening pulse pressure. When his airway, breathing, and circulation are stabilized, perform a neurologic examination.

History

Try to obtain history information from the patient, if he's lucid, and from his family. Did the patient complain of headache, dizziness, nausea, vision or hearing disturbances, weakness, fatigue, or other problems before his LOC decreased? Has his family noticed changes in the patient's behavior, personality, memory, or temperament? Also, ask

Glasgow Coma Scale

You've probably head terms such as *lethargic, obtunded,* and *stuporous* used to describe a progressive decrease in a patient's level of consciousness. However, the Glasgow Coma Scale provides a more accurate, less subjective method of recording such changes, grading consciousness in relation to eye opening and motor and verbal responses.

To use the Glasgow Coma Scale, test the patient's ability to respond to verbal, motor, and sensory stimulation. The scoring system doesn't determine exact level of consciousness, but it does provide an easy way to describe the patient's basic status and helps to detect and interpret changes from baseline findings. A decreased reaction score in one or more categories may signal an impending neurologic crisis. A score of 7 or less indicates severe neurologic damage.

TEST	REACTION	SCORE
Eyes	Open spontaneously	4
	Open to verbal command	3
	Open to pain	2
	No response	1
Best motor response	Obeys verbal command	6
	Localizes painful stimulus	5
	Flexion-withdrawal	4
	Flexion-abnormal (decorticate rigidity)	3
	Extension (decerebrate rigidity)	2
	No response	1
Best verbal response	Oriented and converses	5
	Disoriented and converses	4
	Inappropriate words	3
	Incomprehensible sounds	2
	No response	1
Total		3 to 15

about a history of neurologic disease, cancer, or recent trauma; drug and alcohol use; and the development of other signs and symptoms. Ask the patient or family if the patient has had a fall or other injury that may account for the decreased LOC.

Because decreased LOC can result from disorders that affect virtually every body system, tailor the remainder of your evaluation according to the patient's associated symptoms.

Common medical causes

◆ ***Adrenal crisis.*** Decreased LOC, ranging from lethargy to coma, may develop within 8 to 12 hours of onset. Early associated findings include progressive weakness, irritability, anorexia, headache, nausea and vomiting, diarrhea, abdominal pain, and fever. Later signs include hypotension; rapid, thready pulse; oliguria; cool, clammy skin; and flaccid extremities. The patient with chronic adrenocortical hypofunction may have hyperpigmented skin and mucous membranes.

♦ ***Brain abscess.*** Decreased LOC varies from drowsiness to deep stupor, depending on abscess size and site. Early signs — constant intractable headache, nausea, vomiting, and seizures — reflect a rising ICP. Typical later features include ocular disturbances (nystagmus, vision loss, and pupillary inequality) and signs of infection such as fever. Other findings may include personality changes, confusion, abnormal behavior, dizziness, facial weakness, aphasia, ataxia, tremor, and hemiparesis.

♦ ***Brain tumor.*** LOC decreases slowly, from lethargy to coma. The patient may also experience apathy, behavior changes, memory loss, decreased attention span, morning headache, dizziness, vision loss, ataxia, and sensorimotor disturbances. Aphasia and seizures are possible, along with signs of hormonal imbalance, such as fluid retention or amenorrhea. In later stages, papilledema, vomiting, bradycardia, and widening pulse pressure also appear. In the final stages, the patient may exhibit a decorticate or decerebrate posture.

♦ ***Cerebral aneurysm (ruptured).*** Somnolence, confusion and, at times, stupor characterize moderate bleeding; deep coma occurs in severe bleeding, which is commonly fatal. Onset is usually abrupt, with sudden, severe headache, nausea, and vomiting. Nuchal rigidity, back and leg pain, fever, restlessness, irritability, occasional seizures, and blurred vision reflect meningeal irritation. The type and severity of other findings vary with the site and severity of the hemorrhage and may include hemiparesis, hemisensory defects, dysphagia, and visual defects.

♦ ***Cerebrovascular accident (CVA).*** LOC changes vary in degree and onset, depending on the lesion's size and location and the presence of edema. *Thrombotic CVA* usually follows multiple transient ischemic attacks. Onset may be abrupt or take several minutes, hours, or days. *Embolic CVA* occurs suddenly, and deficits reach their peak almost at once. Deficits associated with a *hemorrhagic CVA* usually develop over minutes or hours.

Associated findings vary with CVA type and severity and may include disorientation; intellectual deficits, such as memory loss and poor judgment; personality changes; and emotional lability. Other possible findings include dysarthria, dysphagia, ataxia, aphasia, apraxia, agnosia, unilateral sensorimotor loss, and visual disturbances. In addition, urine retention, incontinence, constipation, headache, vomiting, and seizures may occur.

♦ ***Diabetic ketoacidosis.*** This life-threatening disorder produces a fairly rapid decrease in LOC, ranging from lethargy to coma. This is commonly preceded by polydipsia, polyphagia, and polyuria. The patient may complain of weakness, anorexia, abdominal pain, nausea, and vomiting. He may also exhibit orthostatic hypotension; fruity breath odor; Kussmaul's respirations; warm, dry skin; and a rapid, thready pulse.

♦ ***Encephalitis.*** Within 24 to 48 hours after onset, the patient may develop LOC changes ranging from lethargy to coma. Other possible findings include abrupt onset of fever, headache, nuchal rigidity, vomiting, irritability, seizures, aphasia, ataxia, hemiparesis, nystagmus, photophobia, myoclonus, and cranial nerve palsies.

♦ ***Encephalopathy.*** In *hepatic encephalopathy,* signs and symptoms develop in four stages. *Prodromal stage:* slight personality changes (disorientation, forgetfulness, slurred speech) and slight tremor.

Impending stage: tremor progressing to asterixis (the hallmark of hepatic encephalopathy), lethargy, aberrant behavior, and apraxia. *Stuporous stage:* stupor and hyperventilation, with the patient noisy and abusive when aroused. *Comatose stage:* coma with decerebrate posture, hyperactive reflexes, positive Babinski's reflex, and fetor hepaticus.

In life-threatening *hypertensive encephalopathy,* LOC progressively decreases from lethargy to stupor to coma. In addition to markedly elevated blood pressure, the patient may experience severe headache, vomiting, seizures, visual disturbances, transient paralysis and, eventually, Cheyne-Stokes respirations.

In *hypoglycemic encephalopathy,* LOC rapidly deteriorates from lethargy to coma. Early signs and symptoms include nervousness, restlessness, and confusion; hunger; alternate flushing and cold sweats; and headache, trembling, and palpitations. Blurred vision progresses to motor weakness, hemiplegia, dilated pupils, pallor, decreased pulse, shallow respirations, and seizures. Flaccidity and decerebrate posture appear late.

Depending on its severity, *hypoxic encephalopathy* produces a sudden or gradual decrease in LOC, leading to coma and brain death. Early on, the patient appears confused and restless, with cyanosis and increased heart and respiratory rates and blood pressure. Later, his respiratory pattern becomes abnormal, and assessment reveals decreased pulse, blood pressure, and deep tendon reflexes (DTRs); Babinski's reflex; absent doll's eye reflex; and fixed pupils.

In *uremic encephalopathy,* LOC decreases gradually from lethargy to coma. Early on, the patient may appear apathetic, inattentive, confused, and irritable and may complain of headache, nausea, fatigue, and anorexia. Other findings may include vomiting, tremors, edema, papilledema, hypertension, cardiac arrhythmias, dyspnea, crackles, oliguria, or Kussmaul's or Cheyne-Stokes respirations.

♦ ***Heatstroke.*** As body temperature increases, LOC gradually decreases from lethargy to coma. Early signs and symptoms include malaise, tachycardia, tachypnea, orthostatic hypotension, muscle cramps, and syncope. The patient may be irritable, anxious, and dizzy and may report severe headache. At onset, his skin is hot, flushed, and diaphoretic; later, when fever exceeds 105° F (40.5° C), the skin becomes hot, flushed, and anhidrotic. Pulse and respiratory rate increase markedly, and blood pressure drops precipitously. Other findings may include vomiting, diarrhea, dilated pupils, or Cheyne-Stokes respirations.

♦ ***Hypernatremia.*** This disorder, life-threatening if acute, causes LOC to deteriorate from lethargy to coma. The patient is irritable and exhibits twitches progressing to seizures. Other associated signs and symptoms may include nausea, malaise, fever, thirst, flushed skin, dry mucous membranes, or weak, thready pulse.

♦ ***Hyperosmolar hyperglycemic nonketotic syndrome.*** LOC decreases rapidly from lethargy to coma. Early findings may include polyuria, polydipsia, weight loss, or weakness. Later, the patient may develop hypotension, poor skin turgor, dry skin and mucous membranes, tachycardia, tachypnea, oliguria, or seizures.

♦ ***Hypokalemia.*** LOC gradually decreases to lethargy; coma is rare. Other possible findings include confusion, nausea, vomiting, diarrhea, and polyuria; weakness, decreased reflexes, and malaise; and dizziness, hypotension, and arrhythmias.

♦ ***Hyponatremia.*** This disorder, life-threatening if acute, produces decreased LOC in late stages. Early nausea and malaise may progress to behavior changes, incoordination and, eventually, seizures and coma.

♦ ***Hypothermia.*** In *severe hypothermia* (temperature below 90° F [32.2° C]), LOC decreases from lethargy to coma. Deep tendon reflexes (DTRs) disappear, and ventricular fibrillation occurs, possibly followed by cardiopulmonary arrest. In *mild to moderate hypothermia,* the patient may experience memory loss and slurred speech in addition to shivering, weakness, fatigue, and apathy. Other early signs include ataxia, muscle stiffness, and hyperactive DTRs; diuresis; tachycardia and decreased respiratory rate and blood pressure; and cold, pale skin. Later, muscle rigidity and decreased reflexes may develop, along with peripheral cyanosis, bradycardia, arrhythmias, severe hypotension, decreased respiratory rate, and oliguria.

♦ ***Intracerebral hemorrhage.*** This life-threatening disorder produces rapid, steady loss of consciousness within hours, commonly accompanied by severe headache, dizziness, nausea, and vomiting. Associated signs and symptoms vary and may include increased blood pressure, irregular respirations, Babinski's reflex, seizures, aphasia, decreased sensations, hemiplegia, decorticate or decerebrate posture, or dilated pupils.

♦ ***Meningitis.*** Confusion and irritability are expected, although stupor, coma, and seizures may occur in severe meningitis. Fever develops early, possibly accompanied by chills. Associated findings include severe headache, nuchal rigidity, hyperreflexia and, possibly, opisthotonos. The patient exhibits Kernig's and Brudzinski's signs and possibly ocular palsies, photophobia, facial weakness, or hearing loss.

♦ ***Seizure disorders.*** *Complex partial seizure* produces decreased LOC, manifested as a blank stare, purposeless behavior (picking at clothing, wandering, lip smacking, or chewing motions), and unintelligible speech. The seizure may be heralded by an aura and followed by several minutes of mental confusion. *Absence seizure* usually involves a brief change in LOC, indicated by blinking or eye rolling, blank stare, and slight mouth movements. *Generalized tonic-clonic seizure* typically begins with a loud cry and sudden loss of consciousness; muscle spasm alternates with relaxation, and tongue biting, incontinence, labored breathing, apnea, or cyanosis may also occur. Consciousness returns after the seizure, but the patient remains confused and may have difficulty talking. He may complain of drowsiness, fatigue, headache, muscle aching, and weakness and may fall into deep sleep. *Atonic seizure* produces sudden unconsciousness for a few seconds. *Status epilepticus,* rapidly recurring seizures without intervening periods of physiologic recovery and return of consciousness, can be life-threatening.

♦ ***Shock.*** Decreased LOC — lethargy progressing to stupor and coma — occurs late in shock. Associated findings include confusion, anxiety, and restlessness; hypotension; tachycardia; weak pulse with narrowing pulse pressure; dyspnea; oliguria; and cool, clammy skin. *Hypovolemic shock* also produces massive or insidious bleeding, either internally or externally. *Cardiogenic shock* may produce chest pain or arrhythmias and signs of heart failure, such as dyspnea, cough, edema, distended neck veins, and weight gain. *Septic shock* may be accompanied by high fever and chills. *Anaphylactic shock* usually involves stridor.

♦ ***Subdural hemorrhage (acute).*** In this potentially life-threatening disorder, agitation and confusion are followed by progressively decreasing LOC from somnolence to coma. The patient may also experience headache, fever, unilateral pupil dilation, decreased pulse and respiratory rates, widening pulse pressure, seizures, hemiparesis, and Babinski's reflex.

♦ ***Thyroid storm.*** LOC decreases suddenly and can progress to coma. Irritability, restlessness, confusion, and psychotic behavior precede the deterioration. Associated signs and symptoms include tremors and weakness; visual disturbances; tachycardia, arrhythmias, and angina; warm, moist, flushed skin; and vomiting, diarrhea, and fever to 105° F (40.5° C).

♦ ***Transient ischemic attack.*** LOC decreases abruptly (with varying severity) and returns to normal gradually within 24 hours. Site-specific findings may include vision loss, nystagmus, aphasia, dizziness, dysarthria, unilateral hemiparesis or hemiplegia, tinnitus, paresthesia, dysphagia, or staggering or incoordinated gait.

♦ ***West Nile encephalitis.*** This brain infection is caused by West Nile virus, a mosquito-borne flavivirus commonly found in Africa, West Asia, and the Middle East. Mild infection is common; signs and symptoms include fever, headache, and body aches, commonly with skin rash and swollen lymph glands. More severe infection is marked by high fever, headache, neck stiffness, stupor, disorientation, coma, tremors, occasional seizures, paralysis and, rarely, death.

Other causes

♦ ***Alcohol.*** Use of alcohol causes varying degrees of sedation, irritability, and incoordination; intoxication frequently causes stupor.

♦ ***Drugs.*** Sedation and other degrees of decreased LOC can result from overdose of barbiturates, other central nervous system depressants, and aspirin.

Special considerations

Reassess the patient's LOC and neurologic status at least hourly. Carefully monitor ICP and intake and output. Ensure airway patency and proper nutrition. Take precautions to help ensure the patient's safety. Keep him on bed rest with the side rails up. Apply restraints only if absolutely necessary because their use may increase his agitation and confusion. Talk to the patient even if he appears comatose; your voice may help reorient him to reality.

Pediatric pointers

The primary cause of decreased LOC in children is head trauma, which commonly results from physical abuse or motor vehicle accident. Other causes include accidental poisoning, hydrocephalus, and meningitis or brain abscess following an ear or respiratory infection. To reduce the parents' anxiety, include them in the child's care. Offer them support and realistic explanations of their child's condition.

LIGHT FLASHES

[Photopsias]

A cardinal symptom of vision-threatening retinal detachment, light flashes can occur locally or throughout the visual field. They may occur in conjunction with floaters or alone. The patient usually reports seeing spots, stars, or lightning-type streaks. Flashes can occur suddenly or gradually and can indicate temporary or permanent vision impairment.

In most cases, light flashes signal the splitting of the posterior vitreous membrane into two layers; the inner layer detaches from the retina and the outer layer remains fixed to it. Light flashes are typically perceived in subdued lighting or even total darkness. The sensation of light flashes may result from vitreous traction on the retina, hemorrhage caused by a tear in the retinal capillary, or strands of solid vitreous floating in a local pool of liquid vitreous.

Emergency interventions

Until retinal detachment is ruled out, restrict the patient's eye and body movement. Retinal tears can commonly be treated with laser or freezing methods if a retinal detachment isn't present.

History and physical examination

Ask the patient when the light flashes began. Can he pinpoint their location, or do they occur throughout the visual field? If the patient is experiencing eye pain or headache, have him describe it. Also, ask if the patient wears or has ever worn corrective lenses, and if he or a family member has a history of eye or vision problems. Also ask if the patient has other medical problems — especially hypertension or diabetes mellitus, which can cause retinopathy and possibly retinal detachment. Obtain an occupational history because light flashes may be related to job stress or eye strain.

Next, perform a complete eye and vision examination, especially if trauma is apparent or suspected. Begin by inspecting the external eye, lids, lashes, and tear puncta for abnormalities and the iris and sclera for signs of bleeding. Observe pupil size and shape. Also, check for reaction to light, accommodation, and consensual light response. Then test visual acuity in each eye. Also test visual fields; document light flashes the patient reports during this test.

Common medical causes

- ***Cytomegalovirus (CMV) retinitis.*** Symptomatic CMV infection normally occurs only in immunocompromised persons. Visual symptoms include floaters, flashes of light that may indicate retinal detachment, blind spots, blurred or decreased vision, and loss of peripheral vision.
- ***Head trauma.*** A patient who has sustained minor head trauma may report "seeing stars" when the injury occurs. He may also complain of localized pain at the injury site, generalized headache, and dizziness. Later, he may develop nausea, vomiting, and decreased level of consciousness.
- ***Migraine headache.*** Light flashes — possibly accompanied by an aura — may herald a classic migraine headache. As these symptoms subside, the patient typically experiences a severe, throbbing, unilateral headache that usually lasts 1 to 12 hours and may be accompanied by paresthesia of the lips, face, or hands; slight confusion; dizziness; photophobia; nausea; and vomiting.
- ***Retinal detachment.*** Light flashes described as floaters or spots are localized in the portion of the visual field where the retina is detaching. With macular involvement, the patient may experience painless vision impairment resembling a curtain covering the visual field.
- ***Vitreous detachment.*** Visual floaters may accompany sudden onset of light flashes. Usually, one eye is affected at a time.

Special considerations

If the patient has retinal detachment, prepare him for reattachment surgery. Explain that, after surgery, he may need to continue wearing eye patches and may have activity and position restrictions until the retina heals completely.

If the patient doesn't have retinal detachment, reassure him that his light flashes are temporary and don't indicate eye damage. They will gradually resolve over a period of time with no permanent alteration in vision. For the patient with a migraine headache, maintain a quiet, darkened environment, encourage sleep, and administer analgesics as ordered.

Pediatric pointers

Children may experience light flashes after minor head trauma.

Ballard scale for calculating gestational age

NEUROMUSCULAR MATURITY

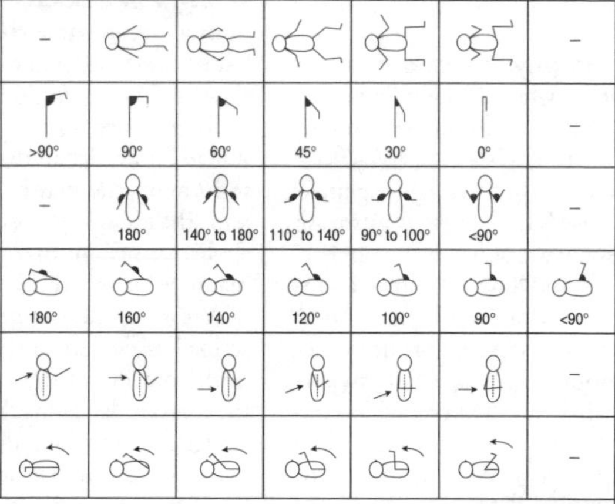

NEUROMUSCULAR MATURITY SIGN	SCORE -1	0	1	2	3	4	5	RECORD SCORE HERE
POSTURE	–						–	
SQUARE WINDOW (Wrist)	>90°	90°	60°	45°	30°	0°	–	
ARM RECOIL	–	180°	140° to 180°	110° to 140°	90° to 100°	<90°	–	
POPLITEAL ANGLE	180°	160°	140°	120°	100°	90°	<90°	
SCARF SIGN							–	
HEEL TO EAR							–	
							TOTAL NEUROMUSCULAR MATURITY SCORE	

PHYSICAL MATURITY

PHYSICAL MATURITY SIGN	SCORE -1	0	1	2	3	4	5	RECORD SCORE HERE
SKIN	Sticky, friable, transparent	Gelatinous, red, translusent	Smooth, pink; visible vessels	Superficial peeling or rash; few visible vessels	Cracking; pale areas; rare visible vessels	Parchment-like; deep cracking; no visible vessels	Leathery, cracked, wrinkled	
LANUGO	None	Sparse	Abundant	Thinning	Bald areas	Mostly bald	–	
PLANTAR SURFACE	Heel-toe 40 to 50 mm: –1; <40 mm: –2	>50 mm; no crease	Faint red marks	Anterior transverse crease only	Creases over anterior two-thirds	Creases over entire sole	–	
BREAST	Imperceptible	Barely perceptible	Flat areola, no bed	Stippled areola; 1- to 2-mm bud	Raised areola; 3- to 4-mm bud	Full areola; 5- to 10-mm bud	–	
EYE AND EAR	Lids fused, loosely: –1; tightly: –2	Lids open; pinna flat, stays folded	Slightly curved pinna; soft, slow recoil	Well-curved pinna; soft but ready recoil	Formed and firm; instant recoil	Thick cartilage; ear stiff	–	
GENITALIA, (Male)	Scrotum flat, smooth	Scrotum empty; faint rugae	Testes in upper canal; rare rugae	Testes descending; few rugae	Testes down; good rugae	Testes pendulous; deep rugae	–	
GENITALIA, (Female)	Clitoris prominent; labia flat	Prominent clitoris; small labia minora	Prominent clitoris; enlarging minora	Majora and minora equally prominent	Majora large; minora small	Majora cover clitoris and minora	–	
							TOTAL PHYSICAL MATURITY SCORE	

Reproduced from Ballard, J.L., "New Ballard Score Expanded to Include Extremely Premature Infants," *Journal of Pediatrics* 119:417-423, 1991, with permission of Mosby-Year Book, Inc.

SCORE

Neuromuscular _____

Physical __________

Total ____________

MATURITY RATING

TOTAL MATURITY SCORE	GESTATIONAL AGE (WEEKS)
−10	20
−5	22
0	24
5	26
10	28
15	30
20	32
25	34
30	36
35	38
40	40
45	42
50	44

GESTATIONAL AGE (Weeks)

By dates __________

By ultrasound ______

By score __________

Low birth weight

Two groups of infants are born weighing less than the normal minimum birth weight of 5.5 lb (2,500 g) — those who are born prematurely (before the 37th week of gestation) and those who are small for gestational age (SGA). The premature infant weighs an appropriate amount for his gestational age and probably would have matured normally if carried to term. Conversely, the SGA infant weighs less than the normal amount for his age, even if carried to term, and his organs are mature. Differentiating the two helps direct the search for a cause. (See *Ballard Scale for calculating gestational age.*)

In the premature infant, low birth weight usually results from a disorder that prevents the uterus from retaining the fetus, interferes with the normal course of pregnancy, causes premature separation of the placenta, or stimulates uterine contractions before term. In the SGA infant, intrauterine growth may be retarded by a disorder that interferes with placental circulation, fetal development, or maternal health. (See *Maternal causes of low birth weight,* page 362.)

Regardless of the cause, low birth weight is associated with higher infant morbidity and mortality; in fact, these infants are 20 times more likely to die within the first month of life. Low birth weight can also signal a life-threatening emergency.

Emergency interventions

Because low birth weight is associated with poorly developed body systems, particularly the respiratory system, your priority is to monitor respiratory status. Be alert for signs of distress, such as apnea, grunting respirations, intercostal or xiphoid retractions, or a respiratory rate exceeding 60 breaths/minute after the first hour of

Maternal causes of low birth weight

If the infant is small for his gestational age, consider these possible maternal causes:
- acquired immunodeficiency syndrome
- alcohol or narcotic abuse
- chronic maternal illness
- cigarette smoking
- hypertension
- hypoxemia
- malnutrition
- toxemia.

If the infant is born prematurely, consider these common maternal causes:
- abruptio placentae
- amnionitis
- cocaine or crack use
- incompetent cervix
- placenta previa
- polyhydramnios
- preeclampsia
- premature rupture of membranes
- severe maternal illness
- urinary tract infection.

life. If you detect any of these signs, prepare to resuscitate the infant. Endotracheal intubation or supplemental oxygen with a hood may be needed.

Monitor the infant's axillary temperature. Decreased fat reserves may keep him from maintaining normal body temperature, and a drop below 97.8° F (36.5° C) exacerbates respiratory distress by increasing oxygen consumption. To maintain normal body temperature, use an overbed warmer or an isolette. (If these are unavailable, use a wrapped rubber bottle filled with warm water, but be careful to avoid hyperthermia.) Cover the infant's head to prevent heat loss.

History and physical examination

As soon as possible, evaluate the infant's neuromuscular and physical maturity to determine gestational age. Follow with a routine neonatal examination.

Common medical causes

- ***Chromosomal aberrations.*** Abnormalities in the number, size, or configuration of chromosomes can cause low birth weight and possibly multiple congenital anomalies in a premature or SGA infant. For example, an infant with trisomy 21 (Down syndrome) may be SGA and have prominent epicanthal folds, a flat-bridged nose, a protruding tongue, palmar simian creases, muscular hypotonia, and an umbilical hernia.
- ***Cytomegalovirus infection.*** Although low birth weight in this disorder is usually associated with premature birth, some infants may be SGA. Assessment at birth reveals these classic signs: petechiae and ecchymoses, jaundice, and hepatosplenomegaly, which increases for several days. The infant also has a high fever, lymphadenopathy, tachypnea, and dyspnea, along with prolonged bleeding at puncture sites.
- ***Placental dysfunction.*** Low birth weight and a wasted appearance occur in an SGA infant. The infant may be symmetrically short or may appear relatively long for his low weight. Additional findings reflect the underlying cause. For example, if maternal hyperparathyroidism caused placental dysfunction, the infant may exhibit muscle jerking and twitching, carpopedal spasm, ankle clonus, vomiting, tachycardia, and tachypnea.
- ***Rubella (congenital).*** Usually, the low-birth-weight infant with this disease is born at term but is SGA. A characteristic "blueberry muffin" rash accompanies cataracts, purpuric lesions, hepatosplenomegaly, and a large anterior fontanel. Abnormal heart sounds, if present, vary with the type of associated congenital heart defect.
- ***Varicella (congenital).*** Low birth weight is accompanied by cataracts and skin vesicles.

Special considerations

To make up for low fat and glycogen stores in the low-birth-weight infant, initiate feedings as soon as examination reveals the presence of peristalsis and the suck, swallow, and gag reflexes, and continue to feed every 2 to 3 hours. Provide gavage or I.V. feeding for sick or very premature infants. Check abdominal girth with each feeding, and check stools for blood because increasing girth and bloody stools may indicate necrotizing enterocolitis. A sepsis workup may be necessary if there are signs of infection associated with low birth weight.

Check the infant's vital signs every 15 minutes for the first hour and at least once every hour thereafter until his condition stabilizes. Be alert for changes in temperature or behavior, feeding problems, or periods of apnea — possible indications of infection. Also, monitor blood glucose levels and watch for signs of hypoglycemia, such as irritability, jitteriness, tremors, seizures, irregular respirations, lethargy, and a high-pitched or weak cry. And, if the infant is receiving supplemental oxygen, carefully monitor arterial blood gas values and the oxygen concentration of inspired air to prevent retinopathy.

Monitor the infant's urine output by weighing diapers before and after voiding. Check urine color, measure specific gravity, and test for the presence of glucose, blood, or protein. Also, watch for changes in the infant's skin color because increasing jaundice may indicate hyperbilirubinemia.

Encourage the parents to participate in their infant's care to strengthen bonding, and allow ample time for their questions.

Lymphadenopathy

Lymphadenopathy — enlargement of one or more lymph nodes — may result from increased production of lymphocytes or reticuloendothelial cells or from infiltration of cells that aren't normally present. This sign may be generalized (involving three or more node groups) or localized. Generalized lymphadenopathy may be caused by an inflammatory process, such as bacterial or viral infection; connective tissue disease; endocrine disorder; or neoplasm. Localized lymphadenopathy most commonly results from infection or trauma affecting the drained area. (See *Reviewing common sites of localized lymphadenopathy,* page 364.)

Normally, lymph nodes are discrete, mobile, nontender and, except in children, nonpalpable. (However, palpable nodes may be normal in adults.) Nodes that exceed 1 cm in diameter are cause for concern. They may be tender, and the skin overlying the lymph node may be erythematous, suggesting a draining lesion. Or, nodes may be hard and fixed, tender or nontender, suggesting a malignant tumor.

History and physical examination

Ask the patient when he first noticed the swelling and if it's located on one side of his body or both. Are the swollen areas sore, hard, or red? Ask the patient if he has recently had an infection or other health problems. Also ask if a biopsy has ever been done on any nodes, as this may indicate a previously diagnosed cancer. Find out if the patient has a family history of cancer.

Palpate the entire lymph node system to determine the extent of lymphadenopathy and to detect other areas of local enlargement. Use the pads of your index and middle fingers to move the skin over underlying tissues at the nodal area. If

Reviewing common sites of localized lymphadenopathy

When you detect an enlarged lymph node, palpate the entire lymph node system to determine the extent of lymphadenopathy. Include the lymph nodes indicated here in your assessment.

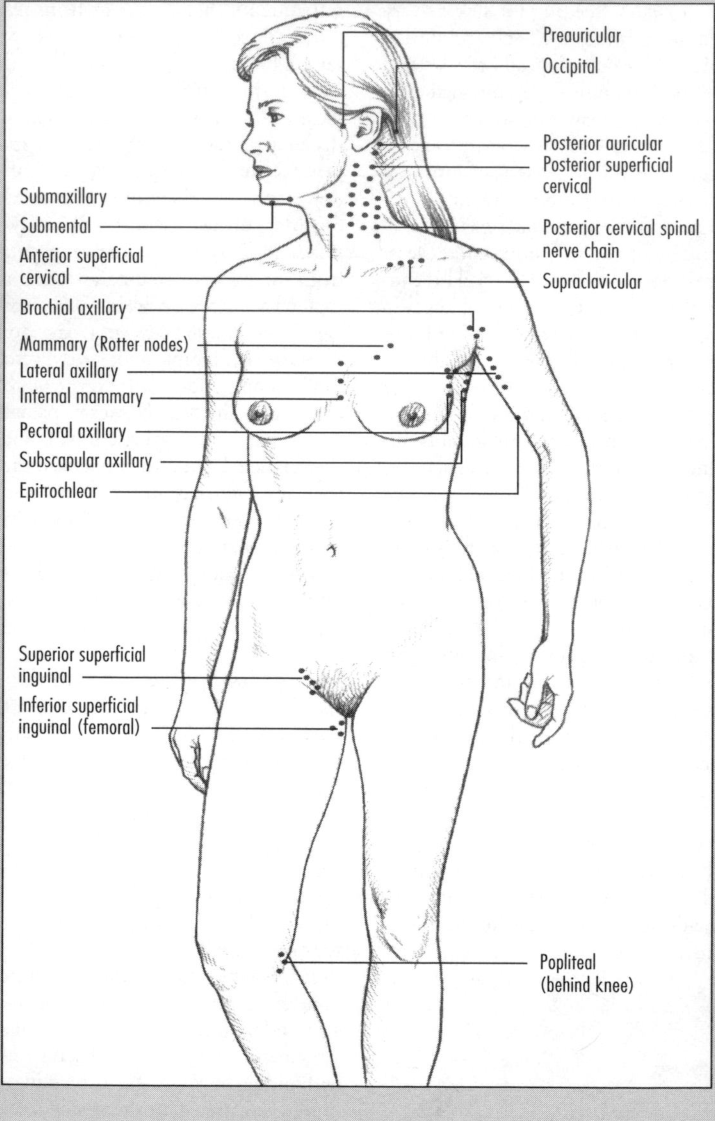

you detect enlarged nodes, note their size in centimeters and whether they're fixed or mobile, tender or nontender, and erythematous or not. Also note their texture: Is the node discrete, or does the area feel matted? If you detect enlarged lymph nodes, check the area drained by that part of the lymph system for signs of infection, such as erythema and swelling or other abnormalities suggestive of a possible malignancy. Also, palpate for and percuss the spleen.

Common medical causes

◆ ***Acquired immunodeficiency syndrome.*** Besides lymphadenopathy, findings include a history of fatigue, night sweats, afternoon fevers, weight loss, and cough with several recurrent infections appearing soon afterward.

◆ ***Brucellosis.*** Generalized lymphadenopathy most commonly affects cervical and axillary lymph nodes, making them tender. This disease usually begins insidiously with easy fatigability, headache, backache, anorexia, and arthralgias; it may also begin abruptly with chills, fever, and diaphoresis.

◆ ***Cytomegalovirus infection.*** Generalized lymphadenopathy occurs in the immunocompromised patient and is accompanied by fever, malaise, rash, and hepatosplenomegaly.

◆ ***Hodgkin's disease.*** The extent of lymphadenopathy reflects the stage of malignancy—from stage I involvement of a single lymph node region to stage IV generalized lymphadenopathy. Common early signs and symptoms include pruritus and, fatigue, weakness, night sweats, malaise, weight loss, and unexplained fever (usually to 101° F [38.3° C]). Also, if mediastinal lymph nodes enlarge, tracheal and esophageal pressure produces dyspnea, cough, and dysphagia.

◆ ***Leptospirosis.*** Lymphadenopathy occurs infrequently in this rare disease. More common findings include sudden onset of fever and chills, malaise, myalgia, headache, nausea and vomiting, and abdominal pain.

◆ ***Leukemia (acute lymphocytic).*** Generalized lymphadenopathy is accompanied by fatigue, malaise, pallor, and low fever. The patient also experiences prolonged bleeding time, swollen gums, weight loss, bone or joint pain, and hepatosplenomegaly.

◆ ***Leukemia (chronic lymphocytic).*** Generalized lymphadenopathy appears early, along with fatigue, malaise, and fever. As the disease progresses, hepatosplenomegaly, severe fatigue, and weight loss occur. Other late findings include bone tenderness, edema, pallor, dyspnea, tachycardia, palpitations, bleeding, anemia, and macular or nodular lesions.

◆ ***Lyme disease.*** Spread by the bite of certain ticks, Lyme disease begins with a skin lesion called erythema chronicum migrans. As the disease progresses, the patient may manifest lymphadenopathy, constant malaise and fatigue, and intermittent headache, fever, chills, and aches. He may develop arthralgias and, eventually, neurologic and cardiac abnormalities.

◆ ***Malignant lymphoma.*** Painless enlargement of one or more peripheral lymph nodes is the most common sign of this disease, with generalized lymphadenopathy characterizing stage IV. Dyspnea, cough, and hepatosplenomegaly occur, along with systemic complaints of fever to 101° F (38.3° C), night sweats, fatigue, malaise, and weight loss.

◆ ***Mononucleosis (infectious).*** Characteristic, painful lymphadenopathy involves cervical, axillary, and inguinal nodes. Commonly, there's posterior cervical adenopathy. Typically, prodromal symptoms, such as headache, malaise, and fatigue, occur 3 to 5 days before the appearance of the classic triad of lymphadenopathy, sore throat, and temperature fluctuations with an evening peak of about 102° F (38.9° C). Hepatosplenomegaly may develop, along with findings of stomatitis, exudative tonsillitis, or pharyngitis.

♦ ***Mycosis fungoides.*** Lymphadenopathy occurs in stage III of this rare, chronic malignant lymphoma and is accompanied by ulcerated brownish red tumors that are painful and itchy.

♦ ***Rheumatoid arthritis.*** Lymphadenopathy is an early, nonspecific finding associated with fatigue, malaise, continuous low fever, weight loss, and vague arthralgias and myalgias. Later, the patient develops joint tenderness, swelling, and warmth; joint stiffness after inactivity (especially in the morning); and subcutaneous nodules on the elbows. Eventually joint deformity, muscle weakness, and atrophy may occur.

♦ ***Sarcoidosis.*** Generalized, bilateral hilar, and right paratracheal forms of lymphadenopathy with splenomegaly are common. Initial findings are arthralgia, fatigue, malaise, weight loss, and pulmonary symptoms. Other findings vary with the site and extent of fibrosis. Typical cardiopulmonary findings include breathlessness, cough, substernal chest pain, and arrhythmias. Musculoskeletal and cutaneous features may include muscle weakness and pain, phalangeal and nasal mucosal lesions, and subcutaneous skin nodules. Common ophthalmic findings include eye pain, photophobia, and nonreactive pupils. Central nervous system involvement may produce cranial or peripheral nerve palsies and seizures.

♦ ***Sjögren's syndrome.*** Lymphadenopathy of the parotid and submaxillary nodes may occur in this rare disorder. Assessment reveals cardinal signs of dry eyes and dry mouth, which may be accompanied by photosensitivity, poor vision, eye fatigue, nasal crusting, and epistaxis.

♦ ***Syphilis (secondary).*** Generalized lymphadenopathy occurs in the second stage and may be accompanied by a macular, papular, pustular, or nodular rash on the arms, trunk, palms, soles, face, and scalp. A palmar rash is a significant diagnostic sign. Headache, malaise, anorexia, weight loss, nausea, vomiting, sore throat, and low fever may occur.

♦ ***Systemic lupus erythematosus.*** Generalized lymphadenopathy commonly accompanies the hallmark butterfly rash, photosensitivity, Raynaud's phenomenon, and joint pain and stiffness. Pleuritic chest pain and cough may appear with systemic findings, such as fever, anorexia, or weight loss.

♦ ***Tuberculous lymphadenitis.*** Lymphadenopathy may be generalized or restricted to superficial lymph nodes. Affected lymph nodes may become fluctuant and drain to surrounding tissue. They may be accompanied by fever, chills, weakness, or fatigue.

♦ ***Waldenström's macroglobulinemia.*** Lymphadenopathy may appear along with hepatosplenomegaly. Associated findings include retinal hemorrhage, pallor, and signs of heart failure, such as neck vein distention and crackles. The patient shows decreased level of consciousness, abnormal reflexes, and signs of peripheral neuritis. Weakness, fatigue, weight loss, epistaxis, and GI bleeding may also occur.

Other causes

♦ ***Drugs.*** Phenytoin may cause generalized lymphadenopathy.

♦ ***Immunizations.*** Typhoid vaccination may also cause generalized lymphadenopathy.

Special considerations

If the patient has fever above 101° F (38.3° C), don't automatically assume that the temperature should be lowered. A patient with a bacterial or viral infection must tolerate the fever, which may assist recovery. Provide antipyretics if the patient is very uncomfortable. Tepid sponge baths or a hypothermia blanket may also be used. Antibiotics or antivirals may also be prescribed for known infections.

Expect to obtain blood for routine blood work, a platelet count, and liver and renal function studies. Prepare the patient for other scheduled diagnostic tests, such as chest X-ray, liver and spleen scan, lymph node biopsy, or lymphography to visualize the lymphatic system. If tests reveal infection, check your facility's policy regarding infection control.

Pediatric pointers

Infection is the most common cause of lymphadenopathy in children. The condition is commonly associated with otitis media and pharyngitis.

Provide antipyretics if the child has a history of febrile seizures.

M

McBurney's sign

A telltale indicator of localized peritoneal inflammation in appendicitis, McBurney's sign is tenderness elicited by palpating the right lower quadrant over McBurney's point. Before McBurney's sign is elicited, the abdomen is inspected for distention and auscultated for hypoactive or absent bowel sounds.

History and physical examination

Ask the patient about abdominal pain. When did it begin? Does coughing, movement, eating, or elimination worsen or help relieve it? Also ask about the development of other signs and symptoms. Ask the patient to point with a finger to the spot where the pain is worst.

Continue light palpation of the patient's abdomen to detect additional tenderness, rigidity, guarding, or pain. Observe the patient's facial expression for signs of pain, such as grimacing or wincing. (See *Eliciting McBurney's sign.*)

Common medical causes

♦ ***Appendicitis.*** McBurney's sign appears within 2 to 12 hours after the onset of appendicitis, after initial pain in the epigastric and periumbilical area shifts to the right lower quadrant (McBurney's point). This persistent point pain increases with walking or coughing. Nausea and vomiting may occur from the start. Boardlike abdominal rigidity and rebound tenderness accompany cutaneous skin sensitivity, fever, constipation or diarrhea, tachycardia, retractive respirations, anorexia, and moderate malaise.

Rupture of the appendix causes sudden cessation of pain. Then, signs of peritonitis develop, such as severe abdominal pain, pallor, hypoactive or absent bowel sounds, diaphoresis, and high fever.

Special considerations

Draw blood for laboratory tests and prepare the patient for abdominal X-rays to confirm appendicitis. Expect to prepare the patient for appendectomy.

Pediatric pointers

McBurney's sign is also elicited in children with appendicitis.

Geriatric pointers

In elderly patients, McBurney's sign (as well as other peritoneal signs) may be decreased or absent.

McMurray's sign

Frequently an indicator of medial meniscal injury, McMurray's sign is a palpable, audible click or pop elicited by manipulating the leg. It results when gentle manipulation of the leg traps torn cartilage and then lets it snap free. Because eliciting this sign forces the surface

EXAMINATION TIP

Eliciting McBurney's sign

To elicit McBurney's signs, position the patient supine with his knees slightly flexed and his abdominal muscles relaxed. Then palpate deeply and slowly in the right lower quadrant over McBurney's point — one-third of the distance from the anterior superior iliac spine to the umbilicus. Point tenderness, a positive McBurney's sign, indicates appendicitis.

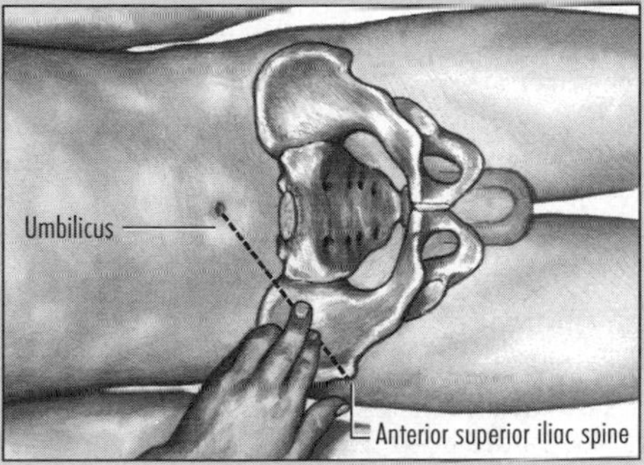

of the tibial plateau against the femoral condyles, such manipulation is contraindicated in patients with suspected fractures of the tibial plateau or femoral condyles.

A positive McMurray's sign augments other findings commonly associated with meniscal injury, such as severe knee pain and decreased range of motion.

History and physical examination

Before McMurray's sign has been elicited, find out if the patient is experiencing acute knee pain. Then ask him to describe any recent knee injury. For example, did his injury place twisting external or internal force on the knee, or did he experience blunt knee trauma from a fall? Also ask about previous knee injury, surgery, or prosthetic replacement or other joint problems, such as arthritis, which could have weakened the knee. Ask if anything aggravates or relieves the pain and if he needs assistance to walk.

Have the patient point to the exact area of pain. Assess the leg's range of motion, both passive and with resistance. Next check for cruciate ligament stability by noting anterior or posterior movement of the tibia on the femur (drawer sign). Finally, measure the quadriceps muscles in both legs for symmetry. (See *Eliciting McMurray's sign*, page 370.)

Common medical causes

♦ ***Meniscal tear.*** In this injury, McMurray's sign can frequently be elicited. Associated signs and symptoms may include acute knee pain at the medial or lateral joint line (depending on injury site) and decreased range of motion or locking of the knee joint. Quadriceps weakening and atrophy frequently occur.

Special considerations

Prepare the patient for knee X-rays, arthroscopy, and arthrography, and obtain previous X-rays for comparison. If trauma precipitated the knee pain and McMurray's sign, an effusion or hemarthrosis may occur. Prepare the patient for aspiration of the joint. Immobilize and apply ice to the knee, and apply a cast or a knee immobilizer.

EXAMINATION TIP

Eliciting McMurray's sign

Eliciting this sign requires special training and gentle manipulation of the patient's leg to avoid extending a meniscal tear or locking the knee. If you have been trained, place the patient in a supine position and flex his affected knee until his heel nearly touches his buttocks. Place your thumb and index finger on either side of the knee joint space and grasp his heel with your other hand. Then rotate the foot and lower leg laterally to test the posterior aspect of the medial meniscus. To test the lateral meniscus, follow the same procedure with medial rotation of the foot and lower leg.

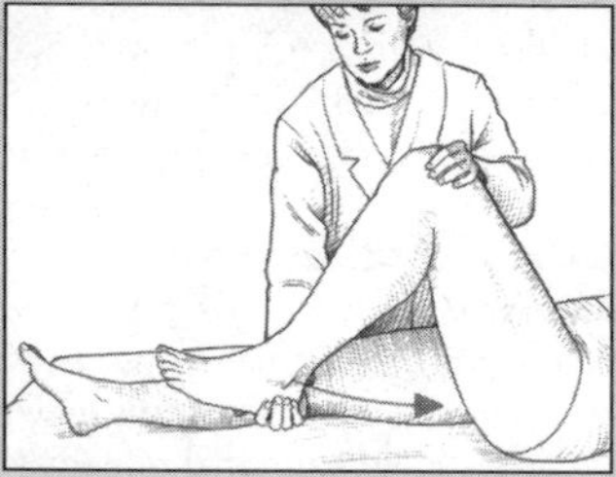

Keeping the foot in a lateral position, extend the knee to a 90-degree angle to test the anterior aspect of the medial meniscus. You can use a median foot position to test the anterior aspect of the lateral meniscus. A palpable or audible click — positive McMurray's sign — indicates a meniscal tear.

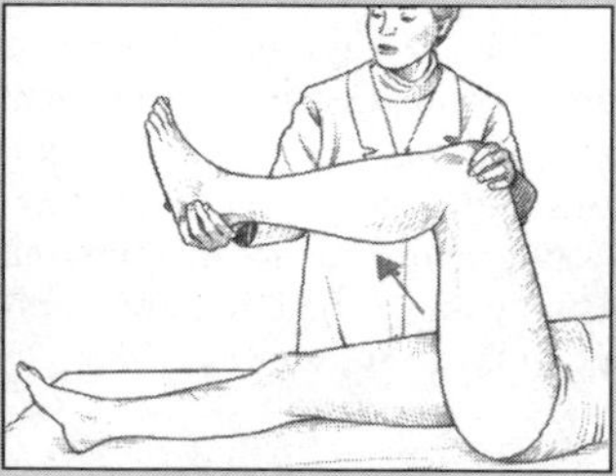

Pediatric pointers

McMurray's sign in adolescents is usually elicited when sports injury has caused a meniscal tear. It may also be elicited in children with congenital discoid meniscus.

Melena

A common sign of upper GI bleeding, melena is the passage of black, tarry stools commonly with a distinctive odor. Characteristic color results from bacterial degradation and the action of hydrochloric acid on the blood as it travels through the GI tract. At least 60 ml of blood is needed to cause this sign. (See *Comparing melena and hematochezia.*)

Severe melena can signal acute bleeding and life-threatening hypovolemic shock. Usually, melena indicates bleeding from the esophagus, stomach, or duodenum, although it can also occur after bleeding from the jejunum, ileum, or ascending colon. In addition, this sign can result from swallowing blood, as in epistaxis; from certain drugs; and from alcohol. Because false melena may be caused by ingestion of lead, iron, bismuth, or licorice (which causes black stools without the presence of blood), all black stools should be tested for occult blood.

Emergency interventions

If the patient is experiencing severe melena, quickly take orthostatic vital signs to detect hypovolemic shock. A decline of 10 mm Hg or more in systolic pressure or an increase of 10 beats or more in pulse rate suggests volume depletion. Quickly look for other signs of shock, such as tachycardia, tachypnea, and cool, clammy skin. Insert a large-gauge I.V. line to administer replacement fluids and allow blood transfusion. Place the patient flat on his back with his head turned to the side and his

Comparing melena and hematochezia

The site, amount, and rate of blood flow through the GI tract determine whether a patient will develop melena (black, tarry stools) or hematochezia (bright red, bloody stools). Usually, melena indicates *upper* GI bleeding, and hematochezia indicates *lower* GI bleeding. However, in some disorders, melena may alternate with hematochezia. This chart helps differentiate these two often-related signs.

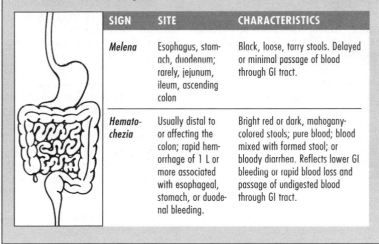

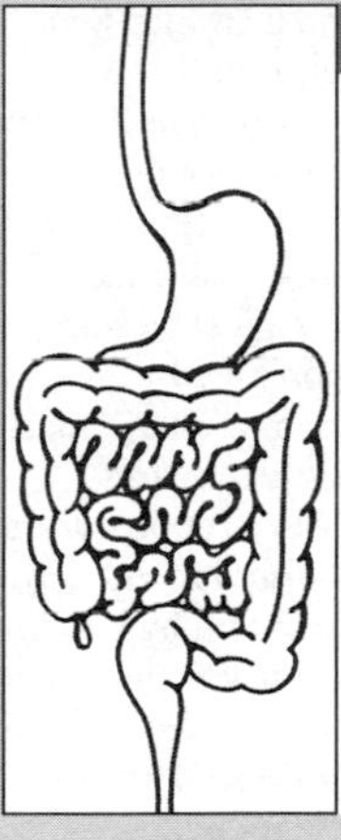

SIGN	SITE	CHARACTERISTICS
Melena	Esophagus, stomach, duodenum; rarely, jejunum, ileum, ascending colon	Black, loose, tarry stools. Delayed or minimal passage of blood through GI tract.
Hematochezia	Usually distal to or affecting the colon; rapid hemorrhage of 1 L or more associated with esophageal, stomach, or duodenal bleeding.	Bright red or dark, mahogany-colored stools; pure blood; blood mixed with formed stool; or bloody diarrhea. Reflects lower GI bleeding or rapid blood loss and passage of undigested blood through GI tract.

feet elevated. Administer supplemental oxygen as needed.

History and physical examination

If the patient's condition permits, ask when he discovered his stools were black and tarry. Ask about the frequency and quantity of bowel movements. Has he had melena before? Ask about other signs and symptoms, notably hematemesis or hematochezia, and about use of anti-inflammatory drugs, alcohol, and other GI irritants. Also, find out if he has a history of GI lesions or ulcers.

Next, inspect the patient's mouth and nasopharynx for evidence of bleeding. Perform an abdominal examination that includes auscultation, palpation, and percussion.

Common medical causes

♦ ***Colon cancer.*** Early tumor growth on the right side of the colon may cause melena accompanied by abdominal aching, pressure, or cramps. As the disease progresses, the patient develops weakness, fatigue, and anemia. Eventually, he also experiences diarrhea or obstipation, anorexia, weight loss, vomiting, and other signs of intestinal obstruction.

When a tumor is on the left side, melena seldom occurs until late in the disease. Early tumor growth commonly causes rectal bleeding with intermittent abdominal fullness or cramping and rectal pressure. As the disease progresses, findings may include obstipation, diarrhea, or pencil-shaped stools. At this stage, bleeding from the colon is signaled by melena or bloody stools.

♦ ***Ebola virus infection.*** Melena, hematemesis, and bleeding from the nose, gums, and vagina may occur late in this disorder. Patients usually report abrupt onset of headache, malaise, myalgia, high fever, diarrhea, abdominal pain, dehydration, and lethargy on the 5th day of exposure. Pleuritic chest pain, dry hacking cough, and pharyngitis have also been noted. A maculopapular rash appears between days 5 and 7.

♦ ***Esophageal cancer.*** Melena is a late sign. Increasing obstruction first causes painless dysphagia, then rapid weight loss. The patient may experience steady chest pain with substernal fullness, nausea, vomiting, or hematemesis. Other findings may include hoarseness, cough (possibly hemoptysis), hiccups, sore throat, and halitosis.

♦ ***Esophageal varices (ruptured).*** This life-threatening disorder can cause melena, hematochezia, and hematemesis. Melena is preceded by signs of shock, such as tachycardia, tachypnea, hypotension, and cool, clammy skin. Agitation or confusion signals developing hepatic encephalopathy.

♦ ***Gastritis.*** Melena and hematemesis are common. The patient may also experience belching, nausea, vomiting, malaise, or mild epigastric or abdominal discomfort that's exacerbated by eating.

♦ ***Mallory-Weiss syndrome.*** Melena and hematemesis follow vomiting. Severe upper abdominal bleeding leads to signs and symptoms of shock, such as tachycardia, tachypnea, hypotension, and cool, clammy skin. The patient may also report epigastric or back pain.

♦ ***Mesenteric vascular occlusion.*** This life-threatening disorder causes slight melena with 2 to 3 days of persistent, mild abdominal pain. Later, abdominal pain becomes severe and may be accompanied by tenderness, distention, guarding, or rigidity. The patient may also experience anorexia, vomiting, fever, or profound shock.

♦ ***Peptic ulcer.*** Melena may signal life-threatening hemorrhage after vascular penetration. The patient may also experience nausea, vomiting, hematemesis, hematochezia, and diffuse epigastric pain that's gnawing, burning, or sharp. With hypovolemic shock come tachycardia, tachypnea, hypotension, dizziness, syncope, and cool, clammy skin.

♦ ***Small-bowel tumors.*** These tumors may bleed and cause melena. Other signs and symptoms may include abdominal pain, distention, and increasing frequency and pitch of bowel sounds.

♦ ***Thrombocytopenia.*** Melena or hematochezia may accompany other manifestations of bleeding tendency: hematemesis, epistaxis, petechiae, ecchymoses, hematuria, vaginal bleeding, and characteristic blood-filled oral bullae. Typically, the patient displays malaise, fatigue, weakness, and lethargy.

♦ ***Typhoid fever.*** Melena or hematochezia occurs late in this disorder and may occur with hypotension and hypothermia. Other late findings may include mental dullness or delirium, marked abdominal distention and diarrhea, marked weight loss, and profound fatigue.

♦ ***Yellow fever.*** Melena, hematochezia, and hematemesis are ominous signs of hemorrhage, a classic feature that occurs with jaundice. Other findings may include fever, headache, nausea, epistaxis, albuminuria, petechiae and mucosal hemorrhage, or dizziness.

Other causes

♦ ***Drugs and alcohol.*** Aspirin, other nonsteroidal anti-inflammatory drugs, and alcohol all can cause gastric irritation and consequent melena.

Special considerations

Monitor vital signs and look closely for signs of hypovolemic shock. For general comfort, encourage bed rest, and keep the patient's perianal area clean and dry to prevent skin irritation and breakdown. Prepare him for diagnostic tests, such as blood studies, gastroscopy or other endoscopic studies, barium swallow, or upper GI series.

Pediatric pointers
Neonates may experience melena neonatorum due to extravasation of blood into the alimentary canal. In older children, melena usually results from peptic ulcer, gastritis, and Meckel's diverticulum.

Geriatric pointers
In elderly patients who have recurrent intermittent GI bleeding without a clear etiology, angiography or exploratory laparotomy should be considered if the risk from continued anemia outweighs the risk associated with the procedures.

MENORRHAGIA

Menorrhagia is prolonged or excessive menstrual bleeding. Bleeding can be perceived as or heavier than normal; blood loss is 80 ml or more per menstrual cycle. Among the causes of menorrhagia are endocrine diseases, hypertension, diabetes mellitus, drug therapy, blood disorders, uterine disorders, and gynecologic procedures.

Emergency interventions
Evaluate hemodynamic status by taking orthostatic vital signs. Insert a large-gauge I.V. line to begin fluid replacement if the patient shows an increase of 10 beats/minute in pulse rate, a decrease of 10 mm Hg in systolic blood pressure, or other signs of hypovolemic shock, such as pallor, tachycardia, tachypnea, or cool, clammy skin. Place the patient in a supine position with her feet elevated, and administer supplemental oxygen as needed. Then prepare the patient for a pelvic examination to help determine the cause of bleeding.

History
If the patient's condition permits, obtain a history. Determine her age at menarche, the duration of menstrual periods, and the interval between them. Establish the date of the patient's last menses, and ask about recent changes in her normal menstrual pattern. Have the patient describe the character and amount of bleeding. For example, how many pads or tampons does she use? Has she noted clots or tissue in the blood? Further, ask about other signs and symptoms before and during the menstrual period.

Next, ask if the patient is sexually active. Does she use a method of birth control? If so, what kind? Could she be pregnant? Be sure to note the number of pregnancies, the outcome of each, and any pregnancy-related complications. Find out the dates of her most recent pelvic examination and Pap smear and the details of previous gynecologic infections or neoplasms. In addition, be sure to ask about previous episodes of abnormal bleeding and the outcome of treatment. If possible, obtain a pregnancy history of the patient's mother, and determine if the patient was exposed in utero to diethylstilbestrol.

Be sure to ask the patient about her general health and medical history. Note particularly if the patient or her family has a history of thyroid, adrenal, or hepatic disease, blood dyscrasias, or tuberculosis because these may predispose to menorrhagia. Also, ask about the patient's past surgical procedures and recent emotional stress. In addition, find out if the patient has undergone X-ray or other radiation therapy.

Common medical causes
- ***Blood dyscrasias.*** Menorrhagia is one of several possible signs of a bleeding disorder. Other possible associated findings include epistaxis, bleeding gums, purpura, hematemesis, hematuria, and melena.
- ***Hypothyroidism.*** Menorrhagia is a frequent early sign and is accompanied by such nonspecific findings as fatigue, cold intolerance, constipation, and weight gain despite anorexia. As hypothyroidism

progresses, intellectual and motor activity decrease; the skin becomes dry, pale, cool, and doughy; the hair becomes dry and sparse; and the nails become thick and brittle. Myalgia, hoarseness, decreased libido, infertility, and delayed deep tendon reflexes commonly occur. Eventually, the patient develops a characteristic dull, expressionless face and edema of the face, hands, and feet. Other possible findings, such as bradycardia or abdominal distention, may occur.

♦ ***Uterine fibroids.*** Menorrhagia is the most common sign, but other forms of abnormal uterine bleeding, as well as dysmenorrhea or leukorrhea, can also occur. Possible related findings include abdominal pain, a feeling of abdominal heaviness, backache, constipation, urinary urgency or frequency, and an enlarged uterus, which usually isn't tender.

Other causes

♦ ***Drugs.*** Use of oral contraceptives may cause sudden onset of profuse, prolonged menorrhagia. Anticoagulants have been associated with excessive menstrual flow. Injectable or implanted contraceptives cause menorrhagia in some women.

♦ **Herb alert** Herbal medicines such as ginseng can cause postmenopausal bleeding.

♦ ***Intrauterine devices.*** Menorrhagia can result from the use of intrauterine contraceptive devices.

Special considerations

Continue to monitor the patient closely for signs of hypovolemia. Monitor intake and output, and estimate uterine blood loss comparing the numbers of sanitary napkins or tampons used during an abnormal period and a normal period. To help decrease blood flow, encourage the patient to rest and to avoid strenuous activities.

Prepare the patient for a pelvic examination if one hasn't already been performed, and obtain blood and urine samples for pregnancy testing.

Pediatric pointers

Irregular menstrual function in young girls may be accompanied by hemorrhage and resulting anemia.

Geriatric pointers

In postmenopausal women, vaginal bleeding can result from hormone therapy or from endometrial atrophy. Malignancy should be ruled out.

METRORRHAGIA

Metrorrhagia — uterine bleeding that occurs between menstrual periods — can range from staining to hemorrhage. It may be the only indication of an underlying gynecologic disorder or can be a result of stress, drug therapy, gynecologic treatments, and intrauterine devices. It's a common sign of slight physiologic bleeding from the endometrium during ovulation.

History

Begin your evaluation by obtaining a thorough menstrual history. Ask the patient her age at menarche and about the duration of menstrual periods, the interval between them, and the average number of tampons or pads she uses. When does metrorrhagia usually occur in relation to her period? Does she experience other signs or symptoms? Find out the date of her last menses, and ask about other recent changes in her normal menstrual pattern. Get details of previous gynecologic problems. If applicable, obtain a contraceptive and obstetric history. Record the dates of her last Papanicolaou test and pelvic examination. Ask if episodes of bleeding coincide with sexual activity. Next, ask about her general health and recent changes. Is she under emotional stress? If possible, obtain a pregnancy history of the patient's mother. Was the patient exposed in utero to diethylstilbestrol? (This drug has been linked to vaginal adenosis.)

Common medical causes

♦ ***Cervicitis.*** This nonspecific infection may cause spontaneous bleeding, spotting, or posttraumatic bleeding. Assessment reveals red, granular, irregular lesions on the external cervix. Purulent vaginal discharge (with or without odor), lower abdominal pain, and fever may occur.

♦ ***Dysfunctional uterine bleeding.*** Abnormal uterine bleeding not caused by pregnancy or a major gynecologic disorder usually occurs as metrorrhagia, although menorrhagia is possible. Bleeding may be profuse or scant, intermittent or constant.

♦ ***Endometrial polyps.*** In most patients, this disorder causes abnormal bleeding—usually intermenstrual or postmenopausal. Some patients remain asymptomatic, however.

♦ ***Endometriosis.*** Metrorrhagia (usually premenstrual) may be the only indication of this disorder, or it may accompany pelvic discomfort and dyspareunia. A tender, fixed adnexal mass may be palpable on bimanual examination.

♦ ***Endometritis.*** This disorder causes metrorrhagia and purulent vaginal discharge. It also causes fever, lower abdominal pain, and abdominal muscle spasm.

♦ ***Gynecologic cancer.*** Metrorrhagia is commonly an early sign of cervical or uterine cancer. Later, the patient may experience weight loss, pelvic pain, fatigue and, possibly, an abdominal mass.

♦ ***Uterine leiomyomas.*** Besides metrorrhagia, these tumors may cause lower abdominal pain that worsens with menses, backache, constipation, and urinary frequency or retention. Tumors are usually nontender.

♦ ***Vaginal adenosis.*** This disorder commonly causes metrorrhagia. Palpation reveals roughening or nodules in affected vaginal areas.

Other causes

♦ ***Drugs.*** Anticoagulants and oral, injectable, or implanted contraceptives may cause metrorrhagia.

♦ **Herb alert** Herbal medicines, such as ginseng, can cause postmenopausal bleeding.

♦ ***Surgery and procedures.*** Cervical conization and cauterization may cause metrorrhagia.

Special considerations

Obtain blood and urine samples for pregnancy testing. A pelvic examination may be indicated. Encourage bed rest to reduce bleeding. Give analgesics for discomfort.

Pediatric pointers

Neonate females may exhibit vaginal bleeding for a few days due to in utero exposure to estrogen. Any other vaginal bleeding should be considered pathologic and investigated immediately.

Geriatric pointers

Vaginal bleeding in postmenopausal woman can be a result of hormone replacement therapy.

Miosis

Miosis—pupillary constriction caused by contraction of the sphincter muscle in the iris—is a normal response to fatigue, increased light, and administration of miotic drugs; part of the eye's accommodation reflex; and part of the aging process (pupil size steadily decreases from adolescence to about age 60). However, it can also stem from ocular or neurologic disorders, trauma, use of systemic drugs, or contact lens overuse.

History and physical examination

Begin by asking the patient if he has experienced other ocular symptoms, and have him describe their onset, duration, and intensity. Does he wear contact lenses? Be sure to ask about trauma, serious systemic disease, and use of topical and systemic medications.

Next, perform a thorough eye examination. Examine and compare both pupils for size (many persons have a normal discrepancy), color, shape, reaction to light, accommodation, and consensual light response. Examine both eyes for additional signs, and then evaluate extraocular muscle function by assessing the six cardinal fields of gaze. Finally, test visual acuity in each eye, with and without correction, paying particular attention to blurred or decreased vision in the miotic eye.

Common medical causes

♦ ***Argyll Robertson pupil.*** This light-near dissociative response is most commonly associated with neurosyphilis. It's usually bilateral, and patients don't experience symptoms directly related to it. Pupils are asymmetrical and irregular; they react poorly to light but constrict normally to a near stimulus.

♦ ***Cerebrovascular arteriosclerosis.*** Miosis is usually unilateral, depending on the site and extent of vascular damage. Other findings may include visual blurring, slurred speech or possibly aphasia, loss of muscle tone, memory loss, vertigo, and headache.

♦ ***Cluster headache.*** Ipsilateral miosis, tearing, conjunctival injection, and ptosis commonly accompany a severe cluster headache, along with facial flushing and sweating, bradycardia, restlessness, and nasal stuffiness or rhinorrhea.

♦ ***Corneal foreign body.*** Miosis in the affected eye occurs with pain, a foreign-body sensation, slight vision loss, conjunctival injection, photophobia, and profuse tearing.

♦ ***Corneal ulcer.*** Miosis in the affected eye appears with moderate pain, visual blurring and possibly some vision loss, and diffuse conjunctival injection.

♦ ***Horner's syndrome.*** Moderate miosis is common in this congenital or acquired syndrome and occurs ipsilaterally to the lesion. Related ipsilateral findings include a sluggish pupillary reflex, slight enophthalmos, moderate ptosis, facial anhidrosis, transient conjunctival injection, and vascular headache. When the syndrome is congenital, the iris on the affected side may appear lighter.

♦ ***Hyphema.*** Usually the result of blunt trauma, hyphema can cause miosis with moderate pain, visual blurring, diffuse conjunctival injection, and slight eyelid swelling. The eyeball may feel harder than normal.

♦ ***Iritis (acute).*** Miosis typically occurs in the affected eye along with decreased pupillary reflex, severe eye pain, photophobia, visual blurring, conjunctival injection and, possibly, pus accumulation in the anterior chamber. It can be traumatic, idiopathic, or associated with systemic disease.

♦ ***Neuropathy.*** Two forms of neuropathy occasionally cause miosis. In *diabetic neuropathy,* related effects may include paresthesia, other sensory disturbances, extremity pain, orthostatic hypotension, impotence, incontinence, and leg muscle weakness and atrophy. In *alcoholic neuropathy,* related effects are progressive, variable muscle weakness and wasting; various sensory disturbances; and hypoactive deep tendon reflexes.

♦ ***Parry-Romberg syndrome.*** This facial hemiatrophy typically causes miosis, sluggish pupillary reflexes, enophthalmos, nystagmus, ptosis, and different-colored irises.

♦ ***Physiologic anisocoria.*** This is a physiologic difference in the size of the two pupils. The patient usually has no symptoms and may not be aware of the difference. Response to light and near vision testing are usually normal. Difference in the size of the pupils is usually less than 2 cm.

♦ ***Pontine hemorrhage.*** Bilateral miosis is characteristic, along with rapid onset of coma, total paralysis, decerebrate posture, absent doll's eye sign, and a positive Babinski's sign.

♦ ***Uveitis.*** *Anterior uveitis* commonly causes miosis in the affected eye, moderate to severe eye pain, severe conjunctival injection, and photophobia. In *posterior uveitis,* miosis is accompanied by gradual onset of eye pain, photophobia, visual floaters, visual blurring, conjunctival injection and, commonly, distorted pupil shape.

Other causes

♦ ***Chemical burns.*** An opaque cornea may make miosis difficult to detect. Chemical burns may also cause moderate to severe pain, diffuse conjunctival injection, inability to keep the eye open, visual blurring, and blistering.

♦ ***Drugs.*** Such topical drugs as acetylcholine, carbachol, demecarium bromide, echothiophate iodide, and pilocarpine are used to treat eye disorders specifically for their miotic effect. Such systemic drugs as barbiturates, cholinergics, cholinesterase inhibitors, clonidine (overdose), guanethidine, opiates, and reserpine also cause miosis, as does deep anesthesia.

Special considerations

Because any ocular abnormality can be a source of fear and anxiety, reassure and support the patient. Clearly explain diagnostic tests ordered, which may include a complete ophthalmologic examination or a neurologic workup.

Pediatric pointers

Miosis occurs frequently in the neonate, simply because he's asleep or sleepy most of the time.

MOUTH LESIONS

Mouth lesions include ulcers (the most common type), cysts, firm nodules, hemorrhagic lesions, papules, vesicles, bullae, and erythematous lesions. They may occur anywhere on the lips, cheeks, hard and soft palate, salivary glands, tongue, gingivae, or mucous membranes. Many are painful and can be readily detected. Some, however, are asymptomatic; when these occur deep in the mouth, they may be discovered only through a complete oral examination. (See *Common mouth lesions,* page 378.) Mouth lesions can result from trauma, infection, systemic disease, drugs, or radiation therapy.

History and physical examination

Begin your evaluation with a thorough history. Ask the patient when the lesions appeared and whether he has noticed pain, odor, or drainage. Also ask about associated complaints, particularly skin lesions. Obtain a complete medication history, including drug allergies, and a complete medical history. Note especially any malignancy, sexually transmitted disease, I.V. drug use, recent infection, or trauma. Ask about his dental history, including oral hygiene habits, frequency of dental examinations, and the date of his most recent dental visit.

Next, perform a complete oral examination, noting lesion sites and character. Examine the patient's lips for color and texture. Inspect and palpate the buccal mucosa and tongue for color, texture, and contour; note especially painless ulcers on the sides or base of the tongue. Hold the tongue with a piece of gauze, lift it, and examine its underside and the floor of the mouth. Depress the tongue with a tongue blade and examine the oropharynx. Inspect teeth and gums, noting missing, broken, or discolored teeth; dental caries; excessive debris; and bleed-

Common mouth lesions

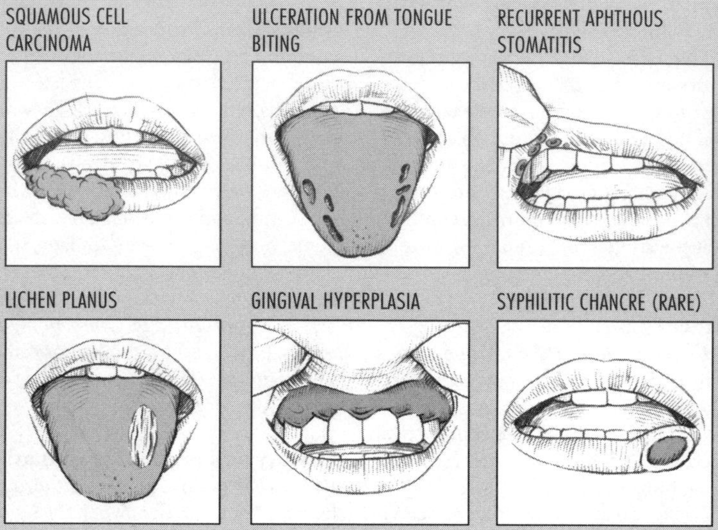

ing, inflamed, swollen, or discolored gums. Palpate the neck for adenopathy, especially in patients over age 45 who smoke tobacco or use alcohol excessively.

Common medical causes

◆ ***Acquired immunodeficiency syndrome (AIDS).*** Oral lesions may represent an early indication of the immunosuppression that's characteristic of this disease. Fungal infections can occur; oral candidiasis is the most common. Bacterial or viral infections of oral mucosa, tongue, gingivae, and periodontal tissue occur. The primary oral neoplasm associated with AIDS is Kaposi's sarcoma, usually found on the hard palate. It may appear initially as an asymptomatic, flat or raised lesion, ranging in color from red to blue to purple. As these tumors grow, they may ulcerate and become painful.

◆ ***Actinomycosis (cervicofacial).*** This chronic fungal infection typically causes small, firm, flat, painful or painless swellings on the oral mucosa and under the skin of the jaw and neck. Swellings may indurate and form abscesses or fistulas with a characteristic purulent yellow discharge.

◆ ***Behçet's syndrome.*** This chronic, progressive syndrome causes small, painful ulcers on the lips, gums, buccal mucosa, and tongue. In severe cases, the ulcers also form on the palate, pharynx, and esophagus. Typically, the ulcers have a reddened border and are covered with a gray or yellow exudate. Similar lesions appear on the scrotum and penis or labia majora; small pustules or papules on the trunk and limbs; and painful erythematous nodules on the shins. Ocular lesions may also develop.

◆ ***Candidiasis.*** This common fungal infection characteristically causes soft, elevated plaques on the buccal mucosa, tongue, and sometimes the palate, gingivae, and floor of the mouth; the plaques may be wiped away. The lesions of *acute atrophic candidiasis* are red and painful. The lesions of *chronic hyperplastic candidiasis* are white and firm. Localized areas of redness, pruritus, and foul odor may be present.

◆ ***Discoid lupus erythematosus.*** Oral lesions are common, typically appearing on the tongue, buccal mucosa, and palate as erythematous areas with white spots and radiating white striae. Associated findings include skin lesions on the face, possibly extending to the neck, ears, and scalp; if the scalp is involved, alopecia may result. Hair follicles are enlarged and filled with scale all over the body.

◆ ***Erythema multiforme.*** This acute inflammatory skin disease causes sudden onset of vesicles and bullae on the lips and buccal mucosa. Also, erythematous macules and papules form symmetrically on the hands, arms, feet, legs, face, and neck and, possibly, in the eyes and on the genitalia. Lymphadenopathy may also occur. Manifestations of visceral involvement include fever, malaise, cough, throat and chest pain, vomiting, diarrhea, myalgias, arthralgias, fingernail loss, blindness, hematuria, and signs of renal failure.

◆ ***Gingivitis (acute necrotizing ulcerative).*** This condition causes a sudden onset of gingival ulcers covered with a grayish white pseudomembrane. Other findings may include tender or painful gingivae, intermittent gingival bleeding, and halitosis.

◆ ***Herpes simplex.*** In primary infection, a brief period of prodromal tingling and itching, accompanied by fever and pharyngitis, is followed by eruption of vesicles on any part of the oral mucosa, especially the tongue, gums, and cheeks. Vesicles form on an erythematous base, then rupture and leave a painful ulcer, followed by a yellowish crust. Other findings include submaxillary lymphadenopathy, increased salivation, halitosis, anorexia, and keratoconjunctivitis.

◆ ***Herpes zoster.*** This common viral infection may cause painful vesicles on the buccal mucosa, tongue, uvula, pharynx, and larynx. Small red nodules commonly erupt unilaterally around the thorax or vertically on the arms and legs and rapidly become vesicles filled with clear fluid or pus; vesicles dry and form scabs about 10 days after eruption. Fever and general malaise accompany pruritus, paresthesia or hyperesthesia, and tenderness along the course of the involved sensory nerve.

◆ ***Inflammatory fibrous hyperplasia.*** This painless nodular swelling of the buccal mucosa typically results from cheek trauma or irritation and is characterized by pink, smooth, pedunculated areas of soft tissue.

◆ ***Leukoplakia, erythroplakia.*** *Leukoplakia* is a white lesion that can't be removed simply by rubbing the mucosal surface — unlike candidiasis. It may occur in response to chronic irritation from dentures or tobacco, or it may represent dysplasia or early squamous cell carcinoma. *Erythroplakia* is red and edematous and has a velvety surface. Ninety percent of all cases of erythroplakia are either dysplasia or cancer.

◆ ***Pemphigoid (benign mucosal).*** This autoimmune disease is characterized by vesicles on the oral mucous membranes, the conjunctiva and, less commonly, the skin. Mouth lesions typically develop months or even years before other manifestations and may occur as desquamative patchy gingivitis or as a vesicobullous eruption. Secondary fibrous bands may lead to dysphagia, hoarseness, and blindness. Recurrent skin lesions include vesicobullous eruptions, usually on the inguinal area and extremities, and an erythematous, vesicobullous plaque on the scalp and face near the affected mucous membranes.

◆ ***Pemphigus.*** This chronic skin disease is characterized by vesicles and bullae that appear in cycles. Bullae on the oral mucosa rupture, leaving painful lesions

that bleed easily. Associated findings include bullae anywhere on the body, denudation of the skin, and pruritus.
◆ ***Pyogenic granuloma.*** Commonly the result of trauma or irritation, this soft, painless nodule, papule, or polypoid mass usually appears on the gingivae but can also erupt on the lips, tongue, or buccal mucosa. The affected area may be smooth or have a warty surface; erythema develops in the surrounding mucosa. The lesions may ulcerate, producing a purulent exudate.
◆ ***Squamous cell carcinoma.*** It may erupt in areas of leukoplakia and is most common on the lower lip, but it may also occur on the edge of the tongue or the floor of the mouth. High-risk factors include chronic smoking and alcohol intake.
◆ ***Stomatitis (aphthous).*** This common disease is characterized by recurrent, painful ulcerations of the oral mucosa, usually on the dorsum of the tongue, gingivae, and hard palate. In *recurrent aphthous stomatitis minor,* the ulcer begins as one or more erosions covered by a gray membrane and surrounded by a red halo. It's commonly found on the buccal and lip mucosa and junction, tongue, soft palate, pharynx, gingivae, and all places not bound to the periosteum. In *recurrent aphthous stomatitis major,* large, painful ulcers commonly occur on the lips, cheek, tongue, and soft palate; they may last up to 6 weeks and leave scars.
◆ ***Systemic lupus erythematosus.*** Oral lesions are common and appear as erythematous areas associated with edema, petechiae, and superficial ulcers with a red halo and a tendency to bleed. Primary effects include nondeforming arthritis, butterfly rash across the nose and cheeks, and photosensitivity.

Other causes
◆ ***Drugs.*** Various chemotherapeutic agents can directly cause stomatitis. Also, allergic reactions to penicillin, sulfonamides, gold, quinine, streptomycin, phenytoin, aspirin, and barbiturates commonly cause lesions to develop and erupt.
◆ ***Radiation therapy.*** This treatment may cause oral lesions.

Special considerations
If the patient's mouth ulcers are painful, provide a topical anesthetic such as lidocaine.

Pediatric pointers
Causes of mouth ulcers in children include chicken pox, measles, scarlet fever, diphtheria, and hand-foot-and-mouth disease. In neonates, mouth ulcers can result from candidiasis or congenital syphilis.

MURMURS

Murmurs are auscultatory sounds heard in the heart chambers or major arteries. They're classified by their timing and duration in the cardiac cycle, auscultatory location, loudness, configuration, pitch, and quality. *Timing* can be characterized as systolic, holosystolic (continuous throughout systole), diastolic, or continuous through systole and diastole; systolic and diastolic murmurs can be further characterized as early, middle, or late. *Location* refers to the area of maximum loudness, such as the apex, the lower left sternal border, or an intercostal space. *Loudness* is graded on a scale of I to VI, with I signifying the faintest audible murmur. *Configuration,* or shape, refers to the nature of loudness — crescendo, decrescendo, crescendo-decrescendo, decrescendo-crescendo, plateau (even), or variable (uneven). The murmur's *pitch* may be high or low. Its *quality* may be described as harsh, rumbling, blowing, scratching, buzzing, musical, or squeaking.

Murmurs can reflect accelerated blood flow through normal or abnormal valves; forward blood flow through a narrowed or irregular valve or into a dilated vessel; blood backflow through an incompetent valve, septal defect, or patent ductus arteriosus; or decreased blood viscosity. Commonly the result of organic heart disease, murmurs occasionally may signal an emergency situation — for example, a loud holosystolic murmur after acute myocardial infarction (MI) may signal papillary muscle rupture or ventricular septal defect (VSD). Murmurs may also follow surgical implantation of a prosthetic valve. (See *When murmurs signal an emergency*.)

EMERGENCY INTERVENTIONS

When murmurs signal an emergency

Although not normally a sign of emergency, murmurs — especially newly developed ones — may signal a serious complication in patients with bacterial endocarditis or recent acute myocardial infarction (MI).

When caring for a patient with known or suspected bacterial endocarditis, carefully auscultate for any new murmurs. Their development along with crackles, distended neck veins, orthopnea, and dyspnea may signal heart failure.

Regular auscultation is also important in a patient who has experienced an acute MI. A loud decrescendo holosystolic murmur at the apex that radiates to the axilla and left sternal border or throughout the chest is significant, particularly in association with a widely split S_2 murmur and an atrial gallop (S_4). This murmur, when accompanied by signs of acute pulmonary edema, usually indicates the development of acute mitral insufficiency due to rupture of the chordae tendineae — a medical emergency.

Some murmurs are innocent, or functional. An *innocent systolic murmur* is generally soft, medium-pitched, and loudest along the left sternal border at the second or third intercostal space. It's exacerbated by physical activity, excitement, fever, pregnancy, anemia, or thyrotoxicosis. Examples include *Still's murmur* in children and *mammary souffle,* commonly heard over either breast during late pregnancy and early postpartum. (See *Detecting congenital murmurs,* pages 382 and 383.)

History and physical examination

If you discover a murmur, try to determine its type through careful auscultation. (See *Identifying common murmurs,* page 384.) Use the bell of your stethoscope for low-pitched murmurs; the diaphragm for high-pitched murmurs.

Next, obtain a patient history. Ask whether the murmur is a new discovery or whether it has been known since birth or childhood. Find out if the patient has experienced associated symptoms, particularly palpitations, dizziness, syncope, chest pain, dyspnea, and fatigue. Explore the patient's medical history, noting especially any incidence of rheumatic fever, heart disease, or heart surgery, particularly prosthetic valve replacement.

Perform a systematic physical examination. Note especially the presence of cardiac arrhythmias, jugular vein distention, and such pulmonary signs as dyspnea, orthopnea, and crackles. Is the patient's liver tender or palpable? Does he have peripheral edema?

Common medical causes

♦ ***Aortic insufficiency***. *Acute aortic insufficiency* typically causes a soft, short diastolic murmur over the left sternal border that's best heard when the patient sits and leans forward and at the end of a forced held expiration. S_2 may be soft or absent. Sometimes, a soft, short midsystolic murmur may also be heard over the second right intercostal space. Associated findings may include tachy-

(Text continues on page 384.)

EXAMINATION TIP

Detecting congenital murmurs

HEART DEFECT	TYPE OF MURMUR
Aorticopulmonary septal defect	◆ *Small defect:* continuous rough or crackling murmur best heard at the upper left sternal border below the left clavicle, possibly accompanied by a systolic ejection click ◆ *Large defect:* harsh systolic murmur heard at the left sternal border
Atrial septal defect	◆ Midsystolic, spindle-shaped murmur of grade II-III intensity with fixed splitting of S_2; heard at upper left sternal border. Large shunts may also produce a low- to medium-pitched early diastolic murmur over the lower left sternal border.
Bicuspid aortic valve	◆ Early systolic, loud, high-pitched ejection sound or click; best heard at the left sternal border and frequently accompanied by a soft, early or midsystolic murmur at the upper right sternal border; aortic component of S_2 usually accentuated at the left sternal border.
Coarctation of the aorta	◆ Usually a systolic ejection click at the base of the heart, at the apex, or occasionally over the carotid arteries; often accompanied by systolic ejection murmur at the base; disorder may also produce a blowing diastolic murmur of aortic insufficiency.
Common atrioventricular canal defects (endocardial cushion defect)	◆ *With competent mitral valve:* midsystolic, spindle-shaped murmur of grade II-III intensity with fixed splitting of S_2; heard at upper left sternal border: may be accompanied by a low- to medium-pitched early diastolic murmur over lower left sternal border. ◆ *With incompetent mitral valve:* early systolic or holosystolic decrescendo murmur at the apex, with a widely split S_2 and often an S_4.
Ebstein's anomaly	◆ Soft, high-pitched holosystolic blowing murmur that increases with inspiration (Carvallo's sigh); best heard over lower left sternal border and xyphoid area; possibly accompanied by a low-pitched diastolic rumbling murmur at the apex. Fixed splitting of S_2, a loud S_4, and a midsystolic click may also be present.
Left ventricular right atrial communication	◆ Holosystolic, grade II-IV decrescendo murmur heard along the lower left sternal border, accompanied by a normal S_2; large shunts also produce a diastolic rumbling murmur over the apex.
Mitral atresia	◆ Nonspecific systolic murmur and diastolic flow rumble at the lower left sternal border; loud and single S_2.

Detecting congenital murmurs *(continued)*

HEART DEFECT	TYPE OF MURMUR
Partial anomalous pulmonary venous connection	◆ Midsystolic, spindle-shaped grade II-III murmur at the upper left sternal border, possibly accompanied by a low- to medium-pitched early diastolic murmur over the left lower sternal order.
Patent ductus arteriosus	◆ Continuous rough or crackling murmur best heard at the upper left sternal border and below the left clavicle.
Pulmonic insufficiency	◆ Early to middiastolic, soft, medium-pitched crescendo-decrescendo murmur best heard at the second or third right intercostal space; increases during inspiration.
Pulmonic stenosis	◆ Early systolic, harsh, grade IV to VI crescendo-decrescendo murmur at the second left intercostal space, possibly radiating along the left sternal border; accompanied by an early systolic click.
Single atrium	◆ Holosystolic regurgitant murmur at the apex, accompanied by a fixed splitting of S_2.
Supravalvular aortic stenosis	◆ Systolic ejection murmur best heard over the second right intercostal space or higher in the episternal notch or over the right lower neck. Aortic closure sound is usually preserved, and no ejection clicks are heard.
Tetralogy of Fallot	◆ Midsystolic murmur with systolic thrill palpable at the left midsternal border; softer murmurs occurring earlier in systole generally indicate a more severe obstruction.
Tricuspid atresia	◆ Variable, depending on associated defects.
Trilogy of Fallot	◆ Systolic, harsh, crescendo-decrescendo murmur, best heard at the upper left sternal border with radiation toward the left clavicle. Pulmonic component of S_2 becomes progressively softer with increasing degrees of obstruction.
Ventricular septal defect	◆ *Small defect:* usually a holosystolic (but may be limited to early or midsystole), grade II to IV decrescendo murmur heard along the lower left sternal border, accompanied by normal S_2. ◆ *Large defect:* a holosystolic murmur at the lower left sternal border and a midsystolic rumbling murmur at the apex, accompanied by increased S_1 at lower left sternal border and increased pulmonic component of S_2.

EXAMINATION TIP

Identifying common murmurs

The timing and configuration of a murmur can help you identify its underlying cause. Learn to recognize the characteristics of these common murmurs.

AORTIC INSUFFICIENCY (CHRONIC)
Thickened valve leaflets fail to close correctly, permitting backflow of blood into the left ventricle

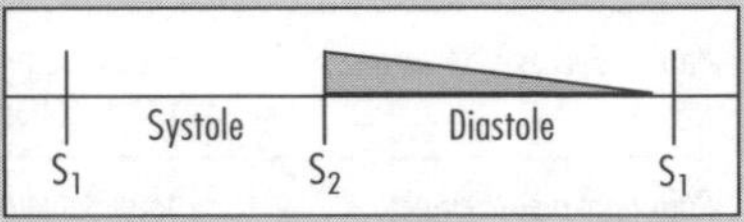

AORTIC STENOSIS
Thickened, scarred, or calcified valve leaflets impede ventricular systolic ejection.

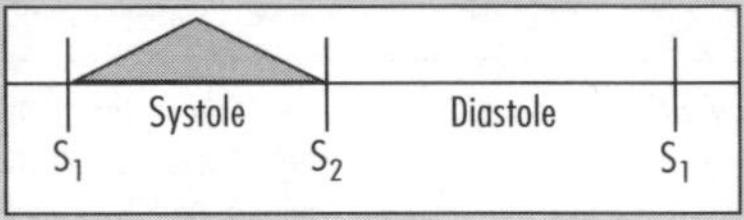

MITRAL VALVE PROLAPSE
Incompetent mitral valve with enlarged posterior leaflet and elongated chordae tendineae bulges into the left atrium.

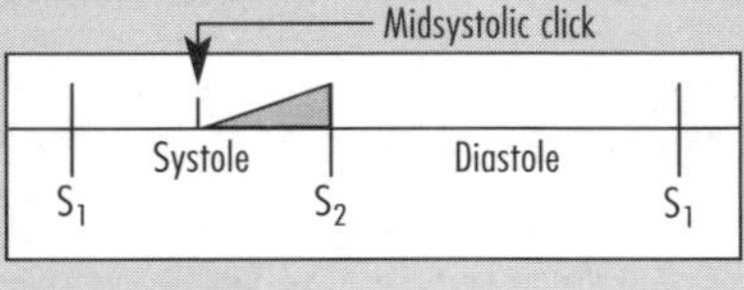

MITRAL INSUFFICIENCY (CHRONIC)
Incompetent mitral valve closure permits backflow of blood into the left atrium.

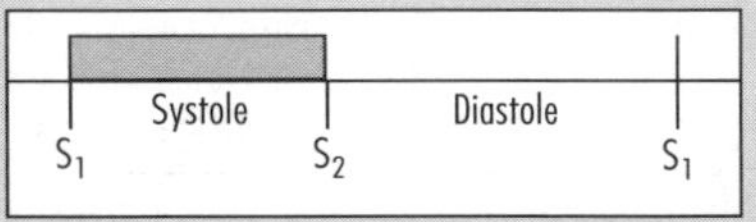

MITRAL STENOSIS
Thickened or scarred valve leaflets cause valve stenosis and restrict blood flow.

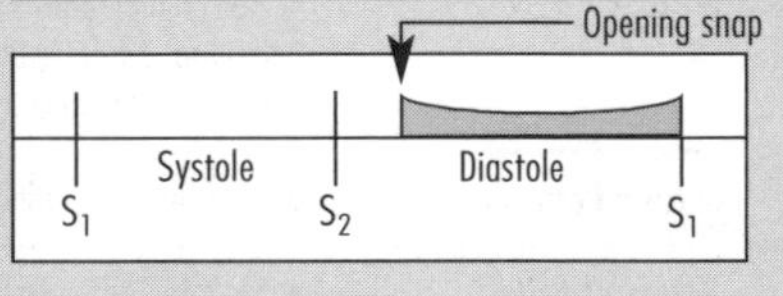

cardia, dyspnea, distended neck veins, crackles, increased fatigue, and pale, cool extremities.

Chronic aortic insufficiency causes a high-pitched, blowing, decrescendo diastolic murmur that's best heard over the second or third right intercostal space or the left sternal border with the patient sitting, leaning forward, and holding his breath after deep expiration. An Austin Flint murmur — a rumbling, middiastolic to late diastolic murmur best heard at the apex — may also be present. Complications may not develop until ages 40 to 50; then, typical findings include palpitations, tachycardia, anginal pain, increased fatigue, dyspnea, orthopnea, and crackles.

♦ ***Aortic stenosis.*** In this valvular disorder, the murmur is systolic, beginning after S_1 and ending at or before aortic valve closure. It's harsh and grating, medium-pitched, and crescendo-decrescendo. Loudest over the second right intercostal space, this murmur may also be heard at the apex, at the suprasternal notch, and over the carotid arteries. In advanced disease, S_2 may be heard as a single sound, with inaudible aortic closure. An early systolic ejection click at the base is typical but is absent when the valve is severely calcified. Associated signs and symptoms usually don't appear until age 30 in congenital aortic stenosis, ages 30 to 65 in stenosis due to rheumatic disease, and after age 65 in calcific aortic stenosis. They may include dizziness, syncope, dyspnea, fatigue, and anginal pain.

♦ ***Cardiomyopathy (hypertrophic).*** This disorder generates a harsh midsystolic murmur, ending at S_2. Best heard over the left sternal border and at the apex, the murmur is commonly accompanied by an audible S_3 or S_4. Major associated symptoms are dyspnea and chest pain; palpitations, dizziness, and syncope may also occur.

♦ ***Mitral insufficiency.*** *Acute mitral insufficiency* is characterized by an early systolic or holosystolic decrescendo murmur at the apex, a widely split S_2, and commonly an S_4. Accompanying findings typically include tachycardia and signs of acute pulmonary edema.

Chronic mitral insufficiency causes a high-pitched, blowing, holosystolic plateau murmur that's loudest at the apex and usually radiates to the axilla or back. Fatigue, dyspnea, and palpitations may also occur.

♦ ***Mitral stenosis.*** In this valvular disorder, the murmur is soft, low-pitched, rumbling, decrescendo-crescendo, and diastolic, accompanied by a loud S_1 and an opening snap — a cardinal sign. It's best heard at the apex with the patient in the left lateral position. In severe stenosis, the murmur of mitral regurgitation may also be heard. Other findings may include hemoptysis, exertional dyspnea and fatigue, and signs of acute pulmonary edema.

♦ ***Mitral valve prolapse.*** This disorder generates a midsystolic to late systolic click with a high-pitched late systolic crescendo murmur, best heard at the apex. Occasionally, multiple clicks may be heard, with or without a systolic murmur. Accompanying findings may include cardiac awareness, migraine headaches, dizziness, weakness, syncope, palpitations, chest pain, dyspnea, severe episodic fatigue, mood swings, or anxiety.

♦ ***Myxomas.*** *A left atrial myxoma* (most common) usually causes a mid-diastolic murmur and a holosystolic murmur that's loudest at the apex, an S_4, an early diastolic thudding sound (tumor plop), and a loud, widely split S_1. Related features may include dyspnea, orthopnea, chest pain, fatigue, weight loss, and syncope.

A *right atrial myxoma* causes a late diastolic rumbling murmur, a holosystolic crescendo murmur, and tumor plop, best heard at the lower left sternal border. Other findings include fatigue, peripheral edema, ascites, and hepatomegaly.

A *left ventricular myxoma* (very rare) causes a systolic murmur best heard at the lower left sternal border, arrhythmias, dyspnea, and syncope. A *right ventricular myxoma* commonly generates a systolic ejection murmur with delayed S_2 and a tumor plop, best heard at the left sternal border. It's accompanied by peripheral edema, hepatomegaly, ascites, dyspnea, and syncope.

♦ ***Papillary muscle rupture.*** In this life-threatening complication of acute MI, a loud holosystolic or decrescendo murmur can be auscultated at the apex. Related findings include severe dyspnea, chest pain, syncope, hemoptysis, tachycardia, and hypotension.

♦ ***Tricuspid insufficiency.*** This valvular abnormality is characterized by a soft, high-pitched, holosystolic blowing murmur that increases with inspiration (Carvallo's sign) and is best heard over the lower left sternal border and the xiphoid area. After a lengthy asymptomatic period, exertional dyspnea and orthopnea may develop as well as neck vein distention, ascites, peripheral cyanosis and edema, and muscle wasting.

♦ ***Tricuspid stenosis.*** This valvular disorder causes a diastolic murmur similar to that of mitral stenosis, but louder with inspiration. S_1 may also be louder. Associated signs and symptoms may include fatigue, distended neck veins, ascites, hepatomegaly, and dyspnea.

Other causes

♦ ***Treatments.*** Prosthetic valve replacement may cause variable murmurs, depending on the location, valve composition, and method of operation.

Special considerations

Prepare the patient for diagnostic tests, such as electrocardiography and echocardiography. Because cardiac abnormality is frightening to the patient, provide emotional support.

Pediatric pointers

Innocent murmurs, such as Still's murmur, are frequently heard in young children and commonly disappear in puberty. Pathognomonic heart murmurs in infants and young children usually result from congenital heart disease, such as atrial and ventricular septal defects. Other murmurs can be acquired, as in rheumatic heart disease.

MUSCLE ATROPHY

[Muscle wasting]

Muscle atrophy results from denervation or prolonged muscle disuse. When deprived of regular exercise, muscle fibers lose both bulk and length, producing a visible loss of muscle size and contour and apparent emaciation or deformity in the affected area. Even slight atrophy usually causes some loss of motion or power.

Atrophy usually results from neuromuscular disease or injury. However, it may also stem from certain metabolic and endocrine disorders and prolonged immobility. Some muscle atrophy also occurs with aging.

History and physical examination

Ask the patient when and where he first noticed the muscle wasting and how it has progressed. Also ask about associated symptoms, such as weakness, pain, loss of sensation, and recent weight loss. Review the patient's medical history for chronic illnesses; musculoskeletal or neurologic disorders, including trauma; and endocrine and metabolic disorders. Ask about use of alcohol and drugs, particularly steroids.

Begin the physical examination by determining the location and extent of atrophy. Visually evaluate small and large muscles. Check all major muscle groups for size, tonicity, and strength. Measure the circumference of all limbs, comparing sides. (See *Measuring limb circumference.*) Check for muscle contractures in all limbs by fully extending joints and noting pain or resistance. Complete the examination by palpating peripheral pulses for quality and rate, assessing sensory function in and around the atrophied area, and testing deep tendon reflexes.

Common medical causes

♦ ***Amyotrophic lateral sclerosis.*** Initial symptoms of this progressive disease include muscle weakness and atrophy that typically begin in one hand, spread to the arm, and then develop in the other hand and arm. Eventually, weakness and atrophy spread to the trunk, neck, tongue, larynx, pharynx, and legs. Progressive respiratory muscle weakness leads to respiratory insufficiency. Other findings include muscle flaccidity, fasciculations, hyperactive deep tendon reflexes, slight leg muscle spasticity, dysphagia, impaired speech, excessive drooling, and depression.

♦ ***Burns.*** Prolonged immobility, fibrous scar tissue formation, pain, and loss of serum proteins from severe burns can limit muscle movement, resulting in atrophy.

◆ ***Hypothyroidism.*** Reversible weakness and atrophy of proximal limb muscles may occur in hypothyroidism. Accompanying findings commonly include muscle cramps and stiffness; cold intolerance; weight gain despite anorexia; mental dullness; dry, pale, cool, doughy skin; puffy face, hands, and feet; and bradycardia.

◆ ***Meniscal tear.*** Quadriceps muscle atrophy, resulting from prolonged knee immobility and muscle weakness, is a classic sign of this traumatic disorder.

◆ ***Multiple sclerosis.*** This degenerative disease may cause arm and leg atrophy as a result of chronic progressive weakness; spasticity and contractures may also develop. Associated signs and symptoms commonly wax and wane and may include diplopia and blurred vision, nystagmus, hyperactive deep tendon reflexes, sensory loss or paresthesia, dysarthria, dysphagia, incoordination, ataxic gait, intention tremors, emotional lability, impotence, or urinary dysfunction.

◆ ***Osteoarthritis.*** This chronic disorder eventually causes atrophy proximal to involved joints as a result of progressive weakness and disuse. Other late signs and symptoms include bony joint deformities, such as Heberden's nodes on the distal interphalangeal joints, crepitus and fluid accumulation, and contractures.

◆ ***Parkinson's disease.*** In this disorder, muscle rigidity, weakness, and disuse may cause muscle atrophy. The patient may exhibit insidious tremors that usually begin in the fingers (pill-rolling tremor), worsen with stress, and ease with purposeful movement and sleep. He may also develop bradykinesia; a characteristic propulsive gait; a high-pitched, monotone voice; masklike facies; drooling; dysphagia; dysarthria; and, occasionally, oculogyric crisis or blepharospasm.

◆ ***Peripheral neuropathy.*** In this disorder, muscle weakness progresses slow-

EXAMINATION TIP

Measuring limb circumference

To ensure accurate and consistent limb circumference measurements, use a consistent reference point each time and measure with a limb in full extension. The diagram below shows the correct reference points for arm and leg measurements.

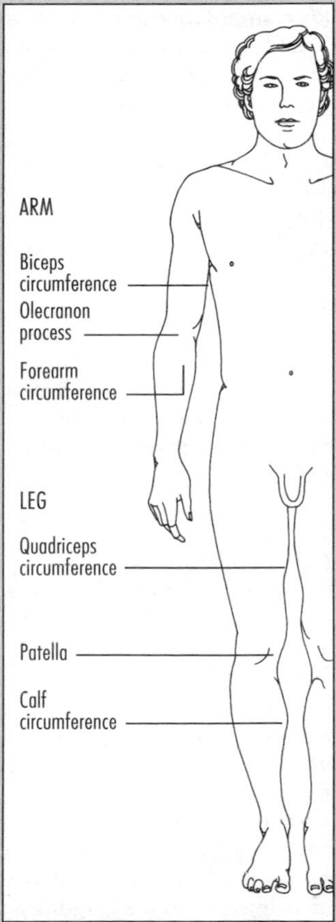

ly to flaccid paralysis and eventually atrophy. Distal extremity muscles are generally affected first. Associated findings may include loss of vibration sense; paresthesia, hyperesthesia, or anesthesia in the hands and feet; mild to sharp, burning pain; anhidrosis; glossy red skin; and diminished or absent deep tendon reflexes.

◆ ***Protein deficiency.*** If chronic, this may lead to muscle weakness and atrophy. Other findings include chronic fatigue, apathy, anorexia, dry skin, peripheral edema, and dull, sparse, dry hair.

◆ ***Rheumatoid arthritis.*** Muscle atrophy occurs in the late stages of this disorder, as joint pain and stiffness decrease range of motion and discourage muscle use.

◆ ***Spinal cord injury.*** Trauma to the spinal cord can cause severe muscle weakness and flaccid, then spastic, paralysis, eventually leading to atrophy. Other signs and symptoms depend on the level of injury but may include respiratory insufficiency or paralysis, sensory losses, bowel and bladder dysfunction, hyperactive deep tendon reflexes, positive Babinski's reflex, sexual dysfunction, priapism, hypotension, and anhidrosis (usually unilateral).

Other causes

◆ ***Drugs.*** Prolonged steroid therapy interferes with muscle metabolism and leads to atrophy, most prominently in the limbs.

◆ ***Immobility.*** Prolonged immobilization from bed rest, casts, splints, or traction may cause muscle weakness and atrophy.

Special considerations

Because contractures can occur as atrophied muscle fibers shorten, help the patient maintain muscle length by encouraging him to perform frequent active range-of-motion exercises. If he can't actively move a joint, provide active-assistive or passive exercises, and apply splints or braces to maintain muscle length. If you find resistance to full extension during exercise, use heat, pain medication, or relaxation techniques to relax the muscle. Then slowly stretch it to full extension. (*Caution:* Don't pull or strain the muscle; you may tear muscle fibers and cause further contracture.) If these techniques fail to correct the contracture, use moist heat, a whirlpool bath, resistive exercises, or ultrasound therapy. If these techniques aren't effective, surgical release of contractures may be necessary.

Prepare the patient for electromyography, nerve conduction studies, muscle biopsy, and X-rays or computed tomography scans.

Pediatric pointers

In young children, profound muscle weakness and atrophy can result from muscular dystrophy. Muscle atrophy may also result from cerebral palsy and poliomyelitis and from paralysis associated with meningocele and myelomeningocele.

MUSCLE FLACCIDITY

[Muscle hypotonicity]

Flaccid muscles are profoundly weak and soft, with decreased resistance to movement, increased mobility, and greater than normal range of motion. The result of disrupted muscle innervation, flaccidity can be localized to a limb or muscle group or generalized over the entire body. Its onset may be acute, as in trauma, or chronic, as in neurologic disease.

Emergency interventions

If the patient's muscle flaccidity results from trauma, ensure that his cervical spine has been stabilized. Quickly determine his respiratory status. If you note signs of respiratory insufficiency—dyspnea, shallow respirations, nasal flaring, and cyanosis—administer oxygen by nasal cannula or mask. Intubation and mechanical ventilation may be necessary.

History and physical examination

If the patient isn't in distress, ask about onset and duration of flaccidity, precipitating factors, and associated symptoms, notably weakness, other muscle changes, and sensory loss or paresthesia.

Examine the affected muscles for atrophy, which indicates a chronic problem. Test muscle strength and check deep tendon reflexes in all limbs.

Common medical causes

◆ ***Amyotrophic lateral sclerosis.*** Progressive muscle weakness and paralysis are accompanied by generalized flaccidity. Typically, these effects begin in one hand, spread to the arm, and then develop in the other hand and arm. Eventually, they spread to the trunk, neck, tongue, larynx, pharynx, and legs. Progressive respiratory muscle weakness leads to respiratory insufficiency. Other findings may include muscle cramps and coarse fasciculations, hyperactive deep tendon reflexes (DTRs), slight leg muscle spasticity, dysphagia, dysarthria, excessive drooling, and depression.

◆ ***Brain lesions.*** Frontal and parietal lobe lesions may cause contralateral flaccidity, weakness or paralysis, and eventually spasticity. Other findings may include hyperactive DTRs, positive Babinski's sign, loss of proprioception, analgesia, anesthesia, and thermanesthesia.

◆ ***Cerebrovascular accident.*** In this type of brain injury, caused by an obstruction of brain blood flow, hypoxic damage to motor areas of the brain can lead to paresis and flaccidity of muscles.

◆ ***Guillain-Barré syndrome.*** Progression of muscle flaccidity is typically symmetrical and ascending, moving from the feet to the arms and facial nerves within 24 to 72 hours of onset. Associated findings include sensory loss or paresthesia, absent deep tendon reflexes, tachycardia (or, less commonly, bradycardia), fluctuating hypertension and orthostatic hypotension, diaphoresis, incontinence, dysphagia, dysarthria, hypernasality, and facial diplegia. Weakness may progress to total motor paralysis and respiratory failure.

◆ ***Huntington's chorea.*** Besides flaccidity, progressive mental status changes and choreiform movements are major symptoms. Others include poor balance, hesitant or explosive speech, dysphagia, impaired respirations, and incontinence.

◆ ***Muscle disease.*** Muscle weakness and flaccidity are features of myopathies and muscular dystrophies.

◆ ***Peripheral nerve trauma.*** Flaccidity, paralysis, and loss of sensation and reflexes in the innervated area can occur.

◆ ***Peripheral neuropathy.*** Flaccidity usually occurs in the legs as a result of chronic progressive muscle weakness and paralysis. It may also cause mild to sharp burning pain, glossy red skin, anhidrosis, and loss of vibration sensation. Paresthesia, hyperesthesia, or anesthesia may affect the hands and feet. DTRs may be hypoactive or absent.

◆ ***Seizure disorder.*** Brief periods of syncope and generalized flaccidity commonly follow a grand mal seizure.

◆ ***Spinal cord injury.*** Spinal shock can result in acute muscle flaccidity or spasticity below the level of injury. Associated signs and symptoms that occur below the level of injury may include paralysis; absent DTRs; analgesia; thermanesthesia; loss of proprioception and vibration, touch, and pressure sensation; and anhidrosis (usually unilateral). Hypotension, bowel and bladder dysfunction, and impotence or priapism may also occur. Injury in the C1 to C5 region can cause respiratory paralysis and bradycardia.

Special considerations

Provide regular, systematic, passive range-of-motion exercises to preserve joint mobility and to increase circulation. Reposition a patient with generalized flaccidity every 2 hours to prevent skin breakdown. Pad bony prominences and other pressure points, and prevent thermal injury by testing bathwater before the patient bathes. Treat isolated flaccidity by supporting the affected limb in a sling or with a splint.

Prepare the patient for diagnostic tests, such as cranial and spinal X-rays or computed tomography scans and electromyography.

Pediatric pointers

Pediatric causes of muscle flaccidity include myelomeningocele, Lowe's disease, Werdnig-Hoffmann disease, and muscular dystrophy. An infant or young child with generalized flaccidity may lie in a froglike position, with hips and knees abducted.

MUSCLE SPASMS

[Muscle cramps]

Muscle spasms are strong, painful contractions. They can occur in virtually any muscle but are most common in the calf and foot. Muscle spasms typically result from simple muscle fatigue, after exercise, and during pregnancy. However, they may also reflect electrolyte imbalances, neuromuscular disorders, or the use of certain drugs. They're commonly precipitated by movement and can usually be relieved by slow stretching.

Emergency interventions

If the patient complains of frequent or unrelieved spasms in many muscles, accompanied by paresthesia in his hands and feet, quickly attempt to elicit Chvostek's and Trousseau's signs. If these signs are present, suspect hypocalcemia. Evaluate respiratory function, watching for the development of laryngospasm; provide supplemental oxygen as necessary, and prepare to intubate the patient and provide mechanical ventilation. Draw blood for calcium levels and arterial blood gas analysis, and insert an I.V. line for administration of a calcium supplement. Monitor cardiac status, and prepare to begin resuscitation if necessary.

History and physical examination

If the patient isn't in distress, ask when the spasms began. How long did they last? How painful were they? Did anything worsen or lessen the pain? Ask about other symptoms, such as weakness, sensory loss, or paresthesia. What activities was the patient performing before the onset of spasms? How frequently during the day does he perform these activities?

Evaluate muscle strength and tone. Then check all major muscle groups, and note whether any movements precipitate spasms. Test the presence and quality of all peripheral pulses, and examine the limbs for color and temperature changes. Test capillary refill time and inspect for edema, especially in the involved area. Finally, test reflexes and sensory function in all extremities.

Common medical causes

♦ ***Amyotrophic lateral sclerosis.*** Muscle spasms may accompany progressive muscle weakness and atrophy that typically begin in one hand, spread to the arm, and then spread to the other hand and arm. Eventually, muscle weakness and atrophy affect the trunk, neck, tongue, larynx, pharynx, and legs. Progressive respiratory muscle weakness leads to respiratory insufficiency. Other findings may include muscle flaccidity progressing to spasticity, coarse fasciculations, hyperactive deep tendon reflexes

(DTRs), dysphagia, impaired speech, excessive drooling, and depression.

♦ ***Arterial occlusive disease.*** Arterial occlusion typically causes spasms and intermittent claudication in the leg, with residual pain. Associated findings are usually localized to the legs and feet and include loss of peripheral pulses, pallor or cyanosis, decreased sensation, hair loss, dry or scaling skin, edema, and ulcerations.

♦ ***Dehydration.*** Sodium loss may cause limb and abdominal cramps. Other findings may include a slight fever, decreased skin turgor, dry mucous membranes, tachycardia, orthostatic hypotension, muscle twitching, seizures, nausea, vomiting, and oliguria.

♦ ***Hypocalcemia.*** The classic feature is tetany — a syndrome of muscle cramps and twitching, carpopedal and facial muscle spasms, and seizures, possibly with stridor. Chvostek's and Trousseau's signs may be elicited. Related findings include paresthesia of the lips, fingers, and toes; choreiform movements; hyperactive DTRs, fatigue; palpitations; and cardiac arrhythmias.

♦ ***Muscle trauma.*** Excessive muscle strain may cause mild to severe spasms. The injured area may be painful, swollen, reddened, or warm.

♦ ***Respiratory alkalosis.*** Acute onset of muscle spasms may be accompanied by twitching and weakness, carpopedal spasms, circumoral and peripheral paresthesia, vertigo, syncope, pallor, and extreme anxiety. In severe alkalosis, cardiac arrhythmias may occur.

♦ ***Spinal injury or disease.*** Muscle spasms can result from spinal injury, such as cervical extension injury or spinous process fracture, or from spinal disease such as infection.

Other causes

♦ ***Drugs.*** Common spasm-producing drugs include diuretics, corticosteroids, and estrogens.

Special considerations

Depending on the cause, help alleviate your patient's spasms by slowly stretching the affected muscle in the direction opposite the contraction. If necessary, administer a mild analgesic.

Diagnostic studies may include serum calcium and sodium levels, thyroid function tests, and blood flow studies or arteriography.

Pediatric pointers

Muscle spasms rarely occur in children. Their presence suggests hypoparathyroidism, osteomalacia, rickets or, rarely, congenital torticollis.

MUSCLE SPASTICITY

[Muscle hypertonicity]

Spasticity is a state of excessive muscle tone manifested by increased resistance to stretching and heightened reflexes. It's commonly detected by evaluating a muscle's response to passive movement; a spastic muscle offers more resistance when the passive movement is performed quickly. Caused by an upper-motor-neuron lesion, spasticity usually occurs in the arm and leg muscles. Long-term spasticity results in muscle fibrosis and contractures. (See *How spasticity develops*, page 392.)

History and physical examination

Once you detect spasticity, ask the patient about its onset, duration, and progression. What, if any, events precipitate onset? Has he experienced other muscular changes or related symptoms? Does his medical history reveal incidence of trauma or degenerative or vascular disease?

Take the patient's vital signs and perform a complete neurologic examina-

How spasticity develops

Motor activity is controlled by pyramidal and extrapyramidal tracts that originate in the motor cortex, basal ganglia, brain stem, and spinal cord. Nerve fibers from the various tracts converge and synapse at the anterior horn in the spinal cord. Together, they maintain segmental muscle tone by modulating the *stretch reflex arc.* This arc, shown in simplified form below, is basically a negative feedback loop in which muscle stretch (stimulation) causes reflexive contraction (inhibition), thus maintaining muscle length and tone.

Damage to certain tracts results in loss of inhibition and disruption of the stretch reflex arc. Uninhibited muscle stretch produces exaggerated, uncontrolled muscle activity, accentuating the reflex arc and eventually resulting in spasticity.

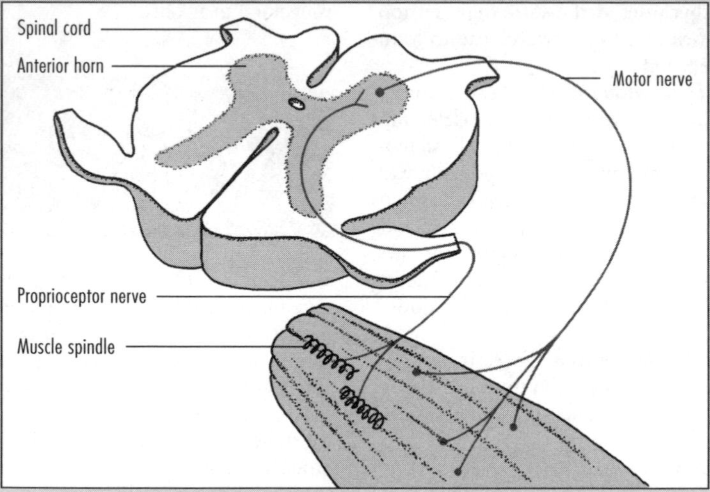

tion. Test reflexes and evaluate motor and sensory function in all limbs. Evaluate muscles for wasting and contractures.

During your examination, keep in mind that generalized spasticity and trismus in a patient with a recent skin puncture or laceration are signs of tetanus. If you suspect this rare disorder, look for signs of respiratory distress. If necessary, provide ventilatory support and monitor the patient closely.

Common medical causes

♦ ***Amyotrophic lateral sclerosis.*** This disorder commonly causes spasticity, spasms, coarse fasciculations, hyperactive deep tendon reflexes, and a Babinski's sign. Earlier effects include progressive muscle weakness and flaccidity that typically begin in the hands and arms and eventually spread to the trunk, neck, larynx, pharynx, and legs; progressive respiratory muscle weakness leads to respiratory insufficiency. Other findings may include dysphagia, dysarthria, excessive drooling, and depression.

◆ ***Cerebrovascular accident.*** Spastic paralysis may develop on the affected side after the acute stage of cerebrovascular accident. Associated findings vary with the site and extent of vascular damage and may include dysarthria, aphasia, ataxia, apraxia, agnosia, ipsilateral paresthesia or sensory loss, vision disturbances, altered level of consciousness (LOC), amnesia and poor judgment, personality changes, emotional lability, bowel and bladder dysfunction, headache, vomiting, and seizures.

◆ ***Epidural hemorrhage.*** Bilateral limb spasticity is a late and ominous sign. Other findings may include a momentary loss of consciousness after head trauma, followed by a lucid interval and then a rapid deterioration in LOC. The patient may also develop unilateral hemiparesis or hemiplegia; seizures; fixed, dilated pupils; high fever; decreased and bounding pulse; widened pulse pressure; elevated blood pressure; irregular respiratory pattern; or decerebrate posture. Babinski's sign can be elicited.

◆ ***Spinal cord injury.*** Spasticity commonly results from cervical high thoracic spinal cord injury, especially from incomplete lesions. Spastic paralysis in the affected limbs follows initial flaccid paralysis; typically, spasticity and muscle atrophy increase for up to 2 years after the injury, then gradually regress to flaccidity. Reflex activity may return after spinal cord shock if the cord hasn't been completely transected, but severe spasticity may persist. Associated signs and symptoms vary with the level of injury but may include respiratory insufficiency or paralysis, sensory losses, bowel and bladder dysfunction, hyperactive deep tendon reflexes, Babinski's sign, sexual dysfunction, priapism, hypotension, anhidrosis, and bradycardia.

◆ ***Tetanus.*** This rare, life-threatening disease causes varying degrees of spasticity. In generalized tetanus, the most common form, early signs and symptoms include jaw and neck stiffness, trismus, headache, irritability, restlessness, low-grade fever with chills, tachycardia, diaphoresis, and hyperactive deep tendon reflexes. As the disease progresses, painful involuntary spasms may spread and cause boardlike abdominal rigidity, opisthotonos, and a characteristic grotesque grin known as risus sardonicus. Reflex spasms may occur in any muscle group with the slightest stimulus. Glottal, pharyngeal, or respiratory muscle involvement can cause death by asphyxia or cardiac failure.

Special considerations

Prepare the patient for diagnostic tests, which may include electromyography, muscle biopsy, or intracranial or spinal magnetic resonance imaging or computed tomography. Administer pain medications and antispasmodics. Passive range-of-motion exercises, splinting, traction, and application of heat may help relieve spasms and prevent contractures. Maintain a calm, quiet environment to help relieve spasms and prevent recurrence, and encourage bed rest. In cases of prolonged, uncontrollable spasticity, as in spastic paralysis, nerve blocks or surgical transection may be necessary for permanent relief.

Pediatric pointers

In children, muscle spasticity may be a sign of cerebral palsy.

MUSCLE WEAKNESS

Muscle weakness is detected by observing and measuring the strength of an individual muscle or muscle group. (See *Testing muscle strength,* pages 394 and 395.) Muscle weakness can result from a malfunction in the cerebral hemispheres, brain stem, spinal cord, nerve roots, peripheral nerves, or myoneural

(Text continues on page 396.)

EXAMINATION TIP

Testing muscle strength

Obtain an overall picture of your patient's motor function by testing strength in 10 selected muscle groups. Ask the patient to attempt normal range-of-motion movements against your resistance. If the muscle group is weak, vary the amount of resistance as necessary to permit accurate assessment. If necessary, position the patient so his limbs don't have to resist gravity, and repeat the test.

ARM MUSCLES

Biceps. With your arm on the patient's hand, have him flex his forearm against your resistance; observe for biceps contraction.

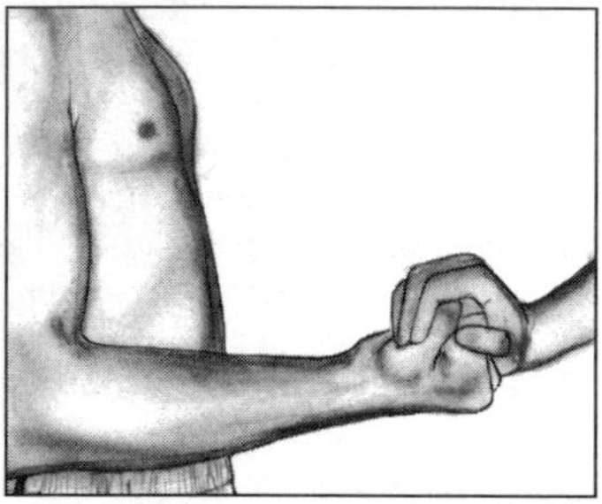

Deltoid muscle. With the patient's arm fully extended, place one hand over his deltoid muscle and the other on his wrist. Ask him to abduct his arm to a horizontal position against your resistance; as he does so, palpate for deltoid contraction.

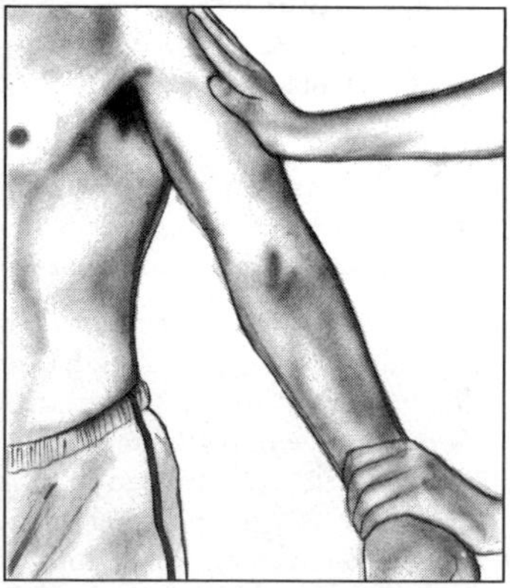

Triceps. Have the patient abduct and hold his arm midway between flexion and extension. Hold and support his arm at the wrist, and ask him to extend it against your resistance. Observe for triceps contraction.

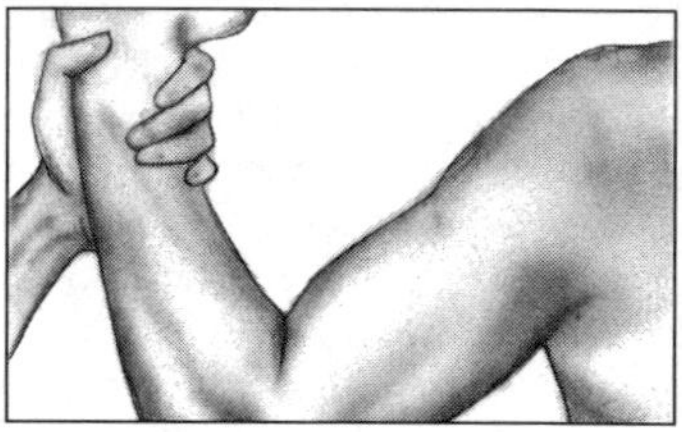

Dorsal interossei. Have the patient extend and spread his fingers, and tell him to try to resist your attempt to squeeze them together.

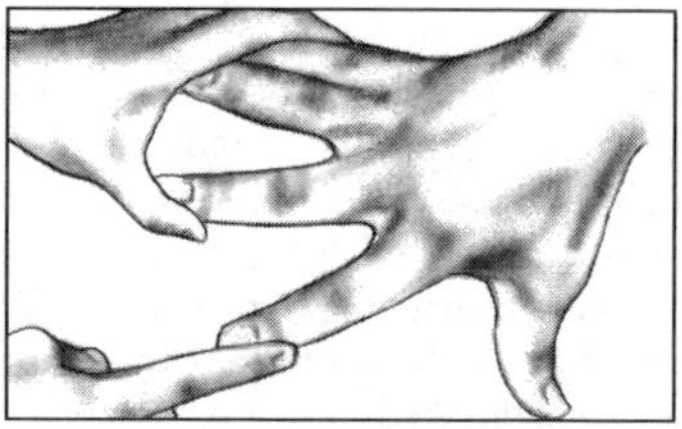

Forearm and hand (grip). Have the patient grasp your middle and index fingers and squeeze as hard as he can.

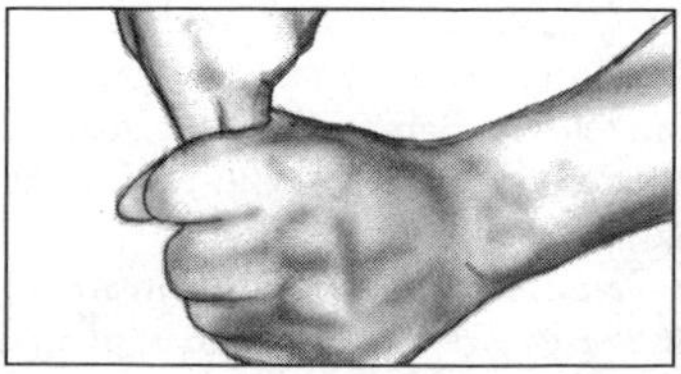

Rate muscle strength on a scale of 0 to 5:
0 = Total paralysis
1 = Visible or palpable contraction but no movement
2 = Full muscle movement with force of gravity eliminated
3 = Full muscle movement against gravity but no movement against resistance
4 = Full muscle movement against gravity; partial movement against resistance
5 = Full muscle movement against both gravity and resistance, normal strength

LEG MUSCLES

Anterior tibial. With the patient's leg extended, place your hand on his foot and ask him to dorsiflex his ankle against your resistance.

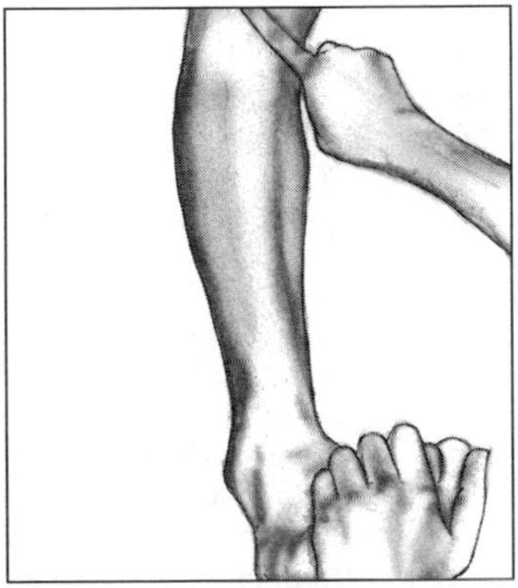

Psoas. While you support his leg, have the patient raise his knee and then flex his hip against your resistance. Observe for psoas muscle contraction.

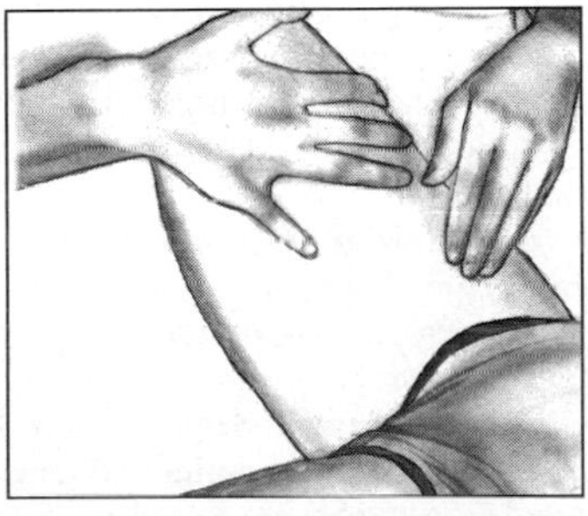

Extensor hallucis longus. With your finger on the patient's great toe, have him dorsiflex the toe against your resistance. Palpate for extensor hallucis contraction.

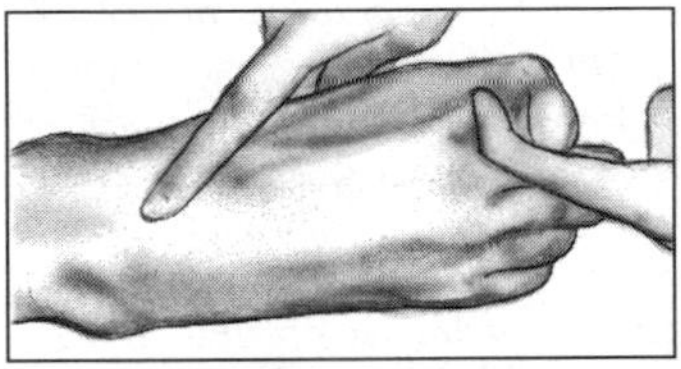

Quadriceps. Have the patient bend his knee slightly while you support his lower leg. Then ask him to extend the knee against your resistance. Palpate for quadriceps contraction.

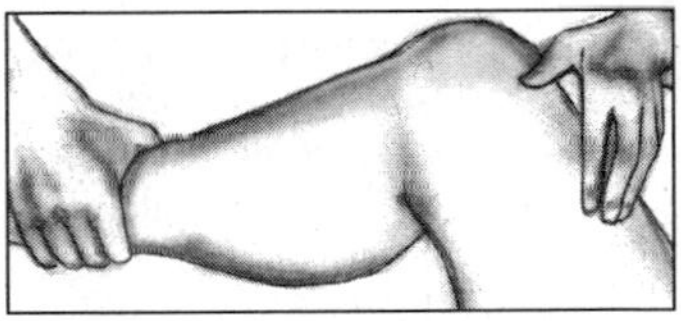

Gastrocnemius. With the patient on his side, support his foot and ask him to plantarflex his ankle against your resistance. Palpate for gastrocnemius contraction.

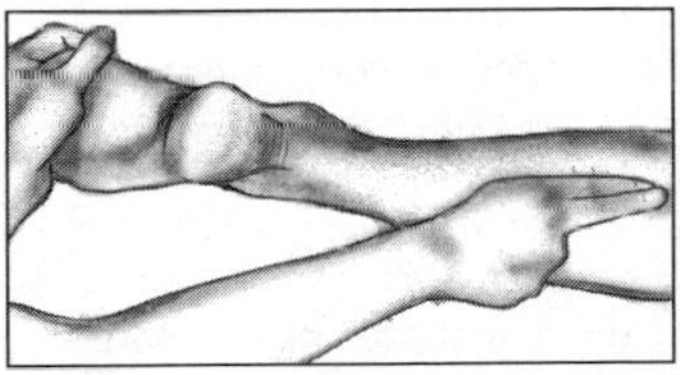

junctions and within the muscle itself. Muscle weakness occurs in certain neurologic, musculoskeletal, metabolic, endocrine, and cardiovascular disorders; as a response to certain drugs; and after prolonged immobilization.

History and physical examination
Begin by determining the location of the patient's muscle weakness. Ask if he has difficulty with specific movements, such as rising from a chair. Find out when he first noticed the weakness; ask him whether it worsens with exercise or as the day progresses. Also ask about related symptoms, especially muscle or joint pain, altered sensory function, and fatigue.

Obtain a medical history, noting especially chronic disease, such as hyperthyroidism; musculoskeletal or neurologic problems, including recent trauma; family history of chronic muscle weakness, especially in males; and alcohol and drug use.

Focus your physical examination on evaluating muscle strength. Test all major muscles bilaterally. When testing, make sure the patient's effort is constant; if it isn't, suspect pain or other reluctance to make the effort. If the patient complains of pain, ease or discontinue testing and have him try the movements again. Remember that the patient's dominant arm, hand, and leg are somewhat stronger than their nondominant counterparts. Besides testing individual muscle strength, test for range of motion at all major joints (shoulder, elbow, wrist, hip, knee, ankle). Also test sensory function in the involved areas, and test deep tendon reflexes bilaterally.

Common medical causes

♦ ***Amyotrophic lateral sclerosis.*** This disorder typically begins with muscle weakness and atrophy in one hand that rapidly spread to the arm and then to the other hand and arm. Eventually, these effects spread to the trunk, neck, tongue, larynx, pharynx, and legs. Progressive respiratory muscle weakness leads to respiratory insufficiency.

♦ ***Anemia.*** Varying degrees of muscle weakness and fatigue are exacerbated by exertion and temporarily relieved by rest. Other signs and symptoms may include pallor, tachycardia, paresthesia, and bleeding tendencies.

♦ ***Brain tumor.*** Signs and symptoms of muscle weakness vary with the location of the tumor. Associated findings include headache, vomiting, diplopia, decreased visual acuity, decreased level of consciousness (LOC), pupillary changes, decreased motor strength, hemiparesis, hemiplegia, diminished sensations, ataxia, seizures, and behavioral changes.

♦ ***Cerebrovascular accident.*** Depending on the site and extent of damage, a cerebrovascular accident may cause contralateral or bilateral weakness of the arms, legs, face, and tongue, possibly progressing to hemiplegia and atrophy. Associated effects may include dysarthria, aphasia, ataxia, apraxia, agnosia, ipsilateral paresthesia or sensory loss, vision disturbances, altered LOC, amnesia and poor judgment, personality changes, bowel and bladder dysfunction, headache, vomiting, and seizures.

♦ ***Guillain-Barré syndrome.*** Rapidly progressive, symmetrical weakness ascends from the feet to the arms and facial nerves and may progress to total motor paralysis and respiratory failure. Associated findings include sensory loss or paresthesia, muscle flaccidity, loss of deep tendon reflexes, tachycardia or bradycardia, fluctuating hypertension and orthostatic hypotension, diaphoresis, bowel and bladder incontinence, facial diplegia, dysphagia, dysarthria, and hypernasality.

♦ ***Herniated disk.*** Pressure on nerve roots leads to muscle weakness, disuse, and ultimately atrophy. The primary symptom is severe lower back pain, possibly radiating to the buttocks, legs, and feet — usually on one side. Diminished reflexes and sensory changes may also occur.

◆ ***Hypercortisolism.*** This disorder may cause limb weakness and eventually atrophy. Related cushingoid features include buffalo hump, moon face, truncal obesity, purple striae, thin skin, acne, elevated blood pressure, fatigue, hyperpigmentation, easy bruising, poor wound healing, and diaphoresis. The male patient may be impotent; the female patient may exhibit hirsutism and menstrual irregularities.

◆ ***Myasthenia gravis.*** Gradually progressive skeletal muscle weakness and fatigue are the cardinal symptoms of this disorder. Typically, weakness is mild upon awakening and worsens during the day. Early signs may include weak eye closure, ptosis, and diplopia; blank, masklike facies; difficulty chewing and swallowing; nasal regurgitation of fluid with hypernasality; and a hanging jaw and bobbing head. Respiratory muscle involvement may eventually lead to respiratory failure.

◆ ***Osteoarthritis.*** This chronic disorder causes progressive muscle disuse and weakness that lead to atrophy.

◆ ***Parkinson's disease.*** Muscle weakness accompanies rigidity in this degenerative disorder. Related findings include a unilateral pill-rolling tremor, propulsive gait, dysarthria, bradykinesia, drooling, dysphagia, masklike facies, and a high-pitched, monotone voice.

◆ ***Peripheral nerve trauma.*** Prolonged pressure on or injury to a peripheral nerve causes muscle weakness and atrophy. Other findings include paresthesia or sensory loss, pain, and loss of reflexes supplied by the damaged nerve.

◆ ***Potassium imbalance.*** In *hypokalemia,* temporary generalized muscle weakness may be accompanied by nausea, vomiting, diarrhea, decreased mentation, leg cramps, diminished reflexes, malaise, polyuria, dizziness, hypotension, and arrhythmias. In *hyperkalemia,* weakness may progress to flaccid paralysis accompanied by irritability and confusion, hyperreflexia, paresthesia or anesthesia, oliguria, anorexia, nausea, diarrhea, abdominal cramps, tachycardia or bradycardia, and arrhythmias.

◆ ***Rheumatoid arthritis.*** Here, muscle weakness may accompany increased warmth, swelling, and tenderness in involved joints; pain; and stiffness, restricting motion.

◆ ***Seizure disorder.*** Temporary generalized muscle weakness may occur after a grand mal seizure; other postictal findings include headache, muscle soreness, and profound fatigue.

◆ ***Spinal trauma and disease.*** Trauma can cause severe muscle weakness, leading to flaccidity or spasticity and, eventually, paralysis. Infection, tumor, and cervical spondylosis or stenosis can also cause muscle weakness.

Other causes

◆ ***Drugs.*** Generalized muscle weakness can result from prolonged corticosteroid use, digoxin toxicity, or excessive doses of dantrolene. Aminoglycoside antibiotics may worsen weakness in patients with myasthenia gravis.

◆ ***Immobility.*** Immobilization in a cast, a splint, or traction can lead to muscle weakness in the involved extremity; prolonged bed rest or inactivity results in generalized muscle weakness.

Special considerations

Provide assistive devices as necessary, and protect the patient from injury. If he has concomitant sensory loss, guard against pressure ulcer formation and thermal injury. With chronic weakness, provide range-of-motion exercises or splint limbs as necessary. Arrange therapy sessions to allow for adequate rest periods, and administer pain medications, as needed.

Prepare the patient for blood tests, muscle biopsy, electromyography, nerve conduction studies, and X-rays or computed tomography scans.

Pediatric pointers
Muscular dystrophy, usually Duchenne's type, is a major cause of muscle weakness in children.

MYDRIASIS

Mydriasis — pupillary dilation caused by contraction of the dilator of the iris — is a normal response to decreased light, strong emotional stimuli, and topical administration of mydriatic and cycloplegic drugs. It can also result from ocular and neurologic disorders, eye trauma, and disorders that decrease level of consciousness (LOC). Keep in mind that mydriasis appears in two ocular emergencies: acute angle-closure glaucoma and traumatic iridoplegia. Mydriasis may be an adverse effect of antihistamines or other drugs.

History and physical examination
Begin by asking the patient about other eye problems, such as pain, blurring, diplopia, or visual field defects. Obtain a health history, focusing on eye or head trauma, glaucoma and other ocular problems, and neurologic and vascular disorders. In addition, obtain a complete medication history.

Next, perform a thorough eye and pupil examination. Inspect and compare the pupils' size, color, and shape, remembering that many people normally have unequal pupils. (See *Grading pupil size.*) Also, test each pupil for light reflex, consensual response, and accommodation. Perform a swinging flashlight test to evaluate a decreased response to direct light coupled with a normal consensual response (Gunn's pupil). Be sure to check the eyes for ptosis, swelling, and ecchymosis. Test visual acuity in both eyes with and without correction. Evaluate extraocular muscle function by checking the six cardinal fields of gaze.

First-time patients and those over age 40 or with a personal or family history of eye health problems need dilated eye examinations. Dilation is important for patients with diabetes, hypertension, sickle cell disease, macular degeneration, or cataracts. People who are highly nearsighted are more prone to retinal detachment and require dilation to identify retinal breaks. Dilated eye examination is also necessary for anyone who has recently had trauma to the head or eye or is experiencing flashes of light, floaters, or a curtain effect. However, certain health and ocular considerations may contraindicate pupil dilation.

Common medical causes
♦ ***Adie's syndrome.*** This disorder is characterized by abrupt unilateral mydriasis, poor or absent pupillary reflexes, visual blurring, and cramplike eye pain. Deep tendon reflexes may be hyperactive or absent.

♦ ***Aortic arch syndrome.*** Bilateral pupillary mydriasis commonly occurs late in this syndrome. Other ocular findings may include visual blurring, transient vision loss, and diplopia. Related findings may include dizziness and syncope; neck, shoulder, and chest pain; bruits; loss of radial and carotid pulses; paresthesia; and intermittent claudication. Blood pressure may be decreased in the arms.

♦ ***Botulism.*** Botulism toxin causes bilateral mydriasis, usually 12 to 36 hours after ingestion. Other early findings are loss of pupillary reflexes, visual blurring, diplopia, ptosis, strabismus and extraocular muscle palsies, anorexia, nausea, vomiting, diarrhea, and dry mouth. Vertigo, hearing loss, hoarseness, hypernasality, dysarthria, dysphagia, progressive muscle weakness, and loss of deep tendon reflexes soon follow.

♦ ***Carotid artery aneurysm.*** Here, unilateral mydriasis may be accompanied by bitemporal hemianopia, decreased visual acuity, hemiplegia, decreased LOC,

EXAMINATION TIP

Grading pupil size

To accurately evaluate pupil size, compare your patient's pupils with the scale shown here. Keep in mind that the maximum constriction may be less than 1 mm and the maximum dilation greater than 9 mm.

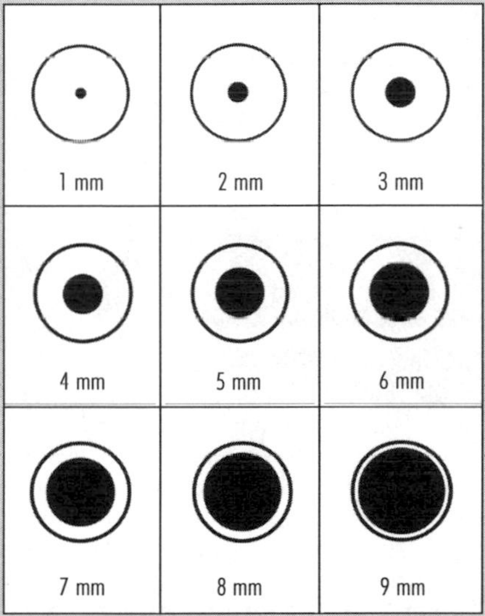

headache, aphasia, behavioral changes, and hypoesthesia.

♦ ***Glaucoma (acute angle-closure).*** This ocular emergency is characterized by moderate mydriasis and loss of pupillary reflex in the affected eye, accompanied by abrupt onset of excruciating pain, decreased visual acuity, visual blurring, halo vision, conjunctival injection, and a cloudy cornea.

♦ ***Oculomotor nerve palsy.*** Unilateral mydriasis is commonly the first sign of this disorder. It's soon followed by ptosis, diplopia, decreased pupillary reflexes, exotropia, and complete loss of accommodation. Focal neurologic signs may accompany signs of increased intracranial pressure.

♦ ***Traumatic iridoplegia.*** Eye trauma commonly paralyzes the sphincter of the iris, causing mydriasis and loss of pupillary reflex; usually, this is transient. Associated findings may include a quivering iris (iridodonesis), ecchymosis, pain, and swelling.

Other causes

♦ ***Drugs.*** Mydriasis can be caused by anticholinergics, antihistamines, sympathomimetics, barbiturates (in overdose), estrogens, and tricyclic antidepressants; it also occurs commonly early in anesthesia induction. Topical mydriatics and cycloplegics, such as phenylephrine, atropine, homatropine, scopolamine, cyclopentolate, and tropicamide, are administered specifically for their mydriatic effects. Other mydriatic drugs include amphetamines or other stimulants, cocaine, glutethimide, Jimson weed, and LSD. A final cause is withdrawal from alcohol or opioids.

♦ ***Surgery.*** Traumatic mydriasis commonly results from ocular surgery.

Special considerations
Diagnostic tests may vary, depending on your findings, but may include a complete ophthalmologic examination and a thorough neurologic workup. Explain diagnostic tests to the patient.

Pediatric pointers
Mydriasis occurs in children as a result of ocular trauma, drugs, Adie's syndrome and, most frequently, increased intracranial pressure.

Myoclonus

Myoclonus — sudden, shocklike contractions of a single muscle or muscle group — occurs in various neurologic disorders and commonly heralds onset of a seizure. These contractions may be isolated or repetitive, rhythmic or arrhythmic, symmetrical or asymmetrical, synchronous or asynchronous, and generalized or focal. They may be precipitated by bright flickering lights, a loud sound, or unexpected physical contact. One type, *intention myoclonus,* is evoked by intentional muscle movement.

Myoclonus occurs normally just before falling asleep and as a part of the natural startle reaction. It also occurs with some poisonings and, rarely, as a complication of hemodialysis.

Emergency interventions
If you observe myoclonus, check for seizure activity. Take vital signs to rule out arrhythmias or a blocked airway. Have resuscitation equipment on hand.

If the patient has a seizure, gently help him lie down. Place a pillow or a rolled towel under his head to prevent concussion. Loosen constrictive clothing, especially around the neck, and turn his head (gently, if possible) to one side to prevent airway occlusion or aspiration of secretions. Insert an oral airway if the teeth aren't already clenched.

Closely monitor the patient and record all observed behaviors. Time the contractions and observe if the contractions start in one muscle group and then progress.

History and physical examination
If the patient is stable, evaluate level of consciousness (LOC) and mental status. Ask about the frequency, severity, location, and circumstances of the myoclonus. Has he ever had a seizure? If so, did myoclonus precede it? Is the myoclonus ever precipitated by a sensory stimulus? During the physical examination, check for muscle rigidity and wasting, and test deep tendon reflexes.

Common medical causes
- ***Alzheimer's disease.*** Generalized myoclonus may occur in advanced stages of this slowly progressive dementia. Other late findings may include mild choreoathetoid movements, muscle rigidity, bowel and bladder incontinence, delusions, and hallucinations.
- ***Creutzfeldt-Jakob disease.*** Diffuse myoclonic jerks appear early in this rapidly progressive dementia. Initially random, they gradually become more rhythmic and symmetrical, commonly occurring in response to sensory stimuli. Associated effects may include ataxia, aphasia, hearing loss, muscle rigidity and wasting, fasciculations, hemiplegia, and vision disturbances or, possibly, blindness.
- ***Encephalitis (viral).*** In this disease, myoclonus is usually intermittent and either localized or generalized. Associated findings vary but may include rapidly decreasing LOC, fever, headache, irritability, nuchal rigidity, vomiting, seizures, aphasia, ataxia, hemiparesis, facial muscle weakness, nystagmus, ocular palsies, and dysphagia.
- ***Encephalopathy***. *Hepatic encephalopathy* occasionally causes myoclonic

jerks in association with asterixis and focal or generalized seizures.

Hypoxic encephalopathy may cause generalized myoclonus or seizures almost immediately after restoration of cardiopulmonary function. The patient may also have a residual intention myoclonus.

Uremic encephalopathy commonly causes myoclonic jerks and seizures. Other signs and symptoms include apathy, fatigue, irritability, headache, confusion, gradually decreasing LOC, nausea, vomiting, oliguria, edema, and papilledema. The patient may also exhibit hypertension, dyspnea, arrhythmias, or abnormal respirations.

◆ ***Epilepsy.*** In *idiopathic epilepsy,* localized myoclonus is usually confined to an arm or leg and occurs singly or in short bursts, typically upon awakening. It's commonly more frequent and severe during the prodromal stage of a major generalized seizure, after which it diminishes in frequency and intensity.

Myoclonic jerks are usually the first signs of *myoclonic epilepsy,* the most common cause of progressive myoclonus. At first, myoclonus is infrequent and localized; but, over a period of months, it becomes more frequent and involves the entire body, disrupting voluntary movement (intention myoclonus). As the disease progresses, myoclonus is accompanied by generalized seizures and dementia.

Other causes

◆ ***Drug withdrawal.*** Myoclonus may be seen in patients with alcohol, narcotic, or sedative withdrawal, and in patients with delirium tremens.

◆ ***Poisoning.*** Acute intoxication with methyl bromide, bismuth, or strychnine may cause an acute onset of myoclonus and confusion.

Special considerations

If your patient's myoclonus is progressive, take seizure precautions. Keep an oral airway, suction equipment, and padded tongue blade at his bedside, and pad the side rails. Because myoclonus may cause falls, remove potentially harmful objects from the patient's environment, and remain with him while he walks. Be sure to instruct the patient and his family about the need for safety precautions.

As needed, administer drugs that suppress myoclonus: ethosuximide, 5-hydroxytryptophan, phenobarbital, clonazepam, or carbidopa. An EEG may be needed to evaluate myoclonus and related brain activity.

Pediatric pointers

Although myoclonus is relatively uncommon in infants and children, it can result from subacute sclerosing panencephalitis, severe meningitis, progressive poliodystrophy, childhood myoclonic epilepsy, and encephalopathies such as Reye's syndrome.

N

NASAL FLARING

Nasal flaring is abnormal dilation of the nostrils. Usually occurring during inspiration, nasal flaring may occasionally occur during expiration or throughout the respiratory cycle. It indicates respiratory dysfunction, ranging from mild difficulty to potentially life-threatening respiratory distress.

Emergency interventions

If you note nasal flaring, quickly evaluate the patient's respiratory status. Inspiratory chest movement, absent breath sounds, cyanosis, diaphoresis, and tachycardia point to complete airway obstruction. As necessary, apply back blows or abdominal thrusts (Heimlich maneuver) to relieve the obstruction. If these don't clear the airway, emergency intubation or tracheostomy and mechanical ventilation may be necessary.

If the patient's airway isn't obstructed but he has difficulty breathing, give oxygen by nasal cannula or face mask. Intubation and mechanical ventilation may be necessary. Insert an I.V. line for fluid and medication access. Begin cardiac monitoring. Obtain a chest X-ray and samples for arterial blood gas and electrolyte studies.

History

Once the patient is stabilized, obtain a pertinent history. Ask about cardiac and pulmonary disorders, such as asthma. Does the patient have allergies? Has he experienced a recent illness, such as a respiratory infection, or trauma?

Common medical causes

♦ ***Adult respiratory distress syndrome (ARDS).*** ARDS causes increased respiratory difficulty, with nasal flaring, dyspnea, tachypnea, diaphoresis, cyanosis, scattered crackles, and rhonchi. Other effects include tachycardia, anxiety, and decreased level of consciousness (LOC).

♦ ***Airway obstruction.*** *Complete obstruction* above the tracheal bifurcation causes sudden nasal flaring, absent breath sounds despite intercostal retractions and marked accessory muscle use, tachycardia, diaphoresis, cyanosis, decreasing LOC and, eventually, respiratory arrest.

Partial obstruction causes nasal flaring with inspiratory stridor, gagging, wheezing, violent cough, marked accessory muscle use, agitation, cyanosis, and hoarseness.

♦ ***Anaphylaxis.*** Severe reactions can cause respiratory distress with nasal flaring, stridor, wheezing, accessory muscle use, intercostal retractions, and dyspnea. Associated signs and symptoms may include nasal congestion, sneezing, pruritus, urticaria, erythema, diaphoresis, angioedema, weakness, hoarseness, dysphagia and, rarely, vomiting, nausea, diarrhea, urinary urgency, and incontinence. Cardiac arrhythmias and signs of shock may occur late.

♦ ***Asthma (acute).*** An asthmatic attack can cause nasal flaring, dyspnea, tachypnea, prolonged expiratory wheezing, accessory muscle use, cyanosis, and a dry or productive cough. Auscultation may reveal rhonchi, crackles, and decreased or absent breath sounds. Other findings include anxiety, tachycardia, and increased blood pressure.

♦ ***Chronic obstructive pulmonary disease.*** This disorder can lead to acute respiratory failure, most commonly secondary to pulmonary infection. Nasal flaring is accompanied by prolonged pursed-lip expiration; accessory muscle use; loose, rattling, productive cough; cyanosis; reduced chest expansion; crackles; rhonchi; wheezing; and dyspnea.

♦ ***Pneumothorax.*** This acute disorder can result in respiratory distress with nasal flaring, dyspnea, tachypnea, shallow respirations, hyperresonance or tympany on percussion, agitation, distended neck veins, tracheal deviation, and cyanosis. Other findings typically include sharp chest pain, tachycardia, hypotension, cold and clammy skin, diaphoresis, and subcutaneous crepitation. Breath sounds may be decreased or absent on the affected side; similarly, chest wall motion may be decreased on the affected side. Similar findings can occur in patients with *hydrothorax, chylothorax, or hemothorax,* depending on the amount of fluid accumulation.

♦ ***Pulmonary edema.*** This disorder typically produces nasal flaring, severe dyspnea, wheezing, and a cough that produces frothy, pink sputum. Other findings may include increased accessory muscle use, tachycardia, cyanosis, hypotension, crackles, distended neck veins, peripheral edema, or decreased LOC.

♦ ***Pulmonary embolus.*** Signs of this potentially life-threatening disorder may include nasal flaring, dyspnea, tachypnea, wheezing, cyanosis, pleural friction rub, or productive cough (possibly hemoptysis). Its other effects include sudden chest tightness or pleuritic pain, tachycardia, hypotension, low-grade fever, syncope, marked anxiety, and restlessness.

Other causes

♦ ***Diagnostic tests.*** Forced inspiration or expiration during pulmonary function tests, such as vital capacity testing, can cause nasal flaring.

♦ ***Treatments.*** Certain respiratory treatments such as deep breathing can cause nasal flaring.

Special considerations

To help ease breathing, place the patient in a high Fowler's position. If he's at risk for aspirating secretions, place him in a modified Trendelenburg's or side-lying position. If necessary, suction frequently to remove oropharyngeal secretions. Administer humidified oxygen to thin secretions and decrease airway drying and irritation. Provide adequate hydration to liquefy secretions. Reposition the patient every hour, and encourage coughing and deep breathing. Avoid administering sedatives or opiates, which can depress the cough reflex or respirations. Continually assess the patient's respiratory status, and check his vital signs every 30 minutes, or as necessary.

Prepare the patient for diagnostic tests, such as chest X-rays, lung scan, pulmonary arteriography, sputum culture, complete blood count, arterial blood gas analysis, and 12-lead electrocardiogram.

Pediatric pointers

Nasal flaring is an important sign of respiratory distress in infants and very young children, who can't verbalize their discomfort. Common causes include airway obstruction, hyaline membrane disease, croup, and acute epiglottiditis. Use of a croup tent may improve oxygenation and humidification for such patients.

Prepare the patient for X-rays or computed tomography scans of the nose, sinuses, or skull. Promote fluid intake to thin secretions, as needed. Give antihistamines, decongestants, analgesics, or antipyretics.

Nausea

Nausea is a sensation of profound revulsion to food or of impending vomiting. Commonly accompanied by autonomic signs—such as hypersalivation, diaphoresis, tachycardia, pallor, and tachypnea, it's closely associated with both anorexia and vomiting.

This common symptom of GI disorders also occurs in fluid and electrolyte imbalance, infection, and metabolic, endocrine, labyrinthine, and cardiac disorders. It's a frequent occurrence during the first trimester of pregnancy. Nausea may also arise from severe pain, anxiety, alcohol intoxication, overeating, or ingestion of distasteful food or liquids. It may be a result of drug therapy, surgery, or radiation.

History and physical examination

Begin by obtaining a complete medical history. Focus on GI, endocrine, and metabolic disorders, recent infections, and cancer or its treatment. Ask about medication use and alcohol consumption. If the patient is a female of childbearing age, ask if she is or could be pregnant. Have the patient describe the onset, duration, and intensity of the nausea and what causes or relieves it. Ask about related complaints, particularly vomiting (color, amount), abdominal pain, anorexia and weight loss, changes in bowel habits or stool character, excessive belching or flatus, and a sensation of bloating.

Inspect the skin for jaundice, bruises, and spider angiomas, and assess skin turgor. Next, inspect the abdomen for distention, auscultate for bowel sounds and bruits, palpate for rigidity and tenderness, and test for rebound tenderness. Palpate and percuss the liver for enlargement. Assess other body systems as appropriate.

Common medical causes

♦ ***Adrenal insufficiency.*** Common GI findings in this endocrine disorder include nausea, vomiting, anorexia, and diarrhea. Other findings may include a weak, irregular pulse, weakness, fatigue, weight loss, bronze skin, hypotension vitiligo, and depression.

♦ ***Appendicitis.*** In acute appendicitis, a brief period of nausea may accompany onset of abdominal pain. Pain typically begins as vague epigastric or periumbilical discomfort and rapidly progresses to severe stabbing pain localized in the right lower quadrant (McBurney's sign). Associated findings usually include abdominal rigidity and tenderness, cutaneous hyperalgesia, fever, constipation or diarrhea, tachycardia, anorexia, moderate malaise, and positive psoas and obturator signs.

♦ ***Cholecystitis (acute).*** Here, nausea commonly follows severe right-upper-quadrant pain that may radiate to the back or shoulders, commonly following meals. Associated findings include mild vomiting, abdominal tenderness and, possibly, rigidity and distention, fever with chills, diaphoresis, and a positive Murphy's sign.

♦ ***Cholelithiasis.*** In this disorder, nausea accompanies attacks of severe right-upper-quadrant or epigastric pain after ingestion of fatty foods. Other associated findings include vomiting, abdominal tenderness and guarding, flatulence, belching, epigastric burning, tachycardia, and restlessness. Occlusion of the common bile duct may cause jaundice, clay-colored stools, fever, and chills.

♦ ***Cirrhosis.*** Insidious early symptoms of cirrhosis typically include nausea and vomiting, anorexia, abdominal pain, and constipation or diarrhea. As the disease progresses, jaundice and hepatomegaly may occur with abdominal distention, spider angiomas, palmar erythema, severe pruritus, dry skin, fetor hepaticus, enlarged superficial abdominal veins, mental changes, and bilateral gynecomastia and testicular atrophy or menstrual irregularities.

♦ ***Diverticulitis.*** Besides nausea, diverticulitis may cause intermittent abdominal pain, constipation or diarrhea, low-grade fever and, commonly, a palpable, tender, firm, fixed mass.

♦ ***Gastritis.*** Nausea is common in this disorder, especially after ingestion of alcohol, aspirin, spicy foods, or caffeine. Vomiting of mucus or blood, epigastric pain, belching, fever, and malaise may occur.

♦ ***Gastroenteritis.*** Usually viral, this disorder causes nausea, vomiting, diarrhea, and abdominal cramping. Fever, malaise, hyperactive bowel sounds, abdominal pain and tenderness, and possible dehydration may also develop.

♦ ***Heart failure.*** This disorder may cause nausea and vomiting, particularly with right-sided heart failure. Associated findings include tachycardia, ventricular gallop, profound fatigue, dyspnea, crackles, peripheral edema, jugular vein distention, ascites, nocturia, and diastolic hypertension.

♦ ***Hepatitis.*** Nausea is an insidious early symptom of viral hepatitis. Vomiting, fatigue, myalgia and arthralgia, headache, anorexia, photophobia, pharyngitis, cough, and fever also occur early in the preicteric phase.

♦ ***Hyperemesis gravidarum.*** Unremitting nausea and vomiting that persist beyond the first trimester are characteristic of this disorder of pregnancy. Vomitus ranges from undigested food, mucus, and bile early in the disorder to a "coffee-ground" appearance in later stages. Associated findings include weight loss, signs of dehydration, headache, and delirium.

♦ ***Intestinal obstruction.*** Nausea occurs frequently, especially in high small-intestinal obstruction. Vomiting may be bilious or fecal; abdominal pain is usually episodic and colicky but can become severe and steady with strangulation. Constipation occurs early in large-intestinal and later in small-intestinal obstruction; obstipation may signal complete obstruction. Bowel sounds are typically hyperactive in partial obstruction and hypoactive or absent in complete obstruction. Abdominal distention and tenderness may be accompanied by visible peristaltic waves or a palpable abdominal mass.

♦ ***Labyrinthitis.*** Nausea and vomiting commonly occur with this acute inner ear inflammation. More significant findings include severe vertigo, progressive hearing loss, nystagmus, tinnitus and, possibly, otorrhea.

♦ ***Ménière's disease.*** This disease causes sudden, brief, recurrent attacks of nausea, vomiting, vertigo, tinnitus, diaphoresis, and nystagmus. It also causes hearing loss and ear fullness.

♦ ***Mesenteric artery ischemia.*** Here, nausea and vomiting may accompany severe cramping abdominal pain, especially after meals. Other findings include diarrhea or constipation, abdominal tenderness and bloating, anorexia, weight loss, and abdominal bruits.

♦ ***Metabolic acidosis.*** This acid-base imbalance may cause nausea and vomiting, anorexia, diarrhea, Kussmaul's respirations, and decreased LOC.

♦ ***Migraine headache.*** Nausea and vomiting may occur in the prodromal stage. Other findings may include photophobia, light flashes, increased sensitivity to noise, light-headedness and, possibly partial vision loss and paresthesia of the lips, face, or hands.

♦ ***Motion sickness.*** In this disorder, nausea and vomiting are brought on by motion or rhythmic movement. Headache, dizziness, fatigue, diaphoresis, hypersalivation, and dyspnea may also occur.

♦ ***Pancreatitis (acute).*** Nausea, usually followed by vomiting, is an early symptom of pancreatitis. Common associated findings include steady, severe pain in the epigastrium or left upper quadrant that may radiate to the back; abdominal tenderness and rigidity; diminished bowel sounds; and fever. Tachycardia, restlessness, hypotension, skin mottling, and cold, sweaty extremities may occur in severe cases.

♦ ***Peptic ulcer.*** In this disorder, nausea and vomiting may follow attacks of sharp or burning epigastric pain. Attacks typically occur when the stomach is empty or after ingestion of alcohol, caffeine, or aspirin; they're relieved by eating or by taking antacids or antisecretory agents. Hematemesis or melena may also occur.

♦ ***Peritonitis.*** Nausea and vomiting usually accompany acute abdominal pain localized to the area of inflammation. Other findings may include high fever with chills, tachycardia, hypoactive or absent bowel sounds, abdominal distention and tenderness (including rebound tenderness), positive obturator sign and obturator weakness, diaphoresis, hypotension, shallow respirations, pale, cold skin, and hiccups.

♦ ***Preeclampsia.*** Nausea and vomiting commonly occur in this disorder of pregnancy, along with rapid weight gain, epigastric pain, generalized edema, elevated blood pressure, oliguria, severe frontal headache, hyperreflexia, and blurred or double vision.

Other causes

♦ ***Drugs.*** Common nausea-producing drugs include antineoplastic agents, opiates, ferrous sulfate, levodopa, oral potassium chloride replacements, estrogens, sulfasalazine, antibiotics, quinidine, anesthetic agents, and digoxin or theophylline overdose.

♦ **Herb alert** Herbal medicines such as ginkgo biloba and St. John's wort can cause adverse effects, including nausea.

♦ ***Radiation and surgery.*** Radiation therapy may cause nausea and vomiting. Postoperative nausea and vomiting are common, especially after abdominal surgery.

Special considerations

If your patient is experiencing severe nausea, prepare him for blood tests to determine fluid and electrolyte status and acid-base balance. Have him breathe deeply to ease his nausea; keep his room air fresh and clean-smelling by removing bedpans and emesis basins promptly after use and by providing adequate ventilation. Because he could easily aspirate vomitus when supine, elevate his head or position him on his side.

Because pain can precipitate or intensify nausea, administer pain medications promptly, as needed. If possible, give medications by injection or suppository to prevent exacerbating nausea. When you administer antiemetics, be alert for abdominal distention and hypoactive bowel sounds, which may indicate gastric retention. If you detect these signs, insert a nasogastric tube, as required.

Pediatric pointers

Nausea, frequently described as stomachache, is one of the most common childhood complaints. Commonly the result of overeating, it can also occur as part of diverse disorders, ranging from acute infections to a conversion reaction caused by fear.

Geriatric pointers

Elderly patients have increased dental caries; tooth loss; decreased salivary gland function, which causes mouth dryness; reduced gastric acid output and motility; and decreased senses of taste and smell. All of these may be factors contributing to nonpathologic nausea.

NECK PAIN

Neck pain may originate from any neck structure, from the meninges and cervical vertebrae to blood vessels, muscles, or lymphatic tissue. This symptom can also be referred from other areas of the body. Its location, onset, and pattern help determine its origin and underlying causes. Neck pain usually results from trauma and degenerative, congenital, inflammatory, metabolic, and neoplastic disorders.

Emergency interventions

If the patient's neck pain is due to trauma, first provide proper cervical spine immobilization, preferably with a long backboard and a Philadelphia collar. (See *Applying a Philadelphia collar.*) Then take vital signs, and perform a quick neurologic evaluation. If he shows signs of respiratory distress, give oxygen. Intubation and mechanical ventilation may be necessary. Ask the patient (or his companion, if the patient can't answer) how the injury occurred. Then examine the neck for abrasions, swelling, lacerations, erythema, and ecchymoses.

Applying a Philadelphia collar

A lightweight molded polyethylene collar designed to hold the neck straight with the chin slightly elevated and tucked in, the Philadelphia cervical collar immobilizes the cervical spine, decreases muscle spasms, and relieves some pain. It also prevents further injury and promotes healing.

When applying the collar, fit it snugly around the patient's neck and attach the Velcro fasteners or buckles at the back. Be sure to check the patient's airway and his neurovascular status to make sure that the collar isn't too tight.

Also make sure that the collar isn't placed too high in front, which can hyperextend the neck. In a patient with a neck sprain, hyperextension may cause the ligaments to heal in a shortened position; in a patient with a cervical spine fracture, it could cause serious neurologic damage.

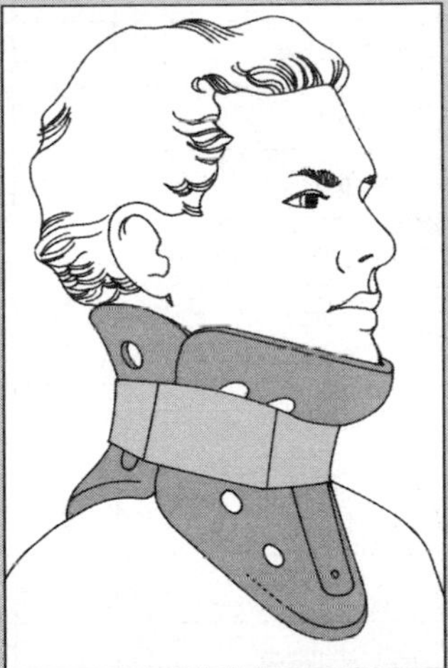

History and physical examination

If the patient hasn't sustained trauma, inquire about the severity and onset of his neck pain. Where in the neck does he feel pain? Does anything relieve or worsen the pain? Ask about the other symptoms, such as headaches. Next, focus on the patient's current and past illnesses and injuries, diet, medication use, and family health history.

Thoroughly inspect the patient's neck, shoulders, and cervical spine for swelling, masses, erythema, and ecchymoses. Assess active range of motion in his neck by having him perform flexion, extension, rotation, and lateral side bending. Note the degree of pain produced by these movements. Examine posture and test muscle strength. Check the sensation in his arms, and assess his hand grasp and arm reflexes. Attempt to elicit

Neck pain: Common causes and associated findings

S&S

CAUSES	MAJOR ASSOCIATED SIGNS AND SYMPTOMS													
	Arm pain	Back pain	Brudzinski's sign	Decreased level of consciousness	Decreased range of motion	Deformity	Dysphagia	Dyspnea	Ecchymoses	Fatigue	Fever	Headache	Hemoptysis	Hoarseness
Ankylosing spondylitis	◆	◆			◆					◆	◆			
Cervical extension injury	◆	◆										◆		
Cervical spine fracture					◆	◆						◆		
Cervical spine tumor					◆									
Cervical spondylosis	◆				◆									
Esophageal trauma							◆						◆	
Herniated cervical disk	◆	◆			◆									
Laryngeal cancer							◆	◆					◆	◆
Lymphadenitis											◆			
Meningitis			◆	◆							◆	◆		
Neck sprain					◆				◆					
Rheumatoid arthritis					◆	◆				◆	◆			
Spinous process fracture					◆	◆								
Subarachnoid hemorrhage			◆	◆								◆		
Thyroid trauma								◆	◆					
Torticollis														
Tracheal trauma							◆	◆					◆	◆

Kernig's sign	Lymphadenopathy	Malaise	Muscle spasms	Nuchal rigidity	Paralysis	Paresthesia	Swelling	Tenderness	Weakness
		◆		◆					
			◆	◆			◆		
					◆				
					◆	◆			◆
						◆			◆
							◆		
						◆			◆
	◆								
	◆	◆						◆	
◆				◆					
			◆	◆			◆		
		◆				◆	◆	◆	◆
			◆				◆	◆	
◆				◆					
							◆		
				◆	◆				

Brudzinski's and Kernig's signs, and palpate the cervical lymph nodes for enlargement. (See *Neck pain: Common causes and associated findings.*)

Common medical causes

◆ ***Ankylosing spondylitis.*** Intermittent, moderate-to-severe neck pain and stiffness with severely restricted range of motion are characteristic of this disorder. Related findings, which occur intermittently, may include lower back pain and stiffness, arm pain, low-grade fever, limited chest expansion, malaise, anorexia, fatigue and, occasionally, iritis.

◆ ***Cervical extension injury.*** Anterior or posterior neck pain may develop within hours or days after a whiplash injury. Anterior pain usually diminishes within several days, but posterior pain persists and may even intensify. Associated findings may include tenderness, swelling and nuchal rigidity, arm or back pain, occipital headache, muscle spasms, visual blurring, and unilateral miosis on the affected side.

◆ ***Cervical spine fracture.*** Fracture at C1 to C4 commonly causes sudden death; survivors may experience severe neck pain that restricts all movement, intense occipital headache, quadriplegia, deformity, or respiratory paralysis.

◆ ***Cervical spine tumor.*** *Metastatic tumors* typically cause persistent neck pain that increases with movement and isn't relieved by rest; *primary tumors* cause mild to severe pain along a specific nerve root. Other findings depend on the site of the lesion and may include paresthesia, arm or leg weakness that progresses to atrophy and paralysis, and bladder or bowel incontinence.

◆ ***Cervical spondylosis.*** This degenerative process causes posterior neck pain that restricts movement and is aggravated by it. Pain may radiate down either arm and may accompany paresthesia and weakness.

ALTERNATIVE THERAPY

Therapeutic touch for neck pain

Therapeutic touch can be used to treat pain and reduce inflammation. This alternative therapy is a combination of body work and visualization in which the practitioner assesses the patient's energy field by slowly moving his hands a few inches over the patient's body. (Therapeutic touch is a misnomer because body contact is rare.) Blocked energy fields, evidenced by a feeling of radiant heat or unusual pressure, indicate an underlying disorder.

Energy fields are believed to be linked to hemoglobin levels in circulating blood. By dissipating the blocked energy to other parts of the body, therapeutic touch is believed to restore the patient's vitality and well-being.

♦ ***Esophageal trauma.*** An esophageal mucosal tear or a pulsion diverticulum may cause mild neck pain, chest pain, edema, hemoptysis, and dysphagia.

♦ ***Herniated cervical disk.*** This disorder characteristically causes variable neck pain that restricts movement and is aggravated by it. It also may cause referred pain, paresthesia and other sensory disturbances, or arm weakness.

♦ ***Laryngeal cancer.*** Neck pain that radiates to the ear develops late in this disorder. The patient may also exhibit dysphagia, dyspnea, hemoptysis, stridor, hoarseness, or cervical lymphadenopathy.

♦ ***Lymphadenitis.*** In this disorder, enlarged and inflamed cervical lymph nodes cause acute pain and tenderness. Fever, chills, and malaise may also occur.

♦ ***Meningitis.*** Neck pain may accompany characteristic nuchal rigidity. Related findings include fever, headache, photophobia, positive Brudzinski's and Kernig's signs, and decreased LOC.

♦ ***Neck sprain.*** *Minor sprains* typically cause pain, slight swelling, stiffness, and restricted range of motion. *Ligament rupture* causes pain, marked swelling, ecchymosis, muscle spasms, and nuchal rigidity with head tilt.

♦ ***Rheumatoid arthritis.*** This disorder usually affects peripheral joints, but it can also involve the cervical vertebrae. Acute inflammation may cause moderate to severe pain that radiates along a specific nerve root; increased warmth, swelling, and tenderness in involved joints; stiffness that restricts range of motion; paresthesia and muscle weakness; low-grade fever; anorexia; malaise; fatigue; and possible neck deformity. Some pain and stiffness remain after the acute phase.

♦ ***Spinous process fracture.*** Fracture near the cervicothoracic junction causes acute pain radiating to the shoulders. Associated findings include swelling, exquisite tenderness, restricted range of motion, muscle spasms, and deformity.

♦ ***Subarachnoid hemorrhage.*** This life-threatening condition may cause moderate to severe neck pain and rigidity, headache, and a decreased LOC. Kernig's and Brudzinski's signs are present.

♦ ***Thyroid trauma.*** Besides mild to moderate neck pain, thyroid trauma may cause local swelling and ecchymosis. If a hematoma forms, it can cause dyspnea.

♦ ***Torticollis.*** In this neck deformity, severe neck pain accompanies recurrent unilateral stiffness and muscle spasms that cause the characteristic head tilt.

♦ ***Tracheal trauma.*** *Fracture of the tracheal cartilage,* a life-threatening condition, causes moderate to severe neck pain and respiratory difficulty. *Torn tracheal mucosa* causes mild to moderate pain and may result in airway occlusion, hemoptysis, hoarseness, or dysphagia.

Special considerations

Promote patient comfort by giving anti-inflammatory drugs and analgesics, as needed. Prepare him for diagnostic tests, such as X-rays, computed tomography scan, blood tests, and cerebrospinal fluid analysis. (See *Therapeutic touch for neck pain.*)

Pediatric pointers

The most common causes of neck pain in children are meningitis and trauma. A rare cause of neck pain is congenital torticollis.

NIPPLE DISCHARGE

Nipple discharge can occur spontaneously or can be elicited by nipple stimulation and doesn't always signal a problem. It's characterized as intermittent or constant, unilateral or bilateral, and by color, consistency, and composition. Its incidence increases with age and parity. Although rare, this sign can occur in men and in nulligravida, regularly menstruating women. It's relatively common and often normal in parous women. A thick, grayish discharge—benign epithelial debris from inactive ducts—can commonly be elicited in middle-aged parous women. Colostrum, a thin, yellowish or milky discharge, is common in the last weeks of pregnancy.

Nipple discharge can be the result of taking medications, such as oral contraceptives, sedatives, or tranquilizers, or it can signal serious underlying disease, particularly when accompanied by other breast changes. Significant causes include endocrine disorders, cancer, certain drugs, and blocked lactiferous ducts.

History and physical examination

Ask the patient when she first noticed the discharge, and determine its duration, extent, quantity, color, and consistency. Has she had other nipple and breast changes, such as pain, tenderness, itching, warmth, changes in contour, and lumps? If she reports a lump, question her about its onset, location, size, and consistency.

Obtain a complete gynecologic and obstetric history, and determine her normal menstrual cycle and the date of her last menses. Ask if she experiences breast swelling and tenderness, bloating, irritability, headaches, abdominal cramping, nausea, or diarrhea before or during menses. Note the number, date, and outcome of her pregnancies and, if she breast-fed, the approximate date of her last lactation. Ask her about her history of breast-related procedures, including therapeutic, diagnostic, and cosmetic. Also, check for risk factors of breast cancer—family history, previous or current malignancies, nulliparity or first pregnancy after age 30, early menarche, or late menopause.

Is the patient taking hormones (oral contraceptive pills or hormone replacement therapy)? Is the discharge spontaneous, or does it have to be expressed? If the discharge becomes bloody, instruct the patient to seek medical evaluation.

Start your physical examination by characterizing the discharge. If the discharge isn't frank, try to elicit it. (See *Eliciting nipple discharge*, page 412.) Then examine the nipples and breasts with the patient in four positions: sitting with her arms at her sides, with her arms overhead, with her hands pressing on her hips; and leaning forward from a standing position so her breasts are suspended. Check for nipple deviation, flattening, retraction, redness, asymmetry, thickening, excoriation, erosion, or cracking. Inspect her breasts for asymmetry, irregular contours, dimpling, erythema, and peau d'orange. With the patient supine, palpate the breasts and axilla for lumps, giving special attention to the areolae. Note the size, location, delineation, consistency, and mobility of any lumps you find.

EXAMINATION TIP

Eliciting nipple discharge

If your patient has a history or evidence of nipple discharge, you can attempt to elicit it during your examination. Position the patient supine, and gently squeeze her nipple between your thumb and index finger; note any discharge through the nipple. Then place your fingers on the areola, as shown, and palpate the entire areolar surface, watching for any discharge through areolar ducts.

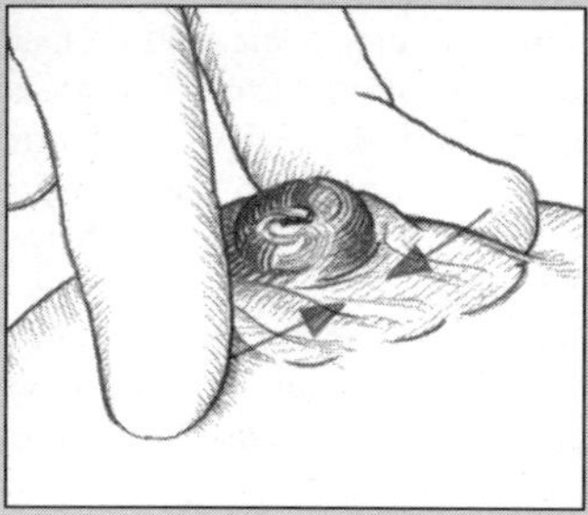

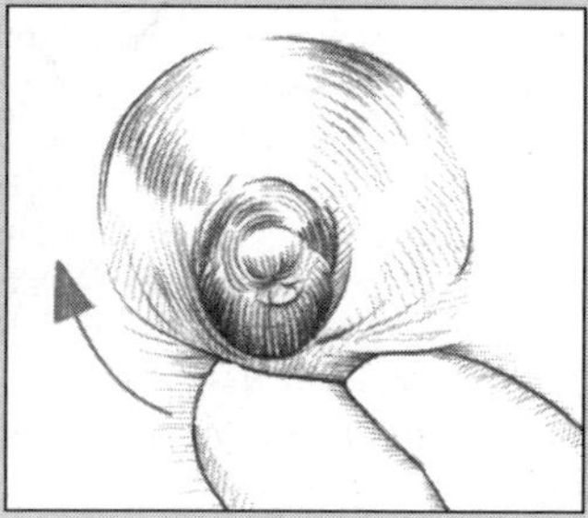

Ductographic mammography may be needed to locate nonpalpable cancer or benign tumor causing the discharge.

Common medical causes

♦ ***Abscess.*** This disorder, most common in lactating women, may produce a thick, purulent discharge from a cracked nipple or infected duct. Associated findings include abrupt onset of high fever with chills; breast pain, tenderness, and erythema; a palpable soft nodule or generalized induration; and possibly nipple retraction.

♦ ***Cancer.*** This may cause bloody, watery, or purulent discharge from a normal-appearing nipple. Characteristic findings include a hard, irregular, fixed lump; erythema; dimpling; peau d'orange; changes in contour; nipple deviation, flattening, or retraction; axillary lymphadenopathy; and possibly breast pain.

♦ ***Choriocarcinoma.*** Galactorrhea (a white or grayish milky discharge) may result from this highly malignant neoplasm, which can follow pregnancy. Other characteristics include persistent uterine bleeding and bogginess after delivery or curettage and vaginal masses.

♦ ***Intraductal papilloma.*** *Single* intraductal papillomas generally affect women nearing menopause. *Multiple* intraductal papillomas are most common in younger women. This disorder is the most common cause and is the predominant sign of unilateral serous, serosanguineous, or bloody nipple discharge — usually from only one duct. Discharge may be intermittent or profuse and constant and can commonly be stimulated by gentle pressure around the areola. Subareolar nodules, breast pain, and tenderness may occur.

♦ ***Mammary duct ectasia.*** A thick, sticky, grayish discharge from multiple ducts may be the first sign of this disorder. The discharge may be bilateral and is usually spontaneous. Other findings include a rubbery, poorly delineated lump beneath the areola, with a blue-green discoloration of the overlying skin; nipple retraction; and redness, swelling, tenderness, and burning pain in the areola and nipple.

♦ ***Paget's disease.*** Denuded skin on the nipple, which is red, intensely itchy and, possibly, eroded or excoriated, produces a serous or bloody discharge. The discharge is usually unilateral.

♦ ***Prolactin-secreting pituitary tumor.*** Bilateral galactorrhea may occur in patients with this tumor. Other findings include amenorrhea, infertility, decreased libido and vaginal secretions, headaches, and blindness.

♦ ***Proliferative (fibrocystic) breast disease.*** This benign disorder occasionally causes a bilateral clear, milky, or straw-colored discharge, which is rarely purulent or bloody. Multiple round, soft, tender nodules are usually palpable in both breasts, although they may occur singly. Usually, nodules are mobile and are located in the upper outer quadrant. Nodule size, tenderness, and discharge increase during the luteal phase of the menstrual cycle. Symptoms then regress after menses.

Other causes

♦ ***Drugs.*** Galactorrhea can be caused by some antihypertensives (reserpine and methyldopa), oral contraceptives, cimetidine, metoclopramide, verapamil, and psychotropic agents, particularly phenothiazines and tricyclic antidepressants.

♦ ***Surgery.*** Chest wall surgery may stimulate the thoracic nerves, causing intermittent bilateral galactorrhea.

Special considerations

Although nipple discharge is usually insignificant, it can be very frightening to the patient. Help relieve the patient's anxieties by clearly explaining the nature and origin of her discharge. Apply a breast binder, which may reduce discharge by eliminating nipple stimulation.

Diagnostic tests may include tissue biopsy (if a breast lump is found), cytologic study of the discharge, ductographic mammography, ultrasonography, transillumination, and serum prolactin.

Pediatric pointers

Nipple discharge in children and adolescents is rare. When it does occur, it's almost always nonpathologic, such as the bloody discharge that sometimes accompanies onset of menarche. Infants of either sex may produce a milky breast discharge beginning 3 days after birth and lasting up to 2 weeks.

Geriatric pointers

In postmenopausal women, breast changes are considered malignant until proven otherwise. Encourage continued regular breast self examination and obtain a history of hormone replacement therapy, including herbal preparations.

NIPPLE RETRACTION

Nipple retraction, the inward displacement of the nipple below the level of surrounding breast tissue, may indicate an inflammatory breast lesion or cancer. It results from scar tissue formation within a lesion or large mammary duct. As the scar tissue shortens, it pulls adjacent tissue inward, causing nipple deviation, flattening, and finally retraction.

History and physical examination

Ask the patient when she first noticed retraction of the nipple. Has she experienced other nipple changes, such as itching, discoloration, discharge, or excoriation? Has she noticed breast pain, lumps, redness, swelling, or warmth? Obtain a history, noting risk factors of breast cancer, such as a family history or previous malignancy.

Carefully examine both nipples and breasts with the patient sitting upright with her arms at her sides, with her hands pressing on her hips, with her arms overhead, and with the patient leaning forward from a standing position so her breasts are suspended. Look for redness, excoriation, and discharge; nipple flattening and deviation; and breast asymmetry, dimpling, or contour differences.

EXAMINATION TIP

Differentiating nipple retraction from inversion

Nipple retraction is commonly confused with nipple inversion, a common abnormality that's often congenital and does not usually signal underlying disease. A *retracted* nipple appears flat and broad, whereas an *inverted* nipple can be pulled out from the sulcus where it hides.

NIPPLE RETRACTION

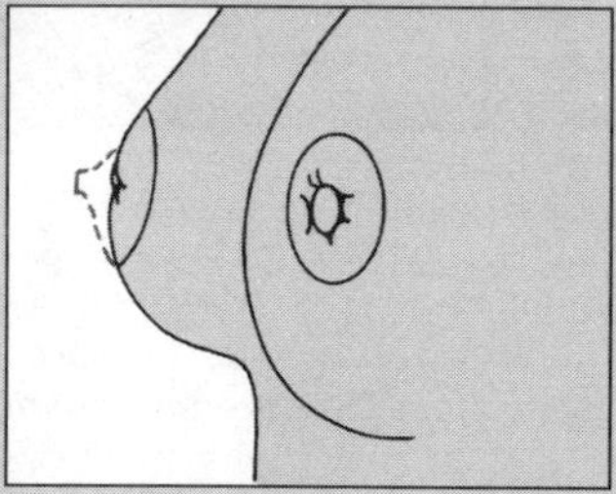

NIPPLE INVERSION

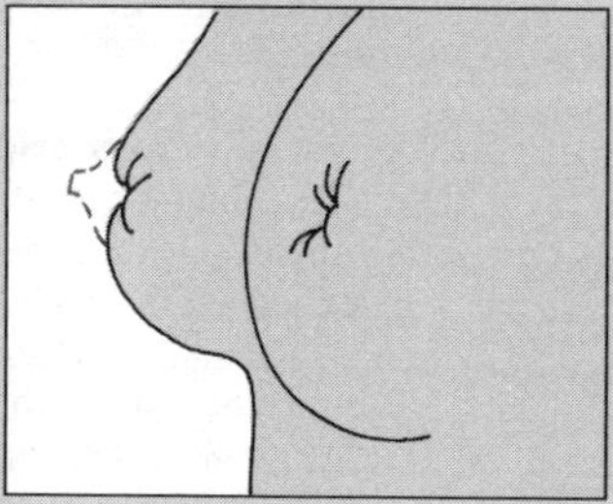

(See *Differentiating nipple retraction from inversion.*)

Try to evert the nipple by gently squeezing the areola. With the patient supine, palpate both breasts for lumps, especially beneath the areola. Mold breast skin over the lump or gently pull it up toward the clavicle, looking for accentuated nipple retraction. Also, palpate axillary lymph nodes.

Common medical causes

- ***Abscess.*** This disorder, most common in lactating women, occasionally causes unilateral nipple retraction. More frequent findings include high fever with chills; breast pain, erythema, and tenderness; breast induration or soft mass; and cracked, sore nipples, possibly with purulent discharge.
- ***Cancer.*** Unilateral nipple retraction is commonly accompanied by a hard, fixed, nontender nodule beneath the areola, as well as other breast nodules. Other nipple changes include itching, burning, erosion, and watery or bloody discharge. Breast changes commonly include dimpling, altered contour, peau d'orange, ulceration, tenderness (possibly pain), redness, and warmth. Axillary lymph nodes may be enlarged.
- ***Mammary duct ectasia.*** Nipple retraction commonly accompanies a poorly defined, rubbery nodule beneath the areola; blue-green skin discoloration; areolar burning, itching, swelling, tenderness, or erythema; and nipple pain with a thick, sticky, grayish, multiductal discharge.
- ***Mastitis.*** In this disorder, nipple retraction, deviation, cracking, or flattening may accompany a firm and indurated or tender, flocculent, discrete breast nodule, warmth, erythema, tenderness, and edema. Fatigue, high fevers, and chills may also be present.

Other causes

- ***Surgery.*** Previous breast surgery may cause underlying scarring and retraction.

Special considerations

Prepare the patient for diagnostic tests, including mammography, cytology of nipple discharge, and biopsy.

Pediatric pointers

Nipple retraction doesn't occur in prepubescent females.

Nocturia

Nocturia — excessive urination at night — may result from disruption of the normal diurnal pattern of urine concentration or from overstimulation of the nerves and muscles that control urination. Normally, more urine is concentrated during the night than during the day. As a result, most persons excrete three to four times more urine during the day and can sleep for 6 to 8 hours during the night without being awakened. In nocturia, the patient may awaken one or more times during the night to empty his bladder and excrete 700 ml or more of urine.

Although nocturia usually results from renal and lower urinary tract disorders, it may result from cardiovascular, endocrine, or metabolic disorders. This common sign may also result from drugs that induce diuresis, particularly when they're taken at night, and from the ingestion of large quantities of fluids, especially caffeinated beverages or alcohol, at bedtime.

History and physical examination

Begin by exploring the history of the patient's nocturia. When did it begin? How often does it occur? Can the patient identify a specific pattern? Precipitating factors? Also, note the volume of urine voided. Ask the patient about change in the color, odor, or consistency of his urine. Has the patient changed his usual pattern or volume of fluid intake? Next, explore associated symptoms. Ask about pain or burning on urination, difficulty initiating a urine stream, costovertebral angle tenderness, and flank, upper abdominal, or suprapubic pain.

Determine if the patient or his family has a history of renal or urinary tract disorders or endocrine and metabolic diseases, particularly diabetes. Is he taking drugs that increase urine output, such as diuretics, cardiac glycosides, and antihypertensives?

Focus your physical examination on palpating and percussing the kidneys, the costovertebral angle, and the bladder. Carefully inspect the urinary meatus. Inspect a urine specimen for color, odor, and the presence of sediment.

Common medical causes

♦ ***Benign prostatic hyperplasia.*** Common in men older than age 50, this disorder causes nocturia when significant urethral obstruction develops. Typically, it causes frequency, hesitancy, incontinence, reduced force and caliber of the urine stream and, possibly, hematuria. Oliguria may also occur. Palpation reveals a distended bladder and an enlarged prostate. The patient may also complain of lower abdominal fullness, perineal pain, and constipation. Obstruction may lead to renal failure.

♦ ***Cystitis.*** All three forms of cystitis may cause nocturia marked by frequent, small voidings and accompanied by dysuria and tenesmus. *Bacterial cystitis* may also cause urinary urgency; hematuria; fatigue; suprapubic, perineal, flank, and lower back pain; and occasionally, low-grade fever. Most common in women between the ages of 25 and 60, *chronic interstitial cystitis* is characterized by Hunner's ulcers — small, punctate, bleeding lesions in the bladder; it also causes gross hematuria. Symptoms resemble bladder cancer, which must be ruled out. *Viral cystitis* also causes urinary urgency, hematuria, and fever.

♦ ***Diabetes insipidus.*** The result of antidiuretic hormone deficiency, this disorder usually causes nocturia early in its course. It's characterized by intermittent voiding of moderate to large amounts of urine. Diabetes insipidus can also cause polydipsia and dehydration.

♦ ***Diabetes mellitus.*** In this early sign of diabetes mellitus, voidings are frequent and large. Associated features include daytime polyuria, polydipsia, polyphagia, frequent urinary tract infections, recurrent yeast infections, vaginitis, weakness, fatigue, weight loss and, possibly, signs of dehydration, such as dry mucous membranes and poor skin turgor.

♦ ***Hypercalcemic nephropathy.*** In this disorder, the patient has intermittent nighttime voiding of moderate to large amounts of urine. Related findings include daytime polyuria, polydipsia, and occasionally, hematuria and pyuria.

♦ ***Prostatic cancer.*** This disorder is usually asymptomatic in early stages. Later, it causes nocturia with infrequent voiding of moderate amounts of urine. Other characteristic effects include dysuria (most common symptom), difficulty initiating a urine stream, bladder distention, urinary frequency, weight loss, pallor, weakness, perineal pain, and constipation. Palpation reveals a hard, irregularly shaped, nodular prostate.

♦ ***Pyelonephritis (acute).*** Nocturia occurs frequently in this inflammatory disorder and is usually characterized by infrequent voiding of moderate amounts of urine. The urine may appear cloudy. Associated signs and symptoms include a high sustained fever with chills, fatigue, unilateral or bilateral flank pain, costovertebral angle tenderness, weakness, dysuria, hematuria, urinary frequency and urgency, and tenesmus. Occasionally, anorexia, nausea, vomiting, diarrhea, and hypoactive bowel sounds may occur.

♦ ***Renal failure (chronic).*** Nocturia occurs relatively early in this disorder and is usually characterized by infrequent voiding of moderate amounts of urine. As the disorder progresses, oliguria or even anuria develops. Other widespread effects of chronic renal failure include fatigue, ammonia breath odor, Kussmaul's respirations, peripheral edema, elevated blood pressure, decreased level of consciousness, confusion, emotional lability, muscle twitching, anorexia, metallic taste in the mouth, constipation or diarrhea, petechiae, ecchymoses, pruritus, yellow- or bronze-tinged skin, nausea, and vomiting.

Other causes

♦ ***Drugs.*** Any drug that mobilizes edematous fluid or causes diuresis (for example, diuretics and cardiac glycosides) may cause nocturia; obviously, this effect depends on when the drug is administered.

Special considerations

Patient care includes maintaining fluid balance, ensuring adequate rest, and providing patient education. Monitor vital signs, intake and output, and daily weight; continue to document the frequency of nocturia, amount, and specific gravity. Plan administration of diuretics for daytime hours, if possible. Also plan rest periods to compensate for sleep lost because of nocturia.

Prepare the patient for diagnostic tests, which may include routine urinalysis, urine concentration and dilution studies, and serum blood urea nitrogen, creatinine, and electrolyte levels.

Pediatric pointers

In children, nocturia may be involuntary; the condition is commonly known as enuresis, or bedwetting. With the exception of prostate disorders, causes of nocturia are generally the same for children and adults. However, children with pyelonephritis are more susceptible to sepsis, which may display as fever, irritability, and poor skin perfusion. In addition, girls may experience vaginal discharge and vulvar soreness or pruritus.

Geriatric pointers

Postmenopausal women have decreased bladder elasticity, but urine output remains constant, resulting in nocturia.

Nuchal rigidity

Frequently an early sign of meningeal irritation, nuchal rigidity is stiffness of the neck that prevents flexion. To elicit this sign, attempt to passively flex the patient's neck and touch his chin to his chest. If nuchal rigidity is present, this maneuver triggers pain and muscle spasms. (Be sure to rule out cervical spinal misalignment, such as a fracture or dislocation, before testing for nuchal rigidity. Severe spinal cord damage could result.) Don't try to perform flexion movement beyond the point of resistance. If the patient has a suspected head or neck injury assume that he has a cervical injury until a cervical spine X-ray has been obtained and a neck injury is ruled out.

Nuchal rigidity may herald life-threatening subarachnoid hemorrhage or meningitis. It may also be a late sign of cervical arthritis, in which joint mobility is gradually lost. The patient may notice nuchal rigidity when he attempts to flex his neck during daily activities.

Emergency interventions

After eliciting nuchal rigidity, attempt to elicit Kernig's and Brudzinski's signs. Quickly evaluate level of consciousness (LOC). Take vital signs. If you note signs of increased intracranial pressure (ICP), such as increased systolic pressure, bradycardia, and widened pulse pressure, start an I.V. line for drug administration and deliver oxygen, as necessary. Draw a specimen for routine blood studies.

History and physical examination

Obtain a patient history, relying on family members if altered LOC prevents the patient from responding. Ask about the onset and duration of neck stiffness, precipitating factors, and associated symptoms, such as headache, fever, nausea and vomiting, or motor and sensory changes. Also ask the patient about recent head or neck surgeries. Check for a history of hypertension, head trauma, recent head or neck surgery, cerebral aneurysm or arteriovenous malformation, endocarditis, recent infection (such as sinusitis or pneumonia), or recent dental work. Then, obtain a complete drug history.

If the patient has no other signs of meningeal irritation, ask about a history of arthritis or neck trauma. Can the patient recall pulling a muscle in his neck? Inspect his hands for swollen, tender joints, and palpate the neck for pain or tenderness.

Common medical causes

♦ ***Cervical arthritis.*** In this disorder, nuchal rigidity develops gradually. Initially, the patient may complain of neck stiffness in the early morning or after a period of inactivity. Stiffness then becomes increasingly severe and frequent. Pain on movement, especially with lateral motion or head turning, is common. Typically, arthritis also affects other joints, especially those in the hands.

♦ ***Encephalitis.*** This viral infection may cause nuchal rigidity accompanied by other signs of meningeal irritation, such as positive Kernig's and Brudzinski's signs. Usually, nuchal rigidity appears abruptly and is preceded by headache, vomiting, and fever. The patient may display a rapidly decreasing LOC, progressing from lethargy to coma within 24 to 48 hours of onset. Associated features include seizures, ataxia, hemiparesis, nystagmus, and cranial nerve palsies, such as dysphagia and ptosis.

♦ ***Meningitis.*** Nuchal rigidity is an early sign in this disorder and is accompanied by other signs of meningeal irritation — positive Kernig's and Brudzinski's signs, hyperreflexia and, possibly, opisthotonos. Other early features include fever with chills, headache, photophobia, and vomiting. Initially, the patient is confused and irritable; later, he may become stuporous and seizure-prone or may slip into coma. Cranial nerve involvement may cause ocular palsies, facial weakness, and hearing loss. An erythematous papular rash occurs in some forms of viral meningitis; a purpuric rash may occur in meningococcal meningitis.

♦ ***Subarachnoid hemorrhage.*** Nuchal rigidity develops immediately after bleeding into the subarachnoid space. Kernig's and Brudzinski's signs may be present on examination. The patient may experience abrupt onset of severe headache, photophobia, fever, nausea and vomiting, dizziness, cranial nerve palsies, and focal neurologic signs, such as hemiparesis or hemiplegia. His LOC deteriorates rapidly, possibly progressing to coma. Signs of increased ICP, such as bradycardia and altered respirations, may also occur.

Special considerations

Prepare the patient for diagnostic tests, such as computed tomography scans, magnetic resonance imaging, and cervical spinal X-rays and lumbar puncture to examine the cerebrospinal fluid.

Monitor vital signs, intake and output, and neurologic status closely. Avoid routine administration of narcotic analgesics because these may mask signs of increasing ICP. Enforce strict bed rest; keep the head of the bed elevated at least 30 degrees to help minimize ICP.

Pediatric pointers

Nuchal rigidity reliably indicates meningeal irritation in children, unless they're paralyzed or comatose.

NYSTAGMUS

Nystagmus refers to the involuntary oscillations of one or—more commonly—both eyeballs. These oscillations are usually rhythmic and may be horizontal, vertical, or rotary. They may be transient or sustained and may occur spontaneously or on deviation or fixation of the eyes. Nystagmus may be dissociated, that is, more pronounced in one eye than the other. Although nystagmus is fairly easy to identify, the patient may be unaware of it unless it affects his vision.

Nystagmus may be classified as jerk or pendular. *Jerk nystagmus* (convergence-retraction, downbeat, vestibular) has a fast component and then a slow—perhaps unequal—corrective component in the opposite direction. *Pendular nystagmus* consists of horizontal (pendular) or vertical (seesaw) oscillations that are equal in both directions and resemble the movements of a clock's pendulum. (See *Classifying nystagmus*.)

Nystagmus is considered a *supranuclear* ocular palsy. That is, it results from pathology in the visual perceptual area, vestibular system, cerebellum, or brain stem rather than in the extraocular muscles or cranial nerve III, IV, or VI. Its causes are varied and include brain stem or cerebellar lesions, multiple sclerosis, encephalitis, labyrinthine disease, and drug toxicity. Occasionally, nystagmus is normal, as in the unconscious patient during the doll's eye test (oculocephalic stimulation) or the cold caloric water test (oculovestibular stimulation).

History and physical examination

Begin by asking the patient how long he's had nystagmus. Does it occur intermittently? Does it affect his vision? Ask about recent infection, especially of the ear or respiratory tract, and about head trauma and cancer. Does the patient or anyone in his family have a history of cerebrovascular accident (CVA)? Then explore associated signs and symptoms. Ask about vertigo, dizziness, tinnitus, nausea or vomiting, numbness, weakness, bladder dysfunction, fever, and apparent movement of the environment (oscillopsia).

Begin the physical examination by assessing the patient's level of conscious-

EXAMINATION TIP

Classifying nystagmus

JERK NYSTAGMUS

Convergence-retraction nystagmus refers to the irregular jerking of the eyes back into the orbit during upward gaze. It can indicate midbrain tegmental damage.

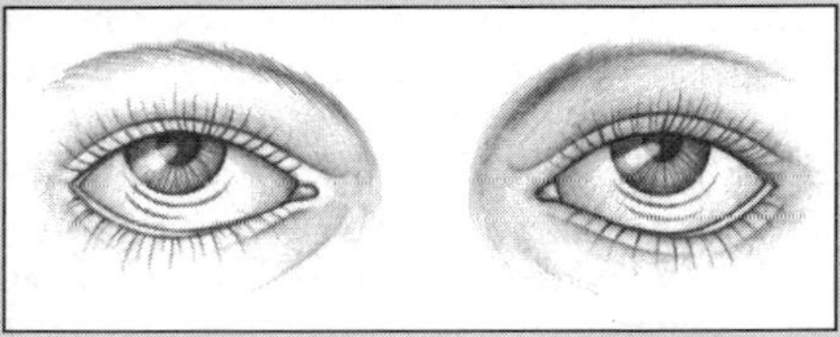

Downbeat nystagmus refers to the irregular downward jerking of the eyes during downward gaze. It can signal lower medullary damage; other causes include cerebellar degeneration, demyelinating disease, hydrocephalus, and anticonvulsant or lithium therapy.

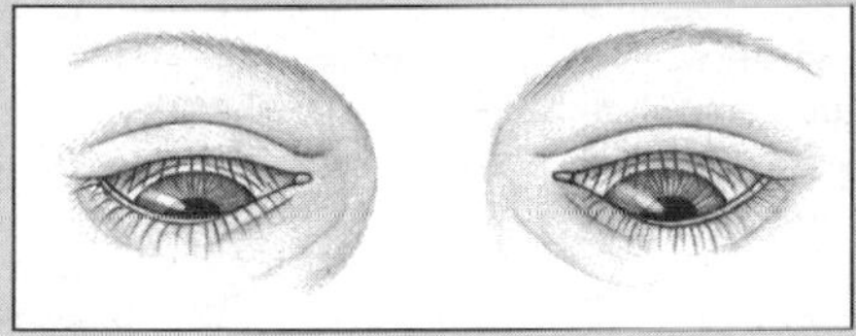

Vestibular nystagmus describes horizontal or rotary movement of the eyes. It suggests vestibular disease or cochlear dysfunction and is frequently elicited or enhanced by specific head positions.

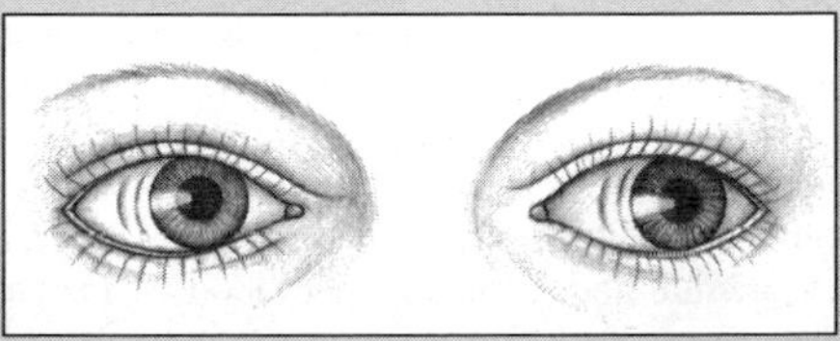

PENDULAR NYSTAGMUS

Horizontal nystagmus refers to oscillations of equal velocity around a center point. It can indicate a congenital loss of visual acuity or multiple sclerosis.

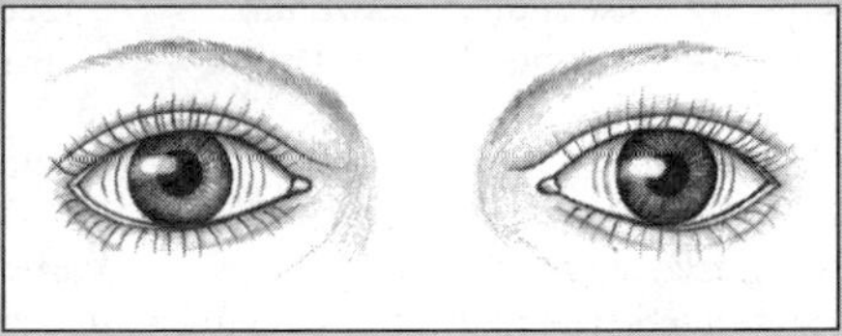

Vertical, or seesaw, nystagmus is the rapid, seesaw movement of the eyes; one eye rises while the other falls. It suggests an optic chiasm lesion in association with a bitemporal hemianopia and midbrain lesions.

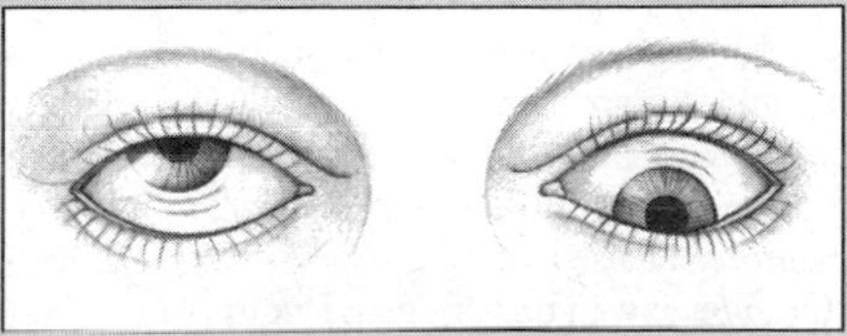

ness (LOC) and vital signs. Be alert for signs of increased intracranial pressure (ICP), such as pupillary changes, drowsiness, elevated systolic pressure, and altered respiratory pattern. Next, assess nystagmus fully by testing extraocular muscle function: Ask the patient to focus straight ahead and then to follow your finger up, down, and in an "X" across his face. Note when nystagmus occurs as well as its velocity and direction. Finally, test reflexes, motor and sensory function, and the cranial nerves. Abnormal spontaneous eye movements that mimic nystagmus — such as ocular flutter, square wave jerks, or opsoclonus (irregular, rapid, horizontal and vertical eye movements) — usually reflect cerebellar disease.

Common medical causes

♦ ***Brain tumor.*** Insidious onset of jerk nystagmus may signal tumors of the brain stem or cerebellum. Associated characteristics include deafness, dysphagia, nausea and vomiting, vertigo, and ataxia. Brain stem compression by the tumor may cause signs of increased ICP, such as altered LOC, bradycardia, widening pulse pressure, and elevated systolic blood pressure.

♦ ***Cerebrovascular accident.*** A CVA involving the posterior inferior cerebellar artery may cause sudden horizontal or vertical jerk nystagmus that may be gaze-dependent. Other findings include dysphagia, dysarthria, loss of pain and temperature sensation on the ipsilateral face and contralateral trunk and limbs, ipsilateral Horner's syndrome (unilateral ptosis, pupillary constriction, and facial anhidrosis), and cerebellar signs, such as ataxia and vertigo. Signs of increased ICP, such as altered LOC, bradycardia, widening pulse pressure, and elevated systolic pressure, may also occur.

♦ ***Encephalitis.*** In this disorder, jerk nystagmus is typically accompanied by altered LOC, ranging from lethargy to coma. Usually, it's preceded by sudden onset of fever, headache, and vomiting. Among other features are nuchal rigidity, seizures, aphasia, ataxia, photophobia, and cranial nerve palsies, such as dysphagia and ptosis.

♦ ***Head trauma.*** Brain stem injury may cause jerk nystagmus, which is usually horizontal. The patient may also display pupillary changes, altered respiratory pattern, coma, and decerebrate posture.

♦ ***Labyrinthitis (acute).*** This inner ear inflammation causes sudden onset of jerk nystagmus, accompanied by dizziness, vertigo, tinnitus, nausea, and vomiting. The fast component of the nystagmus is toward the unaffected ear. Gradual sensorineural hearing loss may also occur.

♦ ***Ménière's disease.*** This inner ear disorder is characterized by acute attacks of jerk nystagmus, severe nausea and vomiting, dizziness, vertigo, progressive hearing loss, tinnitus, and diaphoresis. Typically, the direction of jerk nystagmus varies from one attack to the next. Attacks may last from 10 minutes to several hours.

Other causes

♦ ***Drugs and alcohol.*** Jerk nystagmus may result from barbiturate, phenytoin, or carbamazepine toxicity or from alcohol intoxication.

Special considerations

Prepare the patient for diagnostic tests, such as electronystagmography and a cerebral computed tomography scan.

Pediatric pointers

In children, pendular nystagmus may be idiopathic, or it may sometimes result from early impaired vision associated with such disorders as optic atrophy, albinism, congenital cataracts, severe astigmatism, corneal opacity, achromatopsia, bilateral macular disease, and aniridia.

O

OCULAR DEVIATION

Ocular deviation refers to abnormal eye movement that may be *conjugate* (both eyes move together) or *disconjugate* (one eye moves differently from the other). This common sign may result from ocular, neurologic, endocrine, or systemic disorders that interfere with the muscles, nerves, or brain centers governing eye movement. Occasionally, it signals a life-threatening disorder, such as ruptured cerebral aneurysm. (See *Ocular deviation: Characteristics and causes*, page 422.)

Normally, eye movement is directly controlled by the extraocular muscles innervated by the oculomotor, trochlear, and abducens nerves (cranial nerves III, IV, and VI). Together, these muscles and nerves direct a visual stimulus to fall on corresponding parts of the retina. Disconjugate ocular deviation may result from unequal muscle tone (*nonparalytic strabismus*) or from muscle paralysis associated with cranial nerve damage (*paralytic strabismus*). Conjugate ocular deviation may result from disorders that affect the centers in the cerebral cortex and brain stem responsible for conjugate eye movement. Typically, such disorders cause *gaze palsy*— difficulty moving the eyes in one or more directions. Only the extraocular muscles are affected in some forms of isolated strabismus, ptosis, Duane syndrome, and congenital fibrosis of the extraocular muscles (CFEOM).

Emergency interventions

If the patient displays ocular deviation, quickly take his vital signs and look for altered level of consciousness (LOC), pupil changes, motor or sensory dysfunction, and severe headache. If possible, ask the patient's family about behavioral changes. Is there a history of recent head trauma? Respiratory support may be necessary. Also, prepare the patient for emergency neurologic tests such as a computed tomography scan.

History and physical examination

If the patient isn't in distress, find out how long he's had the ocular deviation. Is it accompanied by double vision, eye pain, or headache? Also, ask if he's noticed associated motor or sensory changes or fever.

Check for a history of hypertension, diabetes, allergies, and thyroid, neurologic, or muscular disorders. Then obtain a thorough ocular history. Has the patient ever had extraocular muscle imbalance, eye or head trauma, or eye surgery?

During the physical examination, observe the patient for partial or complete ptosis. Does he spontaneously tilt his head or turn his face to compensate for ocular deviation? Check for eye redness or periorbital edema. Assess visual acu-

Ocular deviation: Characteristics and causes

CRANIAL NERVE AND EXTRAOCULAR MUSCLES INVOLVED	CHARACTERISTICS	PROBABLE CAUSES
Oculomotor nerve (III), medial rectus, superior rectus, inferior rectus, and inferior oblique muscles	Inability to focus the eye upward, downward, inward, and outward; drooping eyelid; and, except in diabetes, a dilated pupil in the affected eye	Cerebral aneurysm, diabetes, brain tumor, temporal lobe herniation from increased intracranial pressure
Trochlear nerve (IV), superior oblique muscle	Loss of downward and outward movement in the affected eye	Head trauma
Abducens nerve (VI), lateral rectus muscle	Loss of outward movement in the affected eye	Brain tumor

ity, then evaluate extraocular muscle function by testing the six cardinal fields of gaze.

Common medical causes

♦ ***Brain tumor.*** The nature of ocular deviation depends on the site and extent of the tumor. Associated signs and symptoms may include headache that's most severe in the morning, behavioral changes, memory loss, dizziness, confusion, vision loss, motor and sensory dysfunction, aphasia and, possibly, signs of hormonal imbalance. The patient's LOC may slowly deteriorate from lethargy to coma. Late signs include papilledema, vomiting, increased systolic blood pressure, widening pulse pressure, and decorticate posture.

♦ ***Cavernous sinus thrombosis.*** In this disorder, ocular deviation may be accompanied by diplopia, photophobia, exophthalmos, orbital and eyelid edema, corneal haziness, diminished or absent pupillary reflexes, or impaired visual acuity. Other features may include high fever, headache, malaise, nausea and vomiting, seizures, or tachycardia. Retinal hemorrhages and papilledema are late signs.

♦ ***Cerebrovascular accident.*** This life-threatening disorder may cause ocular deviation, depending on the site and extent of the stroke. Accompanying features are also variable and may include altered LOC, contralateral hemiplegia and sensory loss, dysarthria, dysphagia, homonymous hemianopia, blurred vision, or diplopia. In addition, the patient may develop urine retention or incontinence or both, constipation, behavioral changes, headache, vomiting, and seizures.

♦ ***Diabetes mellitus.*** A leading cause of isolated CN III palsy, especially in the middle-aged patient with long-standing mild disease, diabetes may cause ocular deviation and ptosis. Typically, the patient also complains of sudden onset of diplopia and pain.

♦ ***Encephalitis.*** This infection causes ocular deviation and diplopia in some patients. Typically, it begins abruptly with fever, headache, and vomiting, followed by signs of meningeal irritation (for example, nuchal rigidity) and of neuronal damage (for example, seizures, aphasia, ataxia, hemiparesis, cranial nerve palsies, photophobia). The patient's LOC may rapidly deteriorate from lethargy to coma within 24 to 48 hours after onset.

◆ ***Head trauma.*** The nature of ocular deviation depends on the site and extent of head trauma. The patient may have visible soft-tissue injury, bony deformity, facial edema, and clear or bloody otorrhea or rhinorrhea. Besides these obvious signs of trauma, he may also develop blurred vision, diplopia, nystagmus, behavioral changes, headache, motor and sensory dysfunction, or a decreased LOC that may progress to coma. Signs of increased intracranial pressure — such as bradycardia, increased systolic pressure, and widening pulse pressure — may also occur.

◆ ***Orbital blowout fracture.*** This fracture may entrap the inferior rectus muscle, resulting in ocular deviation and limited extraocular movement. Typically, the patient's upward gaze is absent; other directions of gaze may be affected if edema is dramatic. The globe may also be displaced downward and inward. Associated signs and symptoms include pain, diplopia, nausea, periorbital edema, and ecchymosis.

◆ ***Orbital tumor.*** Ocular deviation occurs as the tumor gradually enlarges. Associated findings include proptosis, diplopia and, possibly, blurred vision.

◆ ***Thyrotoxicosis.*** This disorder may cause exophthalmos — proptotic or protruding eyes — which, in turn, causes limited extraocular movement and ocular deviation. Usually, the patient's upward gaze weakens first, followed by diplopia. Other features are lid retraction, a wide-eyed staring gaze, excessive tearing, edematous eyelids and, sometimes, inability to close the eyes. Cardinal features of thyrotoxicosis include tachycardia, palpitations, weight loss despite increased appetite, diarrhea, tremors, an enlarged thyroid, dyspnea, nervousness, diaphoresis, heat intolerance, and an atrial or ventricular gallop.

Special considerations

Continue to monitor the patient's vital signs and neurologic status if you suspect an acute neurologic disorder. Take seizure precautions, if necessary. Also, prepare the patient for diagnostic tests, such as blood studies, orbital and skull X-rays, and computed tomography scan.

Pediatric pointers

In children, the most common cause of ocular deviation is congenital esotropia. Clinical manifestations include amblyopia, large angle of esodeviations, refractive errors, apparent abduction deficit, dissociated vertical deviation, or inferior oblique overaction. Normally, children achieve binocular vision by age 3 to 4 months. Although severe strabismus is readily apparent, mild strabismus must be confirmed by tests for misalignment, such as the corneal light reflex test and the cover test. Testing is crucial — early corrective measures help preserve binocular vision and cosmetic appearance. Also, mild strabismus may indicate retinoblastoma, a tumor that may be asymptomatic before age 2, except for a characteristic whitish reflex in the pupil.

OLIGOMENORRHEA

In most women, menstrual bleeding occurs every 24 to 32 days. Although some variation is normal, menstrual bleeding at intervals of greater than 36 days may indicate oligomenorrhea — abnormally infrequent menstrual bleeding characterized by three to six menstrual cycles per year. When menstrual bleeding does occur, it's usually profuse, prolonged (up to 10 days), and laden with clots and tissue. Occasionally, scant bleeding or spotting occurs between these heavy menses.

Oligomenorrhea may develop suddenly, or it may follow a period of gradually lengthening cycles. Although oligomenorrhea may alternate with normal menstrual bleeding, it can progress to secondary amenorrhea (greater than 3 months between cycle and menstrual bleeding).

Because oligomenorrhea is frequently associated with anovulation, it's common in infertile, early postmenarchal, and perimenopausal women. Usually, this sign reflects abnormalities of the hormones that govern normal endometrial function. It may result from ovarian, hypothalamic, pituitary, and other metabolic disorders, and from the effects of certain drugs. It may also result from emotional or physical stress — such as sudden weight change, debilitating illness, or rigorous physical training.

History and physical examination

After asking the patient how old she is, find out when menarche occurred. Has she ever experienced normal menstrual cycles? When did she begin having abnormal cycles? Ask her to describe the pattern of bleeding. How many days does the bleeding last, and how frequently does it occur? Does her menstrual flow contain clots and tissue fragments? Note the date of her most recent menstrual bleeding. Obtain her reproductive history including birth control methods, gynecologic procedures, and pregnancies.

Next, determine if she's having symptoms of ovulatory bleeding. Does she experience mild, cramping abdominal pain about 14 days before she bleeds? Is the bleeding accompanied by premenstrual symptoms, such as breast tenderness, irritability, bloating, weight gain, nausea, and diarrhea? Does she have cramping or pain with bleeding?

Ask about previous gynecologic disorders such as ovarian cysts. If the patient is breast-feeding, has she experienced problems with milk production? If she hasn't been breast-feeding recently, has she noticed milk leaking from her breasts? Ask about recent weight gain or loss. Is the patient less than 80% of her ideal weight? If so, does she claim that she's overweight? Ask if she's exercising more vigorously than usual.

Screen for metabolic disorders by asking about excessive thirst, frequent urination, or fatigue. Has the patient been jittery or had palpitations? Ask about headache, dizziness, and impaired peripheral vision. Complete the history by finding out what drugs the patient is taking.

Begin the physical examination by taking the patient's vital signs and weighing her. Inspect for increased facial hair growth, sparse body hair, male distribution of fat and muscle, acne, and clitoral enlargement. Note if the skin is abnormally dry or moist, and check hair texture. Also, be alert for signs of psychological or physical stress.

Common medical causes

♦ ***Adrenal hyperplasia.*** In this disorder, oligomenorrhea may occur with signs of androgen excess, such as clitoral enlargement and male distribution of hair, fat, and muscle mass.

♦ ***Anorexia nervosa.*** Anorexia nervosa may cause sporadic oligomenorrhea or amenorrhea. Its cardinal symptom, though, is a morbid fear of being fat associated with loss of more than 20% of ideal body weight. Typically, the patient displays dramatic skeletal muscle atrophy and loss of fatty tissue; dry or sparse scalp hair; lanugo on the face and body; and blotchy or sallow, dry skin. Other symptoms include constipation, decreased libido, and sleep disturbances.

♦ ***Diabetes mellitus.*** Oligomenorrhea may be an early sign in this disorder. In juvenile-onset diabetes, the patient may have never had normal menses. Associated findings include excessive hunger, polydipsia, polyuria, weakness, fatigue, dry mucous membranes, poor skin turgor, irritability and emotional lability, and weight loss.

♦ ***Hypothyroidism.*** Besides oligomenorrhea, this disorder may result in fatigue; forgetfulness; cold intolerance; unexplained weight gain; constipation; bradycardia; decreased mental acuity; dry, flaky, inelastic skin; puffy face, hands, and feet; hoarseness; periorbital edema; ptosis; dry, sparse hair; and thick, brittle nails.

♦ ***Prolactin-secreting pituitary tumor.*** Oligomenorrhea or amenorrhea may be the first sign of a prolactin-secreting pituitary tumor. Accompanying findings include unilateral or bilateral galactorrhea, infertility, loss of libido, and sparse pubic hair. Headache and visual field disturbances — such as diminished peripheral vision, blurred vision, diplopia, and hemianopia — signal tumor expansion.

♦ ***Thyrotoxicosis.*** This disorder may cause oligomenorrhea along with reduced fertility. Cardinal findings include irritability, weight loss despite increased appetite, dyspnea, tachycardia, palpitations, diarrhea, tremors, diaphoresis, heat intolerance, an enlarged thyroid and, possibly, exophthalmos.

Other causes

♦ ***Drugs.*** Drugs that increase androgen levels — such as corticosteroids, corticotropin, anabolic steroids, danazol, and injectable and implanted contraceptives — may cause oligomenorrhea. Oral contraceptives may be associated with delayed resumption of normal menses when their use is discontinued; however, 95% of women resume normal menses within 3 months. Other drugs that may cause oligomenorrhea include phenothiazine derivatives, amphetamines, and antihypertensive drugs, which increase prolactin levels.

Special considerations

Prepare the patient for diagnostic tests, such as blood hormone levels, thyroid studies, or pelvic imaging studies.

Pediatric pointers

Teenage girls may experience oligomenorrhea associated with immature hormonal function. However, prolonged oligomenorrhea or the development of amenorrhea may signal congenital adrenal hyperplasia or Turner's syndrome.

Geriatric pointers

Oligomenorrhea in the perimenopausal woman usually indicates impending onset of menopause.

OLIGURIA

A cardinal sign of renal and urinary tract disorders, oliguria is clinically defined as urine output of less than 400 ml per 24 hours. Typically, this sign occurs abruptly and may herald serious — possibly life-threatening — hemodynamic instability. Its causes can be classified as prerenal (decreased renal blood flow), intrarenal (intrinsic renal damage), or postrenal (urinary tract obstruction); the pathophysiology differs for each classification. (See *How oliguria develops,* pages 426 and 427.) Oliguria associated with a prerenal or postrenal cause is usually promptly reversible with treatment, although it may lead to intrarenal damage if untreated. However, oliguria associated with an intrarenal cause is usually more persistent and may be irreversible.

History and physical examination

Begin by asking the patient about his usual daily voiding pattern, including frequency and amount. When did he first notice changes in this pattern and in the color, odor, or consistency of his urine? Ask about pain or burning on urination. Note his normal daily fluid intake. Has he recently been drinking more or less than usual? Has he had recent episodes of diarrhea or vomiting that might cause fluid loss? Next, explore associated complaints, especially fatigue, loss of appetite, thirst, dyspnea, chest pain, or recent weight gain.

How oliguria develops

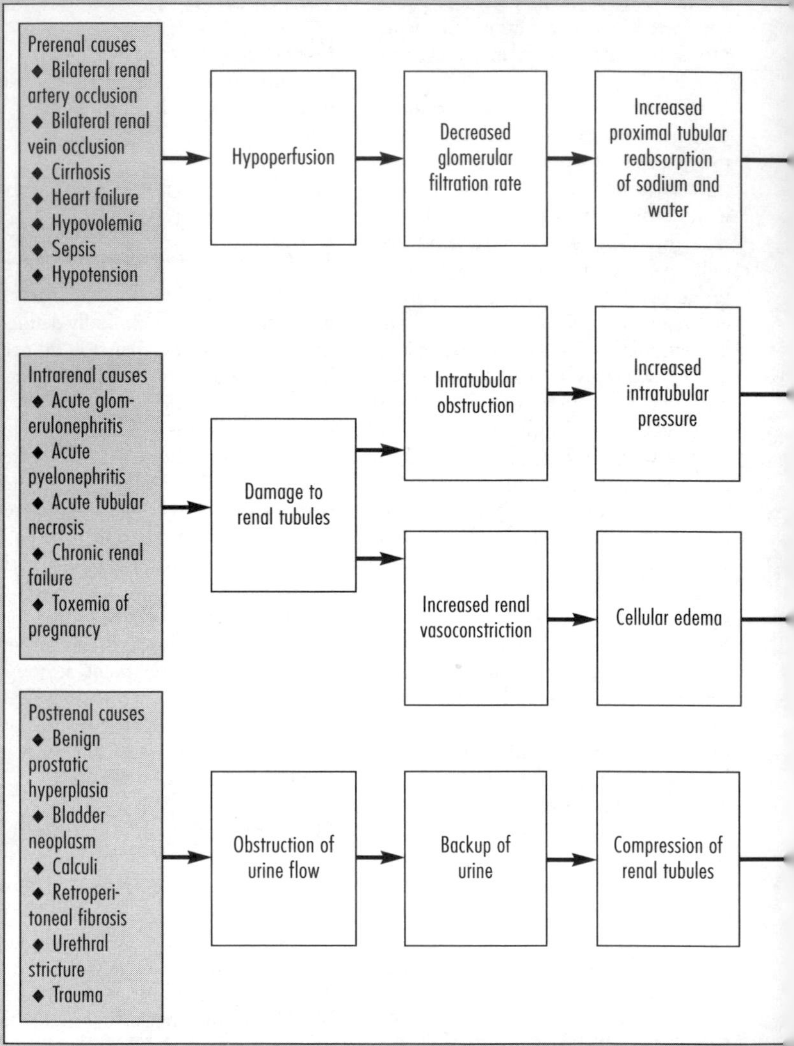

Check for a history of renal, urinary tract, or cardiovascular disorders. Note recent traumatic injury, surgery associated with significant blood loss, and recent blood transfusions. Was the patient exposed to nephrotoxic agents, such as heavy metals, organic solvents, anesthetics, or radiographic contrast media? Next, obtain a drug history.

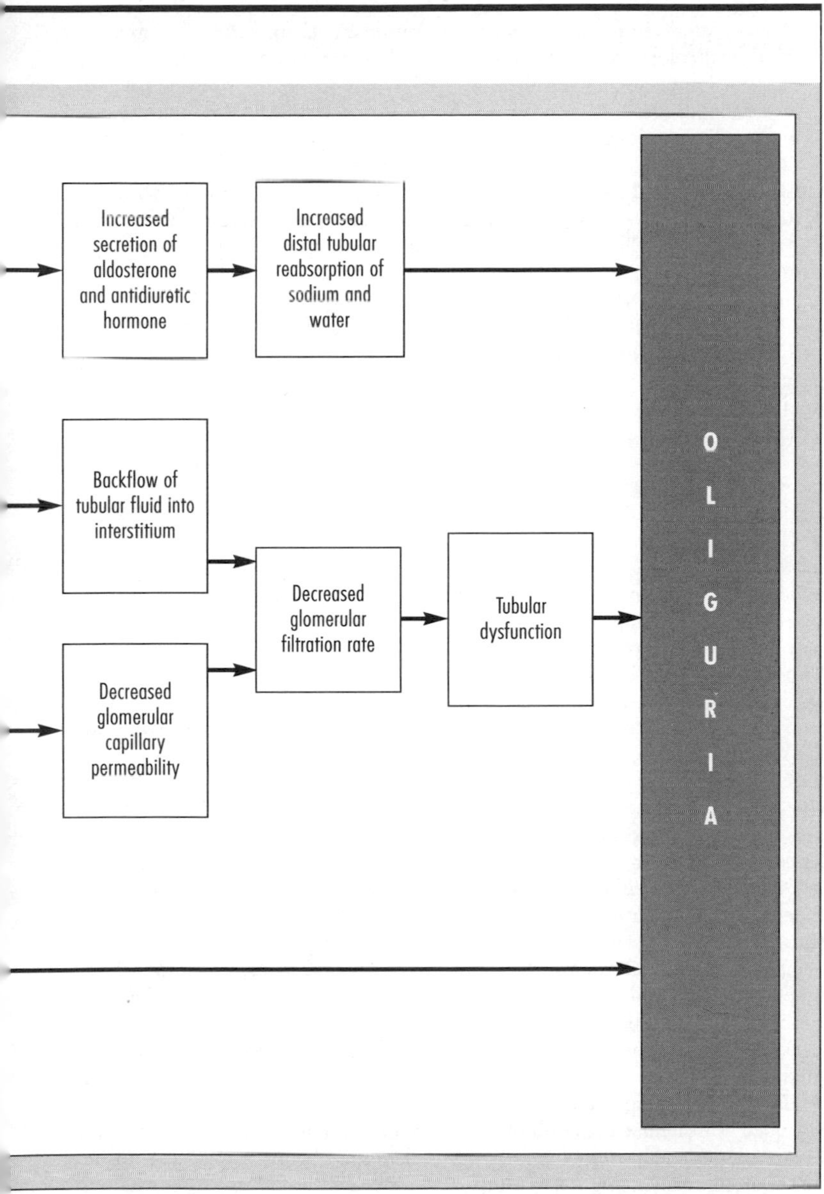

Begin the physical examination by taking the patient's vital signs and weighing him. Assess his overall appearance for edema. Palpate both kidneys for tenderness and enlargement, and percuss for costovertebral angle (CVA) tenderness. Also, inspect the flank area for edema or erythema. Auscultate the heart and lungs for abnormal sounds and the flank area for renal artery bruits.

Obtain a urine sample and inspect it for abnormal color, odor, or sediment. Use reagent strips to test for glucose, protein, and blood. Also, use a urinometer to measure specific gravity.

Common medical causes

♦ ***Acute tubular necrosis (ATN).*** An early sign of ATN, oliguria may occur abruptly (in shock) or gradually (in nephrotoxicity). Usually, it persists for about 2 weeks, followed by polyuria. Related features may include signs of hyperkalemia (muscle weakness, cardiac arrhythmias); uremia (anorexia, confusion, lethargy, twitching, seizures, pruritus, Kussmaul's respirations); and heart failure (edema, jugular vein distention, crackles, dyspnea).

♦ ***Calculi.*** Oliguria or anuria may result when stones lodge in the kidneys, ureters, bladder outlet, or urethra. Associated signs and symptoms include urinary frequency and urgency, dysuria, and hematuria or pyuria. Usually, the patient experiences renal colic — excruciating pain that radiates from the CVA to the flank, the suprapubic region, and the external genitalia. This pain may be accompanied by nausea, vomiting, hypoactive bowel sounds, abdominal distention and, occasionally, fever and chills.

♦ ***Glomerulonephritis (acute).*** This disorder causes oliguria or anuria. Other features are mild fever, fatigue, gross hematuria, generalized edema, elevated blood pressure, headache, nausea and vomiting, flank and abdominal pain, and signs of pulmonary congestion (dyspnea, productive cough).

♦ ***Heart failure.*** Oliguria may occur in left-sided heart failure as a result of low cardiac output and decreased renal perfusion. Accompanying signs and symptoms include dyspnea, fatigue, weakness, peripheral edema, distended jugular veins, tachycardia, tachypnea, crackles, and a dry or productive cough. In advanced heart failure, the patient may also develop orthopnea, cyanosis, clubbing, ventricular gallop, diastolic hypertension, cardiomegaly, or hemoptysis.

♦ ***Hypovolemia.*** Any disorder that decreases circulating fluid volume can cause oliguria. Associated findings may include orthostatic hypotension, apathy, lethargy, fatigue, gross muscle weakness, anorexia, nausea, profound thirst, dizziness, sunken eyeballs, poor skin turgor, and dry mucous membranes.

♦ ***Pyelonephritis (acute).*** Accompanying the sudden onset of oliguria in this disorder are high fever with chills, fatigue, flank pain, CVA tenderness, weakness, nocturia, dysuria, hematuria, urinary frequency and urgency, and tenesmus. The urine may appear cloudy. Occasionally, the patient also experiences anorexia, nausea, diarrhea, and vomiting.

♦ ***Renal failure (chronic).*** Oliguria is a major sign of end-stage chronic renal failure. Associated findings reflect progressive uremia and may include fatigue, weakness, irritability, uremic fetor, ecchymoses and petechiae, peripheral edema, elevated blood pressure, confusion, emotional lability, drowsiness, coarse muscle twitching, muscle cramps, peripheral neuropathies, anorexia, metallic taste in the mouth, nausea and vomiting, constipation or diarrhea, stomatitis, pruritus, pallor, or yellow- or bronze-tinged skin. Eventually, seizures, coma, and uremic frost may develop.

♦ ***Renal vein occlusion (bilateral).*** This disorder occasionally causes oliguria accompanied by acute lower back and flank pain, CVA tenderness, fever, pallor, hematuria, enlarged and palpable kidneys, edema and, possibly, signs of uremia.

♦ ***Toxemia of pregnancy.*** In severe preeclampsia, oliguria may be accompanied by elevated blood pressure, dizziness, diplopia, blurred vision, epigastric pain, nausea and vomiting, irritability, and severe frontal headache. Typically, the oliguria is preceded by generalized edema and sudden weight gain of more than 3 lb (1.4 kg) per week during the second trimester or more than 1 lb (0.45 kg) per week during the third trimester. If preeclampsia progresses to eclampsia, the patient develops seizures and may slip into coma.

♦ ***Urethral stricture.*** This disorder causes oliguria accompanied by chronic urethral discharge, urinary frequency and urgency, dysuria, pyuria, and diminished urine stream. As obstruction worsens, urine extravasation may lead to formation of urinomas and urosepsis.

Other causes

♦ ***Diagnostic studies.*** Contrast media used in radiographic studies may cause nephrotoxicity and oliguria.

♦ ***Drugs.*** Oliguria may result from drugs that cause decreased renal perfusion (diuretics), nephrotoxicity (most notably, aminoglycosides, chemotherapeutics), urine retention (adrenergic and anticholinergic agents), or urinary obstruction associated with precipitation of urinary crystals (sulfonamides, acyclovir).

♦ ***Trauma.*** Crush injuries that release myoglobin from damaged muscles may lead to acute renal failure and oliguria.

Special considerations

Monitor vital signs, intake and output, and daily weight. Depending on the cause of the oliguria, fluids are normally restricted to between 600 ml and 1 L more than the patient's urine output for the previous day. However, you may encourage fluid intake if he's hypokalemic. Provide a diet low in sodium, potassium, and protein.

Laboratory tests may be necessary to determine if the oliguria is reversible. Such tests may include serum blood urea nitrogen and creatinine levels, urea and creatinine clearance, urine sodium levels, and urine osmolality. Abdominal X-rays, ultrasonography, computed tomography scan, and a renal scan may be required.

Pediatric pointers

In the neonate, oliguria may result from edema or dehydration. Major causes include congenital heart disease, respiratory distress syndrome, sepsis, congenital hydronephrosis, acute tubular necrosis, and renal vein thrombosis. Common causes of oliguria in children between ages 1 and 5 are acute poststreptococcal glomerulonephritis and hemolytic-uremic syndrome. After age 5, causes of oliguria are similar to those in adults.

Geriatric pointers

In elderly patients, oliguria may result from gradual progression of an underlying disorder. It may also result from overall poor muscle tone secondary to inactivity, poor fluid intake, or infrequent voiding attempts.

Opisthotonos

A sign of severe meningeal irritation, opisthotonos is characterized by a strongly arched, rigid back; hyperextended neck; bent-back heels, and flexed arms and hands. (See *Recognizing opisthotonos,* page 430.) Usually, this posture occurs spontaneously and continuously; however, it may be aggravated by movement. Presumably, opisthotonos represents a protective reflex because it immobilizes the spine, alleviating the pain associated with meningeal irritation. Occasionally, opisthotonos occurs in achondroplastic dwarfism, although not necessarily as an indicator of meningeal irritation.

Emergency interventions

If the patient is stuporous or comatose, quickly evaluate his vital signs. Employ resuscitative measures, as appropriate. Place the patient in a bed, with rails raised and padded, or in a crib.

History and physical examination

If the patient's condition permits, obtain a history. Consult with a relative of the young child or infant. Ask about a history of cerebral aneurysm or arteriove-

EXAMINATION TIP

Recognizing opisthotonos

In this characteristic posture, the back is severely arched and the neck is hyperextended. The heels bend back on the legs, and the arms and hands flex rigidly at the joints, as shown.

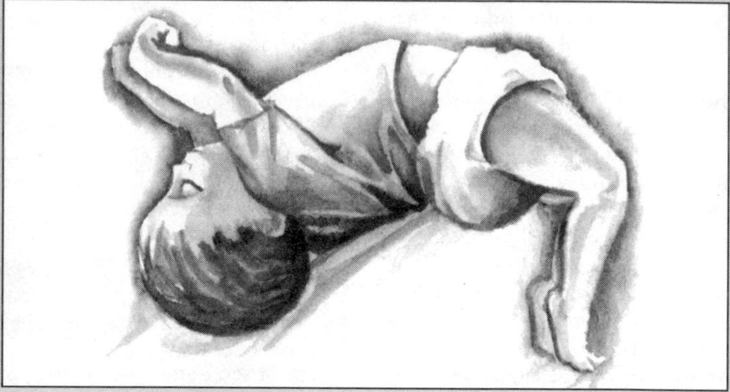

nous malformation and about hypertension. Note recent infection that may have spread to the nervous system. Explore associated findings, such as headache, chills, and vomiting.

Focus the physical examination on the patient's neurologic status. Evaluate level of consciousness (LOC) and test sensorimotor and cranial nerve function. Then check for Brudzinski's and Kernig's signs and for nuchal rigidity.

Common medical causes

♦ ***Arnold-Chiari syndrome.*** Here, opisthotonos typically occurs with the classic manifestations of hydrocephalus—enlarged head; thin, shiny scalp with distended veins; and underdeveloped neck muscles. Other usual findings are a high-pitched cry, abnormal leg muscle tone, anorexia, vomiting, nuchal rigidity, irritability, noisy respirations, and a weak sucking reflex.

♦ ***Meningitis.*** In this infection, opisthotonos accompanies other signs of meningeal irritation, including nuchal rigidity, positive Brudzinski's and Kernig's signs, and hyperreflexia. Meningitis also causes cardinal signs of infection (moderate to high fever with chills and malaise) and of increased intracranial pressure (headache, vomiting and, eventually, papilledema). Other features include irritability; photophobia; diplopia, deafness, and other cranial nerve palsies; and decreased LOC that may progress to seizures and coma.

♦ ***Subarachnoid hemorrhage.*** This disorder may cause opisthotonos with other signs of meningeal irritation, such as nuchal rigidity and positive Kernig's and Brudzinski's signs. Focal signs of hemorrhage, such as severe headache, hemiplegia or hemiparesis, aphasia, photophobia, and other vision problems may also occur. As intracranial pressure rises, the patient may develop bradycardia, elevated blood pressure, altered respiratory pattern, seizures, and vomiting. His LOC may rapidly deteriorate, resulting in coma; then, decerebrate posture may alternate with opisthotonos.

◆ ***Tetanus.*** The initial sign of this life-threatening infection is trismus, or tonic contraction of the muscles of mastication (chewing). Eventually, muscle spasms may affect the abdomen, producing boardlike rigidity; the back, opisthotonos; or the face, risus sardonicus. Spasms of the respiratory muscles occur, causing respiratory distress. Tachycardia, diaphoresis, hyperactive deep tendon reflexes, or seizures may develop.

Other causes

◆ ***Antipsychotics.*** Phenothiazines and other antipsychotic drugs may cause opisthotonos, usually as part of an acute dystonic reaction. This usually can be treated with I.V. diphenhydramine.

Special considerations

Assess neurologic status and check vital signs frequently. Make the patient as comfortable as possible; place him in a side-lying position with pillows for support. If meningitis is suspected, institute respiratory isolation. Lumbar puncture may be ordered to identify pathogens and analyze cerebrospinal fluid. If subarachnoid hemorrhage is suspected, prepare the patient for a computed tomography scan or magnetic resonance imaging.

Pediatric pointers

Opisthotonos is far more common in children—especially infants—than in adults. It's also more exaggerated in children because of nervous system immaturity.

ORTHOPNEA

Orthopnea—difficulty breathing in the supine position—is a common symptom of cardiopulmonary disorders that cause dyspnea. It's commonly a subtle symptom; the patient may complain that he can't catch his breath when lying down, or he may mention that he sleeps most comfortably in a reclining chair or propped up by pillows. Derived from this complaint is the common classification as two- or three-pillow orthopnea.

Orthopnea presumably results from increased hydrostatic pressure in the pulmonary vasculature related to gravitational effects in the supine position. It may also be related to a disease process, such as chronic obstructive pulmonary disease (COPD), that alters the normal mechanics of breathing. In COPD, the supine position inhibits anterior chest expansion and increases dyspnea. Orthopnea may be aggravated by obesity, which restricts diaphragmatic excursion. Assuming the upright position relieves orthopnea by placing much of the pulmonary vasculature above the left atrium, which reduces mean hydrostatic pressure, and by enhancing diaphragmatic excursion, which increases inspiratory volume.

History and physical examination

Begin by asking about a history of cardiopulmonary disorders, such as myocardial infarction, rheumatic heart disease, valvular disease, emphysema, or chronic bronchitis. Does the patient smoke? If so, how much? Explore associated symptoms, noting especially complaints of cough, nocturnal or exertional dyspnea, fatigue, weakness, loss of appetite, or chest pain.

When examining the patient, check for other signs of increased respiratory effort, such as accessory muscle use, shallow respirations, and tachypnea. Also, note barrel chest. Inspect the patient's skin for pallor or cyanosis, and the fingers for clubbing. Observe and palpate for edema, and check for jugular vein distention. Auscultate the lungs and heart.

Common medical causes

- ***COPD.*** This disorder typically causes orthopnea and other dyspneic complaints, accompanied by accessory muscle use, tachypnea, tachycardia, and paradoxical pulse. Auscultation may reveal diminished breath sounds, rhonchi, crackles, and wheezing. The patient may also exhibit a dry or productive cough with copious sputum. Other features include anorexia, weight loss, and edema. Barrel chest, cyanosis, and clubbing are usually late signs.
- ***Left-sided heart failure.*** If heart failure is acute, orthopnea may begin suddenly; if chronic, it may become constant. The earliest symptom is progressively severe dyspnea. Other common early symptoms include Cheyne-Stokes respirations, paroxysmal nocturnal dyspnea, fatigue, weakness, and a cough that may occasionally produce clear or blood-tinged sputum. Tachycardia, tachypnea, and crackles may also occur.

  Other late findings may include cyanosis, ventricular gallop, and hemoptysis. Left-sided heart failure may also lead to signs of shock, such as hypotension, thready pulse, and cold, clammy skin.
- ***Mediastinal tumor.*** Orthopnea, an early sign of this disorder, results from pressure of the tumor against the trachea, bronchus, or lung when the patient lies down. However, many patients are asymptomatic until the tumor enlarges. Then, it may cause retrosternal chest pain, dry cough, hoarseness, dysphagia, stertorous respirations, palpitations, or cyanosis. Examination reveals suprasternal retractions on inspiration, bulging of the chest wall, tracheal deviation, dilated jugular and superficial chest veins, and edema of the face, neck, and arms.

Special considerations

To relieve orthopnea, place the patient in semi-Fowler's or high Fowler's position; if this doesn't help, have the patient lean over a bedside table with his chest forward. If necessary, administer oxygen via nasal cannula. (Remember that patients with COPD require a low flow rate of 1 to 3 L/minute.) Diuretics may be needed to reduce lung fluid.

An ECG, chest X-ray, and pulmonary function tests may be necessary for further evaluation.

Pediatric pointers

Common causes of orthopnea in children include heart failure, croup syndrome, cystic fibrosis, and asthma. Sleeping in an infant seat may improve symptoms for a young child.

Geriatric pointers

If the elderly patient is using more than one pillow at night, consider such noncardiogenic pulmonary reasons as gastroesophageal reflux disease, arthritis or, simply, the need for greater comfort.

ORTHOSTATIC HYPOTENSION

[Postural hypotension]

In orthostatic hypotension, the patient's blood pressure drops 15 to 20 mm Hg or more — with or without an increase in the heart rate of at least 20 beats per minute — when he rises from a supine to a sitting or standing position. (Blood pressure should be measured 2 minutes after the patient changes his position.) This common sign indicates failure of compensatory vasomotor responses to adjust to position changes. It's typically associated with light-headedness, syncope, or blurred vision and may occur in a hypotensive, normotensive, or hypertensive patient. Although frequently a nonpathologic sign in the elderly, orthostatic hypotension may result from prolonged bed rest, fluid and electrolyte imbalance, endocrine or systemic disorders, and the effects of drugs.

To detect orthostatic hypotension, take and compare blood pressure readings with the patient supine, sitting, and standing.

Emergency interventions

If you detect orthostatic hypotension, quickly check for tachycardia, altered level of consciousness (LOC), and pale, clammy skin. If these signs are present, suspect hypovolemic shock. Insert a large-gauge I.V. catheter for fluid or blood replacement. Take the patient's vital signs every 15 minutes, and monitor his intake and output.

History and physical examination

If the patient is in no danger, obtain a history. Ask the patient if he frequently experiences dizziness, weakness, or fainting when he stands. Also ask about associated symptoms, particularly fatigue, orthopnea, impotence, nausea, headache, abdominal or chest discomfort, and GI bleeding. Then obtain a complete drug history.

Begin the physical examination by checking the patient's skin turgor. Palpate peripheral pulses and auscultate the heart and lungs. Finally, test muscle strength and observe the patient's gait for unsteadiness.

Common medical causes

◆ ***Adrenal insufficiency.*** This disorder typically begins insidiously, with progressively severe signs and symptoms. Orthostatic hypotension may be accompanied by fatigue, muscle weakness, anorexia, nausea and vomiting, weight loss, abdominal pain, irritability, and a weak, irregular pulse. Another common feature is hyperpigmentation — bronze coloring of the skin — which is especially prominent on the face, lips, gums, tongue, buccal mucosa, elbows, palms, knuckles, waist, and knees. Diarrhea, constipation, decreased libido, amenorrhea, syncope, and enhanced taste, smell, or hearing may also occur.

◆ ***Alcoholism.*** Chronic alcoholism can cause peripheral neuropathy, which can present as orthostatic hypotension. Other symptoms include impotence, numbness, tingling, nausea, vomiting, changes in bowel habits, and bizarre behavior.

◆ ***Amyloidosis.*** Orthostatic hypotension is commonly associated with amyloid infiltration of the autonomic nerves. Associated signs and symptoms vary widely and may include anginal chest pain, tachycardia, dyspnea, orthopnea, fatigue, and cough.

◆ ***Hyperaldosteronism.*** This disorder typically causes orthostatic hypotension associated with sustained hypertension. Most other clinical effects of hyperaldosteronism result from hypokalemia, which increases neuromuscular irritability and causes muscle weakness, intermittent flaccid paralysis, fatigue, headache, paresthesia and, possibly, tetany with positive Trousseau's and Chvostek's signs. The patient may also exhibit vision disturbances, nocturia, polydipsia, or personality changes.

◆ ***Hyponatremia.*** In this disorder, orthostatic hypotension is typically accompanied by headache, profound thirst, tachycardia, nausea and vomiting, abdominal cramps, muscle twitching and weakness, fatigue, oliguria or anuria, cold clammy skin, poor skin turgor, irritability, seizures, and decreased LOC. Cyanosis, thready pulse, and eventually vasomotor collapse may occur in severe sodium deficit. Common causes include adrenal insufficiency, hypothyroidism, syndrome of inappropriate antidiuretic hormone secretion, and use of thiazide diuretics.

◆ ***Hypovolemia.*** Mild to moderate hypovolemia may cause orthostatic hypotension associated with apathy, fatigue, muscle weakness, anorexia, nausea, or profound thirst. The patient may also develop dizziness, oliguria, sunken eyeballs, poor skin turgor, or dry mucous membranes.

Other causes

◆ ***Drugs.*** Certain drugs may cause orthostatic hypotension by reducing circulating blood volume, causing blood vessel dilatation, or depressing the sympathetic nervous system. These drugs include antihypertensives (especially guanethidine and the initial dose of prazosin), tricyclic antidepressants, phenothiazines, levodopa, nitrates, monoamine oxidase inhibitors, morphine, bretylium, and spinal anesthesia. Large doses of diuretics can also cause orthostatic hypotension.

◆ ***Treatments.*** Orthostatic hypotension is commonly associated with prolonged bed rest (24 hours or longer). It may also result from sympathectomy, which disrupts normal vasoconstrictive mechanisms.

Special considerations

Monitor the patient's fluid balance by carefully recording his intake and output and weighing him daily. To help minimize orthostatic hypotension, advise the patient to change his position gradually. Elevate the head of the patient's bed, and help him to a sitting position with his feet dangling over the side of the bed. If he can tolerate this position, have him sit in a chair for brief periods. Immediately return him to bed if he becomes dizzy or pale, or displays other signs of hypotension.

Always keep the patient's safety in mind; never leave him unattended while he's sitting or walking. Evaluate his need for assistive devices, such as a cane or walker.

Prepare the patient for diagnostic tests, such as hematocrit, serum electrolyte and drug levels, urinalysis, 12-lead electrocardiogram, and chest X-ray.

Pediatric pointers

Because normal blood pressure is lower in children than in adults, familiarize yourself with normal age-specific values to detect orthostatic hypotension. From birth to age 3 months, normal systolic pressure is 40 to 80 mm Hg; from age 3 months to 1 year, 80 to 100 mm Hg; and from age 1 to 12, 100 mm Hg plus 2 mm Hg for every year over age 1. Diastolic blood pressure is first heard at about age 4; it's normally 60 mm Hg at this age and gradually increases to 70 mm Hg by age 12.

The causes of orthostatic hypotension in children may be the same as those in adults.

Geriatric pointers

Elderly patients commonly experience autonomic dysfunction, which can present as orthostatic hypotension. Postprandial hypotension occurs 45 to 60 minutes after a meal and has been documented in up to one-third of nursing home residents.

ORTOLANI'S SIGN

Ortolani's sign — a click or popping sensation that's felt and commonly heard when a neonate's hip is flexed 90 degrees and abducted — is an indication of developmental dysplasia of the hip; it results when the femoral head enters or exits the acetabulum. Screening for this sign is an important part of neonatal care because early detection and treatment of developmental dysplasia of the hip improves the infant's chances of growing with a correctly formed, functional joint.

History and physical examination

During assessment for Ortolani's sign, the infant should be relaxed and lying supine. (See *Detecting developmental dysplasia of the hip.*) After eliciting Ortolani's sign, evaluate the infant for asymmetrical gluteal folds, limited hip abduction, and unequal leg length.

EXAMINATION TIP

Detecting developmental dysplasia of the hip

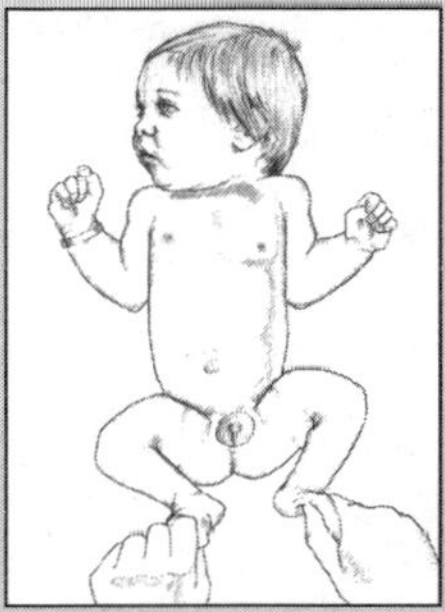

When assessing the neonate, attempt to elicit Ortolani's sign to detect developmental dysplasia of the hip. Begin by placing the infant supine with knees and hips flexed. Observe for symmetry.

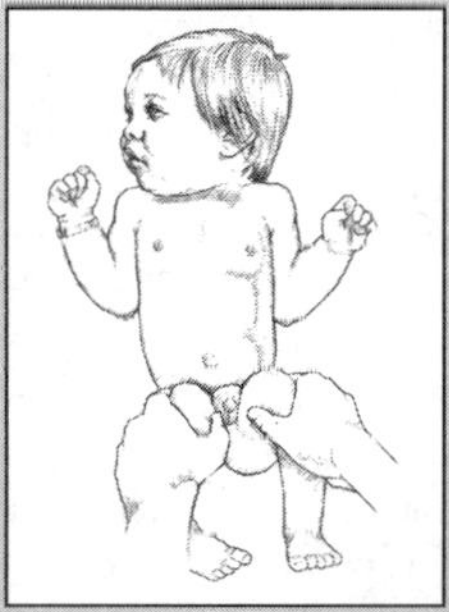

Place your hands on the infant's knees, with your index fingers along his lateral thighs. Then raise his knees to a 90-degree angle with his back.

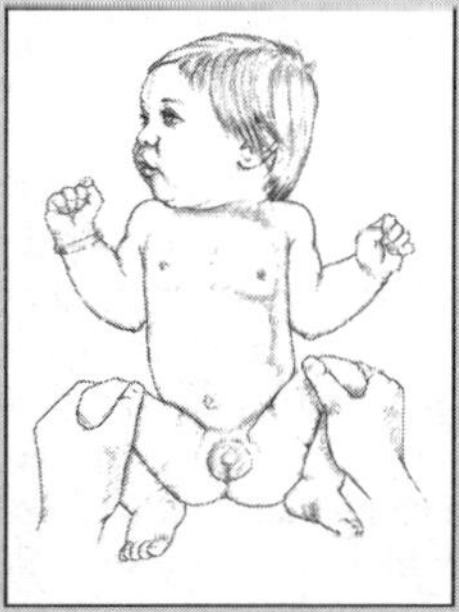

Abduct the infant's thighs so that the lateral aspect of each knee lies almost flat on the table. If the infant has a dislocated hip, you'll feel and often hear a click or popping sensation (Ortolani's sign) as the head of the femur moves out of the acetabulum. The infant may also give a sudden cry of pain.

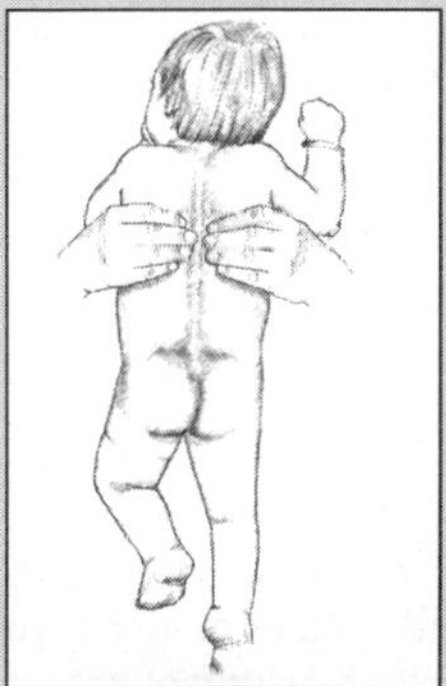

If you elicit a positive Ortolani's sign, look for other signs of developmental dysplasia of the hip. Observe for asymmetry of the infant's gluteal or thigh folds.

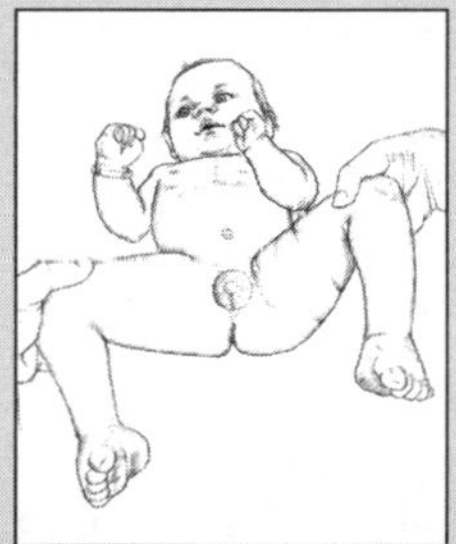

Flex the infant's hips to detect limited abduction.

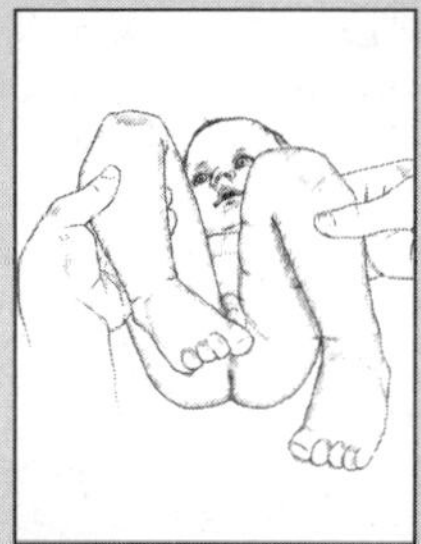

Flex the infant's knees, and observe for apparent shortening of the femur.

Common medical causes

♦ ***Developmental dysplasia of the hip.*** Most common in females and in Native Americans, this disorder causes Ortolani's sign, which may be accompanied by limited hip abduction and unequal gluteal folds. Usually, the infant with developmental hip dysplasia has no gross deformity or pain.

In complete dysplasia, the affected leg may appear shorter, or the affected hip may appear more prominent.

A strong relationship between hip dysplasia and methods of handling the infant has been demonstrated. For instance, the high incidence of developmental hip dysplasia in Inuit and Navajo Indians may be related to their practice of wrapping neonates in blankets or strapping them to cradleboards. In cultures where mothers carry infants on their backs or hips, such as in the Far East or Africa, hip dysplasia is rarely seen.

Special considerations

Ortolani's sign can be elicited only during the first 4 to 6 weeks of life; this is also the optimum time for effective corrective treatment. If treatment is delayed, developmental dysplasia of the hip may cause degenerative hip changes, lordosis, joint malformation, and soft-tissue damage. Various methods of abduction can be used to produce a stable joint. These methods include double-diapering as well as use of soft splinting devices or a plaster hip spica cast.

OTORRHEA

Otorrhea—drainage from the ear—may be bloody (otorrhagia), purulent, clear, or serosanguineous. Its onset, duration, and severity provide clues to the underlying cause. This sign may result from disorders that affect the external ear canal or the middle ear, including allergy, infection, neoplasms, trauma, and collagen diseases. Otorrhea may occur alone or with other symptoms, such as ear pain.

History and physical examination

Begin your evaluation by asking the patient when the otorrhea began, noting how he recognized it. Did he clean the drainage from deep within the ear canal, or did he wipe it from the auricle? Have him describe the color, consistency, and odor of the drainage. Is it clear, purulent, or bloody? Does it occur in one or both ears? Is it continuous or intermittent? If the patient wears cotton in his ear to absorb the drainage, ask how often he changes it.

Then explore associated otologic symptoms, especially pain. Is there tenderness on movement of the pinna or tragus? Ask about vertigo, which is absent in disorders of the external ear canal. Also ask about tinnitus.

Next, check the patient's medical history for recent upper respiratory infection or head trauma. Ask how he cleans his ears and if he's an avid swimmer. Note a history of cancer, dermatitis, or immunosuppressive therapy.

Focus the physical examination on the patient's external ear, middle ear, and tympanic membrane. (If his symptoms are unilateral, examine the uninvolved ear first.) Inspect the external ear, and apply pressure on the tragus and mastoid area to elicit tenderness. Then insert an otoscope, using the largest speculum that will comfortably fit into the ear canal. If necessary, clean cerumen, pus, or other debris from the canal. Observe for edema, erythema, crusts, or polyps. Inspect the tympanic membrane, which should look like a shiny, pearl-gray cone. Note color changes, perforation, absence of the normal light reflex (a cone of light appearing toward the bottom of the drum), or a bulging membrane.

Next, test hearing acuity. Have the patient occlude one ear while you whisper some common two-syllable words toward the unoccluded ear. Stand behind him so he doesn't read your lips, and ask him to repeat what he heard. Perform the test on the other ear using different words. Then use a tuning fork to perform the Weber and Rinne tests.

Complete your assessment by palpating the patient's neck and his preauricular, parotid, and postauricular (mastoid) areas for lymphadenopathy. Also, test the function of cranial nerves VII, IX, X, and XI.

Common medical causes

◆ ***Aural polyps.*** These polyps may cause foul, purulent, and perhaps blood-streaked discharge. If they occlude the external ear canal, polyps may cause partial hearing loss.

◆ ***Cerebrospinal fluid (CSF) otorrhea.*** CSF otorrhea is the escape of CSF through the external auditory canal and requires a communication between the subarachnoid space and the pneumatized areas of the temporal bone. A tympanic membrane perforation or defect in the external ear canal must be present to divert CSF flow from the eustachian tube (which would result in rhinorrhea or postnasal drainage). The flow rate may be small, intermittent, positional, or steady. The bloody drainage may seem thin or it may be clear. CSF otorrhea can be due to accidental trauma (most common), surgical trauma, or nontraumatic causes such as tumors, congenital anomalies, osteitis, or osteomyelitis. Accompanying symptoms may include hearing loss, sensation of pressure in the ear, dizziness, or meningitis.

◆ ***Epidural abscess.*** In this disorder, profuse, creamy otorrhea is accompanied by steady, throbbing ear pain; fever; and temporal or temporoparietal headache on the ipsilateral side.

◆ ***Myringitis (infectious).*** In *acute infectious myringitis,* small, reddened, blood-filled blebs erupt in the external ear canal, on the tympanic membrane and, occasionally, in the middle ear. Spontaneous rupture of these blebs causes serosanguineous otorrhea. Other features include severe ear pain, tenderness over the mastoid process and, rarely, fever and hearing loss. *Chronic infectious myringitis* causes purulent otorrhea, pruritus, and gradual hearing loss.

◆ ***Otitis externa.*** *Acute otitis externa,* commonly known as swimmer's ear, usually causes purulent, yellow, sticky, foul-smelling otorrhea. Inspection may reveal white-green debris in the external ear canal. Associated findings include edema, erythema, pain, and itching of the auricle and external ear canal; severe tenderness with movement of the mastoid, tragus, mouth, or jaw; tenderness and swelling of surrounding nodes; and partial conductive hearing loss. The patient may also develop a low-grade fever and a headache ipsilateral to the affected ear.

Chronic otitis externa usually causes scanty, intermittent otorrhea that may be serous or purulent and possibly foul-smelling. Its primary symptom, though, is itching. Related findings include edema and slight erythema.

Life-threatening *malignant otitis externa* causes debris in the ear canal, which may build up against the tympanic membrane, causing severe pain that's especially acute during manipulation of the tragus or auricle. Most common in diabetics and immunosuppressed patients, this fulminant bacterial infection may also cause pruritus, tinnitus and, possibly, unilateral hearing loss.

◆ ***Otitis media.*** In *acute otitis media,* rupture of the tympanic membrane causes bloody, purulent otorrhea and relieves continuous or intermittent ear pain. Typically, conductive hearing loss worsens over several hours.

In *acute suppurative otitis media,* the patient may also exhibit signs and symptoms of upper respiratory infection — sore throat, cough, nasal discharge, and headache. Other features may include dizziness, fever, nausea, and vomiting.

Chronic otitis media causes intermittent, purulent, foul-smelling otorrhea frequently associated with perforation of the tympanic membrane. Conductive hearing loss occurs gradually and may be accompanied by pain, nausea, or vertigo.

♦ ***Trauma.*** Bloody otorrhea may result from trauma, such as a blow to the external ear, a foreign body in the ear, or barotrauma. Usually, the bleeding is minimal or moderate; it may be accompanied by partial hearing loss.

♦ ***Tumor (malignant).*** *Squamous cell carcinoma of the external ear* causes purulent otorrhea with itching; deep, boring ear pain; hearing loss; and, in late stages, facial paralysis. In *squamous cell carcinoma of the middle ear,* blood-tinged otorrhea occurs early, typically accompanied by hearing loss on the affected side. Pain and facial paralysis are late features.

Special considerations

Apply warm, moist compresses, heating pads, or hot water bottles to the patient's ears to relieve inflammation and pain. Use cotton wicks to gently clean the draining ear or to apply topical drugs. Keep eardrops at room temperature; instillation of cold eardrops may cause vertigo.

Pediatric pointers

When you examine or clean a child's ear, remember that the auditory canal lies horizontally and that the pinna must be pulled *downward* and *backward.* Restrain a child during an ear procedure by having him sit on a parent's lap with the ear to be examined facing you. Have him put one arm around the parent's waist and the other down at his own side, and then ask the parent to hold the child in place. Or, if you are alone with the child, you can have him lie on his abdomen with his arms at his sides and his head turned so the affected ear faces the ceiling. Bend over him, restraining his upper body with your elbows and upper arms.

Otitis media is the most common cause of otorrhea in infants and young children. Children are also likely to insert foreign bodies into their ears, resulting in infection, pain, and purulent discharge.

Otorrhea is the most common complication associated with tympanostomy tubes. It's commonly the result of water contamination or of a new episode of acute otitis media. Parents of children with tubes should be cautioned that ear drainage may be an infection and that the normal symptom of "ear pain" will be absent. Most infections will respond to cleaning and topical antibiotics. The pathogens in children under age 3 are similar to those in acute otitis media.

PQ

Pallor

Pallor is abnormal paleness or loss of skin color, which may develop suddenly or gradually. Although generalized pallor affects the entire body, it's most apparent on the face, conjunctiva, oral mucosa, and nail beds. Localized pallor commonly affects a single limb.

How easily pallor is detected varies with skin color and the thickness and vascularity of subcutaneous tissue. At times, it's merely a subtle lightening of skin color that may be difficult to detect in dark-skinned persons; sometimes it's evident only on the conjunctiva and oral mucosa.

Pallor may result from decreased peripheral or total oxyhemoglobin concentrations. The former reflects diminished peripheral blood flow associated with peripheral vasoconstriction or arterial occlusion or with low cardiac output. The latter usually results from anemia, the chief cause of pallor. (Transient peripheral vasoconstriction may occur on exposure to cold, causing nonpathologic pallor.) (See *How pallor develops,* page 440.)

Emergency interventions

If generalized pallor suddenly develops, quickly look for signs of shock, such as tachycardia, hypotension, oliguria, and decreased level of consciousness. Prepare to infuse fluids or blood rapidly. Keep emergency resuscitation equipment nearby.

History and physical examination

If the patient's condition permits, take a complete history. Does the patient or anyone in his family have a history of anemia? What about chronic disorders that might cause pallor, such as renal failure, heart failure, or diabetes? Ask about the patient's diet, particularly his intake of green vegetables.

Then explore the pallor more fully. Find out when the patient first noticed it. Is pallor constant or intermittent? Does it occur when he's exposed to the cold? Does it occur when he's under emotional stress? Explore associated signs and symptoms, such as dizziness, fainting, orthostasis, weakness and fatigue on exertion, chest pain, palpitations, menstrual irregularities, or loss of libido. If the pallor is confined to one or both legs, ask the patient if walking is painful. Do his legs feel cold or numb? If the pallor is confined to his fingers, ask about tingling and numbness.

Start the physical examination by taking the patient's vital signs. Be sure to check for orthostatic hypotension. Auscultate the heart for gallops and murmurs and the lungs for crackles. Check the patient's skin temperature — cold extremities commonly occur with vasoconstriction or arterial occlusion. Also, note skin ulceration. Finally, palpate pe-

How pallor develops

Pallor may result from decreased concentrations of peripheral oxyhemoglobin or decreased total oxyhemoglobin. The chart below illustrates the progression to pallor.

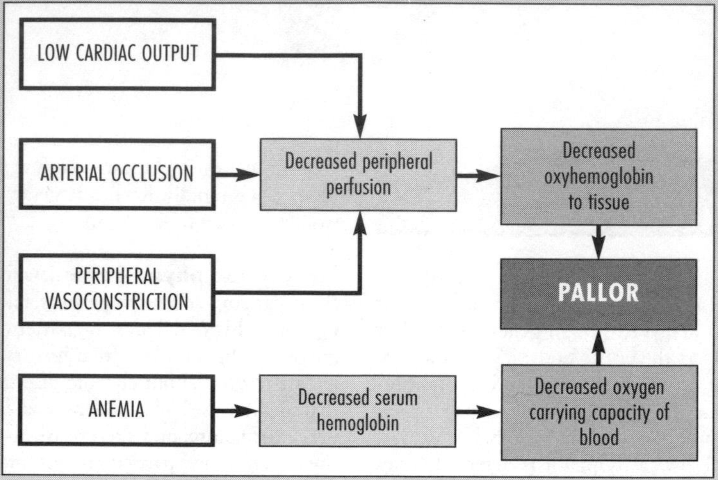

ripheral pulses. An absent pulse in a pale extremity may indicate arterial occlusion, whereas a weak pulse may indicate low cardiac output.

Common medical causes

♦ ***Anemia.*** Typically, pallor develops gradually in this disorder. The patient's skin may also appear sallow or grayish. Other effects may include fatigue, dyspnea, tachycardia, bounding pulse, atrial gallop, systolic bruit over the carotid arteries and, possibly, crackles and bleeding tendencies.

♦ ***Arterial occlusion (acute).*** Pallor develops abruptly in the extremity with the occlusion, which usually results from an embolus. A line of demarcation develops, separating the cool, pale, cyanotic, and mottled skin below the occlusion from the normal skin above it. Accompanying the pallor may be severe pain, intense intermittent claudication, paresthesia, or paresis in the affected extremity. Absent pulses and diminished capillary refill below the occlusion are also characteristic.

♦ ***Arterial occlusive disease (chronic).*** In this disorder, pallor is specific to an extremity — usually one leg but, occasionally, both legs or an arm. It develops gradually from obstructive arteriosclerosis or a thrombus and is aggravated by elevating the extremity. Associated findings include intermittent claudication, weakness, cool skin, diminished pulses in the extremity and, possibly, ulceration and gangrene.

♦ ***Frostbite.*** Pallor is localized to the frostbitten area, such as the feet, hands, or ears. Typically, the area feels cold, waxy and, perhaps, hard in deep frostbite. The skin doesn't blanch and sensation may be absent. As the area thaws, the skin turns purplish blue. Blistering and gangrene may follow if the frostbite was severe.

◆ ***Orthostatic hypotension.*** In this condition, pallor occurs abruptly when the patient rises from a recumbent position to a sitting or standing position. A precipitous drop in blood pressure, an increase in heart rate, and dizziness are also characteristic. At times, the patient loses consciousness for several minutes.

◆ ***Raynaud's disease.*** Pallor of the fingers after exposure to cold or stress is a hallmark of this disease. Typically, the fingers abruptly turn pale, then cyanotic; with rewarming, they become red and paresthetic. In chronic disease, ulceration may occur.

◆ ***Shock.*** Two forms of shock initially cause acute onset of pallor and cool, clammy skin. In *hypovolemic shock,* other early signs include restlessness, thirst, slight tachycardia, and tachypnea. As shock progresses, the skin becomes increasingly clammy, pulse becomes more rapid and thready, and hypotension develops with narrowing pulse pressure. Other signs may include oliguria, subnormal body temperature, and decreased level of consciousness. In *cardiogenic shock,* the signs and symptoms are similar but usually more profound.

Special considerations

If the patient has *chronic generalized* pallor, prepare him for blood studies and, possibly, bone marrow biopsy. The patient with *localized* pallor may require arteriography to accurately determine the cause.

When pallor results from low cardiac output, administer blood and fluid replacements and diuretic, cardiotonic, or antiarrhythmic drugs, as needed. Frequently monitor the patient's vital signs, intake and output, electrocardiogram, and hemodynamic status.

Pediatric pointers

In children, pallor stems from the same causes as it does in adults. It can also stem from congenital heart defects or chronic lung disease.

PALPITATIONS

Defined as a conscious awareness of one's heartbeat, palpitations are usually felt over the precordium or in the throat or neck. The patient may describe them as pounding, jumping, turning, fluttering, flopping, or as missing or skipping beats. Palpitations may be regular or irregular, fast or slow, paroxysmal or sustained.

Although frequently insignificant, this common symptom may result from cardiac or metabolic disorders or from the effects of certain drugs. Nonpathologic palpitations may occur when a prosthetic valve is newly implanted because the valve's clicking sound heightens the patient's awareness of his heartbeat. Transient palpitations may accompany emotional stress, such as fright, anger, or anxiety; physical stress, such as exercise or fever; or use of stimulants, such as tobacco and caffeine.

To help characterize the palpitations, ask the patient to simulate their rhythm by tapping his finger on a hard surface. An irregular "skipped beat" rhythm points to premature ventricular contractions, whereas an episodic racing rhythm that ends abruptly suggests paroxysmal atrial tachycardia.

Emergency interventions

If the patient complains of palpitations, ask him about dizziness and shortness of breath. Then inspect for pale, cool, clammy skin. Take the patient's vital signs, noting hypotension and irregular or abnormal pulse. If these signs are present, suspect cardiac arrhythmia. Prepare to begin cardiac monitoring and, if necessary, to deliver electroshock therapy. Start an I.V. line to administer antiarrhythmic drugs, if needed.

History and physical examination

If the patient isn't in distress, perform a complete cardiac history and physical examination. Ask about cardiovascular or pulmonary disorders, which may cause arrhythmias. Does the patient have a history of hypertension or hypoglycemia? Be sure to obtain a drug history. Has the patient recently started cardiac glycoside therapy? In addition, ask about caffeine, tobacco, and alcohol consumption.

Then explore associated symptoms, such as weakness, fatigue, and anginal pain. Finally, auscultate for gallops, murmurs, and abnormal breath sounds.

Common medical causes

♦ ***Anxiety attack (acute).*** In this disorder, palpitations may be accompanied by diaphoresis, facial flushing, trembling, or an impending sense of doom. Almost invariably, the patient hyperventilates, which may lead to dizziness, weakness, and syncope. Other typical findings include tachycardia, precordial pain, shortness of breath, restlessness, and insomnia.

♦ ***Cardiac arrhythmias.*** Paroxysmal or sustained palpitations may be accompanied by dizziness, weakness, and fatigue. The patient also may experience an irregular, rapid, or slow pulse rate; decreased blood pressure; confusion; pallor; oliguria; or diaphoresis.

♦ ***Hypertension.*** The patient's blood pressure typically exceeds 140/90 mm Hg; he may be asymptomatic or may complain of sustained palpitations alone or with headache, dizziness, tinnitus, or fatigue. He also may experience nausea and vomiting, seizures, or decreased level of consciousness (LOC).

♦ ***Hypocalcemia.*** Typically, this disorder causes palpitations, weakness, and fatigue. It progresses from paresthesia to muscle contraction and carpopedal spasms. The patient also may exhibit muscle twitching, hyperactive deep tendon reflexes, chorea, or positive Chvostek's and Trousseau's signs.

♦ ***Mitral prolapse.*** This valvular disorder may cause paroxysmal palpitations accompanied by sharp, stabbing, or aching precordial pain. The hallmark of this disorder, though, is a midsystolic click followed by an apical systolic murmur. Associated signs and symptoms may include dyspnea, dizziness, severe fatigue, migraine headache, anxiety, paroxysmal tachycardia, crackles, and peripheral edema.

♦ ***Mitral stenosis.*** Early features of this valvular disorder typically include sustained palpitations accompanied by dyspnea and fatigue on exertion. Auscultation also reveals a loud S_1, or opening snap, and a rumbling diastolic murmur at the apex. Patients also may experience related effects, such as an atrial gallop and, in advanced mitral stenosis, orthopnea, dyspnea at rest, paroxysmal nocturnal dyspnea, and atrial fibrillations.

♦ ***Thyrotoxicosis.*** A characteristic symptom in this disorder, sustained palpitations may be accompanied by tachycardia, dyspnea, weight loss despite increased appetite, diarrhea, tremors, nervousness, diaphoresis, heat intolerance and, possibly, exophthalmos and an enlarged thyroid. In addition, the patient may experience an atrial or ventricular gallop.

Other causes

♦ ***Drugs.*** Palpitations may result from drugs that precipitate cardiac arrhythmias or increase cardiac output such as cardiac glycosides, sympathomimetics such as cocaine, ganglionic blockers, and atropine.

♦ **Herb alert** Herbal drugs such as ginseng and ephedra (ma huang) may cause adverse effects, including palpitations and an irregular heartbeat.

Special considerations

Prepare the patient for diagnostic tests, such as an electrocardiogram and Holter monitoring. Remember that even mild palpitations may cause the patient much concern. Maintain a quiet, comfortable environment to minimize anxiety and perhaps decrease palpitations.

Pediatric pointers
Palpitations in children commonly result from fever or congenital heart defects, such as patent ductus arteriosus or septal defects. Because children frequently can't describe this complaint, focus your attention on objective measurements, such as cardiac monitoring, physical examination, and laboratory tests.

PAPULAR RASH

A papular rash consists of small, raised, circumscribed — and perhaps discolored (red to purple) — lesions known as papules. It may erupt anywhere on the body in various configurations and may be acute or chronic. Papular rashes characterize many cutaneous disorders; they may also result from allergy and from infectious, neoplastic, and systemic disorders. (To compare papules with other skin lesions, see *Recognizing common skin lesions*, page 444.)

History and physical examination
Your first step is to evaluate the papular rash fully: note its color, configuration, and location on the patient's body. Find out when it erupted. Has the patient noticed changes in the rash since then? Is it itchy or burning? Painful or tender? Also, have him describe associated signs and symptoms, such as fever, headache, or GI distress.

Next, obtain a medical history, including allergies; previous rashes or skin disorders; infections;, childhood diseases; sexual history, including sexually transmitted diseases (STDs); and cancers. Has the patient recently been bitten by an insect or rodent or exposed to anyone with an infectious disease? Finally, obtain a complete drug history.

Common medical causes
◆ ***Acne vulgaris.*** In this disorder, rupture of enlarged comedones causes inflamed — and perhaps painful and pruritic — papules, pustules, nodules, or cysts on the face and sometimes on the shoulders, chest, and back.
◆ ***Dermatomyositis.*** Gottron's papules — flat, violet-colored lesions on the dorsa of the finger joints — are pathognomonic of this disorder, as is the dusky lilac discoloration of periorbital tissue and lid margins (heliotrope edema). These signs may be accompanied by a transient, erythematous, macular rash in a malar distribution on the face and sometimes on the scalp, forehead, neck, upper torso, and arms. This rash may be preceded by symmetrical muscle soreness and weakness in the pelvis, upper extremities, shoulders, neck and, possibly, the face.
◆ ***Follicular mucinosis.*** In this cutaneous disorder, perifollicular papules or plaques are accompanied by prominent alopecia.
◆ ***Fox-Fordyce disease.*** This chronic disorder is marked by pruritic papules on the axillae, pubic area, and areolae associated with apocrine sweat gland inflammation. Sparse hair growth in these areas is also common.
◆ ***Granuloma annulare.*** This benign, chronic disorder causes papules that usually coalesce to form plaques. The papules spread peripherally to form a ring with a normal or slightly depressed center. They usually appear on the feet, legs, hands, or fingers and may be pruritic or asymptomatic.
◆ ***Human immunodeficiency virus (HIV) infection.*** Acute infection with the HIV retrovirus typically causes a generalized maculopapular rash. Other symptoms include fever, malaise, sore throat, and headache. Lymphadenopathy and hepatosplenomegaly may also occur. Most patients don't recall these symptoms of acute infection.

EXAMINATION TIP

Recognizing common skin lesions

MACULE
A small (usually less than 1 cm in diameter), flat blemish or discoloration; it can be brown, tan, red, or white and has same texture as surrounding skin

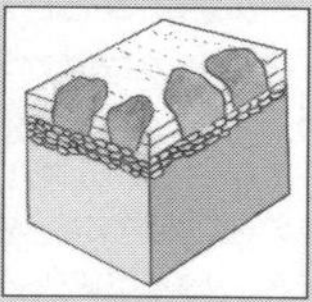

BULLA
A raised, thin-walled blister greater than 0.5 cm in diameter; contains clear or serous fluid

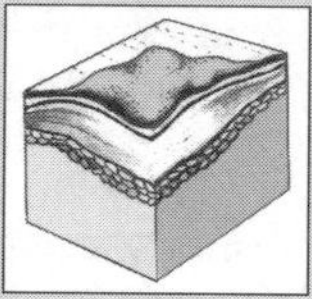

VESICLE
A small (less than 0.5 cm in diameter), thin-walled, raised blister; contains clear, serous, purulent, or bloody fluid

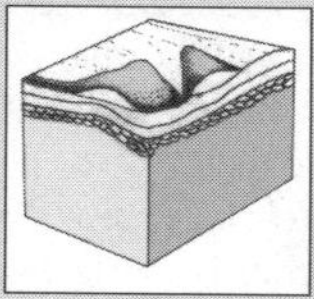

PUSTULE
A circumscribed, pus- or lymph-filled, elevated lesion that may be firm or soft, white or yellow; varies in diameter

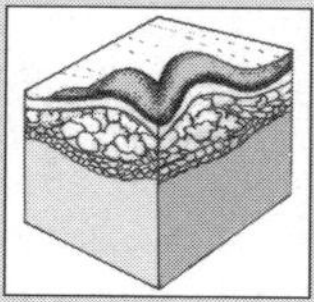

WHEAL
A slightly raised, firm lesion of variable size and shape, surrounded by edema; skin may be red or pale

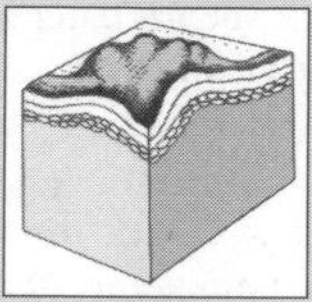

NODULE
A small, firm, circumscribed, elevated lesion approximately 1 to 2 cm in diameter; possible skin discoloration

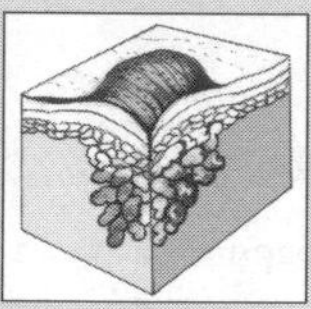

PAPULE
A small, solid lesion less than 1 cm in diameter, with red to purple discoloration

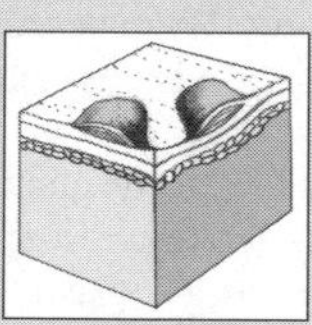

TUMOR
A solid, raised mass usually larger than 2 cm in diameter with possible skin discoloration

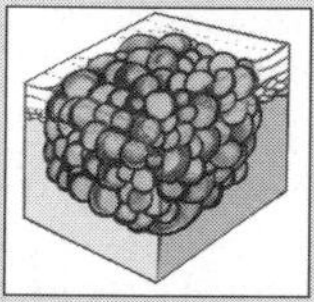

♦ ***Kaposi's sarcoma.*** This neoplastic disorder is characterized by purple or blue papules or macules on the extremities, ears, and nose. These lesions decrease in size with firm pressure and then return to their original size within 10 to 15 seconds. They may become scaly and ulcerate with bleeding. Two variants — classic and acute generalized — affect the elderly and patients with acquired immunodeficiency syndrome (AIDS).

♦ ***Lichen planus.*** Discrete, flat, angular or polygonal, violet papules, commonly marked with white lines or spots, are characteristic of this disorder. The papules may be linear or coalesce into plaques and usually appear on the lumbar region, genitalia, ankles, anterior tibiae, and wrists. Lesions usually develop first on the buccal mucosa as a lacy network of white or gray threadlike papules or plaques. Pruritus, distorted fingernails, and atrophic alopecia commonly occur.

♦ ***Mononucleosis (infectious).*** A maculopapular rash that resembles rubella is an early sign of this infection in 10% of patients. The rash is typically preceded by headache, malaise, and fatigue. It may be accompanied by sore throat, cervical lymphadenopathy, and fluctuating temperature with an evening peak of 101° to 102° F (38.3° to 38.9° C). Splenomegaly and hepatomegaly may also develop.

♦ ***Necrotizing vasculitis.*** In this systemic disorder, crops of purpuric but otherwise asymptomatic papules are typical. Some patients also develop low-grade fever, headache, myalgia, arthralgia, or abdominal pain.

♦ ***Pityriasis rosea.*** This disorder begins with an erythematous "herald patch" — a slightly raised, oval lesion about 2 to 6 cm in diameter that may appear anywhere on the body. A few days to weeks later, yellow to tan or erythematous patches with scaly edges appear on the trunk, arms, and legs, commonly erupting along body cleavage lines in a characteristic "pine tree" pattern. These pruritic patches are about 0.5 to 1 cm in diameter and typically improve with sun exposure.

♦ ***Polymorphic light eruption.*** Abnormal reactions to light may cause papular, vesicular, or nodular rashes on sun-exposed areas. Other symptoms may include pruritus, headache, or malaise.

♦ ***Psoriasis.*** This common chronic disorder begins with small, erythematous papules on the scalp, chest, elbows, knees, back buttocks, or genitalia. These papules are sometimes pruritic and painful. Eventually they enlarge and coalesce, forming elevated, red, scaly plaques covered by characteristic silver scales, except in moist areas such as the genitalia. These scales may flake off easily or thicken, covering the plaque. Associated features include pitted fingernails and arthralgia.

♦ ***Rosacea.*** This hyperemic disorder is characterized by persistent erythema, telangiectasia, and recurrent eruption of papules and pustules on the forehead, malar areas, nose, and chin. Eventually, eruptions recur more frequently and erythema deepens. Rhinophyma may occur in severe cases.

♦ ***Seborrheic keratosis.*** Benign skin tumors begin as small, yellow-brown papules on the chest, back, or abdomen that eventually enlarge and become deeply pigmented. However, in blacks, these papules may remain small and affect only the malar part of the face (dermatosis papulosa nigra).

♦ ***Syringoma.*** This adenoma of the sweat glands causes a yellowish or erythematous papular rash on the face (especially the eyelids), neck, and upper chest.

♦ ***Systemic lupus erythematosus (SLE).*** This disorder is characterized by a "butterfly rash" of erythematous maculopapules or discoid plaques that appears in a malar distribution across the nose and cheeks. Similar rashes may appear elsewhere, especially on exposed body areas. Other cardinal features include photosensitivity and nondeforming arthritis, especially in the hands, feet, and large joints. Among common effects are patchy alopecia, mucous membrane ulceration, low-grade or spiking fever, chills, lymphadenopathy, anorexia, weight loss, abdominal pain, diarrhea or constipation, dyspnea, tachycardia, hematuria, headache, and irritability.

Other causes

♦ ***Drugs.*** Transient maculopapular rashes, usually on the trunk, may accompany reactions to many drugs, including antibiotics, such as tetracycline, ampicillin, cephalosporins, or sulfonamides; benzodiazepines such as diazepam; lithium; phenylbutazone; gold salts; allopurinol; isoniazid; or salicylates.

Special considerations
Apply cool compresses or an antipruritic lotion. Administer antihistamines for allergic reactions and antibiotics for infection.

Pediatric pointers
Common causes of papular rashes in children are infectious diseases, such as molluscum contagiosum or scarlet fever; scabies; insect bites; allergies and drug reactions; or miliaria, depending on the depth of sweat gland involvement.

Geriatric pointers
In bedridden elderly patients, the first sign of pressure ulcers is commonly an erythematous area, sometimes with firm papules. If not properly managed, these lesions progress to deep ulcers and can lead to death.

PARALYSIS

Paralysis, the total loss of voluntary motor function, results from severe cortical or pyramidal tract damage. It can occur in cerebrovascular disorders, degenerative neuromuscular disease, trauma, tumors, or central nervous system infection. Acute paralysis may be an early indicator of a life-threatening disorder, such as Guillain-Barré syndrome, in which ascending paralysis is typically seen.

Paralysis can be local or widespread, symmetrical or asymmetrical, transient or permanent, and spastic or flaccid. It's commonly classified according to location and severity as paraplegia (sometimes transient paralysis of the legs), quadriplegia (permanent paralysis of the arms, legs, and body below the level of the spinal lesion), or hemiplegia (unilateral paralysis of varying severity and permanence). Incomplete paralysis with profound weakness (paresis) may precede total paralysis in some patients.

Emergency interventions
If paralysis has developed suddenly, suspect trauma or an acute vascular insult. After ensuring that the patient's spine is properly immobilized, quickly determine his level of consciousness (LOC) and take his vital signs. Elevated systolic blood pressure, widening pulse pressure, and bradycardia may signal increasing intracranial pressure (ICP). If possible, elevate the patient's head 30 degrees to decrease ICP.

Evaluate respiratory status, and be prepared to administer oxygen, insert an artificial airway, or provide intubation and mechanical ventilation, as needed. To help determine the nature of the patient's injury, ask him for an account of the precipitating events. If he can't respond, try to find an eyewitness.

History and physical examination
If the patient is in no immediate danger, perform a complete neurologic assessment. Start with the history, relying on family members for information if necessary. Ask about the onset, duration, intensity, and progression of paralysis and about the events preceding its development. Focus medical history questions on the incidence of degenerative neurologic or neuromuscular disease, recent infectious illness, sexually transmitted disease, cancer, or recent injury. Explore related symptoms, noting fever, headache, vision disturbances, dysphagia, nausea and vomiting, bowel or bladder dysfunction, muscle pain or weakness, and fatigue.

Next, perform a complete neurologic examination, testing cranial nerve, motor, and sensory function and deep tendon reflexes. Assess strength in all major muscle groups, and note muscle atrophy. (See *Testing muscle strength,* pages 394 and 395.) Document all findings to serve as a baseline.

Common medical causes

◆ ***Amyotrophic lateral sclerosis.*** This invariably fatal disorder causes spastic or flaccid paralysis in the body's major muscle groups, eventually progressing to total paralysis. Early findings include progressive muscle weakness, fasciculations, and muscle atrophy, commonly beginning in the arms and hands. Cramping and hyperreflexia are also common. Involvement of respiratory muscles and the brain stem causes dyspnea and possibly respiratory distress. Progressive cranial nerve paralysis causes dysarthria, dysphagial drooling, choking, and difficulty chewing.

◆ ***Bell's palsy.*** Bell's palsy, a disease of cranial nerve VII, causes transient, unilateral facial muscle paralysis. The affected muscles sag and eyelid closure is impossible. Other signs include increased tearing, drooling, and a diminished or absent corneal reflex.

◆ ***Brain abscess.*** Advanced abscess in the frontal or temporal lobe can cause hemiplegia accompanied by other late findings, such as ocular disturbances, unequal pupils, decreased LOC, ataxia, tremors, or signs of infection.

◆ ***Brain tumor.*** A tumor affecting the motor cortex of the frontal lobe may cause contralateral hemiparesis that progresses to hemiplegia. Onset is gradual but paralysis is permanent without treatment. In early stages, frontal headache and behavioral changes may be the only indicators. Eventually, seizures, aphasia, and signs of increased ICP (decreased LOC and vomiting) develop.

◆ ***Cerebrovascular accident (CVA).*** A CVA involving the motor cortex can cause contralateral paresis or paralysis. Onset may be sudden or gradual, and paralysis may be transient or permanent. Associated signs and symptoms vary widely and may include headache, vomiting, seizures, decreased LOC and mental acuity, dysarthria, dysphagia, ataxia, contralateral paresthesia or sensory loss, apraxia, agnosia, aphasia, vision disturbances, emotional lability, or bowel and bladder dysfunction.

◆ ***Conversion disorder.*** Hysterical paralysis, a classic symptom of conversion disorder, is characterized by the loss of voluntary movement with no obvious physical cause. It can affect any muscle group, appears and disappears unpredictably, and may be associated with histrionic behavior (manipulative, dramatic, vain, irrational) or a strange indifference.

◆ ***Encephalitis.*** Variable paralysis develops in the late stages of this disorder. Earlier signs and symptoms include rapidly decreasing LOC (possibly coma), fever, headache, photophobia, vomiting, signs of meningeal irritation (nuchal rigidity, Kernig's and Brudzinski's signs), aphasia, ataxia, nystagmus, ocular palsies, myoclonus, and seizures.

◆ ***Guillain-Barré syndrome.*** This syndrome is characterized by a rapidly developing but reversible, ascending paralysis. It commonly begins as leg muscle weakness and progresses symmetrically, sometimes affecting even the cranial nerves, producing dysphagia, nasal speech, and dysarthria. Respiratory muscle paralysis may be life-threatening. Other effects may include transient paresthesia, orthostatic hypotension, tachycardia, diaphoresis, or bowel and bladder incontinence.

◆ ***Head trauma.*** After cerebral injury cerebral edema and increased ICP can cause paralysis. Onset is usually sudden. Location and extent vary, depending on the injury. Associated findings also vary but may include decreased LOC; sensory disturbances, such as paresthesia and loss of sensation; headache; blurred or double vision; nausea and vomiting; and focal neurologic disturbances.

◆ ***Multiple sclerosis.*** In this disorder, paralysis commonly waxes and wanes until the later stages, when it may become permanent. Its extent can range from monoplegia to quadriplegia. In most patients, visual and sensory disturbances (paresthesia) are the earliest symptoms.

Later findings are widely variable and may include muscle weakness and spasticity, nystagmus, hyperreflexia, intention tremor, gait ataxia, dysphagia, dysarthria, impotence, or constipation. Urinary frequency, urgency, and incontinence may occur.

♦ ***Myasthenia gravis.*** In this neuromuscular disease, profound muscle weakness and abnormal fatigability may cause paralysis of certain muscle groups. Paralysis is usually transient in early stages but becomes more persistent as the disease progresses. Associated findings depend on the areas of neuromuscular involvement; they may include weak eye closure, ptosis, diplopia, lack of facial mobility, dysphagia, nasal speech, or frequent nasal regurgitation of fluids. Neck muscle weakness may cause the patient's jaw to drop and his head to bob. Respiratory muscle involvement can lead to respiratory distress — dyspnea, shallow respirations, and cyanosis.

♦ ***Parkinson's disease.*** Tremors, bradykinesia, and lead-pipe or cogwheel rigidity are the classic signs of Parkinson's disease. Extreme rigidity can progress to paralysis, particularly in the extremities. In most cases, paralysis resolves with prompt treatment of the disease.

♦ ***Peripheral neuropathy.*** Typically, this syndrome causes muscle weakness that may lead to flaccid paralysis and atrophy. Related effects may include paresthesia, loss of vibration sensation, hypoactive or absent deep tendon reflexes, neuralgia, and skin changes, such as anhidrosis.

♦ ***Rabies.*** This acute disorder causes progressive flaccid paralysis, vascular collapse, coma, and death within 2 weeks after contact with an infected animal. Prodromal signs and symptoms — fever; headache; hyperesthesia; paresthesia, coldness, and itching at the bite site; photophobia; tachycardia; shallow respirations; and excessive salivation, lacrimation, and perspiration — develop almost immediately. Within 2 to 10 days, a phase of excitement begins, marked by agitation, cranial nerve dysfunction (pupil changes, hoarseness, facial weakness, ocular palsies), tachycardia or bradycardia, cyclic respirations, high fever, urine retention, drooling, and hydrophobia.

♦ ***Seizure disorders.*** Seizures, particularly focal seizures, can cause transient local paralysis (Todd's paralysis). Any part of the body may be affected, although paralysis tends to occur contralateral to the site of the irritable focus.

♦ ***Spinal cord injury.*** Complete spinal cord transection results in permanent spastic paralysis below the level of injury. Reflexes may return after resolution of spinal shock. Partial transection causes variable paralysis and paresthesia, depending on the location and extent of injury. (See *Understanding spinal cord syndromes.*)

♦ ***Spinal cord tumors.*** Paresis, pain, paresthesia, and variable sensory loss may occur along the nerve distribution pathway served by the affected cord segment. Eventually, these symptoms may progress to spastic paralysis with hyperactive deep tendon reflexes (or hyporeflexia if the tumor is in the cauda equina) and, perhaps, bladder and bowel incontinence. Untreated paralysis is permanent.

♦ ***Subarachnoid hemorrhage.*** This potentially life-threatening disorder can cause sudden paralysis. The condition may be temporary, resolving with decreasing edema, or permanent, if tissue destruction has occurred. Other acute effects are severe headache, mydriasis, photophobia, aphasia, sharply decreased LOC, nuchal rigidity, vomiting, and seizures.

♦ ***Syringomyelia.*** This degenerative spinal cord disease causes segmental paresis, leading to flaccid paralysis of the hands and arms. Reflexes are absent, and loss of pain and temperature sensation is distributed over the neck, shoulders, and arms in a capelike pattern.

♦ ***Transient ischemic attack (TIA).*** Episodic TIAs may cause transient unilateral paresis or paralysis accompanied by paresthesia, blurred or double vision,

Understanding spinal cord syndromes

When a patient's spinal cord is incompletely severed, he experiences partial motor and sensory loss. Most incomplete cord lesions fit into one of the following syndromes.

ANTERIOR CORD SYNDROME
Anterior cord syndrome usually results from flexion injury, causes motor paralysis and loss of pain and temperature sensation below the level of injury. Touch, proprioception, and vibration sensation are usually preserved.

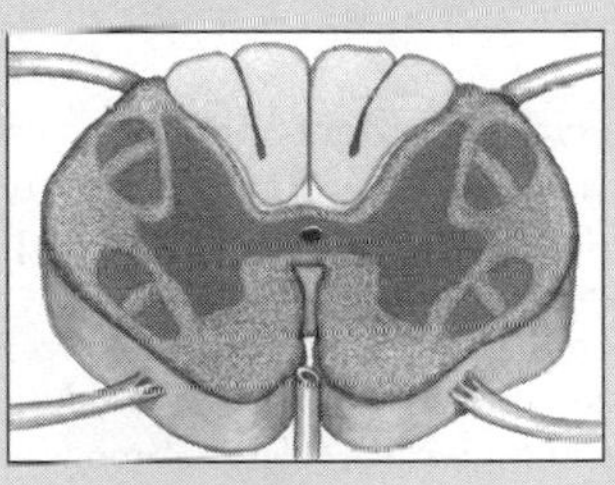

BROWN-SÉQUARD CORD SYNDROME
Flexion, rotation, or penetration injury can cause Brown-Séquard cord syndrome. It's characterized by unilateral motor paralysis and loss of pain ipsilateral to injury and contralateral loss of temperature sensation.

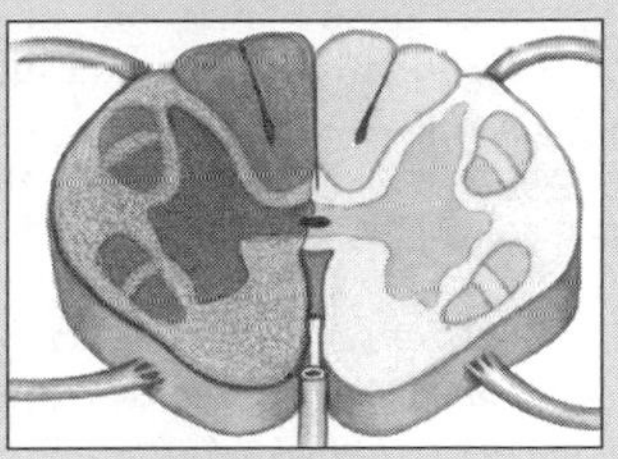

CENTRAL CORD SYNDROME
Hyperextension or flexion injury causes central cord syndrome. Motor loss is variable and greater in the arms than in the legs; sensory loss is usually slight.

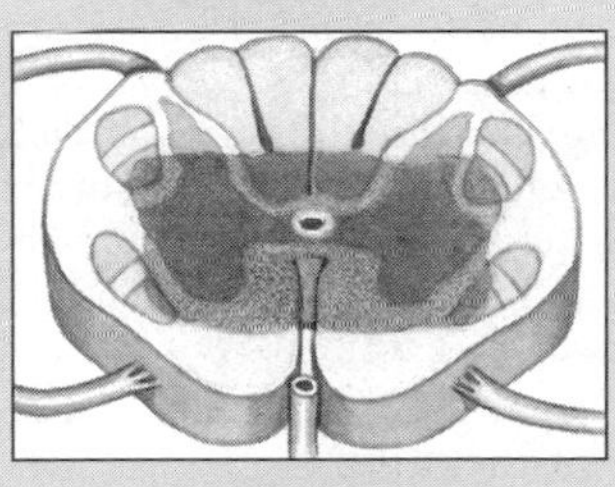

POSTERIOR CORD SYNDROME
Produced by a cervical hyperextension injury, posterior cord syndrome causes only a loss of proprioception and loss of light touch sensation. Motor function remains intact.

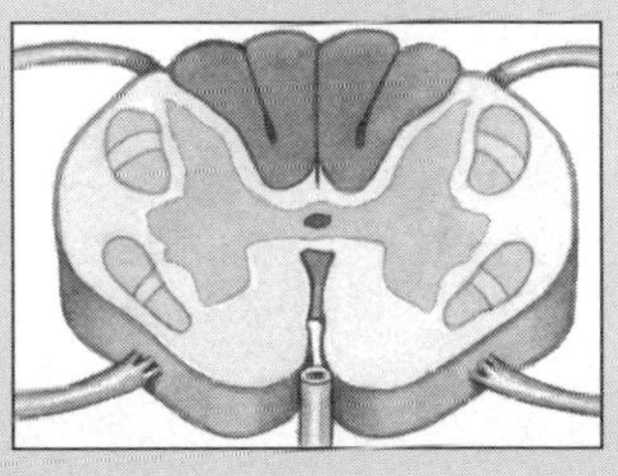

dizziness, aphasia, dysarthria, decreased LOC, and other site-dependent effects.

◆ ***West Nile encephalitis.*** This brain infection is caused by West Nile virus, a mosquito-borne flavivirus endemic to Africa, the Middle East, and western Asia. Mild infections are common and include fever, headache, and body aches, commonly with skin rash and swollen lymph glands. More severe infections are marked by headache, high fever, neck stiffness, stupor, disorientation, coma, tremors, occasional seizures, paralysis and, rarely, death.

Other causes

♦ ***Drugs.*** Therapeutic use of neuromuscular blocking agents, such as pancuronium or curare, causes paralysis.

♦ ***Electroconvulsive therapy.*** This therapy can cause acute but transient, paralysis.

Special considerations

Because a paralyzed patient is particularly susceptible to complications of prolonged immobility, provide frequent position changes, meticulous skin care, and frequent chest physiotherapy. He may benefit from passive range-of-motion exercises to maintain muscle tone, application of splints to prevent contractures, and the use of footboards or other devices to prevent footdrop. If his cranial nerves are affected, the patient will have difficulty chewing and swallowing. Provide a liquid or soft diet, and keep suction equipment on hand in case aspiration occurs. Feeding tubes or total parenteral nutrition may be necessary in severe paralysis. Paralysis and accompanying vision disturbances may make ambulation hazardous; provide a call light and show the patient how to call for help. As appropriate, arrange for physical, speech, or occupational therapy.

Pediatric pointers

Besides the obvious causes — trauma, infection, or tumors — children may contract paralysis from hereditary and congenital disorders, such as Tay-Sachs disease, Werdnig-Hoffmann disease, spina bifida, or cerebral palsy.

PARESTHESIA

Paresthesia is an abnormal sensation or combination of sensations — commonly described as numbness, prickling, or tingling — felt along peripheral nerve pathways. These sensations generally aren't painful; unpleasant or painful sensations are termed *dysesthesias.* Paresthesia may develop suddenly or gradually and may be transient or permanent.

A common symptom of many neurologic disorders, paresthesia may also result from certain systemic disorders or drug effects. It may reflect damage or irritation of the parietal lobe, thalamus, spinothalamic tract, or spinal or peripheral nerves — the neural circuit that transmits and interprets sensory stimuli.

History and physical examination

First, explore the paresthesia. When did the abnormal sensations begin? Have the patient describe their character and distribution. Also, ask about associated signs and symptoms, such as sensory loss and paresis or paralysis. Next, take a medical history, including neurologic, cardiovascular, metabolic, renal, and chronic inflammatory disorders, such as arthritis or lupus. Has the patient recently sustained a traumatic injury or had surgery or invasive procedures that may have damaged peripheral nerves?

Focus the physical examination on the patient's neurologic status. Assess his level of consciousness (LOC) and cranial nerve function. Test muscle strength and deep tendon reflexes (DTRs) in limbs affected by paresthesia. Systematically evaluate light touch, pain, temperature, vibration, and position sensation. Also, note skin color and temperature and palpate pulses.

Common medical causes

♦ ***Arterial occlusion (acute).*** In this disorder, sudden paresthesia and coldness may develop in one or both legs with a saddle embolus. Paresis, intermittent claudication, and aching pain at rest are also characteristic. The extremity becomes mottled with a line of temperature and color demarcation at the level of occlusion. Pulses are absent below the occlusion, and capillary refill is diminished.

♦ ***Arteriosclerosis obliterans.*** This disorder causes paresthesia, intermittent claudication (most common symptom), diminished or absent popliteal and pedal pulses, pallor, paresis, and coldness in the affected leg.

◆ ***Arthritis.*** Rheumatoid or osteoarthritic changes in the cervical spine may cause paresthesia in the neck, shoulders, and arms. The lumbar spine occasionally is affected, causing paresthesia in one or both legs and feet.

◆ ***Brain tumor.*** Tumors affecting the sensory cortex in the parietal lobe may cause progressive contralateral paresthesia accompanied by agnosia, apraxia, agraphia, homonymous hemianopia, or loss of proprioception.

◆ ***Buerger's disease.*** In this smoking-related inflammatory occlusive disorder, exposure to cold makes the feet cold, cyanotic, and numb; after prolonged exposure, they redden, become hot, and tingle. Intermittent claudication, which is aggravated by exercise and relieved by rest, is also common. Other findings include weak peripheral pulses, migratory superficial thrombophlebitis and, later, ulceration, muscle atrophy, and gangrene.

◆ ***Cerebrovascular accident (CVA).*** Although contralateral paresthesia may occur in CVA, sensory loss is more common. Associated features vary with the artery affected and may include contralateral hemiplegia, decreased LOC, or homonymous hemianopia.

◆ ***Diabetes mellitus.*** Diabetic neuropathy can cause paresthesia with a burning sensation in the hands and legs. Other findings may include insidious, permanent anosmia, fatigue, polyuria, polydipsia, weight loss, or polyphagia.

◆ ***Guillain-Barré syndrome.*** In this syndrome, transient paresthesia may precede muscle weakness, which usually begins in the legs and ascends to the arms and facial nerves. Weakness may progress to total paralysis. Other clinical features may include dysarthria, dysphagia, nasal speech, orthostatic hypotension, bladder and bowel incontinence, diaphoresis, tachycardia and, possibly, signs of life-threatening respiratory muscle paralysis.

◆ ***Head trauma.*** Unilateral or bilateral paresthesia may occur when head trauma causes a concussion or contusion; however, sensory loss is more common. Other findings may include variable paresis or paralysis, decreased LOC, headache, blurred or double vision, nausea and vomiting, dizziness, or seizures.

◆ ***Herniated disk.*** Herniation of a lumbar or cervical disk may cause acute or gradual onset of paresthesia along the distribution pathways of affected spinal nerves. Other neuromuscular effects include severe pain, muscle spasms, and weakness that may progress to atrophy unless herniation is relieved.

◆ ***Herpes zoster.*** An early symptom of this disorder, paresthesia occurs in the dermatome supplied by the affected spinal nerve. Within several days, this dermatome is marked by a pruritic, erythematous, vesicular rash associated with sharp, shooting, or burning pain.

◆ ***Hyperventilation syndrome.*** Usually triggered by acute anxiety, this syndrome may cause transient paresthesia in the hands, feet, and perioral area, accompanied by agitation, vertigo, syncope, pallor, muscle twitching and weakness, carpopedal spasm, or cardiac arrhythmias.

◆ ***Migraine headache.*** Paresthesia in the hands, face, and perioral area may herald an impending migraine headache. Other prodromal symptoms may include scotomas, hemiparesis, confusion, dizziness, or photophobia. These effects may persist during the characteristic throbbing headache and continue after it subsides.

◆ ***Multiple sclerosis (MS).*** In this disorder, demyelination of the sensory cortex or spinothalamic tract may cause paresthesia — commonly one of the earliest symptoms. Like other effects of MS, paresthesia commonly waxes and wanes until the later stages, when it may become permanent. Associated findings may include muscle weakness, spasticity, and hyperreflexia.

♦ ***Peripheral nerve trauma.*** Injury to any of the major peripheral nerves may cause paresthesia — commonly dysesthesias — in the area supplied by that nerve. Paresthesia begins shortly after trauma and may be permanent. Other effects may be flaccid paralysis or paresis, hyporeflexia, and variable sensory loss.

♦ ***Peripheral neuropathy.*** This syndrome may cause progressive paresthesia in all extremities. The patient also commonly displays muscle weakness, which may lead to flaccid paralysis and atrophy; loss of vibration sensation; diminished or absent DTRs; neuralgia; and cutaneous changes, such as glossy, red skin and anhidrosis.

♦ ***Rabies.*** Paresthesia, coldness, and itching at the site of an animal bite herald the prodromal stage of rabies. Other prodromal effects are fever, headache, photophobia, hyperesthesia, tachycardia, shallow respirations, and excessive salivation, lacrimation, and perspiration.

♦ ***Raynaud's disease.*** Exposure to cold or stress makes the fingers turn pale, cold, and cyanotic; with rewarming, they become red and paresthetic. Ulceration may occur in chronic cases.

♦ ***Seizure disorders.*** Seizures originating in the parietal lobe usually cause paresthesia of the lips, fingers, and toes. The paresthesias may act as auras that precede tonic-clonic seizures.

♦ ***Spinal cord injury.*** Paresthesia may occur in partial spinal cord transection, after spinal shock resolves. It may be unilateral or bilateral, occurring at or below the level of the lesion. Associated sensory and motor loss is variable. (See *Understanding spinal cord syndromes,* page 449.) Spinal cord injuries may be associated with paresthesia on head flexion (Lhermitte's sign).

♦ ***Spinal cord tumors.*** Paresthesia, paresis, pain, and sensory loss along nerve pathways served by the affected cord segment are manifestations of such tumors. Eventually, paresis may cause spastic paralysis with hyperactive DTRs (or hyporeflexia if the tumor is in the cauda equina) and, possibly, bladder and bowel incontinence.

♦ ***Systemic lupus erythematosus.*** This disorder may cause paresthesia but its primary clinical features include nondeforming arthritis (usually of hands, feet, and large joints), photosensitivity, and a "butterfly rash" across the nose and cheeks.

♦ ***Tabes dorsalis.*** In this disorder, paresthesia — especially of the legs — is a common late symptom. Other effects include ataxia, loss of proprioception and pain and temperature sensation, absent deep tendon reflexes, Charcot's joints, Argyll Robertson pupils, incontinence, and impotence.

♦ ***Transient ischemic attack (TIA).*** Paresthesia typically occurs abruptly in a TIA and is limited to one arm or another isolated part of the body. It usually lasts about 10 minutes and is accompanied by paralysis or paresis. Associated findings may include decreased LOC, dizziness, unilateral vision loss, nystagmus, aphasia, dysarthria, tinnitus, facial weakness, dysphagia, or ataxic gait.

Other causes

♦ ***Drugs.*** Phenytoin, chemotherapeutic agents (such as vincristine, vinblastine, and procarbazine), D-penicillamine, isoniazid, nitrofurantoin, chloroquine, and parenteral gold therapy may cause transient paresthesia that disappears when the drug is discontinued.

♦ ***Radiation therapy.*** Long-term radiation therapy eventually may cause peripheral nerve damage, resulting in paresthesia.

Special considerations

Because paresthesia is commonly accompanied by patchy sensory loss, teach the patient safety measures. For example, have him test bathwater with a thermometer and smoke cigarettes carefully to avoid burning his fingers.

Pediatric pointers

Although children may experience paresthesia associated with the same causes as adults, they're frequently unable to describe this symptom. Nevertheless, hereditary polyneuropathies are usually first recognized in childhood.

PAROXYSMAL NOCTURNAL DYSPNEA

Typically dramatic and terrifying to the patient, this sign refers to an attack of dyspnea that abruptly awakens the patient. An attack commonly causes diaphoresis, coughing, wheezing, and chest discomfort. It abates after the patient sits up or stands for several minutes but may recur every 2 to 3 hours.

Paroxysmal nocturnal dyspnea is a sign of left-sided heart failure. It can reflect decreased respiratory drive, impaired left ventricular function, enhanced reabsorption of interstitial fluid, and increased thoracic blood volume. All of these pathophysiologic mechanisms can cause dyspnea to worsen when the patient lies down.

History and physical examination

Begin by exploring the patient's complaint of dyspnea. Does he have dyspneic attacks only at night or at other times as well, such as after exertion or while sitting down? If so, what type of activity triggers the attack? Does he experience coughing, wheezing, fatigue, or weakness during an attack? Find out if he has a history of lower extremity edema. Ask if he sleeps with his head elevated and, if so, on how many pillows. Obtain a cardiopulmonary history. Does the patient or a family member have a history of myocardial infarction, coronary artery disease, or hypertension? Does he have chronic bronchitis, emphysema, or asthma? Has the patient had cardiac surgery?

Next perform a physical examination. Begin by taking the patient's vital signs and forming an overall impression of his appearance. Is he noticeably cyanotic or edematous? Auscultate the lungs for crackles and wheezing and the heart for gallops and arrhythmias.

Common medical causes

♦ ***Left-sided heart failure.*** Dyspnea — on exertion, during sleep, and eventually even at rest — is an early sign of left-sided heart failure. This sign is characteristically accompanied by Cheyne-Stokes respirations, diaphoresis, weakness, wheezing, and a persistent, nonproductive cough or a cough that produces clear or blood-tinged sputum. As the patient's condition worsens, he develops tachycardia, tachypnea, pulsus alternans (commonly initiated by a premature beat), a ventricular gallop, crackles, and peripheral edema.

In advanced left-sided heart failure, the patient may also exhibit severe orthopnea, cyanosis, clubbing, hemoptysis, and cardiac arrhythmias as well as signs and symptoms of shock, such as hypotension, weak pulse, and cold, clammy skin.

Special considerations

Prepare the patient for diagnostic tests, such as chest X-ray, echocardiography, exercise electrocardiography, and cardiac blood pool imaging. If the hospitalized patient experiences paroxysmal nocturnal dyspnea, assist him to a sitting position or help him walk around the room. If necessary, provide supplemental oxygen. Try to calm him because anxiety can exacerbate dyspnea.

Pediatric pointers

In a child, paroxysmal nocturnal dyspnea usually stems from congenital heart defects that precipitate ventricular failure. Help relieve the child's dyspnea by elevating his head and calming him.

PEAU D'ORANGE

Usually a late sign of breast cancer, peau d'orange (orange-peel skin) is the edematous thickening and pitting of breast skin. This slowly developing sign can also occur with breast or axillary lymph node infection, erysipelas, or Graves' disease. Its striking orange-peel appearance stems from lymphatic edema around deepened hair follicles. (See *Recognizing peau d'orange.*)

History and physical examination

Ask the patient when she first detected peau d'orange. Has she noticed lumps, pain, or other breast changes? Does she have related symptoms, such as malaise, achiness, and weight loss? Is she lactating, or has she recently weaned her infant? Has she had previous breast surgery or axillary surgery that might have impaired lymphatic drainage of a breast?

In a well-lit examining room, observe the patient's breasts. Estimate the extent of the peau d'orange and check for erythema. Assess the nipples for discharge, deviation, retraction, dimpling, and cracking. Gently palpate the area of peau d'orange, noting abnormal warmth, redness, or induration. Then palpate the entire breast, noting fixed or mobile lumps, and the axillary lymph nodes, noting enlargement. Finally, take the patient's temperature.

Common medical causes

♦ ***Breast abscess.*** Usually affecting lactating women with milk stasis, this infectious disorder causes peau d'orange, malaise, breast tenderness and erythema, and a sudden fever that may be accompanied by shaking chills. A cracked nipple may cause a purulent discharge, and an indurated or palpable soft mass may be present.

♦ ***Breast cancer.*** *Lymphedema* associated with advanced breast cancer is the most likely cause of peau d'orange, which usually begins in the dependent part of the breast or the areola. Palpation typically reveals a firm, immobile mass that adheres to the skin above the area of peau d'orange. Inspection of the breasts may reveal changes in contour, size, or symmetry. Inspection of the nipples may reveal deviation, erosion, retraction, and a thin and watery, bloody, or purulent discharge. The patient may report a burning and itching sensation in the nipples as well as a sensation of warmth or heat in the breast. Breast pain may occur but it isn't a reliable indicator of cancer.

EXAMINATION TIP

Recognizing peau d'orange

In peau d'orange, the skin appears to be pitted (as shown below). This condition usually reflects the presence of late-stage breast cancer.

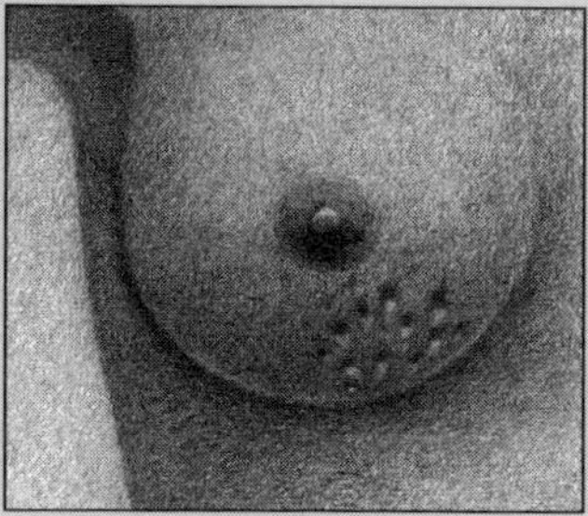

Special considerations

Because peau d'orange usually signals advanced breast cancer, provide emotional support for the patient. Encourage her to express her fears and concerns. Clearly explain expected diagnostic tests, such as mammography and breast biopsy.

Geriatric pointer

Postmenopausal women should be instructed to continue regular self breast examination. Ask the patient about use of hormone replacement therapy (HRT) including herbal preparations.

PERICARDIAL FRICTION RUB

Commonly transient, a pericardial friction rub is a scratching, grating, or crunching sound that occurs when two inflamed layers of the pericardium slide over one another. Ranging from faint to loud, this abnormal sound is best heard along the lower left sternal border during deep inspiration. It indicates pericarditis, which can result from acute infection, cardiac or renal disorders, postpericardiotomy syndrome, or the use of certain drugs.

Occasionally, a pericardial friction rub can resemble a murmur (See *Pericardial friction rub or murmur?*) or a pleural friction rub (see *Comparing auscultation findings,* pages 456 and 457). However, the classic pericardial friction rub has three components. (See *Understanding pericardial friction rubs,* page 458.)

EXAMINATION TIP

Pericardial friction rub or murmur?

Is the sound you hear a pericardial friction rub or a murmur? Here's how to tell. The classic pericardial friction rub has three sound components, which are related to the phases of the cardiac cycle. In some patients, however, the rub's presystolic and early diasystolic sounds may be audible, causing the rub to resemble the murmur of mitral stenosis and regurgitation.

If you don't detect the classic three-component sound, you can distinguish a pericardial friction rub from a murmur by auscultating again and asking yourself these questions.

How deep is the sound?
A pericardial friction rub usually sounds superficial; a murmur sounds deeper in the chest.

Does the sound radiate?
A pericardial friction rub usually doesn't radiate; a murmur may radiate widely.

Does the sound vary with inspiration or changes in patient position?
A pericardial friction rub is usually loudest during inspiration and is best heard when the patient leans forward. A murmur varies in timing and duration with both factors.

History and physical examination

Obtain a complete medical history, noting especially cardiac dysfunction. Has the patient recently had a myocardial infarction or cardiac surgery? Has he ever had pericarditis or a rheumatic disorder, such as rheumatoid arthritis or systemic lupus erythematosus? Does he have chronic renal failure or an infection? If the patient complains of chest pain, ask him to describe its character and location. What relieves the pain? What worsens it?

Take the patient's vital signs, noting especially hypotension, tachycardia, irregular pulse, tachypnea, and fever. Inspect for jugular vein distention, edema,

(Text continues on page 458.)

EXAMINATION TIP

Comparing auscultation findings

During auscultation, you may detect a pleural friction rub, a pericardial friction rub, or crackles — three abnormal sounds that are often confused. Use this chart to help clarify auscultation findings.

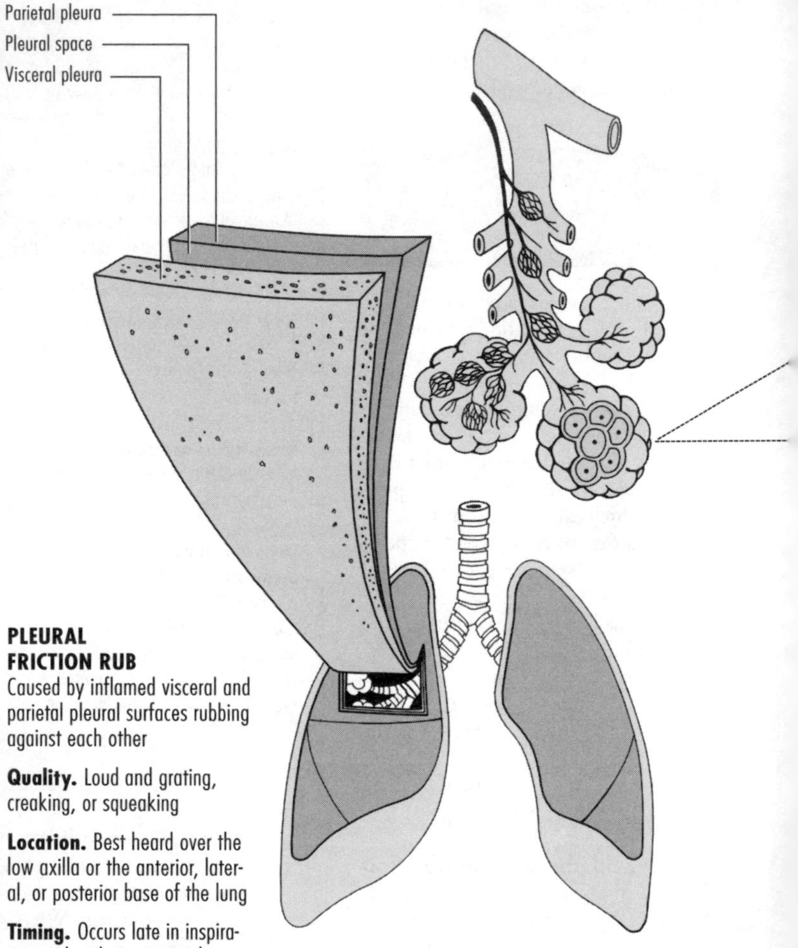

PLEURAL FRICTION RUB
Caused by inflamed visceral and parietal pleural surfaces rubbing against each other

Quality. Loud and grating, creaking, or squeaking

Location. Best heard over the low axilla or the anterior, lateral, or posterior base of the lung

Timing. Occurs late in inspiration and early expiration but ceases when the patient holds his breath; persists during coughing

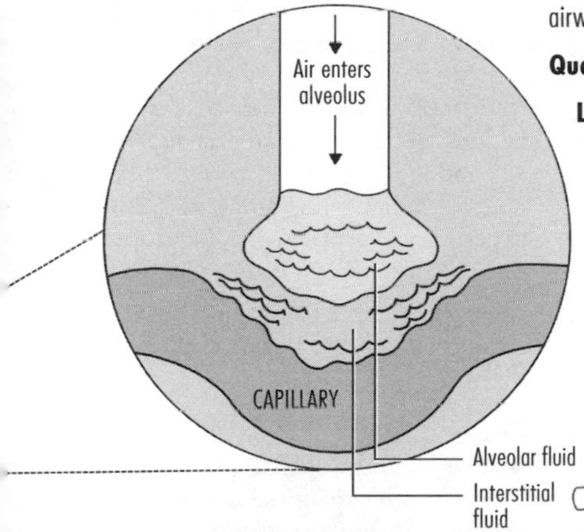

CRACKLES
Caused by air suddenly entering fluid-filled airways

Quality. Nonmusical clicking or rattling

Location. Best heard in less distended and more dependent areas of the lungs, usually at the bases

Timing. Occurs chiefly during inspiration

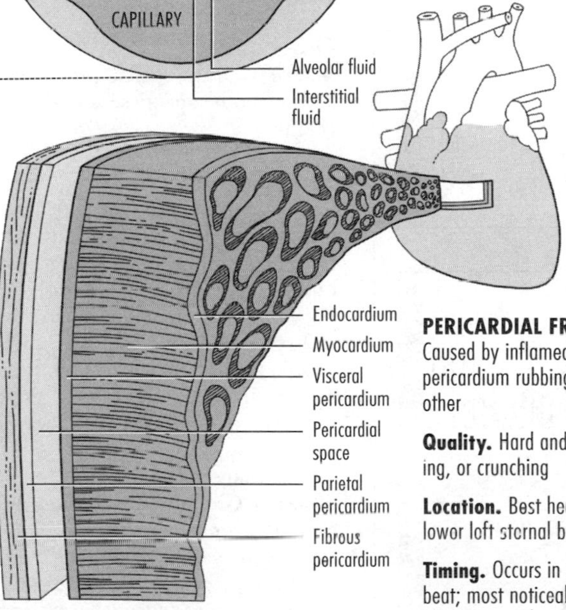

PERICARDIAL FRICTION RUB
Caused by inflamed layers of the pericardium rubbing against each other

Quality. Hard and grating, scratching, or crunching

Location. Best heard along the lower left sternal border

Timing. Occurs in relation to heartbeat; most noticeable during deep inspiration and continues even when the patient holds his breath

EXAMINATION TIP

Understanding pericardial friction rubs

Complete, or classic, pericardial friction rub is triphasic. Its three sound components are linked to phases of the cardiac cycle. The *presystolic* component (A) reflects atrial systole; it precedes the first heart sound (S_1). The *systolic* component (B), usually the loudest, reflects ventricular systole; it occurs between the first and second heart sounds (S_2). The *early diastolic* component (C) reflects ventricular diastole; it follows S_2.

Sometimes, the early diastolic component merges with the presystolic component, producing a dysphasic to-and-fro sound on auscultation. In other patients, auscultation may detect only one component — a monophasic rub, typically during ventricular systole.

TRIPHASIC RUB

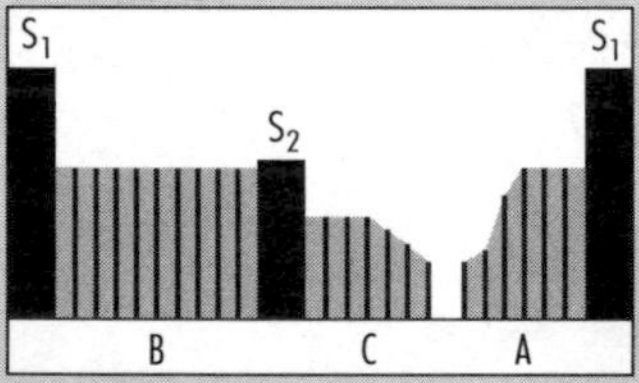

DIPHASIC RUB

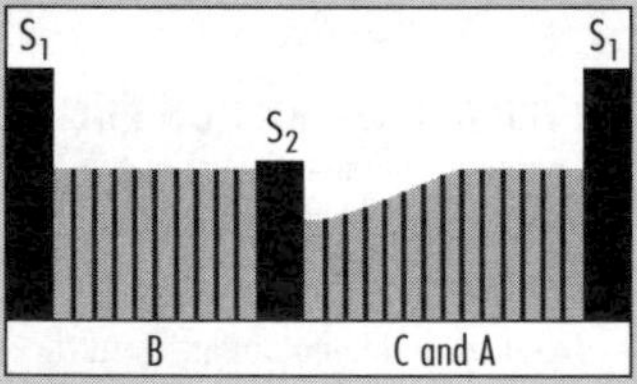

MONOPHASIC RUB

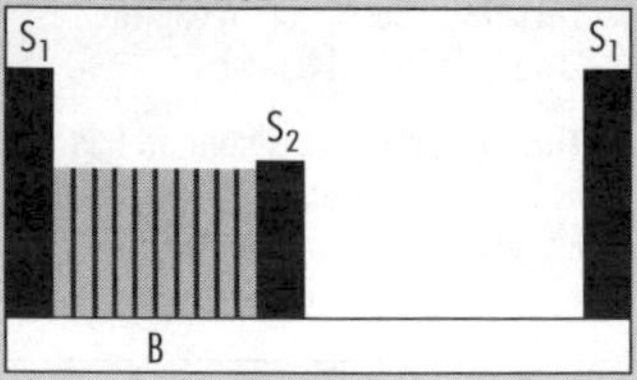

ascites, and hepatomegaly. Auscultate the lungs for crackles.

Common medical causes

◆ ***Pericarditis.*** A pericardial friction rub is the hallmark of *acute pericarditis.* This disorder also causes sharp precordial or retrosternal pain that usually radiates to the left shoulder and neck. The pain worsens when the patient breathes deeply, coughs, or lies flat and, possibly, when he swallows. It abates when he sits up and leans forward. The patient may also develop fever, dyspnea, tachycardia, or arrhythmias.

In *chronic constrictive pericarditis,* a pericardial friction rub develops gradually and is accompanied by signs of decreased cardiac filling and output, such as peripheral edema, ascites, jugular vein distention on inspiration (Kussmaul's sign), and hepatomegaly. Dyspnea, orthopnea, pulsus paradoxus, or chest pain may also occur.

Other causes

◆ ***Drugs.*** Drugs, such as procainamide and chemotherapeutics, can cause pericarditis.

Special considerations

Continue to monitor the patient's cardiovascular status. If the pericardial friction rub disappears, be alert for signs of cardiac tamponade: pallor; cool, clammy skin; hypotension; tachycardia; tachypnea; pulsus paradoxus; and increased jugular vein distention. If these signs occur, prepare the patient for pericardiocentesis to prevent cardiovascular collapse.

Make sure that the patient gets adequate rest. Give anti-inflammatory drugs, antiarrhythmics, diuretics, or antimicrobials to treat the underlying cause. If necessary, prepare him for a pericardiectomy to promote adequate cardiac filling and contraction.

Pediatric pointers

Bacterial pericarditis may develop during the first 2 decades of life, usually before age 6. Although a pericardial friction rub may occur, other signs and symptoms—fever, tachycardia, dyspnea, chest pain, jugular vein distention, and hepatomegaly—more reliably indicate this life-threatening disorder. A pericardial friction rub may also occur after surgery to correct congenital cardiac anomalies. However, it usually vanishes without development of pericarditis.

PERISTALTIC WAVES, VISIBLE

In intestinal obstruction, peristalsis temporarily increases in strength and frequency as the intestine contracts to force its contents past the obstruction. As a result, visible peristaltic waves may roll across the abdomen. Typically, these waves appear suddenly and vanish quickly because increased peristalsis overcomes the obstruction or the GI tract becomes atonic. Peristaltic waves are best detected by stooping at the supine patient's side and inspecting the abdominal contour.

Visible peristaltic waves may also reflect normal stomach and intestinal contractions in thin patients or in malnourished patients with abdominal muscle atrophy.

History and physical examination

After you observe peristaltic waves, collect pertinent history data. For example, ask about a history of pyloric ulcer, stomach cancer, or chronic gastritis, any of which can lead to pyloric obstruction. Also ask about conditions leading to intestinal obstruction, such as intestinal tumors or polyps, gallstones, chronic constipation, or a hernia. Has the patient had recent abdominal surgery? Be sure to obtain a drug history.

Determine if the patient has related symptoms. Spasmodic abdominal pain, for example, accompanies small-bowel obstruction, whereas colicky pain accompanies pyloric obstruction. Is the patient experiencing nausea and vomiting? If he has vomited, ask about the consistency, amount, and color of the vomitus. Lumpy vomitus may contain undigested food particles; green or brown vomitus may contain bile or fecal matter.

Next, with the patient supine, inspect the abdomen for distention, surgical scars and adhesions, or visible loops of bowel. Auscultate for bowel sounds, noting high-pitched, tinkling sounds. Then jar the patient's bed (or roll the patient from side to side) and auscultate for a succussion splash—a splashing sound in the stomach from retained secretions due to pyloric obstruction. Palpate the abdomen for rigidity and tenderness, and percuss for tympany. Check the skin and mucous membranes for dryness and poor skin turgor, which indicate dehydration. Take the patient's vital signs, noting especially tachycardia and hypotension, which indicate hypovolemia.

Common medical causes

♦ ***Large-bowel obstruction.*** Visible peristaltic waves in the upper abdomen are an early sign of this obstruction. Obstipation, however, may be the earliest finding. Other characteristic signs and symptoms develop more slowly than in small-bowel obstruction. These may include nausea, colicky abdominal pain (milder than in small-bowel obstruction), gradual and eventually marked abdominal distention, and hyperactive bowel sounds.

♦ ***Pyloric obstruction.*** Peristaltic waves may be detected in a swollen epigastrium or in the left upper quadrant, usually beginning near the left rib margin and rolling from left to right. Related findings include vague epigastric discomfort or colicky pain after eating, nausea, vomiting, anorexia, and weight loss. Auscultation reveals a loud succussion splash.

◆ ***Small-bowel obstruction.*** Early signs of mechanical obstruction of the small bowel include peristaltic waves rolling across the upper abdomen and intermittent, cramping periumbilical pain. Associated signs and symptoms include nausea, vomiting of bilious or, later, fecal material, and constipation; in partial obstruction, diarrhea may occur. Hyperactive bowel sounds and slight abdominal distention also occur early.

Special considerations

Because visible peristaltic waves are commonly an early sign of intestinal obstruction, monitor the patient's status and prepare him for diagnostic evaluation and treatment. Withhold food and fluids, and explain the purpose and procedure of abdominal X-rays and barium studies, which can confirm obstruction.

If tests confirm obstruction, nasogastric suctioning may be performed to decompress the stomach and small bowel. Provide frequent oral hygiene, and watch for a thick, swollen tongue and dry mucous membranes, which indicate dehydration. Monitor vital signs and intake and output frequently.

Pediatric pointers

In infants, visible peristaltic waves may indicate pyloric stenosis. In small children, peristaltic waves may be visible normally because of the protuberant abdomen, or visible waves may indicate bowel obstruction stemming from congenital anomalies, volvulus, or swallowing of a foreign body.

Geriatric pointers

In elderly patients who present with visible peristaltic waves, always evaluate for fecal impaction, which is a common problem in this age group. Also, obtain a detailed medication history; antidepressants and antipsychotics can predispose patients to constipation and bowel obstruction.

PHOTOPHOBIA

A common symptom, photophobia is an abnormal sensitivity to light or intolerance to light. The patient may be sensitive to sunlight, fluorescent light, or incandescent light. In many patients, photophobia simply indicates increased eye sensitivity without underlying pathology. For example, it can stem from excessive wearing of contact lenses or use of poorly fitted lenses. But, in others, this symptom can result from systemic disorders, ocular disorders such as iritis or corneal inflammation, trauma, or the use of certain drugs.

History and physical examination

If your patient reports photophobia, find out when it began and how severe it is. Did it follow eye trauma, a chemical splash, or exposure to the rays of a sun lamp? If photophobia results from trauma, avoid manipulating the eye. Ask the patient about eye pain and have him describe its location, duration, and intensity. Does he have a sensation of a foreign body in his eye? Does he have other signs and symptoms, such as increased tearing and vision changes?

Next, take the patient's vital signs and assess his neurologic status. Follow this with a careful eye examination, inspecting the eyes' external structures for abnormalities. Examine the conjunctiva and sclera, noting especially their color. Characterize the amount and consistency of any discharge. Then check pupillary reaction to light. Evaluate extraocular muscle function by testing the six cardinal fields of gaze, and test visual acuity in both eyes.

During your assessment, keep in mind that photophobia can accompany life-threatening meningitis, although it isn't a cardinal sign of meningeal irritation. (See *Photophobia: Common causes and associated findings*, page 462.)

Common medical causes

◆ ***Burns.*** In *chemical burns,* photophobia and eye pain may be accompanied by erythema and blistering on the face and lids, miosis, diffuse conjunctival injection, and corneal changes. The patient experiences blurred vision and may be unable to keep his eyes open. In *ultraviolet radiation burns,* photophobia occurs with moderate to severe eye pain. These symptoms develop about 12 hours after exposure to the rays of a welding arc or sun lamp.

◆ ***Conjunctivitis.*** When conjunctivitis affects the cornea, it causes photophobia. Other common findings include conjunctival injection, increased tearing, a foreign-body sensation, a feeling of fullness around the eyes, and eye pain, burning, and itching. *Allergic conjunctivitis* is distinguished by a stringy eye discharge and milky red injection. *Bacterial conjunctivitis* tends to cause a copious, mucopurulent, flaky eye discharge that may make the eyelids stick together and brilliant red conjunctiva. *Fungal conjunctivitis* causes a thick, purulent discharge, extreme redness, and crusted, sticky eyelids. *Viral conjunctivitis* causes copious tearing with little discharge and enlargement of the preauricular lymph nodes.

◆ ***Corneal abrasion.*** A common finding with corneal abrasion, photophobia is usually accompanied by excessive tearing, conjunctival injection, visible corneal damage, and a foreign-body sensation in the eye. Blurred vision and eye pain may also occur.

◆ ***Corneal ulcer.*** This vision-threatening disorder causes severe photophobia and eye pain that's aggravated by blinking. Impaired visual acuity may accompany blurring, eye discharge, and sticky eyelids. Conjunctival injection may occur even though the cornea appears white and opaque. A *bacterial ulcer* may also cause an irregularly shaped corneal ulcer and unilateral pupillary constriction. A *fungal ulcer* may be surrounded by progressively clearer rings.

◆ ***Iritis (acute).*** Severe photophobia may result from this disorder, along with marked conjunctival injection, moderate to severe eye pain, and blurred vision. The pupil may be constricted and may respond poorly to light.

◆ ***Keratitis (interstitial).*** This corneal inflammation causes photophobia, eye pain, blurred vision, dramatic conjunctival injection, and grayish pink corneas. Keratitis may occur from several causes, including viral (HSV, for example), bacterial (for example, pseudomonal, pneumococcal), or fungal.

◆ ***Meningitis (acute bacterial).*** A common symptom of this disorder, photophobia may occur with other signs of meningeal irritation, such as nuchal rigidity, hyperreflexia, and opisthotonos. Brudzinski's and Kernig's signs can be elicited. Fever, an early finding, may be accompanied by chills. Related effects may include headache, vomiting, ocular palsies, facial weakness, pupillary abnormalities, or hearing loss. In severe meningitis, seizures may occur with stupor progressing to coma.

◆ ***Migraine headache.*** Photophobia and noise sensitivity are prominent features of a common migraine. Typically severe, this aching or throbbing headache may also cause fatigue, blurred vision, nausea, and vomiting.

◆ ***Retinal detachment.*** When the retina separates from the choroid, symptoms typically include acute visual loss, flashing lights, floaters, photophobia, or a shade over the vision in one eye.

◆ ***Uveitis.*** Both anterior and posterior uveitis can cause photophobia. Typically, *anterior uveitis* also causes moderate to severe eye pain, severe conjunctival injection, and a small, nonreactive pupil. *Posterior uveitis* develops slowly, causing visual floaters, eye pain, pupil distortion,

Photophobia: Common causes and associated findings

	MAJOR ASSOCIATED SIGNS AND SYMPTOMS										
CAUSES	Conjunctival injection	Corneal changes	Eye discharge	Eye pain	Foreign-body sensation	Nuchal rigidity	Pupillary changes	Tearing, increased	Vision changes	Visual floaters	Vomiting
Burns (chemical)	◆	◆		◆	◆		◆	◆	◆		
Burns (ultraviolet)	◆	◆		◆	◆			◆			
Conjunctivitis	◆		◆	◆	◆			◆			
Corneal abrasion	◆	◆		◆	◆			◆	◆		
Corneal ulcer	◆	◆	◆	◆			◆		◆		
Iritis (acute)	◆			◆			◆		◆		
Keratitis (interstitial)	◆	◆		◆					◆		
Meningitis (acute bacterial)						◆	◆				◆
Migraine headache									◆		◆
Retinal detachment									◆	◆	
Scleritis	◆			◆				◆			
Uveitis (posterior)	◆			◆			◆		◆	◆	

conjunctival injection, and blurred vision.

Other causes

◆ ***Drugs.*** Mydriatics — such as phenylephrine, atropine, scopolamine, cyclopentolate, and tropicamide — can cause photophobia due to ocular dilation. Amphetamines, furosemide, quinine, tetracycline, doxycycline, cocaine, and ophthalmic antifungal drugs — such as trifluridine, vidarabine, and idoxuridine — can also cause photophobia.

Special considerations

Promote the patient's comfort by darkening the room and telling him to close both eyes. If photophobia persists at home, suggest that he wear dark glasses. Prepare the patient for diagnostic tests, such as corneal scraping and slit-lamp examination. Discontinue offending medications as appropriate. Light sensitivity is frequently a natural defense when the eye is traumatized.

Pediatric pointers

Suspect photophobia in any child who squints, rubs his eyes frequently, or wears sunglasses indoors and outside. Congenital disorders such as albinism and childhood diseases, such as measles and rubella, can cause photophobia.

PLEURAL FRICTION RUB

Commonly resulting from pulmonary disorders or trauma, this loud, coarse, grating, creaking, or squeaking sound may be auscultated over one or both lungs during late inspiration or early expiration. It's heard best over the low axilla or the anterior, lateral, or posterior bases of the lung fields with the patient upright. Sometimes intermittent, it may resemble crackles or a pericardial friction rub. (See *Comparing auscultation findings*, pages 456 and 457.)

A pleural friction rub develops when inflammation of the visceral and parietal pleural linings causes congestion and edema. The resultant fibrinous exudate covers both pleural surfaces, displacing the fluid that's normally between them and causing the surfaces to rub together.

Emergency interventions

When you detect a pleural friction rub, quickly look for signs of respiratory distress: shallow or decreased respirations; crowing, wheezing, or stridor; dyspnea; increased accessory muscle use; intercostal or suprasternal retractions; cyanosis; and nasal flaring. Check for hypotension, tachycardia, and a decreased level of consciousness.

If you detect signs of distress, open and maintain an airway. Endotracheal intubation and supplemental oxygen may be necessary. Insert a large-gauge I.V. line to deliver drugs and fluids. Elevate the patient's head 30 degrees. Monitor cardiac status constantly, and check vital signs frequently.

History and physical examination

If the patient isn't in severe distress, explore related symptoms. Find out if he has had chest pain. If so, ask him to describe its location and severity. How long does the pain last? Does it radiate to his shoulder, neck, or upper abdomen? Does the pain worsen with breathing, movement, coughing, or sneezing? Does it abate if he splints his chest, holds his breath, or exerts pressure or lies on the affected side? A pleural friction rub is commonly accompanied by chest pain near the site where the rub is auscultated. The pain is usually sharp and worsens on inspiration.

Ask the patient about a history of rheumatoid arthritis, respiratory or cardiovascular disorders, recent trauma, asbestos exposure, or radiation therapy. If he smokes, obtain a history in pack-years.

Characterize the pleural friction rub by auscultating the lungs with the patient sitting upright and breathing deeply and slowly through his mouth. Is the rub unilateral or bilateral? Also, listen for absent or diminished breath sounds, noting their location and timing in the respiratory cycle. Do abnormal breath sounds clear with coughing? Observe for clubbing and pedal edema, which may indicate a chronic disorder. Then palpate for decreased chest motion and percuss for flatness or dullness.

Common medical causes

♦ ***Asbestosis.*** Besides a pleural friction rub, this disorder may cause dyspnea on exertion, cough, chest pain, and crackles. Clubbing is a late sign.

♦ ***Lung cancer.*** A pleural friction rub may be heard in the affected area of the lung. Other effects may include a cough (possibly with hemoptysis), dyspnea, chest pain, weight loss, anorexia, fatigue, clubbing, fever, or wheezing.

♦ ***Pleurisy.*** A pleural friction rub occurs early in this disorder. However, the cardinal symptom is sudden, intense, usually unilateral, pain in the lower and lateral parts of the chest. Deep breathing, coughing, or thoracic movement aggravates the pain. Decreased breath sounds and inspiratory crackles may be heard over the painful area. Other findings include dyspnea, tachypnea, tachycardia, cyanosis, fever, or fatigue.

♦ ***Pneumonia (bacterial).*** A pleural friction rub occurs in this disorder, which usually starts with a dry, painful, hacking cough that rapidly becomes productive. Related effects develop suddenly; these include shaking chills, high fever, headache, dyspnea, pleuritic chest pain, tachypnea, tachycardia, grunting respirations, nasal flaring, dullness to percussion, and cyanosis. Auscultation reveals decreased breath sounds and fine crackles or bronchial breath sounds and abnormal voice sounds if consolidation occurs.

♦ ***Pulmonary embolism.*** An embolism can cause a pleural friction rub over the affected area of the lung. Usually, the first symptom is sudden dyspnea that may be accompanied by anginal or unilateral pleuritic chest pain. Other clinical features include a nonproductive cough or a cough that produces blood-tinged sputum, tachycardia, tachypnea, low-grade fever, restlessness, and diaphoresis. Less-common findings include massive hemoptysis, chest splinting, leg edema and, with a large embolus, cyanosis, syncope, and jugular vein distention. Crackles, diffuse wheezing, decreased breath sounds, and signs of circulatory collapse may also occur.

♦ ***Systemic lupus erythematosus.*** Pulmonary involvement can cause a pleural friction rub, hemoptysis, dyspnea, pleuritic chest pain, and crackles. More characteristic effects include a butterfly rash, nondeforming joint pain and stiffness, and photosensitivity. Fever, anorexia, weight loss, or lymphadenopathy may also occur.

♦ ***Tuberculosis (pulmonary).*** *I*n this disorder, a pleural friction rub may occur over the affected part of the lung. Early signs and symptoms include weight loss, night sweats, low-grade fever in the afternoon, malaise, dyspnea, anorexia, and easy fatigability. Progression of the disorder usually causes pleuritic pain, fine crackles over the upper lobes, and a productive cough with blood-streaked sputum. Advanced tuberculosis can cause chest retraction, tracheal deviation, and dullness to percussion.

Other causes

♦ ***Treatments.*** Thoracic surgery and radiation therapy can cause pleural friction rubs.

Special considerations

Continue to monitor the patient's respiratory status and vital signs. If the patient's persistent dry, hacking cough tires him, administer antitussives. (Avoid giving narcotics, which can further depress respirations.) Administer oxygen and antibiotics. Prepare the patient for diagnostic tests such as chest X-rays.

Pediatric pointers

Auscultate for a pleural friction rub in a child who has grunting respirations, reports chest pain, or protects his chest by holding it or lying on one side. A pleural friction rub in a child is usually an early sign of pleurisy.

Geriatric pointers

In elderly patients, the intensity of pleuritic chest pain may mimic that of cardiac-related chest pain.

Polydipsia

Polydipsia refers to excessive thirst, a common symptom associated with endocrine disorders and certain drugs. It may reflect decreased fluid intake, increased urine output, or excessive loss of water and salt.

History and physical examination

Find out how much fluid the patient drinks each day. How often and how much does he typically urinate? Does the need to urinate awaken him at night? Determine if he or anyone in his family has diabetes or kidney disease. What medications does he use? Has his lifestyle changed recently? If so, have these changes upset him?

If the patient has polydipsia, take his blood pressure and pulse when he is in the supine and standing positions. A decrease of 10 mm Hg in systolic pressure and a pulse rate increase of 10 beats/minute from the supine to the standing position may indicate hypovolemia. If you detect these changes, ask the patient about recent weight loss. Check for signs of dehydration, such as dry mucous membranes and decreased skin turgor. Infuse I.V. replacement fluids as needed.

Common medical causes

♦ ***Diabetes insipidus.*** This disorder characteristically causes polydipsia and may also cause excessive voiding of dilute urine and mild to moderate nocturia. Fatigue and signs of dehydration occur in severe cases.

♦ ***Diabetes mellitus.*** Polydipsia is a classic finding in this disorder — a consequence of the hyperosmolar state. Other characteristic findings include polyuria, polyphagia, nocturia, weakness, fatigue, and weight loss. Signs of dehydration may occur.

♦ ***Hypercalcemia.*** As this disorder progresses, the patient develops polydipsia, polyuria, nocturia, constipation, paresthesia and, occasionally, hematuria and pyuria. Severe hypercalcemia can progress quickly to vomiting, decreased level of consciousness, and renal failure. Depression, mental lassitude, and increased sleep requirements are common.

♦ ***Hypokalemia.*** This electrolyte imbalance can cause nephropathy, resulting in polydipsia, polyuria, and nocturia. Related hypokalemic effects include muscle weakness or paralysis, fatigue, decreased bowel sounds, hypoactive deep tendon reflexes, and arrhythmias.

♦ ***Psychogenic polydipsia.*** This uncommon disorder causes polydipsia and polyuria, usually without nocturnal awakening. This condition may be associated with any psychiatric disorder but occurs more frequently in schizophrenia. Signs of psychiatric disturbances, such as anxiety or depression, are typical. Other findings may include headache, blurred vision, weight gain, edema, elevated blood pressure or, occasionally, stupor and coma. Signs of heart failure may follow overhydration.

♦ ***Renal disorders (chronic).*** Chronic renal disorders, such as glomerulonephritis or pyelonephritis, damage the kidneys, causing polydipsia and polyuria. Associated signs and symptoms may include nocturia, weakness, elevated blood pressure, pallor or, in later stages, oliguria.

♦ ***Sheehan's syndrome.*** Polydipsia, polyuria, and nocturia occur in this syndrome of postpartum pituitary necrosis. Other features include fatigue, failure to lactate, amenorrhea, decreased pubic and axillary hair growth, and reduced libido.

♦ ***Sickle cell anemia.*** As nephropathy develops, polydipsia and polyuria occur. They may be accompanied by abdominal pain and cramps, arthralgia and, occasionally, lower extremity skin ulcers or bone deformities such as kyphosis and scoliosis.

Other causes

◆ ***Drugs.*** Diuretics and demeclocycline may cause polydipsia. Phenothiazines and anticholinergics can cause dry mouth, making the patient so thirsty that he drinks compulsively.

Special considerations

Carefully monitor the patient's fluid balance by recording his total intake and output. Weigh the patient at the same time each day, in the same clothing, and using the same scale. Regularly check blood pressure and pulse in the supine and standing positions to detect orthostatic hypotension, which may indicate hypovolemia. Because thirst is usually the body's way of compensating for water loss, give the patient ample liquids.

Pediatric pointers

In children, polydipsia usually stems from diabetes insipidus or diabetes mellitus. Rare causes include pheochromocytoma, neuroblastoma, and Prader-Willi syndrome. However, some children develop habitual polydipsia that's unrelated to any disease.

POLYPHAGIA

[Hyperphagia]

Polyphagia refers to voracious or excessive eating of food. This common symptom can be persistent or intermittent, resulting primarily from endocrine and psychological disorders or from the use of certain drugs. Depending on the underlying cause, polyphagia may or may not cause weight gain.

History and physical examination

Begin your evaluation by asking the patient what he has eaten and drunk within the past 24 hours. (If he easily recalls this information, ask about the 2 previous days' intake for a broader view of his dietary habits.) Note the frequency of meals and the amount and types of food eaten. Find out if the patient's eating habits have changed recently. Has he always had a large appetite? Does his overeating alternate with periods of anorexia? Ask about conditions that may trigger overeating, such as stress, depression, or the time before menstruation. Does the patient actually feel hungry, or does he eat simply because food is available? Does he ever vomit or have a headache after overeating?

Explore related signs and symptoms. Has the patient recently gained or lost weight? Does he feel tired, nervous, or excitable? Has he experienced heat intolerance, dizziness, or palpitations? Diarrhea or increased thirst or urination? Obtain a complete drug history, including use of laxatives or enemas.

During the physical examination, weigh the patient. Tell him his current weight, and watch for expression of disbelief or anger. Inspect the skin to detect dryness or poor turgor. Palpate the thyroid for enlargement.

Common medical causes

◆ ***Anxiety.*** Polyphagia may result from mild to moderate anxiety or emotional stress. Mild anxiety typically causes restlessness, sleeplessness, irritability, repetitive questioning, and constant seeking of attention and reassurance. The patient with moderate anxiety may also have selective inattention and difficulty concentrating. Other effects of anxiety may include muscle tension, diaphoresis, GI distress, palpitations, tachycardia, or urinary or sexual dysfunction.

◆ ***Bulimia nervosa.*** Most common in women ages 18 to 29, bulimia nervosa causes polyphagia that alternates with self-induced vomiting, fasting, or diarrhea. The patient typically has normal or less than normal weight but has a morbid fear of obesity. She appears depressed, has low self-esteem, and conceals her overeating.

♦ ***Diabetes mellitus.*** In this disorder, polyphagia occurs with weight loss, polydipsia, and polyuria. It's accompanied by nocturia, weakness, fatigue, and signs of dehydration, such as dry mucous membranes and poor skin turgor.

♦ ***Premenstrual syndrome.*** Appetite changes, typified by food cravings and binges, are common in this syndrome. Abdominal bloating, the most common associated finding, may occur with behavioral changes, such as depression and insomnia. Headache, paresthesia, and other neurologic symptoms may also occur. Related findings include diarrhea or constipation, edema and temporary weight gain, palpitations, back pain, breast swelling and tenderness, oliguria, and easy bruising.

Other causes

♦ ***Drugs.*** Corticosteroids, tricyclic antidepressants, and cyproheptadine may increase appetite, causing weight gain.

Special considerations

Offer the patient with polyphagia emotional support, and help him understand its underlying cause. As needed, refer the patient and his family for psychological counseling.

Pediatric pointers

In children, polyphagia commonly results from juvenile diabetes. In infants 6 to 18 months of age, it may signal a malabsorptive disorder, such as celiac disease. However, polyphagia may occur normally in a child who is experiencing a sudden growth spurt.

Polyuria

A relatively common sign, polyuria is the daily production and excretion of more than 3,000 ml of urine. It's usually reported by the patient as increased urination, especially when it occurs at night. Polyuria is aggravated by overhydration, consumption of caffeine or alcohol, and excessive ingestion of salt, glucose, or other hyperosmolar substances.

Polyuria most commonly results from the use of certain drugs, such as diuretics, and from psychological, neurologic, and renal disorders. It can reflect central nervous system dysfunction that diminishes or suppresses secretion of antidiuretic hormone (ADH), which regulates fluid balance. Or, when ADH levels are normal, it can reflect renal impairment. In both of these pathophysiologic mechanisms, the renal tubules fail to reabsorb sufficient water.

History and physical examination

Because the patient with polyuria is at risk for developing hypovolemia, evaluate fluid status first. Take vital signs, noting especially increased body temperature, tachycardia, and orthostatic hypotension. Inspect for dry skin and mucous membranes, decreased skin turgor and elasticity, and reduced perspiration. Is the patient unusually tired or thirsty? Has he recently lost more than 5% of his body weight? If you detect these effects of hypovolemia, you'll need to infuse replacement fluids.

If the patient doesn't display signs of hypovolemia, explore the frequency and pattern of the polyuria. When did it begin? How long has it lasted? Was it precipitated by a certain event? Ask the patient to describe the pattern and amount of his daily fluid intake. Check for a history of visual deficits, headaches, or head trauma, which may precede diabetes insipidus. Also check for a history of urinary tract obstruction, diabetes mellitus, renal disorders, chronic hypokalemia or hypercalcemia, and psychiatric disorders (both past and present). Find out the schedule and dosage of any drugs the patient is currently taking.

Polyuria: Common causes and associated findings

CAUSES	MAJOR ASSOCIATED SIGNS AND SYMPTOMS									
	Anorexia	Blood pressure increase	Dyspnea	Edema	Fatigue	Headache	Hematuria	Level of consciousness, altered	Mucous membrane dryness	Nocturia
Acute tubular necrosis				♦						♦
Diabetes insipidus					♦				♦	♦
Diabetes mellitus					♦				♦	♦
Glomerulonephritis (chronic)	♦	♦	♦	♦	♦	♦	♦			♦
Postobstructive uropathy				♦					♦	♦
Psychogenic polydipsia		♦		♦		♦		♦		

Perform a neurologic examination, noting especially a change in the patient's level of consciousness. Then palpate the bladder and inspect the urethral meatus. Obtain a urine specimen and check its specific gravity. (See *Polyuria: Common causes and associated findings*.)

Common medical causes

♦ ***Acute tubular necrosis.*** During the diuretic phase of this disorder, polyuria of less than 8 L/day gradually subsides after 8 to 10 days. Urine specific gravity (1.010 or less) increases as polyuria subsides. Related findings include weight loss, decreasing edema, and nocturia.

♦ ***Diabetes insipidus.*** Polyuria of about 5 L/day with a specific gravity of 1.005 or less is common, although extreme polyuria — up to 30 L/day — occasionally occurs. Polyuria is commonly accompanied by polydipsia, nocturia, fatigue, and signs of dehydration, such as poor skin turgor and dry mucous membranes.

♦ ***Diabetes mellitus.*** In this disorder, polyuria seldom exceeds 5 L/day, and urine specific gravity typically exceeds 1.020. The patient usually reports polydipsia, polyphagia, weight loss, weakness, frequent urinary tract infections and yeast vaginitis, fatigue, and nocturia. The patient may also display signs of dehydration.

♦ ***Glomerulonephritis (chronic).*** Polyuria gradually progresses to oliguria in this disorder. Urine output is usually less than 4 L/day; specific gravity is about 1.010. Related GI effects include anorexia, nausea, and vomiting. The patient may experience drowsiness, fatigue, edema, headache, elevated blood pressure, and

	Personality changes	Polydipsia	Polyphagia	Vomiting	Weakness	Weight gain	Weight loss
							◆
		◆					
		◆	◆		◆		◆
				◆			
							◆
	◆	◆				◆	

dyspnea. Nocturia, hematuria, frothy or malodorous urine, and mild to severe proteinuria may occur.

◆ ***Postobstructive uropathy.*** After resolution of a urinary tract obstruction, polyuria—usually more than 5 L/day with a specific gravity of less than 1.010—occurs for several days before gradually subsiding. Bladder distention and edema may occur with nocturia and weight loss. Occasionally, signs of dehydration appear.

◆ ***Psychogenic polydipsia.*** Most common in women over age 30, this disorder usually causes dilute polyuria of 3 to 15 L/day, depending on fluid intake. The patient may appear depressed and have a headache and blurred vision. She may develop weight gain, edema, elevated blood pressure and, occasionally, stupor or coma. In severe overhydration, she may display signs of heart failure.

Other causes

◆ ***Diagnostic tests.*** Transient polyuria can result from radiographic tests that use contrast media.

◆ ***Drugs.*** Diuretics characteristically cause polyuria. Cardiotonic drugs, vitamin D, demeclocycline, phenytoin, lithium, methoxyflurane, and propoxyphene can also cause polyuria.

Special considerations

Maintaining an adequate fluid balance is your primary concern when the patient has polyuria. Record intake and output accurately, and weigh him daily. Closely monitor the patient's vital signs to detect fluid imbalance, and encourage him to drink adequate fluids. Review his medications, and recommend modification where possible to help control symptoms.

Prepare the patient for serum electrolyte, osmolality, blood urea nitrogen, and creatinine studies to monitor fluid and electrolyte status and for a fluid deprivation test to determine the cause of polyuria.

Pediatric pointers

The major causes of polyuria in children are congenital nephrogenic diabetes insipidus, medullary cystic disease, polycystic renal disease, and distal renal tubular acidosis.

Because a child's fluid balance is more delicate than an adult's, check his urine specific gravity at each voiding, and be alert for signs of dehydration. These include a decrease in body weight; decreased skin turgor; pale, mottled, or gray skin; dry mucous membranes; decreased urine output; and absence of tears when crying.

PRIAPISM

A urologic emergency, priapism is a persistent, painful erection that's unrelated to sexual excitation. This relatively rare sign may begin during sleep and appear to be a normal erection but it may last for several hours or days. It's usually accompanied by a severe, constant, dull aching in the penis. Despite the pain, the patient may be too embarrassed to seek medical help and may try to achieve detumescence through continued sexual activity.

Priapism occurs when the veins of the corpora cavernosa fail to drain correctly, resulting in persistent engorgement of the tissues. Without prompt treatment, penile ischemia and thrombosis occur. In about half of all cases, priapism is idiopathic and develops without apparent predisposing factors. Secondary priapism results from blood disorders, neoplasms, trauma, and the use of certain drugs.

Emergency interventions

If the patient has priapism, apply an ice pack to the penis, administer analgesics, and insert an indwelling urinary catheter to relieve urine retention. Procedures to remove blood from the corpora cavernosa, such as irrigation and surgery, may be required.

History and physical examination

When the patient's condition permits, ask him when the priapism began. Is it continuous or intermittent? Has he had a prolonged erection before? If so, what did he do to relieve it? How long did he remain detumescent? Does he have pain or tenderness when he urinates? Has he noticed changes in sexual function?

Explore the patient's medical history. If he reports sickle cell anemia, find out about factors that could precipitate a crisis, such as dehydration and infection. Ask if he has recently suffered genital trauma, and obtain a thorough drug history.

Examine the patient's penis, noting its color and temperature. Check for loss of sensation, and look for signs of infection, such as redness or drainage. Finally, take his vital signs, particularly noting fever.

Common medical causes

♦ ***Cerebrovascular accident (CVA).*** A CVA may cause priapism but sensory loss and aphasia may prevent the patient from noticing or describing it. Other findings depend on the CVA's location and extent but may include contralateral hemiplegia, seizures, headache, dysarthria, dysphagia, ataxia, apraxia, and agnosia. Visual deficits include homonymous hemianopia, blurring, decreased acuity, and diplopia. Urine retention or incontinence, fecal incontinence, constipation, and vomiting may also occur.

♦ ***Penile cancer.*** Cancer that exerts pressure on the corpora cavernosa can cause priapism. Usually, the first sign is a painless ulcerative lesion or an enlarging warty growth on the glans or foreskin; accompanying signs include localized pain, a foul-smelling discharge from the prepuce, a firm lump near the glans, and lymphadenopathy. Later findings may include bleeding, dysuria, urine retention, or bladder distention. Phimosis and poor hygiene have been linked to the development of penile cancer.

♦ ***Sickle cell anemia.*** In this congenital disorder, painful priapism can occur without warning, usually on awakening. The patient may have a history of priapism, impaired growth and development, and increased susceptibility to infection. Related findings include tachycardia, pallor, weakness, hepatomegaly, dyspnea, joint swelling, joint or bone aching, chest pain, fatigue, murmurs, leg ulcers and, possibly, jaundice and gross hematuria.

In sickle cell crisis, signs and symptoms of sickle cell anemia may worsen and other symptoms, such as abdominal pain and low-grade fever, may appear.

◆ ***Spinal cord injury.*** In this condition, the patient may be unaware of the onset of priapism. Related effects depend on the extent and level of the injury and may include autonomic signs such as bradycardia.

Other causes

◆ ***Drugs.*** Priapism can result from the use of phenothiazines, thioridazine, trazodone, androgenic steroids, anticoagulants, or some antihypertensives. It may also occur after an intracorporeal injection of papaverine, a common treatment for impotence.

Special considerations

Prepare the patient for blood tests to help determine the cause of priapism. If he requires surgery, keep his penis flaccid postoperatively by applying a pressure dressing. At least once every 30 minutes, inspect the glans for signs of vascular compromise, such as coolness or pallor.

Pediatric pointers

In neonates, priapism can result from hypoxia but is usually resolved with oxygen therapy. Priapism is more likely to develop in children with sickle cell disease than in adults with the disease.

PRURITUS

Commonly provoking scratching in an attempt to gain relief, this unpleasant itching sensation affects the skin, certain mucous membranes, and the eyes. Most severe at night, pruritus may be exacerbated by increased skin temperature, poor skin turgor, local vasodilation, dermatoses, and stress.

The most common symptom of dermatologic disorders, pruritus may also result from local or systemic disorders or from drug use. Physiologic pruritus, such as pruritic urticarial papules and plaques of pregnancy, may occur in primigravidas late in the third trimester. Pruritus can also stem from emotional upset or contact with skin irritants.

History and physical examination

If the patient reports pruritus, have him describe its onset, frequency, and intensity. If pruritus occurs at night, ask him whether it prevents him from falling asleep or awakens him after he falls asleep. (Generally, pruritus related to dermatoses prevents—but doesn't disturb—sleep.) Is the itching localized or generalized? When is it most severe? How long does it last? Is there a relationship to activities (physical exertion, bathing, applying makeup, or use of perfumes)?

Ask the patient how he cleans his skin. In particular, look for excessive bathing, harsh soaps, contact allergy, and excessively hot water. Does he have occupational exposure to known skin irritants such as glass fiber insulation or chemicals? Ask about the patient's general health and what medications he takes (new medications are suspect). Has he recently traveled abroad? Does he have pets? Does anyone else in the house report itching? Does exercise, stress, fear, depression, or illness seem to aggravate the itching? Ask about contact with skin irritants, previous skin disorders, and related symptoms. Then obtain a complete drug history.

Examine the patient for signs of scratching, such as excoriation, purpura, scabs, scars, or lichenification. Look for primary lesions to help confirm dermatoses.

Common medical causes

◆ ***Anemia (iron deficiency).*** This disorder occasionally causes pruritus. Initially asymptomatic, anemia can later cause dyspnea on exertion, fatigue, listlessness, pallor, irritability, headache, tachycardia, poor muscle tone and, possibly, murmurs. Chronic anemia causes spoon-shaped and brittle nails, cracked mouth corners, a smooth tongue, and dysphagia.

♦ ***Conjunctivitis.*** All forms of conjunctivitis cause eye itching, burning, and pain along with photophobia, conjunctival injection, a foreign-body sensation, excessive tearing, and a feeling of fullness around the eye. *Allergic conjunctivitis* may also cause milky redness and a stringy eye discharge. *Bacterial conjunctivitis* typically causes brilliant redness and a mucopurulent, flaky discharge that may make the eyelids stick together. *Fungal conjunctivitis* causes a thick, purulent discharge and crusting and sticking of the eyelid. *Viral conjunctivitis* may cause copious tearing — but little discharge — and preauricular lymph node enlargement.

♦ ***Dermatitis.*** Several types of dermatitis can cause pruritus accompanied by a skin lesion. *Atopic dermatitis* begins with intense, severe pruritus and an erythematous rash on dry skin at flexion points (antecubital fossa, popliteal area, and neck). During a flare-up, scratching may cause edema, scaling, or pustules. In chronic atopic dermatitis, lesions may progress to dry, scaly skin with white dermatographia, blanching, and lichenification.

Mild irritants and allergies can cause *contact dermatitis*, with itchy small vesicles that may ooze and scale and are surrounded by redness. A severe reaction can cause marked localized edema.

Dermatitis herpetiformis, most common in men between ages 20 and 50, initially causes intense pruritus and stinging. Eight to 12 hours later, symmetrically distributed lesions form on the buttocks, shoulders, elbows, and knees. Sometimes, they also form on the neck, face, and scalp. These lesions are erythematous and papular, bullous, or pustular.

♦ ***Hepatobiliary disease.*** An important diagnostic clue to liver and gallbladder disease, pruritus is commonly accompanied by jaundice and may be generalized or localized to the palms and soles. Other characteristics may include right-upper-quadrant pain, clay-colored stools, chills and fever, flatus, belching and a bloated feeling, epigastric burning, or bitter fluid regurgitation. Later, liver disease may cause mental changes, ascites, bleeding tendencies, spider angiomas, palmar erythema, dry skin, fetor hepaticus, enlarged superficial abdominal veins, bilateral gynecomastia, testicular atrophy or menstrual irregularities, or hepatomegaly.

♦ ***Herpes zoster.*** Within 2 to 4 days of fever and malaise, pruritus, paresthesia or hyperesthesia, and severe, deep pain from cutaneous nerve involvement develop on the trunk or the arms and legs in a dermatome distribution. Up to 2 weeks after initial symptoms, red, nodular skin eruptions appear on the painful areas and become vesicular. About 10 days later, the vesicles rupture and form scabs.

♦ ***Leukemia (chronic lymphocytic).*** Pruritus is an uncommon finding in this disorder. More characteristic effects include fatigue, malaise, generalized lymphadenopathy, fever, hepatomegaly, splenomegaly, weight loss, pallor, bleeding, and palpitations.

♦ ***Lichen simplex chronicus.*** Persistent rubbing and scratching cause localized pruritus and a circumscribed scaling patch with sharp margins. Later, the skin thickens and papules form.

♦ ***Myringitis (chronic).*** This disorder causes pruritus, a purulent discharge, and gradual hearing loss in the affected ear.

♦ ***Pediculosis (lice).*** A prominent symptom, pruritus occurs in the area of infestation. *Pediculosis capitis* (head lice) may also cause scalp excoriation from scratching; matted, foul-smelling, lusterless hair; or occipital or cervical lymphadenopathy; oval, gray-white nits may be visible on hair shafts.

Pediculosis corporis (body lice) initially causes small red papules (usually on the shoulders, trunk, or buttocks), which become urticarial from scratching. Later, rashes or wheals may develop. Untreated, pediculosis corporis causes dry, discolored, thickly encrusted, scaly skin with bacterial infection and scarring. In severe cases, it causes headache, fever, and malaise.

In the patient with *pediculosis pubis* (pubic lice), scratching commonly causes skin irritation. Nits or adult lice and erythematous, itching papules may appear in pubic hair or hair around the anus, abdomen, or thighs.

◆ ***Pityriasis rosea.*** This disorder typically causes mild to severe pruritus that's aggravated by a hot bath or shower. It usually begins with an erythematous herald patch — a slightly raised, oval lesion about 2 to 6 cm in diameter. After a few days or weeks, scaly yellow-tan or erythematous patches erupt on the trunk and extremities and persist for 2 to 6 weeks. Occasionally, these patches are macular, vesicular, or urticarial.

◆ ***Psoriasis.*** Pruritus and pain are common in psoriasis. This skin disorder typically begins with small erythematous papules that enlarge or coalesce to form red elevated plaques with silver scales on the scalp, chest, elbows, knees, back buttocks, or genitals. Nail pitting may occur.

◆ ***Scabies.*** Typically, scabies causes localized pruritus that awakens the patient. It may become generalized and persist up to 2 weeks after treatment. Threadlike lesions several millimeters long are associated with a swollen nodule or red papule. In males, nodular lesions may form on the glans penis, penile shaft, or scrotum. In females, lesions may form on the wrists, elbows, axillae, waistline, or nipples. Excoriation from scratching is common.

◆ ***Tinea pedis.*** This fungal infection causes severe foot pruritus, pain with walking, scales and blisters between the toes, or a dry, scaly squamous inflammation on the entire sole.

◆ ***Urticaria.*** Extreme pruritus and stinging occur as transient erythematous or whitish wheals form on the skin or mucous membranes. Prickly sensations typically precede the wheals, which may affect any part of the body and may range from pinpoint to palm-sized or larger.

◆ ***Vaginitis.*** This disorder frequently causes localized pruritus and a foul-smelling vaginal discharge that may be purulent, white or gray, and curdlike. Perineal pain and urinary dysfunction may also occur.

Other causes

◆ ***Bedbug bites.*** Typically, bedbug bites cause itching and burning and clusters of purpuric spots over the ankles and lower legs.

◆ ***Drug hypersensitivity.*** When mild and localized, an allergic reaction to such drugs as penicillin and sulfonamides can cause pruritus, erythema, an urticarial rash, and edema. However, in a severe drug reaction, anaphylaxis may occur.

◆ **Herb alert** Ingesting pulp from the fruit of the Ginkgo tree can cause rapid formation of vesicles and severe itching.

Special considerations

Administer topical corticosteroids, antihistamines, or tranquilizers, as ordered. If the patient doesn't have a localized infection or skin lesions, suspect a systemic disease and prepare him for a complete blood count and differential, erythrocyte sedimentation rate, protein electrophoresis, and radiologic studies.

Pediatric pointers
Many adult disorders also cause pruritus in children but they may affect different parts of the body. For instance, scabies may affect the head in infants but not in adults. Pityriasis rosea may affect the face, hands, and feet of adolescents.

Some childhood diseases, such as measles or chicken pox, can cause pruritus. Hepatic diseases can also cause pruritus in children as bile salts accumulate on the skin.

PSOAS SIGN

A positive psoas sign — increased abdominal pain when the patient moves his leg against resistance — indicates direct or reflexive irritation of the psoas muscles. This sign, which can be elicited on the right or left side, usually suggests appendicitis but may also signal localized abscesses. It's elicited in a patient with abdominal or lower back pain *after* completion of an abdominal examination to prevent spurious assessment findings. (See *Eliciting a psoas sign*.)

Emergency interventions
If you elicit a positive psoas sign in a patient with abdominal pain, suspect appendicitis. Quickly check the patient's vital signs, and prepare him for surgery: Explain the procedure, restrict food and fluids, and withhold analgesics, which can mask symptoms. Administer I.V. fluids to prevent dehydration but *don't* give cathartics or enemas, which can cause a ruptured appendix and lead to peritonitis.

Check for Rovsing's sign by deeply palpating the patient's *left* lower quadrant. The sign is positive if he reports pain in the *right* lower quadrant, indicating peritoneal irritation.

Common medical causes
♦ ***Appendicitis.*** An inflamed retrocecal appendix can cause a positive right psoas sign. Early epigastric and periumbilical pain disappears only to worsen and localize in the right lower quadrant. This pain also worsens with walking or coughing. Related findings include nausea and vomiting, abdominal rigidity and rebound tenderness, and constipation or diarrhea. Fever, tachycardia, retractive respirations, anorexia, or malaise may also occur. If the appendix ruptures, additional findings may include sudden, severe pain followed by signs of peritonitis, such as hypoactive or absent bowel sounds, high fever, or boardlike abdominal rigidity. A positive obturator sign may also be evident.

♦ ***Retroperitoneal abscess.*** After a lower retroperitoneal infection, an iliac or lumbar abscess can cause a positive right or left psoas sign and fever. An *iliac abscess* causes iliac or inguinal pain that may radiate to the hip, thigh, flank, or knee; a tender mass in the lower abdomen or groin may be palpable. A *lumbar abscess* usually causes back tenderness and spasms on the affected side with a palpable lumbar mass; a tender abdominal mass without back pain may occur.

Special considerations
Monitor vital signs to detect complications, such as pain extension along fascial planes in the abdomen, thigh, hip, subphrenic spaces, mediastinum, and pleural cavities, and peritonitis. Promote patient comfort by helping with position changes. For example, have the patient lie down and flex his right leg and then sit upright.

Prepare the patient for diagnostic tests, such as electrolyte studies and abdominal X-rays.

Pediatric pointers
Elicit a psoas sign by asking the child to raise his head while you exert pressure

EXAMINATION TIP

Eliciting a psoas sign

You can use two techniques to elicit a psoas sign in an adult with abdominal pain. With either technique, increased abdominal pain is a positive result, indicting psoas muscle irritation from an inflamed appendix or a localized abscess.

With the patient supine, instruct her to move her flexed left leg against your hand to test for a left psoas sign. Then, perform this maneuver on the right leg to test for a right psoas sign.

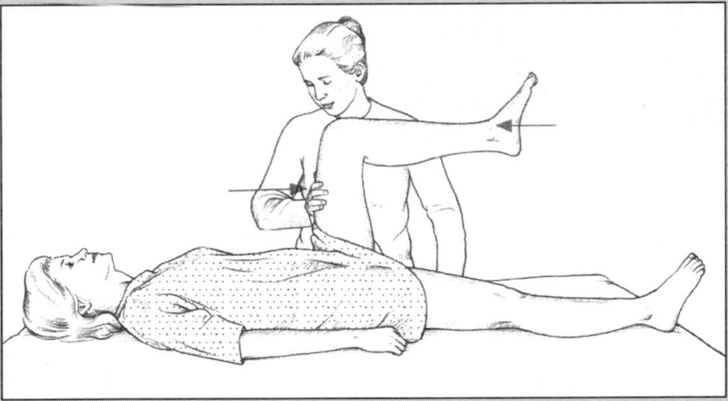

Turn the patient on her right side, then instruct her to push her left leg upward from the hip against your hand to test for a left psoas sign. Next, turn the patient onto her left side, and repeat this maneuver to test for a right psoas sign.

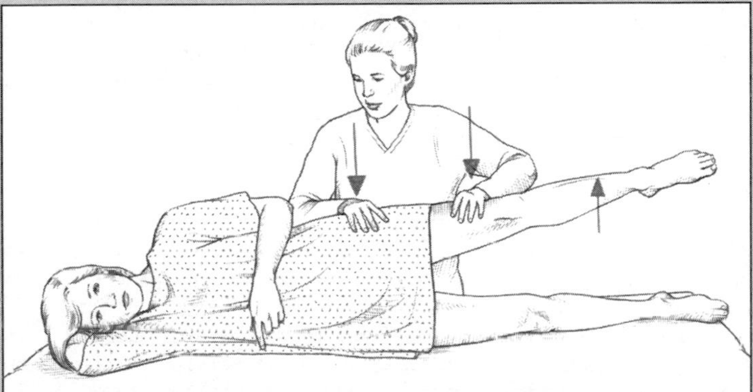

on his forehead. Resulting right-lower-quadrant pain usually indicates appendicitis.

Geriatric pointers

In elderly patients, the psoas sign and other peritoneal signs may be decreased or absent. Be sure to differentiate pain elicited through psoas maneuvers from musculoskeletal or degenerative joint pain.

PSYCHOTIC BEHAVIOR

Psychotic behavior reflects an inability or unwillingness to recognize and acknowledge reality and to relate with others. It may begin suddenly or insidiously, progressing from vague complaints of fatigue, insomnia, or headache to withdrawal, social isolation, and preoccupation with certain issues.

Various behaviors together or separately can constitute psychotic behavior. These include delusions, illusions, hallucinations, bizarre language, and perseveration. *Delusions* are persistent beliefs that have no basis in reality or in the patient's knowledge or experience such as delusions of grandeur. *Illusions* are misinterpretations of external sensory stimuli such as a mirage in the desert. In contrast, *hallucinations* are sensory perceptions that don't result from external stimuli. *Bizarre language* reflects a communication disruption. It can range from echolalia (purposeless repetition of a word or phrase) and clang association (repetition of words or phrases that sound similar) to neologisms (creation and use of words whose meaning only the patient knows). *Perseveration,* a persistent verbal or motor response, may reflect organic brain disease. Motor changes include inactivity, excessive activity, and repetitive movements.

History and physical examination

Because the patient's behavior can make it difficult—or potentially dangerous—to obtain pertinent information, conduct the interview in a calm, safe, and well-lit room. Provide enough personal space to avoid threatening or agitating the patient. Ask him to describe his problem and any circumstances that may have precipitated it. Obtain a drug history, focusing on antipsychotics, and explore his use of alcohol, noting duration of use and amount. (See *Drugs that can cause psychotic behavior.*) Ask about recent illnesses or accidents.

As the patient talks, watch for cognitive, linguistic, or perceptual abnormalities such as delusions. Do thoughts and actions seem to match? Look for unusual gestures, posture, gait, tone of voice, and mannerisms. Does the patient appear to be responding to external stimuli? For example, is he looking around the room?

Interview the patient's family. Which family members does he seem closest to? How does the family describe the patient's relationships, communication patterns, and role? Has a family member ever been hospitalized for psychiatric or emotional illness? Ask about the patient's compliance with his medication regimen.

Finally, evaluate the patient's environment, educational and employment history, and socioeconomic status. Are community services available? How does the patient spend his leisure time? Does he have friends? Has he ever had a close emotional relationship?

When performing the physical examination, explain each step to the patient in short, simple sentences. Always ask before touching the patient.

Common medical causes

◆ ***Neurochemical imbalances.*** Psychotic behavior may result from a lack of dopamine, a neurotransmitter in the brain. Antipsychotic drugs block the postsynaptic dopamine receptors, thus making dopamine more available in the synapse.

Drugs that can cause psychotic behavior

Certain drugs can cause psychotic behavior and other psychiatric signs and symptoms, ranging from depression to violent behavior. Usually, these effects occur during therapy and resolve when the drug is discontinued. If your patient is receiving one of these common drugs and exhibits the behavior described below, the dosage may have to be changed or another drug may have to be substituted.

DRUG	PSYCHIATRIC SIGNS AND SYMPTOMS
albuterol	Hallucination, paranoia
alprazolam	Anger, hostility
amantadine	Visual hallucinations, nightmares
asparaginase	Confusion, depression, paranoia
atropine and anticholinergics	Auditory, visual, and tactile hallucinations; memory loss; delirium; fear; paranoia
bromocriptine	Mania, delusions, sudden relapse of schizophrenia, paranoia, aggressive behavior
cardiac glycosides	Paranoia, euphoria, amnesia, visual hallucinations
cimetidine	Hallucinations, paranoia, confusion, depression, delirium
clonidine	Delirium, hallucinations, depression
corticosteroids (prednisone, corticotropin, cortisone)	Mania, catatonia, depressions, confusions, paranoia, hallucinations
cycloserine	Anxiety, depressions, confusions, paranoia, hallucinations
dapsone	Insomnia, agitation, hallucinations
diazepam	Suicidal thoughts, rage, hallucinations, depression
disopyramide	Agitation, paranoia, auditory and visual hallucinations, panic
disulfiram	Delirium, auditory hallucinations, paranoia, depression
indomethacin	Hostility, depression, paranoia, hallucinations
lidocaine	Disorientation, hallucinations, paranoia
methyldopa	Severe depression, amnesia, paranoia, hallucinations
methysergide	Depersonalization, hallucinations

(continued)

Drugs that can cause psychotic behavior *(continued)*

DRUG	PSYCHIATRIC SIGNS AND SYMPTOMS
propranolol	Severe depression, hallucinations, paranoia, confusion
thyroid hormones	Mania, hallucinations, paranoia
vincristine	Hallucinations

♦ ***Organic disorders.*** Alcohol withdrawal syndrome, cerebral hypoxia, and nutritional disorders can cause psychotic behavior. Other causes include endocrine disorders such as adrenal dysfunction, severe infections such as encephalitis, and neurologic causes, such as Alzheimer's disease or other dementias.

♦ ***Psychiatric disorders.*** Psychotic behavior usually occurs in bipolar disorder, personality disorders, schizophrenia, or posttraumatic stress disorder.

Other causes

♦ ***Drugs.*** Certain drugs can cause psychotic behavior. However, almost any drug can provoke psychotic behavior as a rare, severe adverse or idiosyncratic reaction.

♦ ***Surgery.*** Postoperative delirium and depression may cause psychotic behavior.

Special considerations

Continuously evaluate the patient's orientation to reality. Help him develop a conception of reality by calling him by his preferred name, telling him your name, describing where he is, and using clocks and calendars.

Encourage the patient to become involved in structured activities. However, if he's nonverbal or incoherent, be sure to spend time with him. For example, sit or walk with him, or talk about the day, the season, the weather, or other concrete topics. Avoid making time commitments that you can't keep: This will only upset the patient and may make him withdraw further.

Refer the patient for psychiatric evaluation. Administer antipsychotics or other drugs, as needed, and prepare him for transfer to a mental health center, if necessary.

Don't overlook the patient's physiologic needs. Check his eating habits to avoid dehydration and malnutrition, and monitor his elimination patterns, especially if he's receiving psychotropic drugs, which can cause constipation.

Pediatric pointers

In children, psychotic behavior may result from early infantile autism, symbiotic infantile psychosis, and childhood schizophrenia — all of which can retard development of language, abstract thinking, and socialization. An adolescent patient who exhibits psychotic behavior may have a history of several days' drug use or lack of sleep or food, which must be corrected before therapy can begin.

Geriatric pointers

Psychotic behavior in elderly people may result from cognitive changes caused by aging. Increased susceptibility to adverse effects of drug therapy makes psychotic symptoms a significant concern in this age group.

PTOSIS
[Blepharoptosis]

Ptosis is the excessive drooping of one or both upper eyelids. It may affect children and adults. This sign can be constant, progressive, or intermittent and unilateral or bilateral. When it's unilateral, it's easy to detect by comparing the eyelids' relative positions. Bilateral or mild ptosis is difficult to detect — the eyelids may be abnormally low, covering the upper part of the iris or even part of the pupil instead of overlapping the iris slightly. Other clues include a furrowed forehead or a tipped-back head — both of which help the patient see under his drooping lids. The patient with severe ptosis may not be able to raise his eyelids voluntarily. Because ptosis can resemble enophthalmos, exophthalmometry may be required.

Classification is important for proper treatment. *Congenital ptosis* results from levator muscle underdevelopment or disorders of the third cranial (oculomotor) nerve. *Acquired ptosis* may result from trauma to or inflammation of these muscles and nerves or from certain drugs, systemic diseases, intracranial lesions, or life-threatening aneurysms. However, the most common cause is advanced age, which reduces muscle elasticity and causes senile ptosis. *Mechanical* ptosis occurs when the mass of a neoplasm or the tethering effect of scar formation prevents the upper lid from opening completely. *Apparent* ptosis occurs when hypotropia gives the appearance of ptosis when the eye looks down beyond the lower lid. Occlusion of the other eye, however, reveals the true condition.

History and physical examination

Ask the patient when he first noticed his drooping eyelid and whether it has worsened or improved. Find out if he has suffered a traumatic eye injury recently. (If he has, avoid manipulating the eye to prevent further damage.) Ask about eye pain or headache, and determine its location and severity. Has the patient experienced vision changes? If so, have him describe them. Obtain a drug history, noting especially chemotherapeutic agents. Ask the patient if he has to tilt his head back to see under the lid or raise his eyebrows repeatedly to try to lift the lids.

Assess the degree of ptosis, and check for eyelid edema, exophthalmos, deviation, and conjunctival injection. Evaluate extraocular muscle function by testing the six cardinal fields of gaze. Carefully examine the pupils' size, color, shape, and reaction to light, and test visual acuity.

Keep in mind that ptosis occasionally indicates a life-threatening condition. For example, sudden unilateral ptosis can herald a cerebral aneurysm. (See *Recognizing unilateral ptosis*, page 480.)

Common medical causes

♦ ***Botulism.*** Acute cranial nerve dysfunction causes hallmark signs of ptosis, dysarthria, dysphagia, and diplopia. Other findings include dry mouth, sore throat, weakness, vomiting, diarrhea, hyporeflexia, and dyspnea.

♦ ***Cerebral aneurysm.*** An aneurysm that compresses the third cranial, or oculomotor, nerve (CN III) can cause sudden ptosis, diplopia, a dilated pupil, and inability to rotate the eye. These may be the first signs of this life-threatening disorder. A ruptured aneurysm typically causes sudden severe headache, nausea, vomiting, and decreased level of consciousness (LOC). Other findings may include nuchal rigidity, back and leg pain, fever, restlessness, irritability, occasional seizures, blurred vision, hemiparesis, sensory deficits, dysphagia, and visual defects.

♦ ***Lacrimal gland tumor.*** This disorder frequently causes mild to severe ptosis, depending on the tumor's size and location. It may also cause brow elevation,

EXAMINATION TIP

Recognizing unilateral ptosis

Unilateral ptosis is easy to detect because you can compare the relative positions of both eyelids. In this illustration, the patient's left eyelid is clearly drooping.

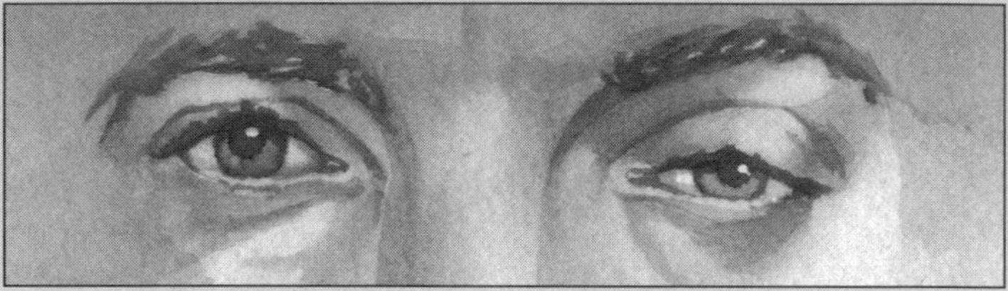

exophthalmos, eye deviation, and eye pain.

♦ ***Myasthenia gravis.*** Commonly the first sign of this disorder, gradual bilateral ptosis may be mild to severe and is accompanied by weak eye closure and diplopia. Other characteristics include muscle weakness and fatigue, which eventually may lead to paralysis. Depending on the muscles affected, other findings may include masklike facies, difficulty chewing or swallowing, dyspnea, or cyanosis.

♦ ***Ocular muscle dystrophy.*** In this disorder, bilateral ptosis progresses slowly to complete eyelid closure. Related signs and symptoms include progressive external ophthalmoplegia and weakness and atrophy of the upper face, neck, trunk, and limb muscles.

♦ ***Ocular trauma.*** Trauma to the nerve or muscles that control the eyelids can cause mild to severe ptosis. Depending on the damage, eye pain, lid swelling, ecchymosis, and decreased visual acuity may also occur.

♦ ***Parry-Romberg syndrome.*** Unilateral ptosis and facial hemiatrophy characterize this disorder. Other signs may include miosis, sluggish pupil reaction to light, enophthalmos, different-colored irises, ocular muscle paralysis, nystagmus, and neck, shoulder, trunk, and extremity atrophy.

Other causes

♦ ***Drugs.*** Vinca alkaloids can cause ptosis.

♦ ***Lead poisoning.*** In this disorder, ptosis usually develops over 3 to 6 months. Other effects include anorexia, nausea, vomiting, diarrhea, colicky abdominal pain, a lead line in the gums, decreased LOC, tachycardia, hypotension and, possibly, irritability and peripheral nerve weakness.

Special considerations

If the patient has decreased visual acuity, orient him to his surroundings. Provide special spectacle frames that suspend the eyelid by traction with a wire crutch. These frames are usually used to help patients with temporary paresis or those who aren't good candidates for surgery.

Prepare the patient for diagnostic studies, such as the Tensilon test and slit-lamp examination. If he needs surgery to correct levator muscle dysfunction, explain the procedure to him.

Pediatric pointers

Astigmatism and myopia may be associated with childhood ptosis. Parents typically discover congenital ptosis when their child is an infant. Usually, the ptosis is unilateral, constant, and accompanied by lagophthalmos, which causes the infant to sleep with his eyes open. If this occurs, teach proper eye care to prevent drying.

EXAMINATION TIP

> **Evaluating peripheral pulses**
>
> The rate, amplitude, and symmetry of peripheral pulses provide important clues to cardiac function and the quality of peripheral perfusion. To gather these clues, palpate peripheral pulses lightly with the pads of your index, middle, and ring fingers, as space permits.
>
> **RATE**
>
> Count all pulses for at least 30 seconds (60 seconds when recording vital signs). The normal rate is between 60 and 100 beats/minute.
>
> **AMPLITUDE**
>
> Palpate the blood vessel during ventricular systole. Describe pulse amplitude by using a scale such as the one below:
>
> 4+ = bounding
> 3+ = normal
> 2+ = difficult to palpate
> 1+ = weak, thready
> 0 = absent
>
> Use a stick figure to easily document the location and amplitude of all pulses.
>
> **SYMMETRY**
>
> Simultaneously palpate pulses (except the carotid pulse) on both sides of the patient's body, and note any inequality. Always assess peripheral pulses methodically, proceeding from the arms to the legs.

PULSE, ABSENT OR WEAK

An absent or weak pulse may be generalized or affect only one extremity. When generalized, this sign is an important indicator of such life-threatening conditions as shock and arrhythmia. Localized loss or weakness of a pulse that's normally strong may indicate acute arterial occlusion, which could require emergency surgery. However, the pressure of palpation may temporarily diminish or obliterate superficial pulses, such as the posterior tibial or the dorsal pedal. Thus, bilateral weakness or absence of these pulses doesn't necessarily indicate underlying pathology. (See *Evaluating peripheral pulses.*)

History and physical examination

If you detect an absent or weak pulse, quickly palpate the remaining arterial pulses to distinguish between localized or generalized loss or weakness. Then quickly check other vital signs, evaluate cardiopulmonary status, and obtain a brief history. Based on your findings, proceed with emergency interventions. (See *Managing an absent or weak pulse*, pages 482 and 483.)

Common medical causes

♦ ***Aortic aneurysm (dissecting).*** When a dissecting aneurysm affects circulation to the innominate, left common carotid, subclavian, or femoral artery, it causes weak or absent arterial pulses distal to the affected area. Absent or diminished pulses occur in 50% of patients with proximal dissection and most commonly involve the brachiocephalic vessels. Pulse deficits are much less common in patients with distal dissection and tend to involve the left subclavian and femoral arteries. Tearing pain usually develops

(Text continues on page 484.)

EMERGENCY INTERVENTIONS

Managing an absent or weak pulse

An absent or weak pulse can result from several life-threatening disorders. Your evaluation and interventions will vary, depending on whether the weak or absent pulse is generalized or localized to one extremity. They'll also depend on associated signs and symptoms. Use the flowchart below to help you establish priorities for managing this emergency successfully.

WEAK OR ABSENT PULSE → Localized to one extremity

▼

Generalized

▼

Patient is confused and restless; has hypotension and cool, pale, clammy skin.

Patient has a history of trauma, possibly with external bleeding, and reports thirst.	Patient has a history of myocardial infarction (MI) or heart failure.	Patient has a history of recent cardiac surgery or catheterization, chest trauma, pericardial effusion, or anticoagulant therapy.	Patient has a history of MI or chronic heart or lung disease.
▼	▼	▼	▼
Check for flat neck veins, low urine output, and narrowed pulse pressure.	Check for distended neck veins, ventricular gallop (S_3), crackles, narrowed pulse pressure.	Check for distended neck veins, pulsus paradoxus, and muffled heart sounds.	Check for irregular heart rate, severe tachycardia, and bradycardia.
▼	▼	▼	▼
If your examination reveals these findings, suspect *hypovolemic shock.*	If your examination reveals these findings, suspect *cardiogenic shock.*	If your examination reveals these findings, suspect *cardiac tamponade.*	If your examination reveals these findings, suspect *arrhythmia.*

▼

Administer oxygen by nasal cannula and insert an I.V. line for fluid infusion. Begin cardiac monitoring and check vital signs every 5 to 15 minutes. A central venous pressure line, an arterial line, or a pulmonary artery catheter may have to be inserted. Be prepared for emergency resuscitation, if necessary.

▼

Anticipate colloid or crystalloid replacement, or both.	Anticipate administering nitroprusside, dopamine, and dobutamine.	Anticipate pericardiocentesis.	Anticipate administering antiarrhythmics or delivering electroshock therapy, or both.

Examine affected extremity for cool, mottled skin and pain.

If your examination reveals these findings suspect *arterial occlusive disease.*

Prepare the patient for diagnostic tests to confirm or rule out arterial occlusion such as ultrasonography. Don't elevate the affected extremity. Start an I.V. line in an unaffected arm or leg and administer heparin or streptokinase, as required. Anticipate preparing the patient for emergency embolectomy or peripheral angioplasty.

Patient has a history of trauma, congenital heart disease, or hypertension and reports severe, tearing chest pain.

Check for pulse quality and blood pressure variation between extremities.

If your examination reveals these findings, suspect *dissecting aortic aneurysm* or *aortic coarctation.*

Patient has a history of severe infection-frequent gram negative, urinary, or respiratory infection.

Check for fever, chills, and widened pulse pressure.

If your examination reveals these findings, suspect *septic shock.*

Patient has a history of an insect sting, drug ingestion, or exposure to another possible allergen.

Check for urticaria, wheezing or stridor, and dyspnea.

If your examination reveals these findings, suspect *anaphylactic shock.*

Patient has history of venous stasis or deep vein thrombosis and reports sharp, substernal chest pain.

Check for dyspnea, crackles, pleural friction rub, and hemoptysis.

If your examination reveals these findings, suspect *pulmonary embolism.*

Administer oxygen by nasal cannula and insert an I.V. line for fluid infusion. Begin cardiac monitoring and check vital signs every 5 to 15 minutes. A central venous pressure line, an arterial line, or a pulmonary artery catheter may have to be inserted. Be prepared for emergency resuscitation, if necessary.

Anticipate preparing the patient for surgery and administering an antihypertensive or nitroprusside.

Anticipate administering antibiotics and vasopressors.

Anticipate emergency intubation or cricothyrotomy and administration of epinephrine.

Anticipate possible intubation and anticoagulant or thrombolytic therapy.

suddenly in the chest and neck and may radiate to the entire back and abdomen. Other findings may include syncope, loss of consciousness, weakness or transient paralysis of the legs or arms, the diastolic murmur of aortic insufficiency, systemic hypotension, and mottled skin below the waist.

♦ ***Aortic arch syndrome (Takayasu's arteritis).*** This syndrome causes weak or abruptly absent carotid pulses and unequal or absent radial pulses. These signs are usually preceded by night sweats, pallor, nausea, anorexia, weight loss, arthralgia, and Raynaud's phenomenon. Other findings may include neck, shoulder, and chest pain; paresthesia; intermittent claudication; bruits; vision disturbances; dizziness; and syncope. If the carotid artery is involved, diplopia and transient blindness may occur.

♦ ***Aortic bifurcation occlusion (acute).*** This rare disorder causes abrupt absence of all leg pulses. The patient reports moderate to severe pain in the legs and, less commonly, in the abdomen, lumbosacral area, or perineum. In addition, his legs are cold, pale, numb, and flaccid.

♦ ***Aortic stenosis.*** In this disorder, the carotid pulse is sustained but weak. Dyspnea, chest pain, and syncope dominate the clinical picture. The patient commonly has an atrial gallop. Other findings may include a harsh systolic ejection murmur, crackles, palpitations, fatigue, and narrowed pulse pressure.

♦ ***Arrhythmias.*** Cardiac arrhythmias may cause generalized weak pulses accompanied by cool, clammy skin. Other findings reflect the arrhythmia's severity and may include hypotension, chest pain, dyspnea, dizziness, or decreased level of consciousness.

♦ ***Arterial occlusion.*** In *acute occlusion*, arterial pulses distal to the obstruction are unilaterally weak and then absent. The affected limb is cool, pale, and cyanotic, with prolonged capillary refill time, and the patient complains of moderate to severe pain and paresthesia. A line of color and temperature demarcation develops at the level of obstruction. Other findings that may occur are varying degrees of limb paralysis and intense intermittent claudication. In *chronic occlusion* associated with arteriosclerosis or Buerger's disease, for example, pulses in the affected limb weaken gradually.

♦ ***Cardiac tamponade.*** Life-threatening cardiac tamponade causes a weak, rapid pulse accompanied by these classic findings: pulsus paradoxus, jugular vein distention, hypotension, and muffled heart sounds. Narrowed pulse pressure, pericardial friction rub, or hepatomegaly may also occur. The patient may appear anxious, restless, and cyanotic and may have chest pain, clammy skin, dyspnea, or tachypnea.

♦ ***Coarctation of the aorta.*** Findings in this disorder include bounding pulses in the arms and neck and decreased pulsations and systolic pulse pressure in the lower extremities.

♦ ***Peripheral vascular disease.*** This disorder causes a weakening and loss of peripheral pulses. The patient complains of aching pain distal to the occlusion that worsens with exercise and abates with rest. The skin feels cool and hair growth is decreased. Impotence may occur in male patients with occlusion in the descending aorta or femoral areas.

♦ ***Pulmonary embolism.*** This disorder causes a generalized weak, rapid pulse. It also may cause abrupt onset of chest pain, tachycardia, apprehension, syncope, diaphoresis, or cyanosis. Acute respiratory effects may include tachypnea, dyspnea, decreased breath sounds, crackles, a pleural friction rub, and a cough—possibly with blood-tinged sputum.

♦ ***Shock.*** In *anaphylactic shock*, pulses become rapid and weak and then uniformly absent within seconds after exposure to an allergen. This is preceded by hypotension, anxiety, restlessness, feelings of doom, intense itching, a pounding headache and, possibly, urticaria.

In *cardiogenic shock*, peripheral pulses are absent and central pulses are weak, depending on the degree of vascular collapse. A drop in systolic blood pressure to 30 mm Hg below baseline, or a sustained reading below 80 mm Hg, causes poor tissue perfusion. Resulting signs include cold, pale, clammy skin; tachycardia; rapid, shallow respirations; oliguria; restlessness; confusion; and obtundation.

In *hypovolemic shock,* depending on the severity of hypovolemia, all pulses in the extremities become weak and then uniformly absent. As shock progresses, remaining pulses become thready and more rapid. Early signs of cardiogenic shock include restlessness, thirst, tachypnea, and cool, pale skin. Late signs include hypotension with narrowing pulse pressure, clammy skin, a drop in urine output to less than 25 ml/hour, confusion, decreased level of consciousness and, possibly, hypothermia.

In *septic shock,* all pulses in the extremities first become weak. Depending on the degree of vascular collapse, pulses may then become uniformly absent. Shock is heralded by chills, sudden fever and, possibly, nausea, vomiting, and diarrhea. Typically, the patient experiences tachycardia, tachypnea, and flushed, warm, dry skin. As shock progresses, he develops thirst, hypotension, anxiety, restlessness, and confusion. Then pulse pressure narrows and the skin becomes cold, clammy, and cyanotic. The patient experiences severe hypotension, oliguria or anuria, respiratory failure, and coma.

◆ ***Thoracic outlet syndrome.*** A patient with this syndrome may develop gradual or abrupt weakness or loss of the pulses in the arms, depending on how quickly vessels in the neck compress. These pulse changes commonly occur after the patient works with his hands above his shoulders, lifts a weight, or abducts his arm. Paresthesia and pain occur along the ulnar distribution of the arm and disappear as soon as the patient returns his arm to a neutral position. In addition, the patient may have asymmetrical blood pressure and cool, pale skin.

Other causes

◆ ***Treatments.*** Localized absent pulse may occur distal to arteriovenous shunts for dialysis.

Special considerations

Continue to monitor the patient's vital signs to detect untoward changes in his condition. Monitor hemodynamic status by measuring daily weight and hourly or daily intake and output and by assessing central venous pressure.

Pediatric pointers

Radial, dorsal pedal, and posterior tibial pulses aren't easily palpable in infants and small children, so be careful not to mistake these normally hard-to-find pulses for weak or absent pulses. Instead, palpate the brachial, popliteal, or femoral pulses to evaluate arterial circulation to the extremities. In children and young adults, weak or absent femoral and more distal pulses may indicate coarctation of the aorta.

PULSE, BOUNDING

Caused by large waves of pressure as blood ejects from the left ventricle with each contraction, a bounding pulse is strong and easily palpable and may be visible over superficial peripheral arteries. It's characterized by regular, recurrent expansion and contraction of the arterial walls and isn't obliterated by the pressure of palpation. (See *Evaluating peripheral pulses*, page 481.) A healthy person develops a bounding pulse during exercise, pregnancy, or periods of anxiety. However, this sign also results from fever or from endocrine, hematologic, or cardiovascular disorders that increase the basal metabolic rate.

History and physical examination

After you detect a bounding pulse, check other vital signs, then auscultate the heart and lungs for abnormal sounds, rates, or rhythms. Ask the patient if he has noticed weakness, fatigue, shortness of breath, or other health changes. Review his medical history for hyperthyroidism, anemia, or cardiovascular disorders, and ask about his use of alcohol.

Common medical causes

- ***Alcoholism (acute).*** Vasodilation of acute alcoholism causes a rapid, bounding pulse and flushed face. An odor of alcohol on the breath and an ataxic gait are common. Other possible findings include hypothermia, bradypnea, labored and loud respirations, nausea, vomiting, diuresis, decreased level of consciousness, and seizures.
- ***Aortic insufficiency.*** Sometimes called a water-hammer pulse, the bounding pulse associated with this condition is characterized by rapid, forceful expansion of the arterial pulse followed by rapid contraction. Widened pulse pressure also occurs. *Acute aortic insufficiency* may cause findings associated with left-sided heart failure and cardiovascular collapse, such as weakness, severe dyspnea, hypotension, a ventricular gallop (S_3), and tachycardia. Additional findings may include pallor, chest pain, palpitations, or strong, abrupt carotid pulsations. The patient may also experience pulsus bisferiens, an early systolic murmur, a murmur heard over the femoral artery during systole and diastole, or a high-pitched diastolic murmur that starts with the second heart sound. An apical diastolic rumble (Austin Flint murmur) may also occur, especially in heart failure. Most patients with *chronic aortic insufficiency* remain asymptomatic until their 40s or 50s, when exertional dyspnea, increased fatigue, orthopnea and, eventually, paroxysmal nocturnal dyspnea may develop.
- ***Febrile disorder.*** Fever can cause a bounding pulse. Accompanying findings reflect the specific disorder.
- ***Thyrotoxicosis.*** This disorder causes a rapid, full, bounding pulse. Associated findings may include tachycardia, palpitations, an S_3 or S_4 gallop, weight loss despite increased appetite, or heat intolerance. The patient also may develop diarrhea, an enlarged thyroid, dyspnea, tremors, nervousness, chest pain, exophthalmos, or signs of cardiovascular collapse. His skin will be warm, moist, and diaphoretic.

Special considerations

Prepare the patient for diagnostic laboratory and radiographic studies. If bounding pulse is accompanied by rapid or irregular heartbeat, you may need to connect the patient to a cardiac monitor for further evaluation.

Pediatric pointers

A bounding pulse can be normal in infants or children because arteries lie close to the skin surface. It can also result from patent ductus arteriosus if the left-to-right shunt is large.

PULSE PRESSURE, NARROWED

Pulse pressure, the difference between systolic and diastolic blood pressures, is measured by sphygmomanometry or intra-arterial monitoring. Normally, systolic pressure exceeds diastolic by about 40 mm Hg. Narrowed pressure — a difference of less than 30 mm Hg — occurs when peripheral vascular resistance increases, cardiac output declines, or intravascular volume markedly decreases. (See *Understanding pulse pressure changes.*)

In conditions that cause mechanical obstruction, such as aortic stenosis, pulse pressure is directly related to the severity of the underlying condition. Usually a late sign, narrowed pulse pressure alone doesn't signal an emergency, even though it commonly occurs in shock and other life-threatening disorders.

Understanding pulse pressure changes

Two major factors affect systolic and diastolic blood pressure and, as a result, pulse pressure:

- the amount of blood that the ventricles eject into the arteries with each beat—known as *stroke volume*
- the arteries' *peripheral resistance* to blood flow.

For example, pulse pressure narrows when systolic pressure falls (lower right), diastolic pressure rises (upper left), or both. These changes reflect decreased stroke volume, increased peripheral resistance, or both.

Pulse pressure widens when systolic pressure rises (upper right), diastolic pressure falls (lower left), or both. These changes reflect increased stroke volume, decreased peripheral resistance, or both.

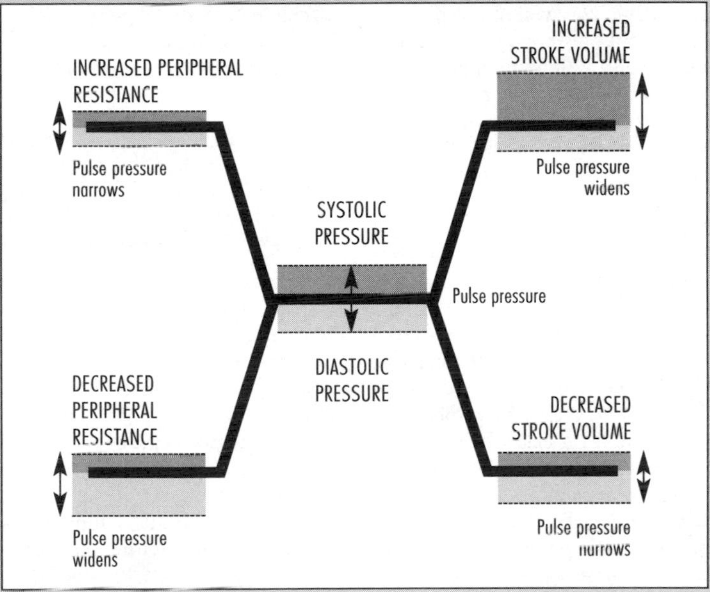

History and physical examination

After you detect a narrowed pulse pressure, check for other signs of heart failure, such as hypotension, tachycardia, dyspnea, distended neck veins, pulmonary crackles, or decreased urine output. Also check for changes in skin temperature or color, strength of peripheral pulses, and level of consciousness (LOC). Auscultate the heart for murmurs. Ask about a history of chest pain, dizziness, or syncope.

Common medical causes

◆ ***Cardiac tamponade.*** In this life-threatening disorder, pulse pressure narrows by approximately 10 to 20 mm Hg. Pulsus paradoxus, neck vein distention, hypotension, and muffled heart sounds are classic. The patient may be anxious, restless, and cyanotic and have clammy skin and chest pain. He may exhibit dyspnea, tachypnea, decreased LOC, and a weak, rapid pulse. Pericardial friction rub or hepatomegaly may also occur.

♦ ***Heart failure.*** Narrowed pulse pressure occurs relatively late and may accompany tachypnea, palpitations, dependent edema, steady weight gain despite nausea and anorexia, chest tightness, slowed mental response, hypotension, diaphoresis, pallor, and oliguria. Assessment reveals a ventricular gallop, inspiratory crackles and, possibly, a tender, palpable liver. Later, dullness develops over the lung bases, and hemoptysis, cyanosis, marked hepatomegaly, and marked pitting edema may occur.

♦ ***Shock.*** In *anaphylactic shock,* pulses become rapid and weak; pulse pressure narrows, and pulses soon become uniformly absent. Within minutes after exposure to an allergen, the patient experiences hypotension, anxiety, restlessness, and feelings of doom, intense itching, a pounding headache and, possibly, urticaria. Other possible findings include dyspnea, stridor, and hoarseness; chest or throat tightness; skin flushing; nausea, abdominal cramps, and urinary incontinence; and seizures.

In *cardiogenic shock,* narrowed pulse pressure occurs relatively late. Typically, peripheral pulses are absent and central pulses are weak. A drop in systolic pressure to 30 mm Hg below baseline, or a sustained reading below 80 mm Hg not attributable to medication, causes poor tissue perfusion. Poor perfusion causes tachycardia; tachypnea; cold, pale, clammy skin; cyanosis; oliguria; restlessness; confusion; and obtundation.

In *hypovolemic shock,* narrowed pulse pressure occurs as a late sign. All peripheral pulses become weak and then uniformly absent. Deepening shock leads to hypotension, urine output of less than 25 ml/hour, confusion, decreased LOC and, possibly, hypothermia.

In *septic shock,* narrowed pulse pressure is a relatively late sign, occurring as all peripheral pulses become weak and then uniformly absent. As shock progresses, the patient exhibits oliguria, thirst, anxiety, restlessness, confusion, and hypotension. Extremities become cool and cyanotic; the skin becomes cold and clammy. In time, he develops severe hypotension, persistent oliguria or anuria, respiratory failure, and coma.

Special considerations

Monitor closely for changes in pulse rate or quality and for hypotension or diminished LOC. Prepare the patient for diagnostic studies to detect valvular heart disease or cardiac tamponade secondary to a pericardial effusion.

Pediatric pointers

In children, narrowed pulse pressure can result from congenital aortic stenosis as well as from disorders that affect adults.

PULSE PRESSURE, WIDENED

Pulse pressure is the difference between systolic and diastolic blood pressures. Normally, systolic pressure is about 40 mm Hg higher than diastolic. Widened pulse pressure — a difference of more than 50 mm Hg — commonly occurs as a physiologic response to fever, hot weather, exercise, anxiety, anemia, or pregnancy. However, it can also result from certain neurologic disorders — especially life-threatening increased intracranial pressure (ICP) — or from cardiovascular disorders that cause backflow of blood into the heart with each contraction such as aortic regurgitation. Widened pulse pressure can easily be identified by monitoring of arterial blood pressure and is commonly detected during routine sphygmomanometric recordings.

Emergency interventions

If the patient's level of consciousness (LOC) is decreased, and you suspect that his widened pulse pressure results from increased ICP, check his vital signs. Maintain a patent airway, and prepare to hyperventilate the patient with a handheld resuscitation bag to help reduce partial pressure of arterial carbon dioxide levels and, thus, ICP. Perform a thorough neurologic examination to serve as a baseline for assessing subsequent changes. Use the Glasgow Coma Scale to evaluate the patient's LOC. (See *Glasgow Coma Scale,* page 354.) Also check cranial nerve function — especially CN III, IV, and VI — and assess pupillary reactions, reflexes, and muscle tone. Insertion of an ICP monitor may be necessary. If you don't suspect increased ICP, ask about chest pain, shortness of breath, weakness, fatigue, and syncope. Check for edema and auscultate for murmurs.

Common medical causes

♦ ***Aortic insufficiency.*** In this disorder, pulse pressure widens progressively as the valve deteriorates, and a bounding pulse and an atrial gallop (S_4) or ventricular gallop (S_3) develop. These signs may be accompanied by chest pain; palpitations; pallor; strong, abrupt carotid pulsations; pulsus bisferiens; and signs of heart failure, such as crackles, dyspnea, and distended neck veins. Auscultation may reveal any of several murmurs, such as early diastolic murmur (common) and Austin Flint murmur.

♦ ***Arteriosclerosis.*** In this disorder, reduced arterial compliance causes progressive widening of pulse pressure, which becomes permanent without treatment of the underlying disorder. This sign is preceded by moderate hypertension and accompanied by signs of vascular insufficiency, such as claudication, angina, and speech and vision disturbances.

♦ ***Febrile disorders.*** Fever can cause widened pulse pressure. Additional symptoms depend on the specific disorder.

♦ ***Increased ICP.*** Widening pulse pressure is an intermediate-to-late sign of increased ICP. Although decreased LOC is the earliest and most sensitive indicator of this life-threatening condition, the onset and progression of widening pulse pressure also parallel rising ICP. (Even a gap of only 50 mm Hg can signal a rapid deterioration in the patient's condition.) Assessment reveals Cushing's triad: bradycardia, hypertension, and respiratory pattern changes. Other findings may include headache, vomiting, impaired or unequal motor movement, vision disturbances such as blurring or photophobia, or pupillary changes.

Special considerations

If the patient displays increased ICP, continually reevaluate his neurologic status and compare your findings carefully with those of previous evaluations. Be alert for restlessness, confusion, unresponsiveness, or decreased LOC. Keep in mind, however, that increasing ICP is commonly signaled by *subtle changes* in the patient's condition rather than the abrupt development of any one sign or symptom.

Pediatric pointers

Increased ICP causes widened pulse pressure in children. Patent ductus arteriosus (PDA) can also cause it but this sign may not be evident at birth. The older child with PDA experiences exertional dyspnea, and pulse pressure widens even further on exertion.

Geriatric pointers

Widened pulse pressure is a more powerful predictor of cardiovascular events in elderly patients than either increased systolic or diastolic blood pressure.

PULSE RHYTHM ABNORMALITY

An abnormal pulse rhythm reflects an underlying cardiac arrhythmia, which may range from benign to life-threatening. (See *Abnormal pulse rhythm: Clue to cardiac arrhythmias,* pages 490 to 493.) Arrhythmias are commonly associated

(Text continues on page 494.)

Abnormal pulse rhythm: Clue to cardiac arrhythmias

An abnormal pulse rhythm may by your only clue that the patient has a cardiac arrhythmia, but this sign doesn't help you pinpoint the specific type of arrhythmia. For that, you need a cardiac monitor or an electrocardiogram (ECG) machine. These devices record the electrical current generated by the heart's conduction system and display this information on an oscillo-

ARRHYTHMIA

Sinus arrhythmia

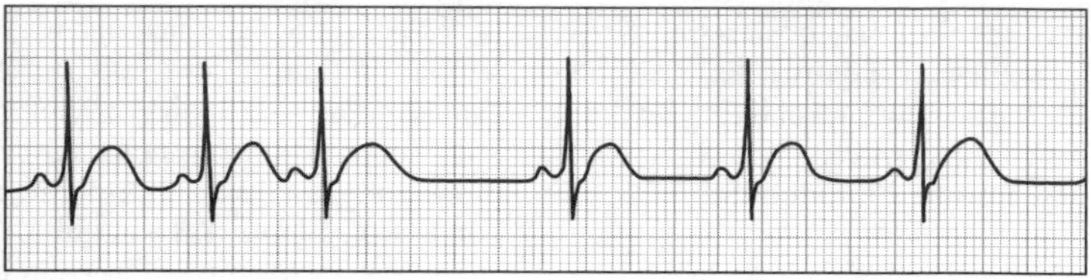

Premature atrial contractions (PACs)

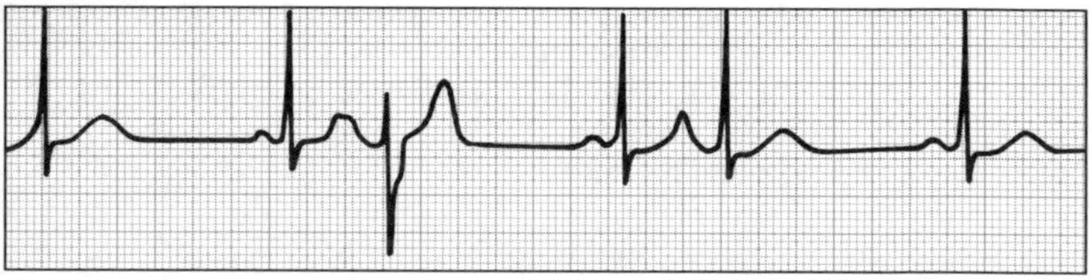

Paroxysmal atrial tachycardia

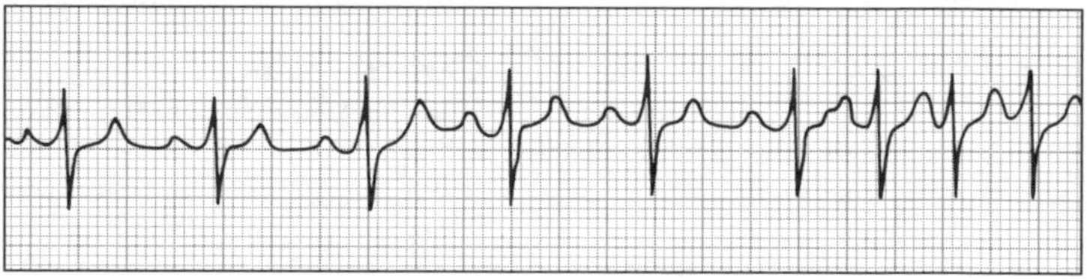

Atrial fibrillation

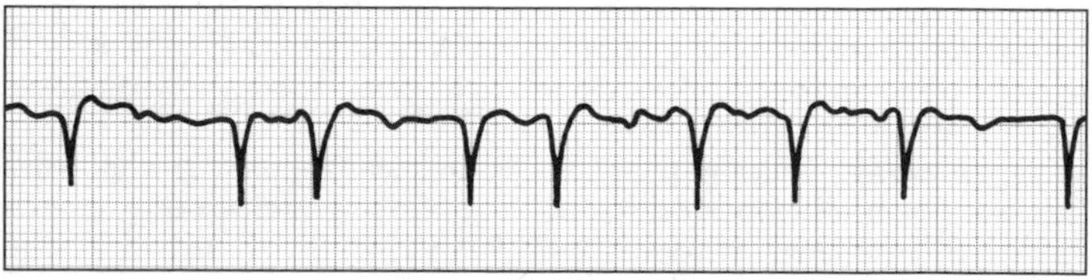

scope screen or a strip-chart recorder. Besides rhythm disturbances, they can identify conduction defects and electrolyte imbalances. The ECG strips below show some common cardiac arrhythmias that can cause abnormal pulse rhythms.

PULSE RHYTHM AND RATE	CLINICAL IMPLICATIONS
Irregular rhythm; fast, slow, or normal rate	◆ Reflex vagal tone inhibition (heart rate increases with inspiration and decreases with expiration) related to normal respiratory cycle ◆ May result from drugs such as in digoxin toxicity ◆ Occurs most commonly in children and young adults
Irregular rhythm during PACs; fast, slow, or normal rate	◆ Occasional PAC may be normal ◆ Isolated PACs indicate atrial irritation—for example, from anxiety or excessive caffeine intake. Increasing PACs may herald other atrial arrhythmias. ◆ May result from heart failure, chronic obstructive pulmonary disease (COPD), or use of cardiac glycosides, aminophylline, or adrenergics
Irregular rhythm at abrupt onset or end of arrhythmia; heart rate exceeding 140 beats/minute	◆ May occur in otherwise normal, healthy persons who are suffering from physical or psychological stress, hypoxia, or digoxin toxicity; who use marijuana; or who consume excessive amounts of caffeine or other stimulants ◆ May be precipitate angina or heart failure
Irregular rhythm; atrial rate exceeding 400 beats/minute; ventricular rate usually 100 to 200 beats/minute	◆ May result from heart failure, COPD, hypertension, sepsis, pulmonary embolism, mitral valve disease, digoxin toxicity (rarely), atrial irritation, postcoronary bypass, or valve replacement surgery ◆ Because atria doesn't contract, preload isn't consistent so cardiac output changes with each beat. Emboli may also result.

(continued)

Abnormal pulse rhythm: Clue to cardiac arrhythmias *(continued)*

ARRHYTHMIA

Premature junctional contractions (PJCs)

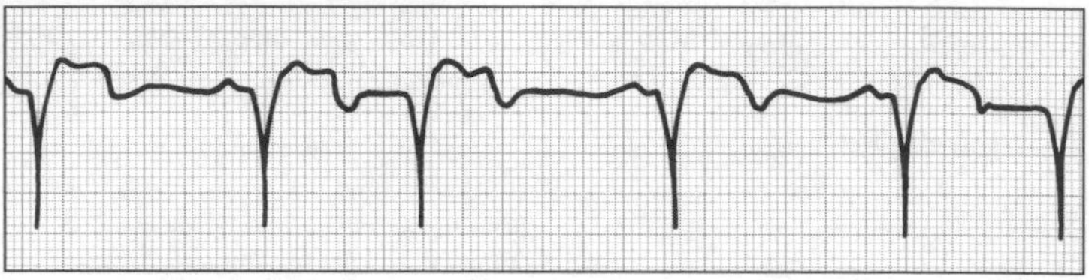

Second-degree atrioventricular (AV) heart block Mobitz Type I (Wenckebach)

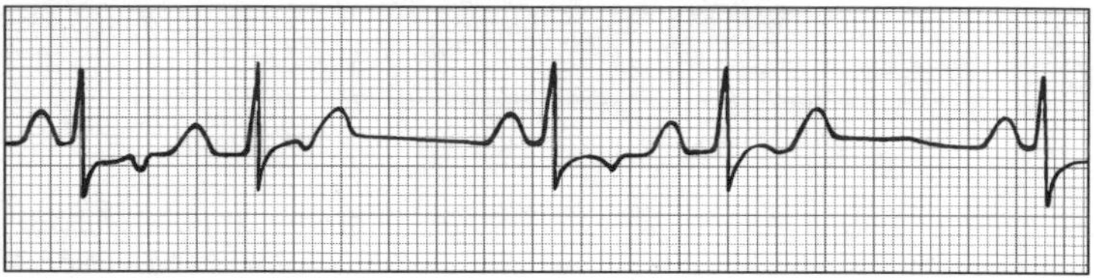

Second-degree AV heart block Mobitz Type II

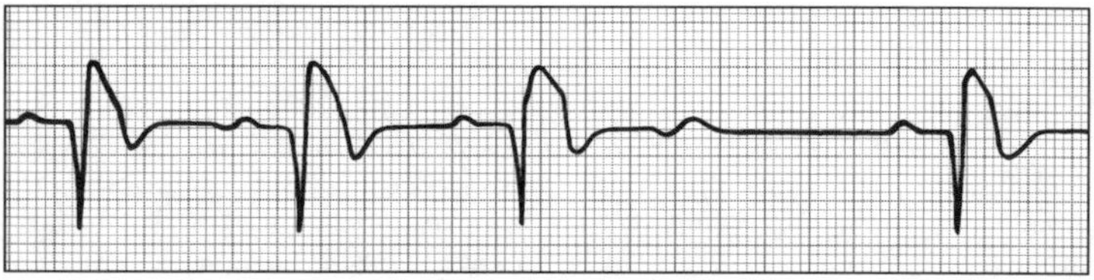

Premature ventricular contractions (multifocal)

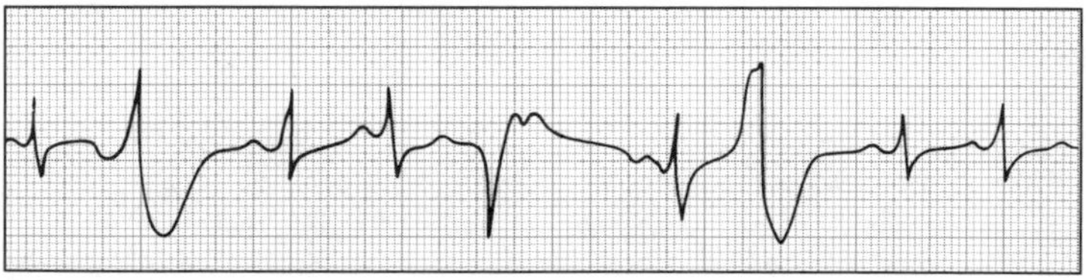

PULSE RHYTHM AND RATE	CLINICAL IMPLICATIONS
Irregular rhythm during PJCs; fast, slow, or normal rate	◆ May result from myocardial infarction (MI) or ischemia, excessive caffeine intake, and most commonly digoxin toxicity (from enhanced automaticity)
Irregular ventricular rhythm; fast, slow, or normal rate	◆ Commonly transient; may progress to complete heart block ◆ May result from inferior wall MI, digoxin or quinidine toxicity, vagal stimulation, electrolyte imbalance, or arteriosclerotic heart disease
Irregular ventricular rhythm; slow or normal rate	◆ May progress to complete heart block ◆ May result from degenerative disease of conduction system, ischemia of AV node in anterior MI, anteroseptal infarction, electrolyte imbalance, or digoxin or quinidine toxicity
Usually irregular rhythm with a long pause after the premature beat; fast, slow, or normal rate	◆ Arise from different ventricular sites or from the same site with changing patterns of conduction ◆ May result from caffeine or stress, alcohol ingestion, myocardial ischemia or infarction, myocardial irritation by pacemaker electrodes, hypocalcemia, hypercalcemia, digoxin toxicity, or exercise

with cardiovascular, renal, respiratory, metabolic, or neurologic disorders or the effects of drugs, diagnostic tests, or treatments. This important finding reflects irregular expansion and contraction of the peripheral arterial walls. It may be persistent or sporadic, rhythmic or arrhythmic. Detected by palpating the radial or carotid pulse, an abnormal rhythm is typically reported first by the patient, who complains of feeling palpitations.

Emergency interventions

Quickly look for signs of reduced cardiac output, such as decreased level of consciousness (LOC), hypotension, or dizziness. Promptly obtain an electrocardiogram (ECG) and possibly a chest X-ray, and begin cardiac monitoring. Insert an I.V. line for administration of emergency cardiac drugs, and give oxygen by nasal cannula or mask. Closely monitor vital signs, pulse quality, and cardiac rhythm because accompanying bradycardia or tachycardia may result in poor tolerance of the abnormal rhythm and cause further deterioration of cardiac output. Keep emergency intubation, cardioversion, and suction equipment handy.

History and physical examination

If the patient's condition permits, ask if he's experiencing pain. If so, find out about onset and location. Does the pain radiate? Ask about a history of heart disease and treatments for arrhythmias. Obtain a medication history and check compliance. Also, ask about caffeine or alcohol use. Digoxin toxicity, cessation of antiarrhythmic drugs, or use of quinidine, sympathomimetics (such as epinephrine), caffeine, or alcohol may cause arrhythmias.

Next, check the patient's apical and peripheral arterial pulses. An apical rate exceeding a peripheral arterial rate indicates a pulse deficit, which may also cause associated signs and symptoms of low cardiac output. Evaluate heart sounds: A long pause between S_1 ("lub") and S_2 ("dub") may indicate a conduction defect. A faint or absent S_1 and an easily audible S_2 may indicate atrial fibrillation or flutter. You may hear the two heart sounds close together on certain beats — suggesting premature atrial contractions — or other variations in heart rate or rhythm. Take the patient's apical and radial pulses while you listen for heart sounds. In some arrhythmias, such as premature ventricular contractions, you may hear the beat with your stethoscope but not feel it over the radial artery when an ineffective contraction has failed to cause a peripheral pulse. Next, count the apical pulse for 60 seconds, noting the frequency of skipped peripheral beats.

Common medical causes

♦ ***Arrhythmias.*** An abnormal pulse rhythm may be the only sign of a cardiac arrhythmia. The patient may complain of palpitations, a fluttering heartbeat, or weak and skipped beats. Pulses may be weak and rapid or slow. Depending on the specific arrhythmia, dull chest pain or discomfort and hypotension may occur. Associated findings, if any, reflect decreased cardiac output. Neurologic findings, for example, include confusion, dizziness, light-headedness, decreased LOC and, sometimes, seizures. Other possible findings include decreased urine output, dyspnea, tachypnea, pallor, and diaphoresis.

Special considerations

The patient may require cardioversion therapy and may need to be sedated beforehand. Prepare the patient for transfer to a cardiac or intensive care unit. If the patient remains in your care, he may require bed rest or help with ambulation. To prevent falls and injury, raise the side rails of his bed and don't leave him unattended while he's sitting or walking. Check vital signs frequently to detect bradycardia, tachycardia, hypertension or hypotension, tachypnea, or dyspnea. Also, monitor intake, output, and daily weight.

Collect blood samples for serum electrolyte, cardiac enzyme, and drug level studies. Prepare the patient for a chest X-ray and a 12-lead ECG. If possible, obtain a previous ECG with which to compare current findings. Prepare the patient for 24-hour Holter monitoring. Explain to the patient the importance of keeping a diary of his activities and symptoms that develop to correlate with the incidence of arrhythmias.

Instruct the patient to avoid tobacco and caffeine, both of which increase arrhythmias. If he has a history of failing to comply with prescribed antiarrhythmic therapy, help him develop strategies to overcome this.

Pulsus alternans

A sign of severe left-sided heart failure, pulsus alternans is a beat-to-beat change in the size and intensity of a peripheral pulse. Although pulse rhythm remains regular, strong and weak contractions alternate. (See *Comparing arterial pressure waves*, pages 496.) An alternation in the intensity of heart sounds or murmurs may accompany this sign.

Pulsus alternans is thought to result from the change in stroke volume that occurs with beat-to-beat alteration in the left ventricle's contractility. Recumbency or exercise increases venous return and reduces the abnormal pulse, which commonly disappears with treatment for heart failure. Rarely, a patient with normal left ventricular function has pulsus alternans but the abnormal pulse seldom persists for more than 10 to 12 beats.

Although most easily detected by sphygmomanometry, pulsus alternans can be detected by palpating the brachial, radial, or femoral artery when systolic pressure varies from beat to beat by more than 20 mm Hg. Because the small changes in arterial pressure that occur during normal respirations may obscure this abnormal pulse, you'll need to have the patient hold his breath during palpation. Apply *light* pressure to avoid obliterating the weaker pulse.

When using a sphygmomanometer to detect pulsus alternans, inflate the cuff 10 to 20 mm Hg above the systolic pressure as determined by palpation, then slowly deflate it. At first, you'll hear only the strong beats. With further deflation, all beats will become audible and palpable and then equally intense. (The difference between this point and the peak systolic level is commonly used to determine the degree of pulsus alternans.) When the cuff is removed, pulsus alternans returns.

Occasionally, the weak beat is so small that no palpable pulse is detected at the periphery. This causes total pulsus alternans, an apparent halving of the pulse rate.

Emergency interventions

Pulsus alternans indicates a critical change in the patient's status. When you detect it, be sure to quickly check other vital signs. Closely evaluate the patient's heart rate, respiratory pattern, and blood pressure. Also, auscultate for a ventricular gallop (S_3) and increased crackles.

Common medical causes

◆ ***Left-sided heart failure.*** In this disorder, pulsus alternans is commonly initiated by a premature beat and is almost always associated with a ventricular gallop. Other findings may include hypotension and cyanosis. Possible respiratory findings include exertional and paroxysmal nocturnal dyspnea, orthopnea, tachypnea, Cheyne-Stokes respirations, hemoptysis, and crackles. Fatigue and weakness are common.

Special considerations

If left-sided heart failure develops suddenly, prepare the patient for transfer to an intensive or cardiac care unit. Meanwhile, elevate the head of his bed to promote respiratory excursion and increase

Comparing arterial pressure waves

The waveforms shown here help differentiate a normal arterial pulse from pulsus alternans and pulsus paradoxus.

NORMAL ARTERIAL PULSE
The percussion wave is a normal arterial pulse and reflects ejection of blood into the aorta (early systole). The tidal wave is the peak of the pulse wave (later systole), and the dicrotic notch marks the beginning of diastole.

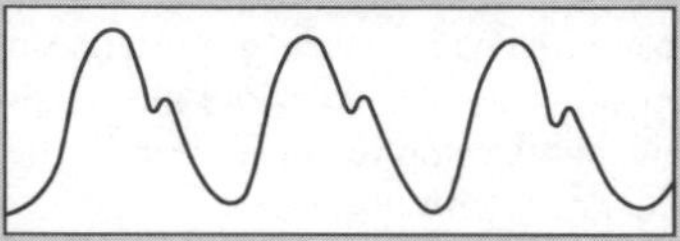

PULSUS ALTERNANS
Pulsus alternans is a beat-to-beat alteration in pulse size and intensity. Although the rhythm of pulsus alternans is regular, the volume varies. If you take the blood pressure of a patient with this abnormality, you'll first heard a loud Korotkoff sound and then a soft sound, continually alternating. Pulsus alternans frequently accompanies states of poor ventricular failure.

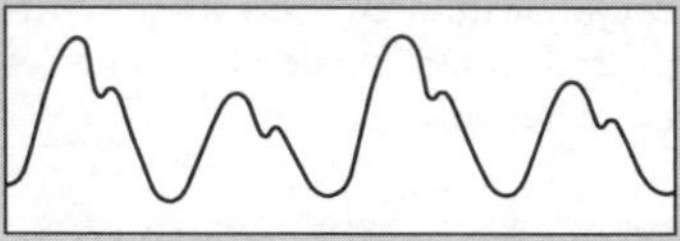

PULSUS PARADOXUS
Pulsus paradoxus is an exaggerated decline in blood pressure during inspiration, resulting from an increase in negative intrathoracic pressure. A pulmonary paradoxus that exceeds 10 mm Hg is considered abnormal and may result from cardiac tamponade, constrictive pericarditis, or severe lung disease.

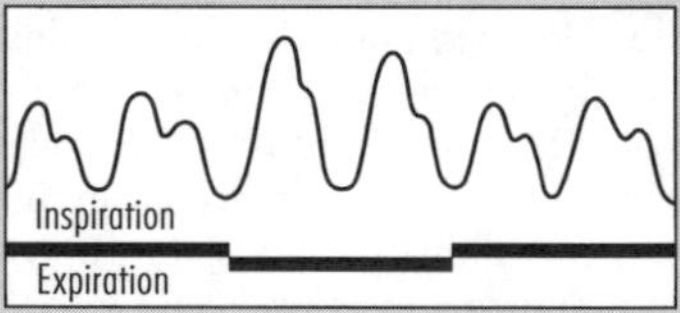

oxygenation. Adjust the patient's current treatment plan to improve cardiac output, reduce the heart's workload, and promote diuresis.

Pediatric pointers

In a child with heart failure, pulsus alternans may be difficult to assess if the child is crying or restless. Try to quiet the child by holding him, if his condition permits.

PULSUS PARADOXUS

Pulsus paradoxus, or paradoxical pulse, is an exaggerated decline in blood pressure during inspiration. Normally, systolic pressure falls less than 10 mm Hg during inspiration. In pulsus paradoxus, however, it falls more than 10 mm Hg. (See *Comparing arterial pressure waves.*) When systolic pressure falls more than 20 mm Hg, the peripheral pulses may be barely palpable or may disappear during inspiration.

Pulsus paradoxus is thought to result from an exaggerated decrease in intrathoracic pressure during inspiration. Normally, systolic pressure drops during inspiration because of blood pooling in the pulmonary system. This, in turn, reduces left ventricular filling and stroke volume. Also, the negative intrathoracic pressure transmits to the aorta. Conditions associated with large intrapleural pressure swings such as asthma or those that reduce left-sided heart filling during inspiration such as pericardial tamponade cause paradoxical pulse.

To accurately detect and measure paradoxical pulse, use a sphygmomanometer or an intra-arterial monitoring device. Inflate the blood pressure cuff 10 to 20 mm Hg beyond the peak systolic pressure. Then deflate the cuff at a rate of 2 mm Hg/second until you hear the first Korotkoff sound during expiration. Note the systolic pressure. As you continue to slowly deflate the cuff, observe the patient's respiratory pattern. If a paradoxical pulse is present, the Korotkoff sounds will disappear with inspiration and return with expiration. Continue to deflate the cuff until you hear Korotkoff sounds during both inspiration and expiration and, again, note the systolic pressure. Subtract this reading from the first one to determine the degree of paradoxical pulse. A difference of more than 10 mm Hg is abnormal.

You can also detect paradoxical pulse by palpating the brachial or femoral pulse over several cycles of slow inspiration and expiration. Marked pulse diminution during inspiration reflects paradoxical pulse. When you check for paradoxical pulse, remember that irregular heart rhythms and tachycardia cause variations in pulse amplitude and must be ruled out before a true paradoxical pulse can be identified.

Emergency interventions

A paradoxical pulse may signal cardiac tamponade — a life-threatening complication of pericardial effusion that occurs when sufficient blood or fluid accumulates to compress the heart. When you detect paradoxical pulse, quickly take the patient's other vital signs. Check for additional signs and symptoms of cardiac tamponade, such as dyspnea, tachypnea, diaphoresis, distended neck veins, tachycardia, narrowed pulse pressure, and hypotension. Emergency pericardiocentesis to aspirate blood or fluid from the pericardial sac may be necessary. Then evaluate the effectiveness of pericardiocentesis by measuring the degree of pulsus paradoxus; it should decrease after aspiration.

Pulsus paradoxus during an asthma attack suggests severe bronchial obstruction. These patients need to be treated aggressively; consider hospital admission.

History and physical examination

If the patient doesn't have cardiac tamponade, find out if he has a history of chronic cardiac or pulmonary disease. Ask about associated signs and symptoms, such as a cough or chest pain. Then auscultate for abnormal breath sounds.

Common medical causes

◆ ***Cardiac tamponade.*** Pulsus paradoxus is a common occurrence in this disorder but it may be difficult to detect if intrapericardial pressure rises abruptly and profound hypotension occurs. In severe tamponade, assessment also reveals these classic findings: hypotension, diminished or muffled heart sounds, and jugular vein distention. Related findings include chest pain, pericardial friction rub, narrowed pulse pressure, anxiety, restlessness, clammy skin, and hepatomegaly. Characteristic respiratory signs and symptoms include dyspnea, tachypnea, and cyanosis; the patient typically sits up and leans forward to facilitate breathing.

If cardiac tamponade develops gradually, paradoxical pulse may be accompanied by weakness, anorexia, and weight loss. The patient may also report chest pain but he doesn't have muffled heart sounds or severe hypotension.

♦ ***Chronic obstructive pulmonary disease (COPD).*** The wide fluctuations in intrathoracic pressure that characterize this disorder cause pulsus paradoxus and possibly tachycardia. Other findings vary but may include dyspnea, tachypnea, wheezing, productive or nonproductive cough, accessory muscle use, barrel chest, and clubbing. The patient may show labored, pursed-lip breathing after exertion or even at rest. He typically sits up and leans forward to facilitate breathing. Auscultation reveals decreased breath sounds, rhonchi, and crackles. Weight loss, cyanosis, or edema may occur.

♦ ***Pericarditis (chronic constrictive).*** Paradoxical pulse can occur in up to 50% of patients with this disorder. Other findings include pericardial friction rub, chest pain, exertional dyspnea, orthopnea, hepatomegaly, and ascites. The patient also exhibits peripheral edema and Kussmaul's sign — distended neck veins that become more prominent on inspiration.

♦ ***Pulmonary embolism (massive).*** Decreased left ventricular filling and stroke volume in massive pulmonary embolism cause pulsus paradoxus as well as syncope and severe apprehension, dyspnea, tachypnea, and pleuritic chest pain. The patient appears cyanotic and has distended neck veins. He may succumb to circulatory collapse, with hypotension and a weak, rapid pulse. Pulmonary infarction may cause hemoptysis, decreased breath sounds, and a pleural friction rub over the affected area.

Special considerations

Prepare the patient for an echocardiogram to visualize cardiac motion and to help identify the causative disorder. In addition, monitor his vital signs and frequently check the degree of paradox. An increase in the degree of paradox suggests recurring or worsening cardiac tamponade or impending respiratory arrest in severe COPD. Vigorous respiratory treatment, such as chest physiotherapy, may avert the need for endotracheal intubation.

Pediatric pointers

Paradoxical pulse commonly occurs in children with chronic pulmonary disease, especially during an acute asthmatic attack. Children with pericarditis may develop pulsus paradoxus due to cardiac tamponade, although this disorder more commonly affects adults. A paradoxical pulse above 20 mm Hg is a reliable indicator of cardiac tamponade in children; a change of 10 to 20 mm Hg is equivocal.

PUPILS, NONREACTIVE

Nonreactive (fixed) pupils fail to constrict in response to light or to dilate when the light is removed. The development of a unilateral or bilateral nonreactive response indicates an important change in the patient's condition; it may signal a life-threatening emergency and possibly brain death. A less-threatening cause is use of certain optic drugs.

Emergency interventions

If the patient is unconscious and develops unilateral or bilateral nonreactive pupils, quickly take his vital signs. Be alert for decerebrate or decorticate posture, bradycardia, elevated systolic blood pressure, widened pulse pressure, and other untoward changes in the patient's condition. Remember, a unilateral dilated, nonreactive pupil may be an early sign of uncal brain herniation. Emergency surgery to try to decrease intracranial pressure (ICP) may be necessary. If the patient isn't already being treated for increased ICP, insert an I.V. line to administer diuretics, osmotics, and corticosteroids. You may also need to begin controlled hyperventilation.

History and physical examination

If the patient isn't unconscious, obtain a brief history. Ask him what type of eyedrops he's using, if any, and when they were last instilled. Also ask if he's experiencing pain, and, if so, try to determine its location, intensity, and duration. Check the patient's visual acuity in both eyes. Then test the pupillary reaction to accommodation: normally, both pupils constrict equally as the patient shifts his glance from a distant to a near object.

To evaluate pupillary reaction to light, first test the patient's *direct light reflex.* Darken the room, and cover one of the patient's eyes. Hold the opposite eyelid open and, using a bright penlight, bring the light toward the patient from the side and shine it directly into his opened eye. If normal, the pupil will promptly constrict. Next, test the *consensual light reflex.* Hold the patient's eyelids open and shine the light into one eye while watching the pupil of the opposite eye. If normal, both pupils will promptly constrict. Repeat both procedures in the opposite eye. A unilateral or bilateral nonreactive response indicates dysfunction of cranial nerves II and III, which mediate the pupillary light reflex. (See *Innervation of direct and consensual light reflexes*, page 500.)

Next, hold a penlight at the side of each eye and examine the cornea and iris for abnormalities. Measure intraocular pressure (IOP) with a tonometer, or estimate IOP by placing your second and third fingers over the patient's closed eyelid (a rock-hard feeling suggests elevated IOP). If the patient has experienced ocular trauma, don't manipulate the affected eye. Ophthalmoscopic and slit-lamp examinations of the eye will be necessary in all patients. After the examination, be sure to cover the affected eye with a protective metal shield but don't let the shield rest on the globe.

Common medical causes

- ***Argyll Robertson pupil.*** In this hallmark of neurosyphilis, the light reflex is absent or abnormal but the near response is intact (light-near dissociation). Both pupils are usually involved but the degree may be asymmetrical.
- ***Botulism.*** Bilateral mydriasis and nonreactive pupils usually appear 12 to 36 hours after ingestion of tainted food. Other early findings include blurred vision, diplopia, ptosis, strabismus, or extraocular muscle palsies, along with anorexia, nausea, vomiting, diarrhea, or dry mouth. Vertigo, deafness, hoarseness, nasal voice, dysarthria, and dysphagia follow. Progressive muscle weakness and absent deep tendon reflexes usually evolve over 2 to 4 days, resulting in severe constipation, paralysis of respiratory muscles, and respiratory distress.
- ***Encephalitis.*** As this disorder progresses, initially sluggish pupils become dilated and nonreactive. Decreased accommodation and other symptoms of cranial nerve palsies, such as dysphagia, develop. Within 48 hours after onset, encephalitis causes a decreased level of consciousness, high fever, headache, vomiting, and nuchal rigidity. Aphasia, ataxia, nystagmus, hemiparesis, or photophobia may occur with seizures.
- ***Glaucoma (acute angle-closure).*** In this ophthalmic emergency, examination reveals a moderately dilated, nonreactive pupil in the affected eye. Conjunctival injection, corneal clouding, or decreased visual acuity also occur. The patient experiences sudden onset of blurred vision, followed by excruciating pain in and around the affected eye. He commonly reports seeing halos around white lights at night. Severely elevated IOP frequently induces nausea and vomiting.
- ***Oculomotor nerve palsy.*** Commonly, the first signs of this oculomotor (CN III) ophthalmoplegia are a dilated, nonreactive pupil and loss of the accommodation reaction. These findings may occur in one eye or both, depending on

EXAMINATION TIP

Innervation of direct and consensual light reflexes

Two reactions — direct and consensual — constitute the pupillary light reflex. Normally, a light shined directly onto the retina of one eye stimulates the parasympathetic nerves to cause brisk constriction of that pupil — the *direct light reflex.* The pupil of the opposite eye also constricts — the *consensual light reflex.*

If the afferent arc is intact the direct response and the consensual should be equal. (Note: the light should not be shined directly into the patient's eye but should be directed from slightly below and upward toward the patient's pupil.)

The optic nerve (CN II) mediates the afferent arc of this reflex from each eye, and the oculomotor nerve (CN III) mediates the efferent arc to both eyes. A nonreactive or sluggish response in one or both pupils indicates dysfunction of these cranial nerves, usually due to degenerative disease of the central nervous system.

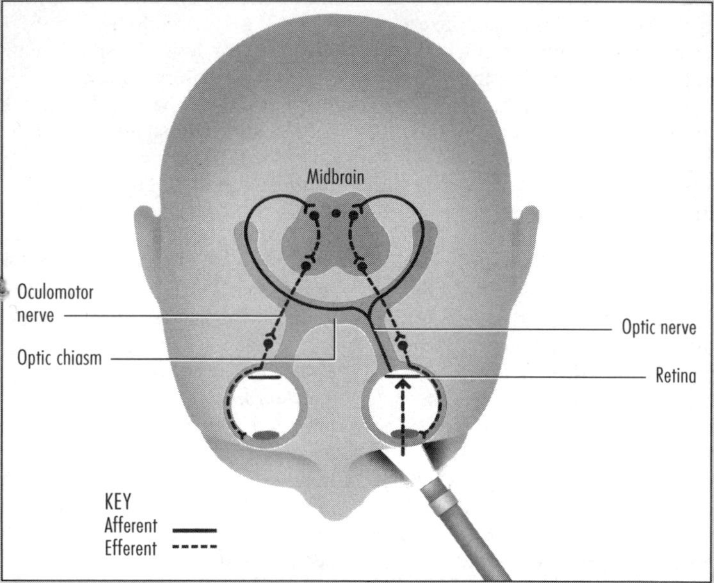

whether the palsy is unilateral or bilateral. Among the causes of total CN III palsy is life-threatening brain herniation. *Central herniation* causes bilateral midposition nonreactive pupils, whereas *uncal herniation* initially causes a unilateral dilated, nonreactive pupil. Other common findings include diplopia, ptosis, outward deviation of the eye, or inability to elevate or adduct the eye. Additional findings depend on the palsy's underlying cause.

♦ ***Uveitis.*** A small, nonreactive pupil that appears suddenly with severe eye pain, conjunctival injection, and photophobia typifies *anterior uveitis.* In *poste-*

rior uveitis, similar features develop insidiously with blurred vision and distorted pupil shape.

Other causes

♦ ***Drugs.*** Instillation of topical mydriatics and cycloplegics may induce a temporarily nonreactive pupil in the affected eye. Opiates, such as heroin and morphine, cause pinpoint pupils with a minimal light response that can be seen only with a magnifying glass. Atropine poisoning causes widely dilated, nonreactive pupils.

Special considerations

If the patient is conscious, monitor his pupillary light reflex to detect changes. If he's unconscious, close his eyes to prevent corneal exposure. (Use tape to secure the eyelids, if needed.)

Pediatric pointers

Children have nonreactive pupils for the same reasons as adults. The most common cause is oculomotor nerve palsy from increased ICP.

Pupils, sluggish

A sluggish pupillary reaction is an abnormally slow pupillary response to light. It can occur in one pupil or both, unlike the normal reaction, which is always bilateral. A sluggish reaction accompanies degenerative disease of the central nervous system and diabetic neuropathy. It can occur normally in the elderly, whose pupils become smaller and less responsive with age.

To assess pupillary reaction to light, first test the patient's *direct light reflex.* Darken the room, and cover one of the patient's eyes while you hold open the opposite eyelid. Using a bright penlight, bring the light toward the patient from the side and shine it directly into his opened eye. If normal, the pupil will promptly constrict. Next, test the *consensual light reflex.* Hold both of the patient's eyelids open, and shine the light into one eye while watching the pupil of the opposite eye. If normal, both pupils will promptly constrict. Repeat both procedures to test light reflexes in the opposite eye. A sluggish reaction in one or both pupils indicates dysfunction of cranial nerves II and III, which mediate the pupillary light reflex. (See *Innervation of direct and consensual light reflexes.*)

History and physical examination

If you detect a sluggish pupillary reaction, determine the patient's visual function. Start by testing visual acuity in both eyes. Then test the pupillary reaction to accommodation; the pupils should constrict equally as the patient shifts his glance from a distant to a near object.

Next, hold a penlight at the side of each eye and examine the cornea and iris for irregularities, scars, and foreign bodies. Measure intraocular pressure (IOP) with a tonometer, or estimate IOP by placing your fingers over the patient's closed eyelid. If the eyeball feels rock-hard, suspect elevated IOP. In addition, ophthalmoscopic and slit-lamp examinations of the eye will need to be performed.

Common medical causes

♦ ***Adie's syndrome.*** This syndrome causes abrupt onset of unilateral mydriasis and a sluggish pupillary response that may progress to a nonreactive response. The patient may complain of blurred vision and cramplike eye pain. Eventually, both eyes may be affected. Musculoskeletal assessment also reveals hypoactive or absent deep tendon reflexes in the arms and legs.

♦ ***Encephalitis.*** This disorder initially causes a bilateral sluggish pupillary response. Later, pupils become dilated and nonreactive, accommodation may diminish, and the patient may display signs of cranial nerve palsies, such as dysphagia and facial weakness. Within 24 to 48 hours after onset, encephalitis causes a decreased level of consciousness (LOC), headache, high fever, vomiting, and nuchal rigidity. Other possible manifestations include aphasia, ataxia, nystagmus, hemiparesis, and photophobia. The patient may exhibit seizure activity and myoclonic jerks.

♦ ***Herpes zoster.*** The patient with herpes zoster affecting the nasociliary nerve may have a sluggish pupillary response. Examination of the conjunctiva reveals follicles. Additional ocular findings include a serous discharge, absence of tears, ptosis, or extraocular muscle palsy.

♦ ***Iritis (acute).*** In this disorder, the affected eye exhibits a sluggish pupillary response and conjunctival injection. The pupil may remain constricted; if posterior synechiae have formed, the pupil will also be irregularly shaped. The patient reports sudden onset of eye pain and photophobia and may also have blurred vision.

♦ ***Myotonic dystrophy.*** In this disorder, sluggish pupillary reaction may be accompanied by lid lag, ptosis, miosis and, possibly, diplopia. Cataract formation may decrease visual acuity. Muscle weakness and atrophy and testicular atrophy may occur.

♦ ***Tertiary syphilis.*** A sluggish pupillary reaction (especially in Argyll Robertson pupils) occurs in the late stage of neurosyphilis, along with marked weakness of the extraocular muscles, visual field defects and, possibly, cataractous changes in the lens. The patient may complain of orbital rim pain, which worsens at night. He may also exhibit lid edema, decreased visual acuity, or exophthalmos. Tertiary lesions appear on the skin and mucous membranes. Liver, respiratory, cardiovascular, or additional neurologic dysfunction may also occur.

♦ ***Wernicke's disease.*** Initially, this disorder causes an intention tremor accompanied by a sluggish pupillary reaction. Later, pupils may become nonreactive. Additional ocular findings include diplopia, gaze paralysis, nystagmus, ptosis, decreased visual acuity, or conjunctival injection. The patient may also exhibit orthostatic hypotension, tachycardia, ataxia, apathy, or confusion.

Pediatric pointers

Children exhibit sluggish pupillary reactions for the same reasons as adults.

PURPURA

Purpura is the extravasation of red blood cells from the blood vessels into the skin, subcutaneous tissue, or mucous membranes. It's characterized by discoloration — usually purplish or brownish red — that's easily visible through the epidermis. Purpuric lesions include petechiae, ecchymoses, and hematomas. (See *Identifying purpuric lesions.*) Purpura differs from erythema in that it doesn't blanch with pressure because it involves blood in the tissues, not just dilated vessels.

Purpura results from damage to the endothelium of small blood vessels, coagulation defects, ineffective perivascular support, capillary fragility and permeability, or a combination of these factors. These faulty hemostatic factors, in turn, can result from thrombocytopenia or other hematologic disorders, invasive procedures or, of course, the use of anticoagulants.

Additional causes are nonpathologic. Purpura can be a consequence of aging, when loss of collagen decreases connective tissue support of superficial skin blood vessels. In an elderly or cachectic person, skin atrophy and inelasticity and loss of subcutaneous fat increase susceptibility to minor trauma, causing purpura to appear along the veins of the forearms, hands, legs, and feet. Prolonged coughing or vomiting can cause crops of petechiae in loose face and neck tissue.

EXAMINATION TIP

Identifying purpuric lesions

Purpuric lesions fall into three categories: petechiae, ecchymoses, and hematomas.

PETECHIAE
Petechiae are painless, round, pinpoint lesions, 1 to 3 cm in diameter. Caused by extravasation of red blood cells into cutaneous tissue, these red or brown lesions usually arise on dependent portions of the body. They appear and fade in crops and can group to form ecchymoses.

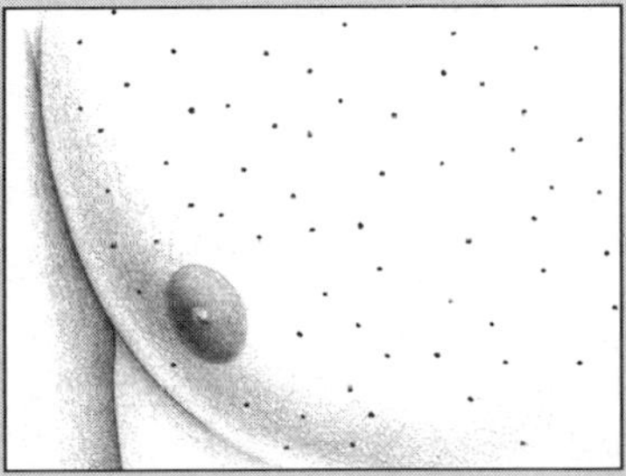

ECCHYMOSES
Ecchymoses, another form of blood extravasation, are larger than petechiae. These purple, blue, or yellow-green bruises vary in size and shape and can arise anywhere on the body as a result of trauma. Ecchymoses usually appear on the arms and legs of patients with bleeding disorders.

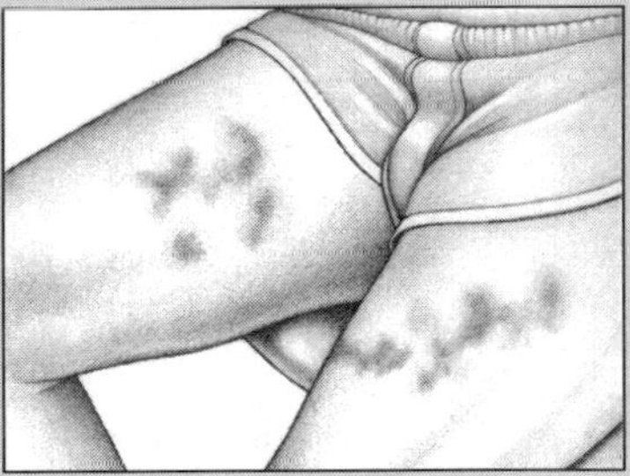

HEMATOMAS
Hematomas are palpable ecchymoses that are painful and swollen. Usually the result of trauma, superficial hematomas are red, whereas deep hematomas are blue. Hematomas often exceed 1 cm in diameter, but their size varies widely.

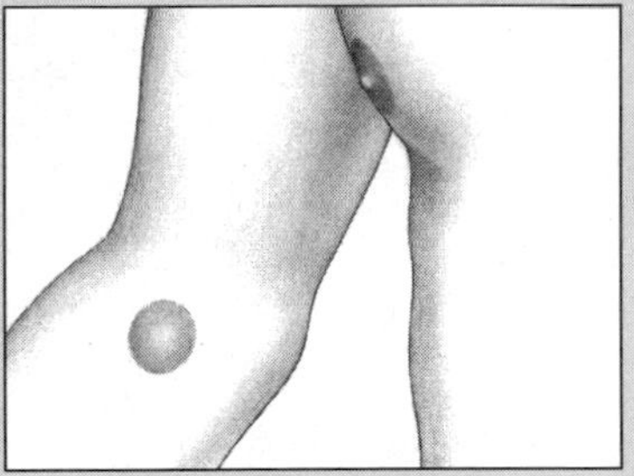

Violent muscle contraction, as occurs in seizures or weight lifting, sometimes results in localized ecchymoses from increased intraluminal pressure and rupture. High fever, which increases capillary fragility, can also cause purpura.

History and physical examination

Ask the patient when he first noticed the lesion and whether he has noticed other lesions on his body. Ask if current lesions have grown in size lately. Does he or his family have a history of bleeding disorders or easy bruising? Find out what medications he's taking, if any, and ask him to describe his diet. Ask about recent trauma, transfusions, or phlebotomy and about the development of associated signs, such as epistaxis, bleeding gums, hematuria, or hematochezia. Also ask about systemic complaints that may suggest infection such as fever. If the patient is female, ask about heavy menstrual flow.

Inspect the patient's entire skin surface to determine the type, size, location, distribution, and severity of purpuric lesions. Also inspect the mucous membranes. Remember that the same mechanisms that cause purpura can also cause internal hemorrhage, although purpura isn't a cardinal indicator of this condition.

Medical causes

♦ ***Autoerythrocyte sensitivity.*** In this syndrome, painful ecchymoses appear either singly or in groups, usually preceded by local itching, burning, or pain. Common associated findings include epistaxis, hematuria, hematemesis, and menometrorrhagia. Abdominal pain, diarrhea, nausea, vomiting, syncope, headache, and chest pain are also common.

♦ ***Disseminated intravascular coagulation.*** This disorder can cause varying degrees of purpura, depending on its severity and underlying cause. Rarely, the patient develops life-threatening *purpura fulminans,* with symmetrical cutaneous and subcutaneous lesions on the arms and legs. He may have cutaneous oozing, hematemesis, or bleeding from incision or needle insertion sites. Other possible findings include acrocyanosis; nausea; dyspnea; seizures; severe muscle, back, or abdominal pain; and signs of acute tubular necrosis such as oliguria.

♦ ***Dysproteinemias.*** In *multiple myeloma,* petechiae and ecchymoses accompany other bleeding tendencies: hematemesis, epistaxis, gum bleeding, or excessive bleeding after surgery. Similar findings occur in *cryoglobulinemia,* which may also cause malignant maculopapular purpura. *Hyperglobulinemia* typically begins insidiously with occasional outbreaks of purpura over the lower legs and feet. These outbreaks eventually become more frequent and extensive, involving the entire lower leg and possibly the trunk. The purpura usually occurs after prolonged standing or exercise and may be heralded by skin burning or stinging. Leg edema, knee or ankle pain, and low-grade fever may precede or accompany the purpura, which gradually fades over 1 or 2 weeks. Persistent pigmentation develops after repeated outbreaks.

♦ ***Easy bruising syndrome.*** This syndrome is characterized by recurrent bruising on the legs, arms, and trunk, either spontaneously or following minor trauma. Bruising may be preceded by pain and is more common in women than in men, especially during menses.

♦ ***Ehlers-Danlos syndrome (EDS).*** Besides petechiae, this syndrome is marked by easy bruising, epistaxis, gum bleeding, hematuria, melena, menorrhagia, and excessive bleeding after surgery. EDS characteristically causes soft, velvety, hyperelastic skin; hyperextensible joints; increased skin and blood vessel fragility; and repeated dislocations of the temporomandibular joint.

♦ ***Idiopathic thrombocytopenic purpura (ITP).*** Chronic ITP typically begins insidiously, with scattered petechiae on the distal arms and legs. Deep-lying ecchymoses may also occur. Other findings include epistaxis, easy bruising, hematuria, hematemesis, or menorrhagia.

♦ ***Leukemia.*** This disease causes widespread petechiae on the skin, mucous membranes, retina, and serosal surfaces. Confluent ecchymoses are uncommon. The patient may also exhibit swollen and bleeding gums, epistaxis, or other bleeding tendencies. Lymphadenopathy and splenomegaly are common.

Acute leukemias also cause severe prostration and high fever and may cause dyspnea, tachycardia, palpitations, or abdominal or bone pain. Confusion, headache, seizures, vomiting, papilledema, or nuchal rigidity may occur late in the disease. *Chronic leukemias* begin insidiously with minor bleeding tendencies, malaise, fatigue, pallor, low-grade fever, anorexia, and weight loss.

◆ ***Myeloproliferative disorders.*** These disorders, which include polycythemia vera, can cause hemorrhage paradoxically accompanied by ecchymoses and ruddy cyanosis. The oral mucosa takes on a deep purplish red hue, and slight trauma causes swollen gums to bleed. Other findings include pruritus, urticaria, and such nonspecific symptoms as lethargy, weakness, fatigue, or weight loss. The patient typically complains of headache, a sensation of fullness in the head, and rushing in the ears; dizziness and vertigo; dyspnea; paresthesia of the fingers; double or blurred vision and scotoma; or epigastric distress. He may also experience intermittent claudication, hypertension, hepatosplenomegaly, or impaired mentation.

◆ ***Systemic lupus erythematosus.*** This chronic inflammatory disorder may cause purpura accompanied by other cutaneous findings, such as scaly patches on the scalp, face, neck, and arms; diffuse alopecia; telangiectasis; urticaria; or ulceration. The characteristic butterfly rash appears in the disorder's acute phase. Common associated signs and symptoms include nondeforming joint pain and stiffness, Raynaud's phenomenon, seizures, psychotic behavior, photosensitivity, fever, anorexia, weight loss, or lymphadenopathy.

◆ ***Thrombotic thrombocytopenic purpura.*** Generalized purpura, hematuria, vaginal bleeding, jaundice, and pallor are among the usual presenting signs and symptoms in this disorder. Most patients have fever, and some also experience fatigue, weakness, headache, nausea, abdominal pain, arthralgias, or hepatosplenomegaly. Possible neurologic effects include seizures, paresthesia, cranial nerve palsies, vertigo, and altered level of consciousness. Renal failure may also occur.

◆ ***Trauma.*** Traumatic injury can cause local or widespread purpura.

Other causes

◆ ***Diagnostic tests.*** Invasive procedures, such as venipuncture or arterial catheterization, may cause local ecchymoses and hematomas due to extravasated blood.

◆ ***Drugs.*** The anticoagulants heparin and Coumadin can cause purpura.

◆ ***Surgery and other procedures.*** Any procedure that disrupts circulation, coagulation, or platelet activity or production may cause purpura. These include pulmonary or cardiac surgery, radiation therapy, chemotherapy, hemodialysis, multiple blood transfusions with platelet-poor blood, or use of plasma expanders such as dextran.

Special considerations

Reassure the patient that purpuric lesions aren't permanent and will fade if the underlying cause can be successfully treated. Warn him not to use cosmetic fade creams or other products in an attempt to reduce pigmentation. If he has a hematoma, apply pressure and cold compresses initially to help reduce bleeding and swelling. After the first 24 hours, apply hot compresses to help speed absorption of blood.

Prepare the patient for diagnostic tests. These may include a peripheral blood smear, bone marrow examination, and blood tests to determine platelet count, bleeding and coagulation times, capillary fragility, clot retraction, one-stage prothrombin time, activated partial thromboplastin time, or fibrinogen levels.

Pediatric pointers

Neonates commonly exhibit petechiae, particularly on the head, neck, and shoulders, after vertex deliveries. Thought to

Assessing for child abuse

When caring for a child with nonpathologic purpuric lesions or other injuries, be sure to assess him for possible abuse. Abuse can be physical, psychological, emotional, or sexual. Be aware that an abuser can be anyone, not just a parent. Risk factors for abusers include high stress level or poor coping skills, lack of social support, and a family history of abuse.

Try to examine the child in private. Suspect child abuse if you detect multiple bruises in various stages of healing. Observe for unusual skin markings or scars that may indicate the object used, such as teeth, a hand, a belt, or a burning cigarette.

The child may have fractures, immersion (or "branding") burns, head trauma, retinal hemorrhages, oral irritation, internal injuries, or genital or rectal trauma. Check the child's records to see if he has been treated for similar injuries in the past. Observe his general appearance. He may seem unkempt, as if neglected, or be dressed inappropriately. The abused child may have a blank look, seem passive or anxious, display erratic or sexual behavior, cling to or move away from parents, or avoid your touch. He may be developmentally delayed.

Note the parents' behavior. They may be uncooperative, evasive, or demanding, or they may not take the child's injuries seriously. The history they give may seem inconsistent with your findings. They may make excuses or blame others, including the child, for the injuries. Remain nonjudgmental even if you suspect abuse. Offer support through referrals to counselors and social workers.

Your priority is the safety of the child. After treating his injuries and collecting evidence when appropriate, make appropriate psychiatric and social support service referrals.

Document your assessment and actions thoroughly and objectively. Become familiar with your institution's protocol for notifying designated authorities because the law requires reporting of all incidents of suspected child abuse.

result from the trauma of birth, these petechiae disappear within a few days. Other causes in infants include thrombocytopenia, vitamin K deficiency, or infantile scurvy.

The most common type of purpura in children is allergic purpura. Other causes in children include trauma, hemophilia, autoimmune hemolytic anemia, Gaucher's disease, thrombasthenia, congenital factor deficiencies, Wiskott-Aldrich syndrome, acute ITP, von Willebrand's disease, or the rare but life-threatening purpura fulminans, which most commonly follows bacterial or viral infection.

As a child grows and tests his motor skills, the risk of accidents multiplies, and ecchymoses and hematomas commonly occur. However, when you assess a child with purpura, be alert for signs of possible child abuse: bruises in different stages of resolution, from repeated beatings; bruise patterns resembling a familiar object, such as a belt, hand, or thumb and finger; and bruises on the face, buttocks, or genitalia, areas unlikely to be injured accidentally. (See *Assessing for child abuse.*)

PUSTULAR RASH

A pustular rash is made up of crops of pustules — vesicles and bullae that fill with purulent exudate. These lesions vary greatly in size and shape and can be generalized or localized to the hair follicles or sweat glands. (See *Recognizing common skin lesions,* page 444.) Pustules can result from skin or systemic disorders, the use of certain drugs, or exposure to skin irritants. For example, people who have been swimming in salt water commonly develop a papulopustular rash under the bathing suit or elsewhere on the body from irritation by sea organisms. Although many pustular lesions are sterile, a pustular rash usually indicates infection. Any vesicular eruption, or even acute contact dermatitis, can become pustular if secondary infection occurs.

History and physical examination

Have the patient describe the appearance, location, and onset of the first pustular lesion. Did another type of skin lesion precede the pustule? Find out how the lesions spread. Ask what medications the patient takes and if he has applied topical medication to his rash. If so, what type and when did he last apply it? Find out if he has a family history of skin disorders. Examine the entire skin surface, noting if it's dry, oily, moist, or greasy. Record the exact location and distribution of the skin lesions and their color, shape, and size.

Medical causes

♦ ***Acne vulgaris.*** Pustules typify inflammatory lesions of this disorder, which is accompanied by papules, nodules, cysts, and open comedones (black heads). Lesions commonly appear on the face, shoulders, back, and chest. Other findings may include pain on pressure, pruritus, and burning. Chronic recurrent lesions cause scars.

♦ ***Blastomycosis.*** This fungal infection causes small, painless, nonpruritic macules or papules that can enlarge to well-circumscribed, verrucous, crusted, or ulcerated lesions edged by pustules. Localized infection may cause only one lesion; systemic infection may cause many lesions on the hands, feet, face, and wrists. Blastomycosis also causes signs of pulmonary infection, such as pleuritic chest pain and a dry, hacking or productive cough with occasional hemoptysis.

♦ ***Folliculitis.*** This bacterial infection of hair follicles causes individual pustules, each pierced by a hair and possibly accompanied by pruritus. "Hot-tub" folliculitis causes pustules on areas covered by a bathing suit.

♦ ***Furunculosis.*** Crops of furuncles (purulent skin lesions involving hair follicles and sebaceous glands) typify this disorder. Furuncles usually begin as small, tender red pustules at the base of hair follicles. They're likely to occur on the face, neck, forearm, groin, axillae buttocks, or legs and to cause local pain, swelling, and redness. The pustules usually remain tense for 2 to 4 days and then become fluctuant. Rupture discharges pus and necrotic material. Then pain subsides but erythema and edema may persist.

♦ ***Impetigo contagiosa.*** This vesiculopustular eruptive disorder, which occurs in nonbullous and bullous forms, is usually caused by streptococci or staphylococci. Vesicles form and break, and exudate dries to form a crust: a thick, yellow crust in streptococcal impetigo and a thin, clear crust in staphylococcal impetigo. Both forms usually cause painless itching.

♦ ***Pompholyx.*** This common recurrent disorder characteristically causes symmetrical vesicular lesions that can become pustular. The lesions appear on the palms and, less commonly, on the soles and may be accompanied by minimal erythema and recurrent pruritus.

♦ ***Pustular miliaria.*** This anhidrotic disorder causes pustular lesions that begin as tiny erythematous papulovesicles at sweat pores. Diffuse erythema may radiate from the lesion. The rash and associated burning and pruritus worsen with sweating.

♦ ***Pustular psoriasis.*** Small vesicles form and eventually become pustules in this disorder. The patient may report pruritus, burning, and pain. Localized pustular psoriasis usually affects the hands and feet. Generalized pustular psoriasis may erupt suddenly in patients with psoriasis, psoriatic arthritis, or exfoliative psoriasis; although rare, this form of psoriasis occasionally is fatal.

♦ ***Rosacea.*** This chronic hyperemic disorder commonly causes telangiectasia with acute episodes of pustules, papules, and edema. Characterized by persistent erythema, rosacea may begin as a flush covering the forehead, malar region, nose, and chin. Intermittent episodes gradually become more persistent, and the skin — instead of returning to its normal color — develops varying degrees of erythema.

♦ ***Scabies.*** Threadlike channels or burrows under the skin characterize this disorder, which can also cause pustules, vesicles, and excoriations. The lesions are a few millimeters long, and a swollen nodule or red papule contains the itch mite. In men, crusted lesions commonly develop on the glans, shaft, or scrotum. In women, lesions may form on the nipples. Lesions also may develop on wrists, elbows, axillae, or waist. Related pruritus worsens with inactivity and warmth.

Other causes

♦ ***Drugs.*** Bromides and iodides commonly cause a pustular rash. Other drug causes include corticotropin, corticosteroids, dactinomycin, trimethadione, lithium, phenytoin, phenobarbital, isoniazid, oral contraceptives, androgens, or anabolic steroids.

Special considerations

Observe wound and skin isolation procedures until infection is ruled out by a Gram stain or culture and sensitivity test of the pustule's contents. If the organism is infectious, don't allow drainage to touch unaffected skin. Instruct the patient to keep his toilet articles and linens separate from those of other family members. Associated pain and itching, altered body image, and the stress of isolation may result in loss of sleep, anxiety, and depression. Give medications to relieve pain and itching, and encourage the patient to express his feelings.

Pediatric pointers

Among the various disorders that cause pustular rash in children are varicella, erythema toxicum neonatorum, candidiasis, impetigo, infantile acropustulosis, or acrodermatitis enteropathica.

R

RACCOON EYES

Raccoon eyes are bilateral periorbital ecchymoses that don't result from facial soft-tissue trauma. Usually an indicator of basilar skull fracture, this sign develops when damage at the time of fracture tears the meninges and causes the venous sinuses to bleed into the arachnoid villi and the cranial sinuses. Raccoon eyes may be the only indicator of a basilar skull fracture, which isn't always visible on skull X-rays. Their appearance signals the need for careful assessment to detect underlying trauma because a basilar skull fracture can injure cranial nerves, blood vessels, and the brain stem. Raccoon eyes can also occur after a craniotomy if the surgery causes a meningeal tear.

History and physical examination

After you detect raccoon eyes, check the patient's vital signs and try to find out when the head injury occurred. (See *Recognizing raccoon eyes,* page 510.) Then evaluate the extent of underlying trauma.

Start by evaluating the patient's level of consciousness (LOC) using the Glasgow Coma Scale. (See *Glasgow Coma Scale,* page 354.) Next, evaluate function of the cranial nerves (CN), especially the CN I (olfactory), CN III (oculomotor), CN IV (trochlear), CN VI (abducens), and CN VII (facial). If the patient's condition permits, also test his visual acuity and gross hearing. Note irregularities in the facial or skull bones, as well as swelling, localized pain, or lacerations of the face and scalp. Check for ecchymoses over the mastoid bone. Inspect the nose and ears for hemorrhage or cerebrospinal fluid (CSF) leakage.

Common medical causes

♦ ***Basilar skull fracture.*** This injury causes raccoon eyes after a head trauma that doesn't involve the orbital area. Associated signs and symptoms vary with the fracture site and may include pharyngeal hemorrhage, epistaxis, rhinorrhea, otorrhea, or a bulging tympanic membrane from blood or CSF. The patient may experience difficulty hearing, headache, nausea, vomiting, cranial nerve palsies, or altered LOC. He may also exhibit a positive Battle's sign.

Other causes

♦ ***Surgery.*** Raccoon eyes occurring after craniotomy may indicate a meningeal tear and bleeding into the sinuses.

Special considerations

Keep the patient on complete bed rest. Perform a neurologic evaluation every hour to reevaluate his LOC. Also, check vital signs hourly; be alert for such changes as bradypnea, bradycardia, hypertension, and fever. To avoid worsening a dural tear, instruct the patient not to blow his nose, cough vigorously, or strain. If otorrhea or rhinorrhea is pre-

Recognizing raccoon eyes

It's usually easy to differentiate raccoon eyes from the "black eyes" associated with facial trauma. Raccoon eyes (shown here) are always bilateral. They develop 2 to 3 days after a closed-head injury that causes basilar skull fracture. In contrast, the periorbital ecchymoses that occur with facial trauma may affect only one eye or both and usually develop within hours of injury.

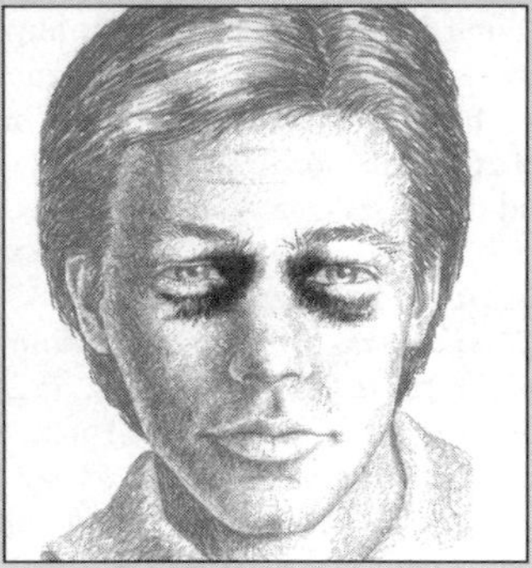

sent, don't attempt to stop the flow. Instead, place a sterile, loose gauze pad under the nose or ear to absorb the drainage. Monitor the amount, check for the halo sign (bluish coloring around the drainage) and test the drainage for glucose to confirm or rule out CSF leakage.

To prevent infection and further tearing of the mucous membranes, never suction or pass a nasogastric tube through the patient's nose. Observe the patient for signs and symptoms of meningitis, such as fever and nuchal rigidity, and expect to administer prophylactic antibiotics.

Prepare the patient for diagnostic tests, such as skull X-ray and, possibly, a computed tomography scan. If the dural tear doesn't heal spontaneously, contrast cisternography to locate the tear may be performed and, possibly, followed by corrective surgery.

Pediatric pointers

Raccoon eyes in children are most commonly caused by a basilar skull fracture from a fall.

REBOUND TENDERNESS

[Blumberg's sign]

A reliable indicator of peritonitis, rebound tenderness is intense, elicited abdominal pain caused by rebound of palpated tissue. (See *Eliciting rebound tenderness.*) The tenderness may be localized, as in an abscess, or generalized, as in perforation of an intra-abdominal organ. Rebound tenderness usually accompanies abdominal pain, tenderness, and rigidity. When a patient has sudden, severe abdominal pain, this sign is usually elicited to detect peritoneal inflammation.

Emergency interventions

If you elicit rebound tenderness in a patient who's experiencing constant, severe abdominal pain, quickly take his vital signs. Insert a large-bore I.V. catheter, and begin administering I.V. fluids. Also insert an indwelling urinary catheter, and monitor intake and output. Give supplemental oxygen as needed, and continue to monitor the patient for signs of shock, such as hypotension and tachycardia.

History and physical examination

If the patient's condition permits, ask him to describe the events that led up to the tenderness. Does movement, exertion, or other activity relieve or aggravate the tenderness? Also, ask about other signs and symptoms, such as nausea and vomiting, fever, or abdominal bloat-

EXAMINATION TIP

Eliciting rebound tenderness

To elicit rebound tenderness, place the patient in a supine position, and push your fingers deeply and steadily into his abdomen (as shown). Then, quickly release the pressure. Pain that results from the rebound of palpated tissue—rebound tenderness—indicates peritoneal inflammation or peritonitis.

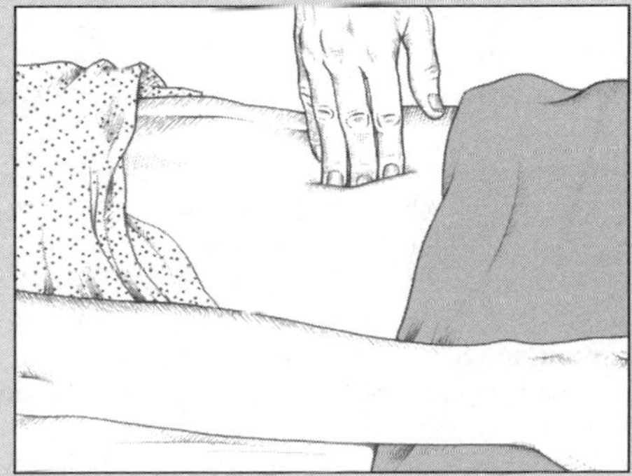

You can also elicit this symptom on a miniature scale by percussing the patient's abdomen lightly and indirectly (as shown). Better still, ask the patient to cough. This allows you to elicit rebound tenderness without having to touch the patient's abdomen and may also increase his cooperation because he won't associate exacerbation of his pain with your actions.

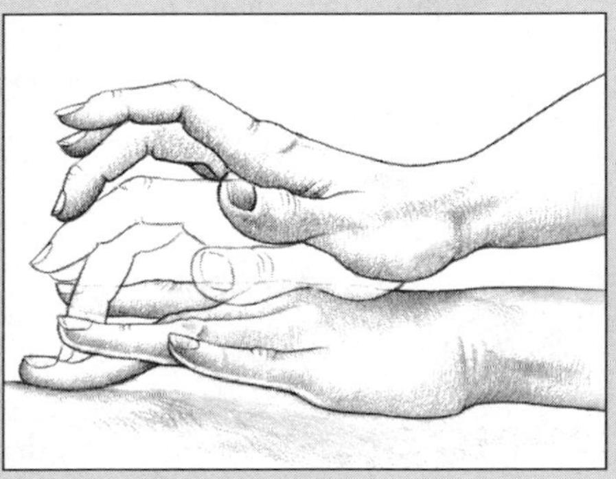

ing or distention. Inspect the abdomen for distention, visible peristaltic waves, and scars. Then auscultate for bowel sounds and characterize their motility. Finally, palpate for associated rigidity or guarding.

Common medical causes

♦ ***Peritonitis.*** In this life-threatening disorder, rebound tenderness is accompanied by sudden and severe abdominal pain, which may be either diffuse or localized. Because movement worsens the patient's pain, he'll usually lie still. Typically, he'll display weakness, pallor, excessive sweating, and cold skin. He may also display hypoactive or absent bowel sounds; tachypnea; nausea and vomiting; abdominal distention, rigidity, and guarding; positive psoas and obturator signs; or a fever of 103° F (39.4° C) or higher. Inflammation of the diaphragmatic peritoneum may cause shoulder pain and hiccups.

Special considerations

Promote comfort by having the patient flex his knees or assume semi-Fowler's position. Be sure to administer analgesics carefully because these drugs could mask associated symptoms. You may administer antiemetics and antipyretics; however, because of decreased intestinal motility and the probability that the patient will have surgery, don't give oral drugs or fluids. Obtain samples of blood, urine, and feces for laboratory testing, and prepare the patient for chest and abdominal X-rays, sonograms, and computed tomography scans. Perform a rectal or pelvic examination.

Pediatric pointers

Eliciting rebound tenderness may be difficult in young children. Be alert for such clues as an anguished facial expression or intensified crying. When you elicit this symptom, use assessment techniques that cause minimal tenderness. For example, have the child hop or jump to allow tissue to rebound gently, and notice if the child clutches at the furniture in pain.

Geriatric pointers

Rebound tenderness may be diminished or absent in the elderly.

RESPIRATIONS, SHALLOW

Respirations are shallow when a diminished volume of air enters the lungs during inspiration. In an effort to obtain enough air, the patient with shallow respirations usually breathes at an accelerated rate. However, as he tires or as his muscles weaken, this compensatory increase diminishes, leading to inadequate gas exchange and such signs as dyspnea, cyanosis, confusion, agitation, loss of consciousness, or tachycardia.

Shallow respirations may develop suddenly or gradually and may last briefly or become chronic. They're a key sign of respiratory distress and neurologic deterioration. Causes include inadequate central respiratory control over breathing, neuromuscular disorders, increased resistance to airflow into the lungs, respiratory muscle fatigue or weakness, voluntary alterations in breathing, and decreased activity from prolonged bed rest.

Emergency interventions

If you observe shallow respirations, be alert for impending respiratory failure or arrest. Is the patient severely dyspneic? Agitated or frightened? Look for signs of airway obstruction. If the patient is choking, perform a series of four back blows, then four abdominal thrusts, to try to expel the foreign object. Use suction if secretions occlude the patient's airway.

If the patient is also wheezing, check for stridor, nasal flaring, and use of accessory muscles. Administer oxygen with a face mask or a handheld resuscitation bag. Attempt to calm the patient.

If the patient loses consciousness, insert an artificial airway and prepare for endotracheal intubation and ventilatory support. Measure his tidal volume and minute volume to determine the need for mechanical ventilation. (See *Measuring lung volumes*.) Check arterial blood gas (ABG) levels, heart rate, and blood pressure. Tachycardia, increased or decreased blood pressure, small minute volume, and deteriorating ABG levels signal the need for intubation and mechanical ventilation.

History and physical examination

If the patient isn't in severe respiratory distress, begin with the history. Ask about chronic illness and surgery or trauma. Has he had a tetanus booster in the past 10 years? Does he have asthma, allergies, or a history of heart failure or vascular disease? Does he have chronic respiratory disorders or infections, or neurologic or neuromuscular disease? Does he smoke? Obtain a medication history and explore the possibility of drug abuse.

Begin the physical examination by assessing the patient's level of consciousness (LOC) and his orientation to time, place, and person. Observe spontaneous movements, and test muscle strength and

EXAMINATION TIP

Measuring lung volumes

Use a Wright respirometer to measure tidal volume (the amount of air inspired with each breath) and minute volume (the volume of air inspired in a minute—or tidal volume multiplied by respiratory rate). You can connect the respirometer to an intubated patients' airway via an endotracheal tube (as shown) or a tracheostomy tube. If the patient isn't intubated, connect the respirometer to a face mask, making sure the seal over the patient's mouth and nose is airtight.

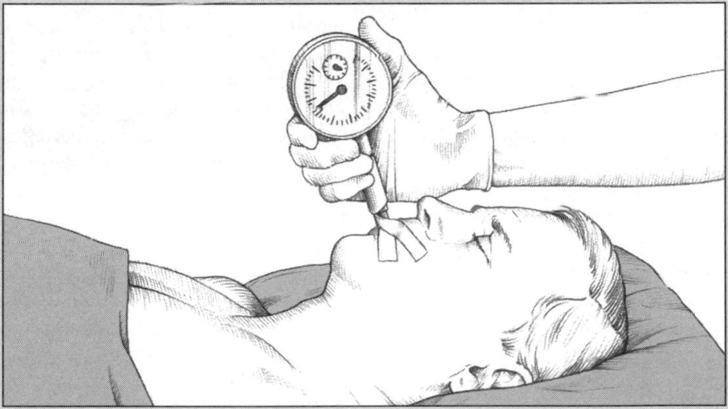

deep tendon reflexes. Next, inspect the chest for deformities and abnormal movements such as intercostal retractions. Inspect the extremities for cyanosis and digital clubbing.

Now, palpate chest expansion and percuss for hyperresonance or dullness. Diaphragmatic chest wall movement is diminished in shallow breathing. Auscultate for diminished, absent, or adventitious breath sounds and for abnormal or distant heart sounds. Do you note peripheral edema? Finally, examine the abdomen for distention, tenderness, and masses.

Common medical causes

◆ ***Adult respiratory distress syndrome.*** Initially, this life-threatening syndrome causes rapid, shallow respirations and dyspnea. Hypoxemia leads to intercostal and suprasternal retractions, diaphoresis, and fluid accumulation, causing rhonchi and crackles. As hypoxemia worsens, the patient exhibits increased breathing difficulty, restlessness, apprehension, decreased LOC, cyanosis, and possibly tachycardia.

◆ ***Amyotrophic lateral sclerosis (ALS).*** Respiratory muscle weakness in this disorder causes progressive shallow respirations. Exertion may result in increased weakness and respiratory distress. ALS initially causes upper extremity muscle weakness and wasting that, within several years, affect the trunk, neck, tongue, and muscles of the larynx, pharynx, and lower extremities. Associated signs and symptoms include muscle cramps and atrophy, hyperreflexia, slight spasticity of the legs, coarse fasciculations of the affected muscle, impaired speech, increased salivation, and difficulty chewing and swallowing.

◆ ***Asthma.*** In this disorder, bronchospasm and hyperinflation of the lungs cause rapid, shallow respirations. In adults, mild persistent signs and symptoms may worsen during severe attacks. Related respiratory effects include wheezing, rhonchi, a dry cough, dyspnea, prolonged expirations, intercostal and supraclavicular retractions on inspiration, nasal flaring, or use of accessory muscles. Chest tightness, tachycardia, and diaphoresis may occur.

◆ ***Atelectasis.*** In this disorder, alveolar collapse and decreased lung expansion cause rapid shallow respirations. Other possible signs and symptoms include a dry cough, dyspnea, tachycardia, anxiety, cyanosis, or diaphoresis. Examination reveals dullness to percussion, decreased breath sounds and vocal fremitus, inspiratory lag, and substernal or intercostal retractions.

◆ ***Bronchiectasis.*** Increased secretions obstruct airflow in the lungs, leading to shallow respirations and a productive cough with copious, foul-smelling, mucopurulent sputum (a classic finding). Other findings include hemoptysis, wheezing, rhonchi, coarse crackles during inspiration, or late-stage clubbing. The patient may complain of weight loss, fatigue, weakness and dyspnea on exertion, fever, malaise, or halitosis.

◆ ***Coma.*** Rapid, shallow respirations result from neurologic dysfunction or restricted chest movement.

◆ ***Emphysema.*** Increased breathing effort causes muscle fatigue, leading to chronic shallow respirations. The patient may also display dyspnea, anorexia, malaise, tachypnea, diminished breath sounds, pursed-lip breathing, accessory muscle use, or barrel chest.

◆ ***Flail chest.*** In this disorder, disruption of the integrity of the chest wall results in rapid, shallow respirations, paradoxical chest wall motion from rib instability, tachycardia, hypotension, ecchymoses, cyanosis, and pain over the affected area.

◆ ***Guillain-Barré syndrome.*** Progressive ascending paralysis causes rapid or progressive onset of shallow respirations. Muscle weakness begins in the lower limbs and extends finally to the face. Associated findings include inability to take a deep breath, paresthesia, dysarthria, diminished or absent corneal reflex, nasal speech, dysphagia, ipsilateral loss of facial muscle control, or flaccid paralysis.

◆ ***Multiple sclerosis.*** Muscle weakness causes progressive shallow respirations. Early features may include diplopia, blurred vision, or paresthesia. Other possible findings are nystagmus, constipation, paralysis, spasticity, hyperreflexia, intention tremor, ataxic gait, dysphagia, dysarthria, urinary dysfunction, impotence, or emotional lability.

◆ ***Myasthenia gravis.*** Progression of this disorder causes respiratory muscle weakness marked by shallow respirations, dyspnea, and cyanosis. Other effects include fatigue, weak eye closure, ptosis, diplopia, or difficulty chewing and swallowing.

◆ ***Pleural effusion.*** In this disorder, restricted lung expansion causes shallow respirations, beginning suddenly or gradually. Other findings include nonproductive cough, weight loss, dyspnea, and pleuritic chest pain. Examination reveals tachycardia, tachypnea, decreased chest motion, flatness to percussion, egophony, decreased or absent breath sounds, or decreased tactile fremitus.

◆ ***Pneumothorax.*** This disorder causes sudden onset of shallow respirations and dyspnea. Related effects are tachycardia; tachypnea; sudden, sharp, severe chest pain (commonly unilateral) worsening with movement; nonproductive cough; accessory muscle use; asymmetrical chest expansion; anxiety; restlessness; hyperresonance or tympany on the affected side; subcutaneous crepitation; decreased vocal fremitus; or diminished or absent breath sounds on the affected side.

◆ ***Pulmonary edema.*** Pulmonary vascular congestion causes rapid, shallow respirations. Early signs and symptoms include dyspnea on exertion, paroxysmal nocturnal dyspnea, and a nonproductive cough. Clinical features also include tachycardia, tachypnea, dependent crackles, and a ventricular gallop. Severe pulmonary edema causes more rapid and labored respirations; widespread crackles; a productive cough with frothy, bloody sputum; worsening tachycardia; arrhythmias; cold, clammy skin; cyanosis; hypotension; or thready pulse.

♦ ***Pulmonary embolism.*** This disorder causes sudden, rapid, shallow respirations and severe dyspnea with anginal or pleuritic chest pain. Other clinical features include tachycardia, tachypnea, a nonproductive cough or a productive cough with blood-tinged sputum, low-grade fever, restlessness, diaphoresis, pleural friction rub, crackles, diffuse wheezing, dullness to percussion, decreased breath sounds, or signs of circulatory collapse. Less common are massive hemoptysis, chest splinting, leg edema, and (with a large embolus) cyanosis, syncope, and distended neck veins.

Other causes

♦ ***Drugs.*** Narcotics, sedatives and hypnotics, tranquilizers, neuromuscular blockers, magnesium sulfate, and anesthetics can cause slow, shallow respirations.

♦ ***Surgery.*** After abdominal or thoracic surgery, pain associated with chest splinting and decreased chest wall motion may cause shallow respirations.

Special considerations

Prepare the patient for diagnostic tests: ABG analysis, pulmonary function tests, chest X-rays, or bronchoscopy.

Position the patient as nearly upright as possible to ease his breathing. Encourage deep breathing and coughing. (Help a postoperative patient splint his incision while coughing.) If he's taking a drug that depresses respirations, follow all precautions, and monitor him closely. Ensure adequate hydration, and use humidification as needed to thin secretions and to relieve inflamed, dry, or irritated airway mucosa. Administer humidified oxygen, bronchodilators, mucolytics, expectorants, or antibiotics.

Turn the patient frequently. He may require chest physiotherapy, incentive spirometry, or intermittent positive-pressure breathing. Monitor for increasing lethargy, which may indicate rising CO_2 levels.

Pediatric pointers

In children, shallow respirations commonly indicate a life-threatening condition. Airway obstruction can occur rapidly; if it does, administer back blows or chest thrusts but not abdominal thrusts, which can damage internal organs.

Possible causes of shallow respirations in infants and children include idiopathic (infant) respiratory distress syndrome, acute epiglottiditis, diphtheria, aspiration of a foreign body, croup, acute bronchiolitis, cystic fibrosis, or bacterial pneumonia.

Observe the child to detect apnea. As needed, use humidification and suction, and administer supplemental oxygen. Give parenteral fluids to ensure adequate hydration. Chest physiotherapy may be required.

Geriatric pointers

Stiffness or deformity of the chest wall associated with aging may cause shallow respirations.

RESPIRATIONS, STERTOROUS

Characterized by a harsh, rattling, or snoring sound, stertorous respirations usually result from the vibration of relaxed oropharyngeal structures during sleep or coma, causing partial airway obstruction. Less commonly, these sounds result from retained mucus in the upper airway.

This common sign occurs in about 10% of normal individuals, especially middle-age, obese men. It may be aggravated by use of alcohol or sedatives before bed, which increases oropharyngeal flaccidity, or by sleeping in the supine position, which allows the relaxed tongue to slip back into the airway. The major pathologic causes of stertorous respirations are obstructive sleep apnea and life-threatening upper airway obstruction associated with an oropharyngeal tumor or with uvular or palatal edema. This obstruction may also occur during the postictal phase of a generalized seizure, when mucus or a relaxed tongue blocks the airway.

Occasionally, stertorous respirations are mistaken for stridor, another sign of upper airway obstruction. However, stridor indicates laryngeal or tracheal obstruction, whereas stertorous respirations signal higher airway obstruction.

History and physical examination

If you detect stertorous respirations, awaken the patient. If the stertorous respirations disappear when the patient awakens, allow him to return to sleep. Observe his breathing pattern for 3 to 4 minutes. Do noisy respirations cease when he turns on his side and recur when he assumes a supine position? Watch carefully for periods of apnea and note their length. When possible, question the patient's partner about his snoring habits. Is she frequently awakened by the patient's snoring? Has she also observed the patient talking in his sleep or sleepwalking? Ask about signs of sleep deprivation, such as personality changes, headaches, daytime somnolence, or decreased mental acuity.

Emergency interventions

If the stertorous breathing doesn't cease when the patient is awake, or if you can't awaken the patient, check the patient's mouth and throat for edema, redness, secretions, or masses. If edema is marked, quickly take vital signs. Observe for signs and symptoms of respiratory distress, such as dyspnea, tachypnea, use of accessory muscles, intercostal muscle retractions, and cyanosis. Elevate the head of the bed 30 degrees to help ease breathing and reduce the edema. Then administer supplemental oxygen by nasal cannula or face mask, and prepare to intubate the patient, perform a tracheostomy, or provide mechanical ventilation. Suction the patient's airway if secretions are causing an obstruction. Insert an I.V. line for fluid and drug access, and begin cardiac monitoring.

Common medical causes

◆ ***Airway obstruction.*** Regardless of its cause, partial airway obstruction may lead to stertorous respirations accompanied by wheezing, dyspnea, tachypnea and, later, intercostal retractions and nasal flaring. If the obstruction becomes complete, the patient abruptly becomes unable to talk and displays diaphoresis, tachycardia, and inspiratory chest movement but absent breath sounds. Severe hypoxemia rapidly ensues, resulting in cyanosis, loss of consciousness, and cardiopulmonary collapse.

◆ ***Obstructive sleep apnea.*** Loud and disruptive snoring is a major characteristic of this syndrome, which commonly affects the obese. Typically, the snoring alternates with periods of sleep apnea, which usually end with loud gasping sounds. Alternating tachycardia and bradycardia may occur.

Episodes of snoring and apnea recur in a cyclic pattern throughout the night. Sleep disturbances, such as somnambulism and talking during sleep, may also occur. Some patients display hypertension and ankle edema. Most awaken in the morning with a generalized headache, feeling tired and unrefreshed. The most common complaint is excessive daytime sleepiness. Lack of sleep may cause depression, hostility, and decreased mental acuity.

Other causes

♦ ***Endotracheal surgery, intubation, or suction.*** These procedures may cause significant palatal or uvular edema, resulting in stertorous respirations.

Special considerations

If airway obstruction is the cause of stertorous breathing, continue to monitor the patient's respiratory status carefully. Administer corticosteroids or antibiotics and cool, humidified oxygen to reduce palatal and uvular inflammation and edema. Laryngoscopy and bronchoscopy (to rule out airway obstruction) or formal sleep studies may be necessary.

Pediatric pointers

In children, the most common cause of stertorous respirations is nasal or pharyngeal obstruction secondary to tonsillar or adenoid hypertrophy or the presence of a foreign body.

Geriatric pointers

Encourage the patient to seek treatment for sleep apnea or significant hypertrophy of the tonsils or adenoids.

RETRACTIONS, COSTAL AND STERNAL

A cardinal sign of respiratory distress in infants and children (although retractions may occur at any age), retractions are visible indentations of the soft tissue covering the chest wall. They may be suprasternal (directly above the sternum and clavicles), intercostal (between the ribs), subcostal (below the lower costal margin of the rib cage), or substernal (just below the xiphoid process). Retractions are usually static and may be mild or severe, producing barely visible to deep indentations.

Normally, infants and young children use abdominal muscles for breathing, unlike older children and adults, who use the diaphragm. When breathing requires extra effort, accessory muscles assist respiration, especially inspiration. Retractions typically accompany accessory muscle use.

Emergency interventions

If you detect retractions in a child, check quickly for other signs of respiratory distress, such as cyanosis, tachypnea, and tachycardia. Also, prepare the child for suctioning, insertion of an artificial airway, and administration of oxygen.

Observe the depth and location of retractions. Also, note the rate, depth, and quality of respirations. Look for accessory muscle use, nasal flaring during inspiration, or grunting during expiration. If the child has a cough, record the color, consistency, and odor of sputum. Note whether the child appears restless or lethargic. Finally, auscultate the child's lungs to detect abnormal breath sounds. (See *Observing retractions,* page 518.)

History and physical examination

If the child's condition permits, ask his parents about his medical history. Was he born prematurely? Was the delivery complicated? Ask about recent signs of an upper respiratory infection, such as a runny nose, cough, and a low-grade fever. How often has the child had respiratory problems during the past year? Has he been in contact with anyone who has had a cold, the flu, or other respiratory ailments? Did he aspirate food, liquid, or a foreign body? Inquire about personal or family history of allergies or asthma. Also, when examining a child, know that crying may accentuate the retractions.

Common medical causes

♦ ***Asthma attack.*** Intercostal and suprasternal retractions may accompany an asthma attack. They're preceded by dyspnea, wheezing, a hacking cough, and

EXAMINATION TIP

Observing retractions

When you observe retractions in infants and children, be sure to note their exact location — an important clue to the cause and severity of respiratory distress. For example, subcostal and substernal retractions usually result from lower respiratory tract disorders, whereas suprasternal retractions usually result from upper respiratory tract disorders.

Mild intercostal retractions alone may be normal. However, intercostal retractions accompanied by subcostal and substernal retractions may indicate moderate respiratory distress. Deep suprasternal retractions typically indicate severe distress.

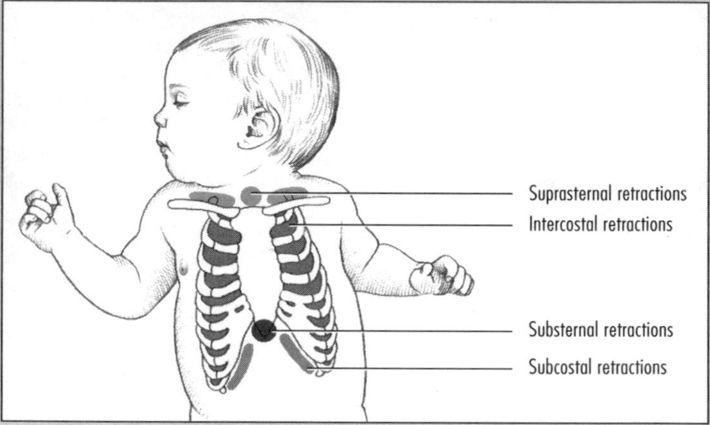

pallor. Related features may include cyanosis or flushing, crackles, rhonchi, diaphoresis, tachycardia, tachypnea, a frightened or anxious expression and, in severe distress, nasal flaring.

♦ ***Epiglottiditis.*** This life-threatening bacterial infection may precipitate severe respiratory distress with suprasternal, substernal, or intercostal retractions; stridor; nasal flaring; cyanosis; and tachycardia. Early features include sudden onset of a barking cough and high fever, sore throat, hoarseness, dysphagia, drooling, dyspnea, or restlessness. The child becomes panicky as edema makes breathing difficult. Total airway occlusion may occur in 2 to 5 hours.

♦ ***Heart failure.*** Usually linked to a congenital heart defect in children, this disorder may cause intercostal and substernal retractions along with nasal flaring, progressive tachypnea, and — in severe respiratory distress — grunting respirations, edema, and cyanosis. Other findings may include productive cough, crackles, jugular vein distention, tachycardia, right-upper-quadrant pain, anorexia, or fatigue.

♦ ***Laryngotracheobronchitis (acute).*** In this viral infection, substernal and intercostal retractions typically follow a low to moderate fever, runny nose, poor appetite, a barking cough, hoarseness, and inspiratory stridor. Associated signs and symptoms may include tachycardia; shallow, rapid respirations; restlessness; irritability; or pale, cyanotic skin.

♦ ***Pneumonia (bacterial).*** This disorder begins with signs of acute infection — such as high fever and lethargy — followed by subcostal and intercostal retractions, nasal flaring, dyspnea, tachypnea, grunting respirations, cyanosis, and a productive cough. Auscultation may reveal diminished breath sounds, scattered crackles, or sibilant rhonchi over the affected lung. GI effects may include vomiting, diarrhea, or abdominal distention.

♦ ***Respiratory distress syndrome.*** Substernal and subcostal retractions are an early sign of this life-threatening syndrome, which affects premature infants shortly after birth. Associated early signs include tachypnea, tachycardia, and expiratory grunting. As respiratory distress worsens, intercostal and suprasternal retractions typically occur, and apnea or irregular respirations replaces grunting. Other effects include nasal flaring, cyanosis, lethargy, and eventual unresponsiveness as well as bradycardia and hypotension. Auscultation may detect crackles over the lung bases on deep inspiration or harsh, diminished breath sounds. Oliguria or peripheral edema may occur.

Special considerations

Continue to monitor the child's vital signs. Keep suction equipment and an appropriate-sized airway at the bedside. Be prepared to administer oxygen. Perform chest physiotherapy with postural drainage to help mobilize and drain excess lung secretions. Bronchodilators and, occasionally, steroids may also be used. Prepare the child for chest X-rays, cultures, and arterial blood gas analysis. Explain the procedures to his parents, and have them calm and comfort the child.

Geriatric pointers

Although retractions may occur at any age, they're more difficult to assess in an older patient who is obese or who has chronic chest wall stiffness or deformity.

Rhinorrhea

Common but rarely serious, rhinorrhea is the free discharge of thin nasal mucus. It can be self-limiting or chronic, resulting from nasal, sinus, or systemic disorders or from a basilar skull fracture. Rhinorrhea can also result from sinus or cranial surgery, excessive use of vasoconstricting nose drops or sprays, or inhalation of an irritant, such as tobacco smoke, dust, or fumes. Depending on the cause, the discharge may be clear, purulent, bloody, or serosanguineous.

History and physical examination

Begin the history by asking the patient if the discharge runs from both nostrils. Is the discharge intermittent or persistent? Did it begin suddenly or gradually? Does the position of his head affect the discharge?

Next, ask the patient to characterize the discharge. Is it watery, bloody, purulent, or foul-smelling? Is it copious or scanty? Does the discharge worsen or improve with the time of day? In addition, find out if the patient is using any medications, especially nose drops or sprays. Has he been exposed to nasal irritants at home or at work? Has he had a recent head injury?

Examine the patient's nose, checking airflow from each nostril. Evaluate the size, color, and condition of the turbinate mucosa (normally pale pink). Note if the mucosa is red, unusually pale, blue, or gray. Then examine the area beneath each turbinate. (See *Using a nasal speculum*, page 520.) Be sure to palpate over the frontal, ethmoid, and maxillary sinuses for tenderness.

To differentiate nasal mucus from cerebrospinal fluid (CSF), collect a small amount of drainage on a glucose test strip. If CSF (which contains glucose) is present, the test will be positive. Finally, using a nonirritating substance, test for anosmia.

EXAMINATION TIP

Using a nasal speculum

To visualize the interior of the nares, you'll need a nasal speculum in the palm of one hand and the penlight in the other hand. Have the patient tilt her head back slightly and rest it against a wall or other firm support, if possible. Insert the speculum blades about ½" (1.3 cm) into the nasal vestibule, as shown. It's important to angle the speculum tip laterally toward the ear to avoid touching the extremely sensitive nasal septum.

Place your index finger on the tip of the patient's nose for stability. Carefully open the speculum blades. Shine the light source in the direction of the nares. Now, inspect the nares. The mucosa should be deep pink. Note discharge, lesions, masses, or mucosal swellings. Check the nasal septum for perforation, bleeding, or crusting. Bluish turbinates suggest allergy. A rounded, elongated projection suggests a polyp.

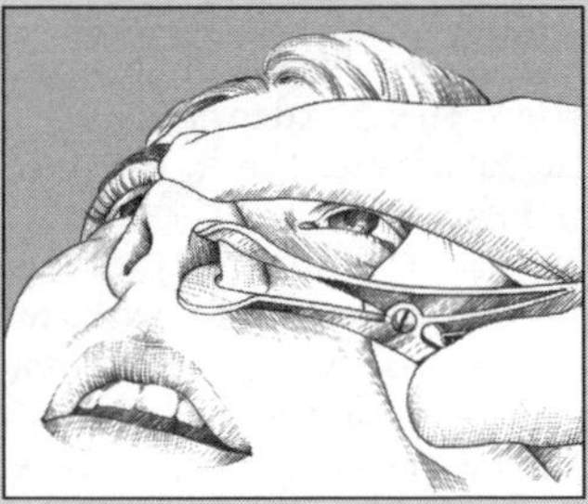

Common medical causes

♦ ***CSF rhinorrhea.*** The roof of the ethmoid and the cribriform plate are the most common trauma sites because bone is thin and the dura is tightly adhered to it in this area. Trauma to this area may cause rhinorrhea immediately or days to weeks later as the wound matures and contracts. Rhinorrhea from tumors and hydrocephalus occurs when increasing intracranial pressure erodes the bone leading to a fistula. Additional symptoms may include an increased flow or "rush of fluid" with forward tilting of the head, a diminished or absent sense of smell, headaches caused by intracranial air, and meningitis. Nontraumatic CSF rhinorrhea is insidious and is most common in females over the age of 30.

♦ ***Common cold.*** An initially watery nasal discharge may become thicker and mucopurulent. Related findings include sneezing, nasal congestion, a dry and hacking cough, sore throat, mouth breathing, or transient loss of smell and taste. In addition, the patient may experience malaise, fatigue, myalgia, arthralgia, a slight headache, dry lips, or a red upper lip and nose.

♦ ***Nasal or sinus tumors.*** Nasal tumors can produce an intermittent, unilateral bloody or serosanguineous discharge that may be purulent and foul smelling. Nasal congestion, postnasal drip, and headache may also occur. In advanced stages, paranasal sinus tumors may cause a cheek mass or eye displacement, facial paresthesia or pain, and nasal obstruction.

♦ ***Rhinitis.*** *Allergic rhinitis* produces an episodic, profuse, watery discharge. (A mucopurulent discharge indicates infection.) Typical associated signs and symptoms include increased lacrimation; nasal congestion; itchy eyes, nose, and throat; postnasal drip; recurrent sneezing; mouth breathing; impaired sense of smell; or frontal or temporal headache. In addition, the turbinates are pale and engorged; the mucosa, pale and boggy.

In *atrophic rhinitis,* the nasal discharge is scanty, purulent, and foul smelling. Nasal obstruction is common, and the crusts may bleed on removal. The mucosa is pale pink and shiny.

In *vasomotor rhinitis,* a profuse and watery nasal discharge accompanies chronic nasal obstruction, sneezing, recurrent postnasal drip, and pale, swollen turbinates. The nasal septum is pink; the mucosa, blue.

◆ ***Sinusitis.*** In acute *sinusitis,* a thick and purulent nasal discharge becomes a purulent postnasal drip that causes throat pain and halitosis. The patient may also experience nasal congestion, severe pain and tenderness over the involved sinuses, fever, headache, or malaise.

In *chronic sinusitis,* the nasal discharge is usually scanty, thick, and intermittently purulent. Nasal congestion and low-grade discomfort or pressure over the involved sinuses can be persistent or recurrent. The patient also may have a chronic sore throat or nasal polyps.

In *chronic fungal sinusitis,* the clinical picture resembles that of chronic bacterial sinusitis. However, some cases — especially in immunocompromised patients — may progress rapidly to exophthalmos, blindness, intracranial extension and, eventually, death.

Other causes

◆ ***Drugs.*** Nasal sprays or drops containing vasoconstrictors may cause rebound rhinorrhea if used longer than 4 to 5 days.

◆ ***Surgery.*** CSF rhinorrhea may occur after sinus or cranial surgery.

Special considerations

You may have to prepare the patient for X-rays of the sinuses or skull and a computed tomography scan. In addition, you may need to administer antihistamines, decongestants, analgesics, or antipyretics. Encourage fluid consumption to thin secretions.

Pregnancy causes physiologic changes that may aggravate rhinorrhea, resulting in eosinophilia and chronic irritable airways.

Pediatric pointers

Rhinorrhea in children may stem from choanal atresia, allergic or chronic rhinitis, acute ethmoiditis, or congenital syphilis. Assume that unilateral rhinorrhea with nasal obstruction is caused by a foreign body in the nose until proven otherwise.

Geriatric pointers

Elderly patients may experience increased adverse effects from medications used to treat rhinorrhea.

RHONCHI

Rhonchi are continuous adventitious breath sounds detected by auscultation. They're usually louder and lower-pitched than crackles — more like a hoarse moan or a deep snore — though they may be described as rattling, sonorous, bubbling, rumbling, or musical. Sibilant rhonchi, or wheezes, are high-pitched.

Rhonchi are heard over large airways, such as the trachea and major bronchial tubes. They occur in pulmonary disorders when air flows through passages that have been narrowed by secretions. The resulting vibration of airway walls produces the rhonchi.

History and physical examination

If you auscultate rhonchi, take the patient's vital signs and be alert for signs of respiratory distress. Characterize the patient's respirations as rapid or slow, shallow or deep, and regular or irregular. Inspect the chest, noting the use of accessory muscles. Is the patient audibly wheezing or gurgling? Auscultate for other abnormal breath sounds, such as crackles and a pleural friction rub. If you detect these sounds, note their location. Are breath sounds diminished or absent? Next, percuss the chest. If the patient has a cough, note its frequency and characterize its sound. If it's productive, examine the sputum for color, odor, consistency, and blood. Note whether the cough is effective in clearing secretions. Do rhonchi clear after coughing?

Ask related questions: Does the patient smoke? If so, obtain a history in pack-years. Has he recently lost weight or felt tired or weak? Does he have asthma or other pulmonary disorders? Is he currently taking prescribed or over-the-counter drugs?

During the examination, keep in mind that thick or excessive secretions, bronchospasm, or inflammation of mucous membranes may lead to airway obstruction. If necessary, suction the patient and keep equipment available for inserting an airway. Keep bronchodilators available to treat bronchospasm.

Common medical causes

♦ ***Asthma.*** An asthma attack typically causes rhonchi, crackles, and wheezing. Other features include apprehension, a dry cough that later becomes productive, prolonged expirations, or intercostal and supraclavicular retractions on inspiration. The patient may also exhibit increased accessory muscle use, nasal flaring, tachypnea, tachycardia, diaphoresis, or flushing or cyanosis.

♦ ***Bronchiectasis.*** This disorder causes lower-lobe rhonchi and crackles, which coughing may help relieve. Its classic sign is a cough that produces mucopurulent, foul-smelling, and possibly bloody sputum. Other findings include fever, weight loss, dyspnea on exertion, fatigue, malaise, halitosis, weakness, or late-stage clubbing.

♦ ***Bronchitis.*** *Acute tracheobronchitis* causes sonorous rhonchi and wheezing due to increased mucus in the airways and bronchospasm. Related findings include chills, sore throat, a low-grade fever of no more than 100° F (37.8° C) in severe illness, muscle and back pain, or substernal tightness. A cough becomes productive as secretions increase.

In *chronic bronchitis,* auscultation may reveal scattered rhonchi, coarse crackles, wheezing, and prolonged expirations. The chronic cough is productive. The patient also displays exertional dyspnea, increased accessory muscle use, barrel chest, cyanosis, tachypnea, and clubbing (a late sign).

♦ ***Pneumonia.*** Bacterial pneumonias can cause rhonchi and a dry cough that later becomes productive. Related signs and symptoms — shaking chills, high fever, myalgias, headache, pleuritic chest pain, tachypnea, tachycardia, dyspnea, cyanosis, diaphoresis, decreased breath sounds, fine crackles — develop suddenly.

♦ ***Pulmonary coccidioidomycosis.*** This disorder causes rhonchi and wheezing. Other features include a cough with fever, occasional chills, pleuritic chest pain, sore throat, headache, backache, malaise, marked weakness, anorexia, hemoptysis, or an itchy macular rash.

Other causes

♦ ***Diagnostic tests.*** Pulmonary function tests or bronchoscopy can loosen secretions and mucus, causing rhonchi.

♦ ***Respiratory therapy.*** This may cause rhonchi from loosened secretions and mucus.

Special considerations

To ease the patient's breathing, place him in semi-Fowler's position, and reposition him every 2 hours. Administer antibiotics, bronchodilators, and expectorants. Also, provide humidification to thin secretions, to relieve inflammation, and to prevent drying. Pulmonary physiotherapy with postural drainage and percussion can also help loosen secretions.

Prepare the patient for diagnostic tests, such as arterial blood gas analysis, pulmonary function studies, sputum analysis, or chest X-rays.

Pediatric pointers

Rhonchi in children can result from bacterial pneumonia, cystic fibrosis, or croup syndrome. Because a respiratory tract disorder may begin abruptly and progress rapidly in an infant or a child, observe closely for signs of airway obstruction.

S

Scotoma

A scotoma is an area of partial or complete blindness within an otherwise normal or slightly impaired visual field. Usually located within the central 30 degrees of the field, the defect ranges from absolute blindness to a barely detectable loss of visual acuity. Typically, the patient can pinpoint the scotoma's location in the visual field. (See *Locating scotomas,* page 524.)

A scotoma can result from retinal, choroid, or optic nerve disorders. A dense scotoma can also be a result of laser treatment near the fovea. A scotoma can be classified as absolute, relative, or scintillating. *Absolute scotoma* is a total inability to see all sizes of test objects used in mapping the visual field. *Relative scotoma* is an ability to see only large test objects. *Scintillating scotoma* is the flash or burst of light commonly seen during a migraine headache.

History and physical examination

First, identify and characterize the scotoma, using such visual field tests as the tangent screen examination, the Goldmann perimeter test, or the automated perimetry test. Two other visual field tests — confrontation testing and the Amsler chart — may also help you identify a scotoma.

Next, test the patient's visual acuity and inspect his pupils for size, equality, and reaction to light. An ophthalmoscopic examination and measurement of intraocular pressure (IOP) are necessary.

Explore the patient's history for eye disorders, vision problems, or chronic systemic disorders. Find out if he takes medications or uses eyedrops.

Common medical causes

♦ ***Chorioretinitis.*** Inflammation of the choroid causes a paracentral scotoma. Ophthalmoscopic examination reveals clouding and cells in the vitreous, subretinal hemorrhage, and neovascularization.

♦ ***Macular degeneration (and congenital macular disorders).*** Any degenerative process or disorder affecting the fovea centralis results in a central scotoma. Ophthalmoscopic examination reveals changes in the macular area. The patient may notice subtle changes in visual acuity, in color perception, and in the size and shape of objects.

♦ ***Optic neuritis.*** Inflammation, degeneration, or demyelination of the optic nerve causes a central, circular, or centrocecal scotoma. The scotoma may be unilateral if one nerve is involved or bilateral of both are affected. It can vary in size, density, and symmetry. The patient may report severe vision loss or blurring, lasting up to 3 weeks, and pain — especially with eye movement. Common ophthalmoscopic findings include hyperemia

Locating scotomas

Scotomas, or "blind spots," are classified according to the affected area of the visual field. The normal scotoma — shown in the temporal region of the right eye — appears in black in all the illustrations.

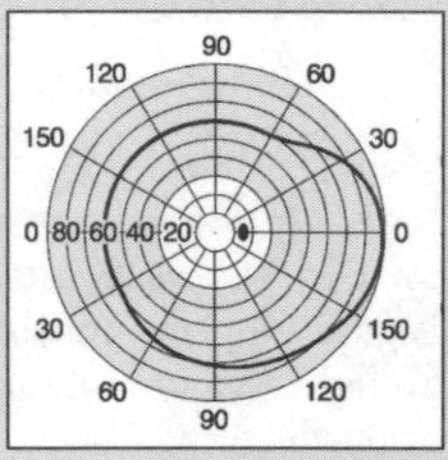

The *normally present scotoma* represents the position of the optic nerve head in the visual field. It appears between 10 and 20 degrees on this chart of the normal visual field.

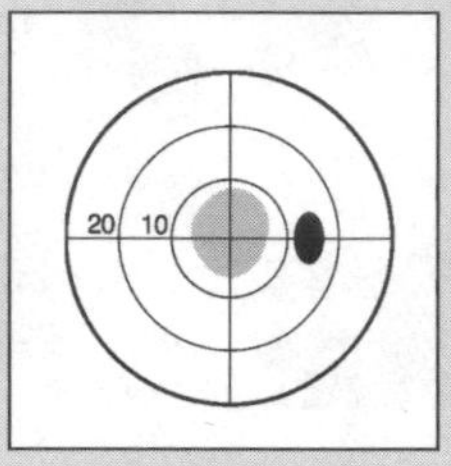

A *central scotoma* involves the point of central fixation. It's always associated with decreased visual acuity.

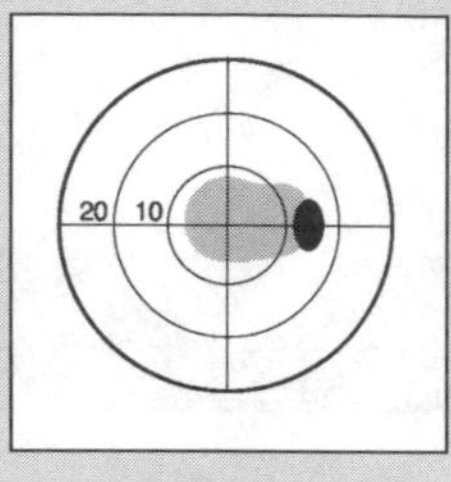

A *centrocecal scotoma* involves the point of central fixation and the area between the blind spot and the fixation point.

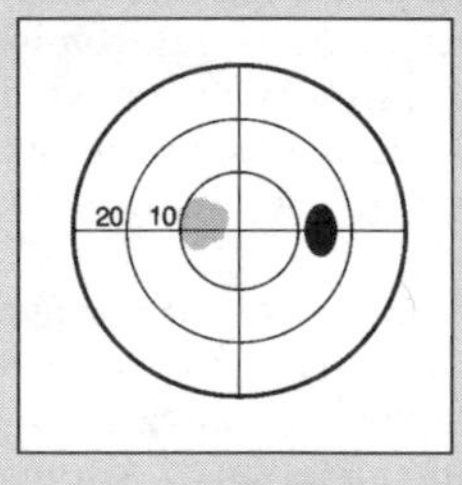

A *paracentral scotoma* affects an area of the visual field that's nasal or temporal to the point of central fixation.

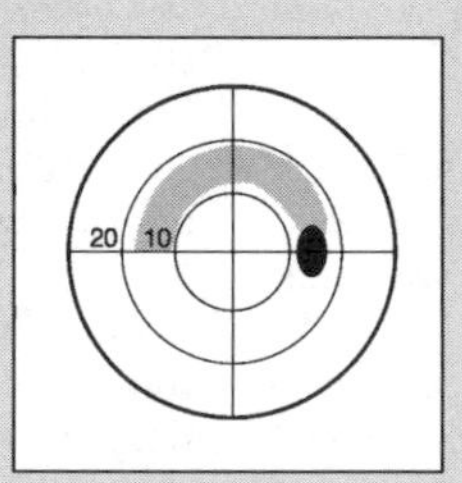

An *arcuate scotoma* arches around the fixation point, ending on the nasal side of the visual field.

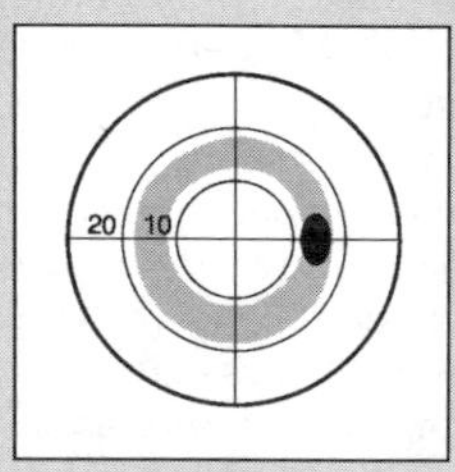

An *annular scotoma* forms a circular defect around the fixation point. It's common in retinal pigmentary degenerations.

of the optic disk, retinal vein distention, blurred disk margins, and filling of the physiologic cup.

♦ ***Retinal pigmentary degenerations.*** These disorders cause premature retinal cell changes leading to cell death. One of these disorders, *retinitis pigmentosa,* initially involves loss of peripheral rods; the resulting annular scotoma progresses concentrically until only a central field of vision (tunnel vision) remains. The earliest symptom — impaired night vision — appears during adolescence. Associated signs include narrowing of the retinal blood vessels and pallor of the optic disk. Eventually, with invasion of the macula, blindness may occur.

Special considerations

For the patient with an arcuate scotoma associated with glaucoma, emphasize regular testing of IOP and visual fields. In addition, teach the patient with a disorder involving the fovea centralis (or the area surrounding it) to periodically use the Amsler chart to detect progression of macular degeneration.

Pediatric pointers

In young children, visual field testing is difficult and requires patience. Confrontation testing is the method of choice.

SCROTAL SWELLING

Scrotal swelling occurs when a condition affecting the testicles, epididymis, or scrotal skin causes edema or a mass; the penis may or may not be involved. Scrotal swelling can affect males of any age. It can be unilateral or bilateral and painful or painless.

The sudden onset of painful scrotal swelling suggests torsion of a testicle or testicular appendages, especially in a prepubescent male. This emergency requires immediate surgery to untwist and stabilize the spermatic cord or to remove the appendage.

Emergency interventions

If severe pain accompanies scrotal swelling, ask when the swelling began. Using a Doppler stethoscope, evaluate blood flow to the testicle. If it's decreased or absent, suspect testicular torsion and prepare the patient for surgery. Withhold food and fluids, insert an I.V. line, and apply an ice pack to the scrotum and elevate it to reduce pain and swelling. An attempt may be made to untwist the cord manually, but even if this is successful, the patient may still require surgery for stabilization.

History and physical examination

If the patient isn't in distress, proceed with the history. Ask about injury to the scrotum, urethral discharge, cloudy urine, increased urinary frequency, and dysuria. Is the patient sexually active? When was his last sexual contact? Find out about recent illnesses, particularly mumps. Does he have a history of prostate surgery or prolonged catheterization? Does changing his body position or level of activity affect the swelling?

Take the patient's vital signs, noting especially fever, and palpate his abdomen for tenderness. Then examine the entire genital area. Assess the scrotum with the patient supine and standing. Note its size and color. Is the swelling unilateral or bilateral? Do you see signs of trauma or bruising? Gently palpate the scrotum for a cyst or a lump. Note especially tenderness or increased firmness. Check the testicles' position in the scrotum. Finally, transilluminate the scrotum to distinguish a fluid-filled cyst from a solid mass (which can't be transilluminated.)

Common medical causes

♦ ***Epididymal cysts.*** Located in the head of the epididymis, these cysts cause painless scrotal swelling.

♦ ***Epididymitis.*** Key features of inflammation are pain, extreme tenderness, and swelling in the groin and scrotum. The patient waddles to avoid pressure on the groin and scrotum during walking. He may have high fever, malaise, urethral discharge and cloudy urine, and lower abdominal pain on the affected side. His scrotal skin may be hot, red, dry, flaky, and thin.

♦ ***Hydrocele.*** Fluid accumulation causes gradual scrotal swelling that's usually painless. The scrotum may be soft and cystic or firm and tense. Palpation reveals a round, nontender scrotal mass.

♦ ***Idiopathic scrotal edema.*** Swelling occurs quickly in this disorder and usually disappears within 24 hours. The affected testicle is pink.

♦ ***Orchitis (acute).*** Mumps may precipitate this disorder, which causes sudden painful swelling of one or both testicles. Related findings include a hot, reddened scrotum, fever of up to 104° F (40° C), chills, lower abdominal pain, nausea, vomiting, and extreme weakness. Urinary signs are usually absent.

♦ ***Scrotal trauma.*** Blunt trauma causes scrotal swelling with bruising and severe pain. The scrotum may appear dark or bluish.

♦ ***Spermatocele.*** This painless or painful cystic mass lies above and behind the testicle and contains opaque fluid and sperm. Its onset may be acute or gradual. Less than 1 cm in diameter, it's movable and can be transilluminated.

♦ ***Testicular torsion.*** Most common before puberty, this urologic emergency causes scrotal swelling; sudden, severe pain; and, possibly, elevation of the affected testicle within the scrotum. It may also cause nausea and vomiting.

♦ ***Testicular tumor.*** Typically painless, smooth, and firm, a testicular tumor causes swelling and a sensation of excessive weight in the scrotum.

♦ ***Torsion of a hydatid of Morgagni.*** Torsion of this small, pea-sized cyst severs its blood supply, causing a hard, painful swelling on the testicle's upper pole.

Other causes

♦ ***Surgery.*** An effusion of blood from surgery can cause a hematocele, leading to scrotal swelling.

Special considerations

Keep the patient on bed rest and give antibiotics. Provide adequate fluids, fiber, and stool softeners. Place a rolled towel between the patient's legs and under the scrotum to help reduce severe swelling. Or, if the patient has mild or moderate swelling, advise him to wear a loose-fitting athletic supporter lined with soft cotton dressings. Administer analgesics for several days to relieve his pain. Encourage sitz baths, and apply heat or ice packs to decrease inflammation.

Prepare the patient for needle aspiration of fluid-filled cysts and other diagnostic tests, such as lung tomography and computed tomography scan of the abdomen, to rule out malignant tumors.

Pediatric pointers

A thorough physical assessment is especially important for children with scrotal swelling, who may be unable to provide history data. In children under 1 year of age, a hernia or hydrocele of the spermatic cord suggests abnormal fetal development. In infants, scrotal swelling may stem from ammonia-related dermatitis if diapers aren't changed often enough. In prepubescent males, it usually results from torsion of the spermatic cord.

Other disorders that can cause scrotal swelling in children include epididymitis (rare before age 10), traumatic orchitis from contact sports, and mumps (most commonly after puberty).

SEIZURES, ABSENCE

Absence seizures are benign, generalized seizures thought to originate subcortically. The patient is physically present, but higher cortical functions are absent during the seizures. These brief episodes of unconsciousness usually last 3 to 20 seconds and can occur 100 or more times a day, commonly causing periods of inattention. Absence seizures usually begin between the ages of 4 and 12 and their frequency typically falls after puberty. Their first sign may be deteriorating schoolwork and behavior. Their cause is unknown.

Absence seizures occur without warning. The patient suddenly stops all purposeful activity and stares blankly ahead, as though daydreaming. Absence seizures may cause automatisms, such as repetitive lip smacking, or mild clonic or myoclonic movements, including mild jerking of the eyelids. The patient may drop objects he's holding, and muscle relaxation may cause him to drop his head or arms or to slump. After the seizure, the patient resumes activity, typically unaware of the episode.

Absence status, a rare form of absence seizure, occurs as a prolonged absence seizure or as repeated episodes of these seizures. Usually not life-threatening, it's most common in patients who have experienced absence seizures.

History and physical examination

If you suspect a patient is having an absence seizure, evaluate its occurrence and duration by reciting a series of numbers and then asking him to repeat them after the attack ends. The patient who has had an absence seizure can't repeat the numbers. Alternatively, if the seizures are occurring within minutes of each other, ask the patient to count for about 5 minutes. He'll stop counting during a seizure and resume when it's over. Look for accompanying automatisms. Find out if the family has noticed a change in behavior or deteriorating schoolwork.

Common medical causes

♦ ***Idiopathic epilepsy.*** Some forms of absence seizure are accompanied by learning disabilities.

Special considerations

Explain the purpose of any diagnostic tests, such as computed tomography scans, magnetic resonance imaging, and electroencephalography. Teach the patient and his family about these seizures and how to recognize their onset, pattern, and duration. Include the child's teacher and school nurse in the teaching process, if possible. If the seizures are being controlled with drug therapy, emphasize the importance of strict compliance.

SEIZURES, COMPLEX PARTIAL

A complex partial seizure occurs when a focal seizure begins in the temporal lobe, limbic system, or frontal lobe and causes a partial alteration of consciousness — usually confusion. Psychomotor seizures can occur at any age, but incidence usually increases during adolescence and adulthood. Two-thirds of patients also have generalized seizures.

An aura — usually a complex hallucination or illusion — typically precedes a psychomotor seizure. The hallucination may be audiovisual (images with sounds), auditory (abnormal or normal sounds or voices from the patient's past), or olfactory (unpleasant smells, such as rotten eggs or burning materials). Other types of auras include sensations of déjà vu, unfamiliarity with surroundings, or depersonalization. Some patients become fearful or anxious, experience lip smacking, or have an unpleasant feeling in the epigastric region that rises toward the chest and throat. The patient usually recognizes the aura and lies down before losing consciousness.

A period of unresponsiveness follows the aura. The patient may experience automatisms (lip smacking, chewing, licking lips, clapping hands), appear dazed and wander aimlessly, perform inappropriate acts (such as undressing in public), be unresponsive, utter incoherent phrases, or (rarely) go into a rage or tantrum. After the seizure, the patient is confused, drowsy, and doesn't remember the seizure. Behavioral automatisms rarely last longer than 5 minutes, but post-seizure confusion and amnesia may persist.

Between attacks, the patient may exhibit slow and rigid thinking, outbursts of anger and aggressiveness, tedious conversation, a preoccupation with naive philosophical ideas, diminished libido, mood swings, and paranoid tendencies.

History

If you witness a complex partial seizure, never attempt to restrain the patient. Instead, lead him gently to a safe area. *(Exception:* Don't approach him if he's angry or violent.) Calmly encourage the patient to sit down, and remain with him until he's fully alert. Always try to protect the patient from injury. After the seizure, ask him if he experienced an aura. Record all your observations and findings.

Common medical causes

♦ ***Brain abscess.*** If the abscess is in the temporal lobe, complex partial seizures commonly occur after the abscess heals. Related problems may include headache, nausea, vomiting, generalized seizures, and a decreased level of consciousness (LOC). The patient may also develop central facial weakness, auditory receptive aphasia, hemiparesis, or ocular disturbances.

♦ ***Head trauma.*** Severe trauma to the temporal lobe (especially from a penetrating injury) can cause complex partial seizure, persisting for months or years. The seizures may decrease in frequency and eventually stop. Head trauma also may cause generalized seizures and behavior and personality changes.

♦ ***Herpes simplex encephalitis.*** The herpes simplex virus commonly attacks the temporal lobe, resulting in complex partial seizures. Other features include fever, headache, coma, or generalized seizures.

♦ ***Temporal lobe tumor.*** Complex partial seizures may be the first sign of this disorder. Other signs and symptoms include headache, pupillary changes, and mental dullness. Increased intracranial pressure may cause a decreased LOC, vomiting and, possibly, papilledema.

Special considerations

After the seizure, remain with the patient to reorient him to his surroundings and to protect him from injury. Keep him in bed until he's fully alert, and remove harmful objects from the area. Offer emotional support to the patient and his family, and teach them how to cope with seizures.

Prepare the patient for diagnostic tests, such as electroencephalography, computed tomography scans, or magnetic resonance imaging.

Pediatric pointers

Complex partial seizures in children may resemble absence seizures. They can result from birth injury, abuse, infection, or cancer. In about one-third of patients, their cause is unknown. They may also be related to childhood febrile seizures or traumatic head injury.

Repeated complex partial seizures commonly lead to generalized seizures. The child may experience a slight aura, which is rarely as clearly defined as those associated with generalized tonic-clonic seizures.

SEIZURES, GENERALIZED TONIC-CLONIC

Like other types of seizures, generalized tonic-clonic seizures are caused by the paroxysmal, uncontrolled discharge of central nervous system neurons, leading to neurologic dysfunction. Unlike most other types of seizures, however, this cerebral hyperactivity isn't confined to the original focus or to a localized area but extends to the entire brain.

A generalized tonic-clonic seizure may begin with or without an aura. As seizure activity spreads to the subcortical structures, the patient loses consciousness, falls to the ground, and may utter a loud cry that's precipitated by air rushing from the lungs through the vocal cords. His body stiffens (tonic phase), then undergoes rapid, synchronous muscle jerking and hyperventilation (clonic phase). Tongue biting, incontinence, diaphoresis, profuse salivation, or signs of respiratory distress may also occur. The seizure usually stops after 2 to 5 minutes. The patient then regains consciousness but is confused. He may complain of headache, fatigue, muscle soreness, or arm and leg weakness.

Generalized tonic-clonic seizures usually occur singly. The patient may be asleep or awake and active. (See *What happens in a generalized tonic-clonic seizure,* page 530.) Possible complications include respiratory arrest due to airway obstruction from secretions, status epilepticus (occurring in 5% to 8% of patients), head or spinal injuries and bruises, Todd's paralysis or, rarely, cardiac arrest. Life-threatening status epilepticus is marked by prolonged seizure activity or by rapidly recurring seizures with no intervening periods of recovery. It's most commonly triggered by abrupt discontinuation of anticonvulsant drugs.

Generalized seizures may be caused by brain tumors, vascular disorders, head trauma, infections, metabolic defects, drug and alcohol withdrawal syndromes, toxins, or genetic defects. Generalized seizures may also result from a focal seizure. The cause of recurring seizures (epilepsy) may be unknown.

Emergency interventions

If you witness the beginning of the seizure, first check the patient's airway, breathing, and circulation, and make sure that the cause isn't asystole or a blocked airway. Stay with the patient and ensure a patent airway. Focus your care on observing the seizure and protecting the patient. Place a towel under his head to prevent injury, loosen his clothing, and move sharp or hard objects out of his way. Never try to restrain the patient or force a hard object into his mouth; you might chip his teeth or fracture his jaw. Only at the start of the ictal phase (start of seizure) can you safely insert a soft object into his mouth.

If possible, turn the patient to one side *during* the seizure to allow secretions to drain. Otherwise, do this at the end of the clonic phase when respirations return. If they fail to return, check for airway obstruction and suction the patient if necessary. Intubation and mechanical ventilation may be needed.

Protect the patient after the seizure by providing a safe area in which he can rest. As he awakens, reassure and reorient him. Check his vital signs and neurologic status. Be sure to carefully record these data and your observations during the seizure.

If the seizure lasts longer than 4 minutes or if a second seizure occurs before full recovery from the first, suspect status epilepticus. Establish an airway, start an I.V. line, give supplemental oxygen, and begin cardiac monitoring. Draw blood for appropriate studies. Turn the patient on his side, with his head in a semidependent position, to drain secretions and prevent aspiration. Periodically turn him to the opposite side, check his arterial blood gas levels for hypoxemia, and administer oxygen by mask, increasing the flow rate if necessary. Administer diazepam or lorazepam by slow I.V. push, repeated two or three times at 10- to 20-minute intervals, to stop the seizures. If the patient isn't a known epileptic, an I.V. bolus of dextrose 50% (50 ml) with thiamine (100 mg) may be ordered. Dextrose may stop the seizures if the patient is hypoglycemic. If his thiamine level is low, also give thiamine to guard against further damage.

If the patient is intubated, expect to insert a nasogastric (NG) tube to prevent vomiting and aspiration. Be aware that if the patient hasn't been intubated, the NG tube itself can trigger the gag reflex and cause vomiting. Be sure to record your observations and the intervals between seizures.

History and physical examination

If you didn't witness the seizure, obtain a description from the patient's companion. Ask when the seizure started and how long it lasted. Did the patient report unusual sensations before the seizure began? Did the seizure start in one area of the body and spread, or did it affect the entire body right away? Did the patient fall on a hard surface? Did his eyes or head turn? Did he turn blue? Did he lose bladder control? Did he have other seizures before recovering?

What happens in a generalized tonic-clonic seizure

BEFORE THE SEIZURE

Prodromal signs and symptoms, such as myoclonic jerks, throbbing headache, or mood changes may occur over several hours or days. The patient may have premonitions of the seizure. For example, he may report an *aura,* such as seeing a flashing light or smelling a characteristic odor.

DURING THE SEIZURE

If a generalized seizure begins with an aura, this indicates that irritability in a specific area of the brain quickly became widespread. Common auras include palpitations, epigastric distress rapidly rising to the throat, head or eye turning, and sensory hallucinations.

Next, *loss of consciousness* occurs as a sudden discharge of intense electrical activity overwhelms the brain's subcortical center. The patient falls and experiences brief, bilateral myoclonic contractures. Air forced through spasmodic vocal cords may produce a piercing, birdlike cry.

During the *tonic phase,* skeletal muscles contract for about 10 to 20 seconds. The patient's eyelids are drawn up, his arms are flexed, and his legs are extended. His mouth opens wide, then snaps shut; he may bite his tongue. His respirations cease because of respiratory muscle spasm, and initial pallor of the skin and mucous membranes (the result of impaired venous return) changes to cyanosis secondary to apnea. The patient arches his back and slowly lowers his arms (as shown below). Other effects include dilated, nonreactive pupils; greatly increased heart rate and blood pressure; increased salivations and tracheobronchial secretions; and profuse diaphoresis.

During the *clonic phase,* lasting about 60 seconds, mild trembling progresses to violent contractures or jerks. Other motor activity includes facial grimaces (with possible tongue biting) or violent expirations of bloody, foamy saliva from clonic contractures of the thoracic cage muscles. Clonic jerks slowly decrease in intensity and frequency. The patient is still apneic.

AFTER THE SEIZURE

The patient's movements gradually cease and he becomes unresponsive to external stimuli. Other postseizure features include stertorous respirations from increased tracheobronchial secretions, equal or unequal pupils (but becoming reactive), and urinary incontinence due to brief muscle relaxation. After about 5 minutes, the patient's level of consciousness increases, and he appears confused and disoriented. His muscle tone, heart rate, and blood pressure return to normal.

After several hours' sleep, the patient awakens exhausted and may have a headache, sore muscles, and amnesia regarding the seizure.

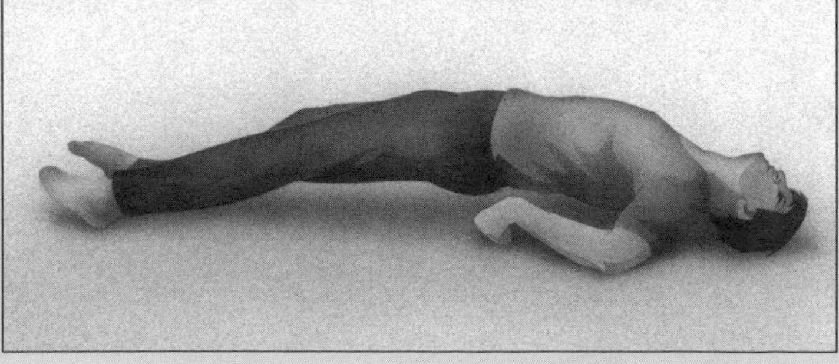

If the patient may have sustained a head injury, observe him closely for loss of consciousness, unequal or nonreactive pupils, and focal neurologic signs. Does he complain of headache and muscle soreness? Is he increasingly difficult to arouse when you check on him at 20-minute intervals? Examine his arms, legs, and face (including tongue) for injury, residual paralysis, or limb weakness.

Next, obtain a history. Has the patient ever had generalized or focal seizures before? If so, do they occur frequently? Do other family members also have them? Is the patient receiving drug therapy? Is he compliant? Also, ask about sleep deprivation, or emotional or physical stress at the time the seizure occurred.

Common medical causes

- ***Brain abscess.*** Generalized seizures may occur in the acute stage of abscess formation or after the abscess disappears. Depending on the size and location of the abscess, decreased level of consciousness (LOC) varies from drowsiness to deep stupor. Early signs and symptoms reflect increased intracranial pressure (ICP); they include constant headache, nausea, vomiting, and focal seizures. Typical later features include ocular disturbances, such as nystagmus, impaired vision, and unequal pupils. Other findings vary with the abscess site but may include aphasia, hemiparesis, abnormal behavior, and personality changes.
- ***Brain tumor.*** Generalized seizures may occur, depending on the tumor's location and type. Other findings include a slowly decreasing LOC, morning headache, dizziness, confusion, focal seizures, vision loss, motor and sensory disturbances, aphasia, and ataxia. Later findings may include papilledema, vomiting, increased systolic blood pressure, widening pulse pressure, and (eventually) decorticate posture.
- ***Cerebrovascular accident (CVA).*** Seizures (focal more commonly than generalized) may occur within 6 months of an ischemic CVA. Associated signs and symptoms vary with the location and extent of brain damage. They include decreased LOC, contralateral hemiplegia, dysarthria, dysphagia, ataxia, unilateral sensory loss, apraxia, agnosia, and aphasia. The patient may also develop visual deficits, memory loss, poor judgment, personality changes, or emotional lability; other possible physical signs include urine retention or incontinence, constipation, headache, or vomiting.
- ***Chronic renal failure.*** End-stage renal failure causes rapid onset of twitching, trembling, myoclonic jerks, and generalized seizures. Related signs and symptoms include anuria or oliguria, fatigue, malaise, irritability, decreased mental acuity, muscle cramps, peripheral neuropathies, anorexia, and constipation or diarrhea. Integumentary effects include skin color changes (yellow, brown, or bronze), pruritus, and uremic frost. Other possible effects include ammonia breath odor, nausea and vomiting, ecchymoses, petechiae, GI bleeding, mouth and gum ulcers, hypertension, and Kussmaul's respirations.
- ***Eclampsia.*** Generalized seizures are a hallmark of this disorder. Related findings include severe frontal headache, nausea and vomiting, vision disturbances, increased blood pressure, peripheral edema, and sudden weight gain. The patient may also exhibit oliguria, irritability, hyperactive deep tendon reflexes (DTRs), or decreased LOC.
- ***Encephalitis.*** An early sign of this disorder, seizures indicate a poor prognosis; they may also occur after recovery as a result of residual damage. Other possible findings include fever, headache, photophobia, nuchal rigidity, vomiting, aphasia, ataxia, hemiparesis, nystagmus, irritability, cranial nerve palsies (causing facial weakness, ptosis, dysphagia), and myoclonic jerks.
- ***Head trauma.*** In severe cases, generalized seizures may occur at the time of injury. (Focal seizures may occur months later.) Severe head trauma may also cause a decreased LOC, leading to coma; soft-

tissue injury of the face, head, or neck; clear or bloody drainage from the mouth, nose, or ears; facial edema; bony deformity of the face, head, or neck; Battle's sign; and lack of response to oculocephalic and oculovestibular stimulation. Motor and sensory deficits and altered respirations also may occur. Examination may reveal signs of increasing ICP, such as decreased response to painful stimuli, nonreactive pupils, bradycardia, increased systolic pressure, and widening pulse pressure. If the patient is conscious, he may exhibit visual deficits, behavioral changes, or headache.

♦ ***Hepatic encephalopathy.*** Generalized seizures may occur late in this disorder. Associated late-stage findings in the comatose patient include fetor hepaticus, asterixis, hyperactive DTRs, and a positive Babinski's sign.

♦ ***Hypoglycemia.*** Generalized seizures usually occur in severe hypoglycemia, accompanied by blurred or double vision, motor weakness, hemiplegia, trembling, excessive diaphoresis, tachycardia, myoclonic twitching, and decreased LOC.

♦ ***Hyponatremia.*** Seizures develop when serum sodium levels fall below 125 mEq/L, especially if the decrease is rapid. Hyponatremia also causes orthostatic hypotension, headache, muscle twitching and weakness, fatigue, oliguria or anuria, cold and clammy skin, decreased skin turgor, irritability, lethargy, confusion, or stupor or coma. Excessive thirst, tachycardia, nausea, vomiting, or abdominal cramps may also occur. Severe hyponatremia may cause cyanosis and vasomotor collapse, with a thready pulse.

♦ ***Hypoparathyroidism.*** Worsening tetany causes generalized seizures. Chronic hypoparathyroidism causes neuromuscular irritability and hyperactive DTRs.

♦ ***Hypoxic encephalopathy.*** Besides generalized seizures, this disorder may cause myoclonic jerks and coma. After recovery, dementia, visual agnosia, choreoathetosis, or ataxia may occur.

♦ ***Neurofibromatosis.*** Multiple brain lesions in this disorder cause focal and generalized seizures. Inspection reveals café-au-lait spots, multiple skin tumors, scoliosis, and kyphoscoliosis. Related findings include dizziness, ataxia, monocular blindness, or nystagmus.

Other causes

♦ ***Arsenic poisoning.*** In addition to generalized seizures, arsenic poisoning may cause a garlicky breath odor, increased salivation, and generalized pruritus. GI effects include diarrhea, nausea, vomiting, and severe abdominal pain. Related effects include diffuse hyperpigmentation; sharply defined edema of the eyelids, face, and ankles; paresthesia of the extremities; alopecia; irritated mucous membranes; weakness; muscle aches; and peripheral neuropathy.

♦ ***Barbiturate withdrawal.*** In chronically intoxicated patients, barbiturate withdrawal may cause generalized seizures 2 to 4 days after the last dose. Status epilepticus is possible.

♦ ***Diagnostic tests.*** Contrast agents used in radiologic tests may cause generalized seizures.

♦ ***Drugs.*** Toxic blood levels of some drugs, such as theophylline, lidocaine, meperidine, penicillins, and cimetidine, may cause generalized seizures. Phenothiazines, tricyclic antidepressants, amphetamines, isoniazid, or vincristine may cause seizures in patients with preexisting epilepsy.

Special considerations

Closely monitor the patient after the seizure for recurring seizure activity. Prepare him for a computed tomography scan or magnetic resonance imaging and electroencephalography.

Pediatric pointers

Generalized seizures are common in children. In fact, 75% to 90% of epileptic patients experience their first seizure before age 20. Many children between ages 3 months and 3 years experience generalized seizures associated with fever; some of these children later develop seizures without fever. Generalized seizures may also stem from inborn errors of metabolism, perinatal injury, brain infection, Reye's syndrome, Sturge-Weber syndrome, arteriovenous malformation, lead poisoning, hypoglycemia, or idiopathic causes. Rarely, the pertussis component of the DPT vaccine causes seizures.

SEIZURES, SIMPLE PARTIAL

Resulting from an irritable focus in the cerebral cortex, simple partial seizures typically last about 30 seconds and don't alter the patient's level of consciousness (LOC). The type and pattern reflect the location of the irritable focus. Simple partial seizures may be classified as *motor,* including jacksonian seizures and epilepsia partialis continua, *or somatosensory,* including visual, olfactory, or auditory seizures.

A *focal motor seizure* is a series of unilateral clonic (muscle jerking) and tonic (muscle stiffening) movements of one part of the body. The patient's head and eyes characteristically turn away from the hemispheric focus — usually the frontal lobe near the motor strip. A tonic-clonic contraction of the trunk or extremities may follow.

A *jacksonian motor seizure* typically begins with a tonic contraction of a finger, the corner of the mouth, or one foot. Clonic movements follow, spreading to other muscles on the same side of the body, moving up the arm or leg, and eventually involving the whole side. Alternatively, clonic movements may spread to the opposite side, becoming generalized and leading to loss of consciousness. In the postictal phase, the patient may experience paralysis in the affected limbs (Todd's paralysis), which usually resolves within 24 hours.

Epilepsia partialis continua causes clonic twitching of one muscle group, usually in the face, arm, or leg. Twitching occurs every few seconds and persists for hours, days, or months without spreading. Spasms affect the distal arm and leg muscles more commonly than the proximal ones; in the face, they affect the corner of the mouth, one or both eyelids or, occasionally, the neck or trunk muscles unilaterally.

A *focal somatosensory seizure* affects a localized body area on one side. Usually, this type of seizure initially causes numbness, tingling, or crawling or "electric" sensations; occasionally, it causes pain or burning sensations in the lips, fingers, or toes. A *visual seizure* involves sensations of darkness or of stationary or moving lights or spots, usually red at first, then blue, green, and yellow. It can affect both visual fields or the visual field on the side opposite the lesion. The irritable focus is in the occipital lobe. In contrast, the irritable focus in an *auditory* or *olfactory seizure* is in the temporal lobe. (See *Body functions affected by focal seizures*, page 534.)

History and physical examination

Be sure to record the patient's behavior in detail; your data may be critical in locating the lesion in the brain. Does the patient turn his head and eyes? If so, to what side? Where does movement first start? Does it spread? Because a partial seizure may become generalized, you'll need to watch closely for loss of consciousness, bilateral tonicity and clonicity, cyanosis, tongue biting, and urinary incontinence.

After the seizure, ask the patient to describe exactly what he remembers, if anything, about the seizure. Check the patient's LOC, and test for residual

Body functions affected by focal seizures

The site of the irritable focus determines which body functions are affected by a focal seizure, as shown in the illustration here.

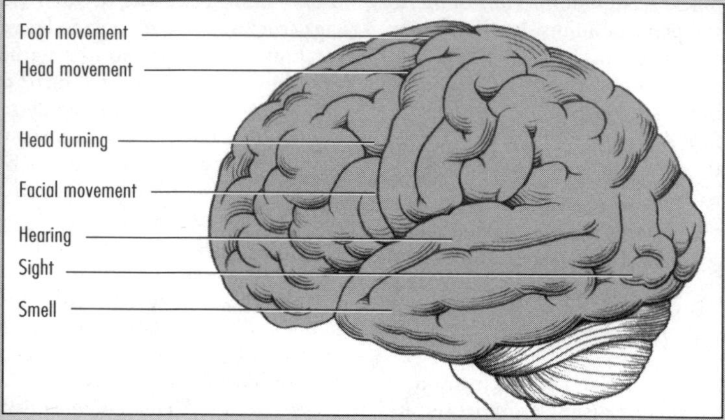

deficits (such as weakness in the involved extremity) and sensory disturbances.

Then obtain a history. Ask the patient what happened before the seizure. Did he recognize its onset? If so, how—by a smell, a visual disturbance, or a sound or visceral phenomenon, such as an unusual sensation in his stomach? How does this seizure compare with others he has had?

In addition, explore fully any history, recent or remote, of head trauma. Also, check for a history of stroke or recent infection, especially with fever, headache, or a stiff neck. Be sure to question the patient about whether he experienced an aura before the onset of the seizures.

Common medical causes

♦ ***Brain abscess.*** Seizures can occur in the acute stage of abscess formation or after resolution of the abscess. Decreased LOC varies from drowsiness to deep stupor. Early signs and symptoms reflect increased intracranial pressure and include a constant, intractable headache, nausea, and vomiting. Later symptoms include ocular disturbances, such as nystagmus, decreased visual acuity, and unequal pupils. Other findings vary according to the abscess site and may include aphasia, hemiparesis, and personality changes.

♦ ***Brain tumor.*** Focal seizures are commonly the earliest indicators of a brain tumor. The patient may report morning headache, dizziness, confusion, vision loss, or motor or sensory disturbances. He may also develop aphasia, generalized seizures, ataxia, decreased LOC, papilledema, vomiting, increased systolic blood pressure, or widening pulse pressure. Eventually, he may assume a decorticate posture.

♦ ***Cerebrovascular accident (CVA).*** A major cause of seizures in patients over age 50, a CVA may induce focal seizures up to 6 months after its onset. Related effects depend on the type and extent of the CVA but may include decreased LOC, contralateral hemiplegia, dysarthria, dysphagia, ataxia, unilateral sensory loss, apraxia, agnosia, or aphasia. A CVA may also cause vision deficits, memory loss, poor judgment, personality changes, emotional lability, headache, urinary incontinence or retention, or vomiting. It may result in generalized seizures.

◆ ***Head trauma.*** Any head injury can cause seizures, but penetrating wounds are characteristically associated with focal seizures. The seizures usually begin 3 to 15 months after injury, decrease in frequency after several years, and eventually stop. The patient may develop generalized seizures and a decreased LOC that may progress to coma.

Special considerations

No emergency care is necessary during a focal seizure, unless it progresses to a generalized seizure. However, you should remain with the patient during the seizure, and reassure him.

Prepare the patient for such diagnostic tests as a computed tomography scan and electroencephalography.

Pediatric pointers

In children more commonly than in adults, focal seizures are likely to spread and become generalized. They typically cause the child's eyes, or his head and eyes, to turn to the side; in neonates, they cause mouth twitching, staring, or both.

Focal seizures in children can result from hemiplegic cerebral palsy, head trauma, child abuse, arteriovenous malformation, or Sturge-Weber syndrome. About 25% of febrile seizures may present as focal seizures.

SETTING-SUN SIGN
[Sunset eyes]

Setting-sun sign refers to the downward deviation of an infant's or young child's eyes as a result of pressure on cranial nerves III, IV, and VI. In this late and ominous sign of increased intracranial pressure (ICP), both eyes are rotated downward, typically revealing an area of sclera above the irises; occasionally, the irises appear to be forced outward. Pupils are sluggish, responding to light unequally.

The infant with increased ICP is typically irritable and lethargic and feeds poorly. Obvious changes in level of consciousness (LOC) may be accompanied by lower extremity spasticity and opisthotonos. Increased ICP typically results from a space-occupying lesion — such as a tumor — or from an accumulation of fluid in the brain's ventricular system, as occurs in hydrocephalus. It also results from intracranial bleeding or cerebral edema.

Setting-sun sign may be intermittent; for example, it may disappear when the infant is upright because this position slightly reduces ICP. The sign may be elicited in a normal infant younger than 4 weeks of age by suddenly changing his head position and in a normal infant up to 9 months of age by shining a bright light into his eyes and removing it quickly.

History and physical examination

If you observe the setting-sun sign in an infant, evaluate his neurologic status; then obtain a brief history from his parents. Has the infant experienced a fall or even a minor trauma? When did this sign appear? Ask about early nonspecific signs of increasing ICP: Has the infant's sucking reflex diminished? Is he irritable, restless, or unusually tired? Does he cry when moved? Is his cry high-pitched? Has he vomited recently?

Next, perform a physical examination, keeping in mind that neurologic responses are primarily reflexive during early infancy. Assess the infant's LOC. Is he awake, irritable, or lethargic? Keeping in mind his age and level of development, try to determine his ability to reach for a bright object or turn toward the sound of a music box. Observe his posture for normal flexion and extension or opisthotonos. Examine muscle tone, and observe for seizure automatisms.

Examine the infant's anterior fontanel for bulging, measure his head circumference, and observe his breathing pattern. (Cheyne-Stokes respirations may accompany increased ICP.) Also, check his pupillary response to light: Unilateral or bilateral dilation occurs as ICP rises. Finally, elicit reflexes that are diminished in increased ICP, especially Moro's reflex. Keep endotracheal intubation equipment available.

Common medical causes

♦ ***Increased ICP.*** Transient or intermittent setting-sun sign commonly occurs late in increased ICP. The infant may have bulging, widened fontanels, increased head circumference, and widened sutures. He may also exhibit decreased LOC, behavioral changes, a high-pitched cry, pupillary abnormalities, and impaired motor movement as ICP increases. Other findings may include increased systolic pressure, widened pulse pressure, bradycardia, changes in breathing pattern, vomiting, and seizures as ICP increases.

Special considerations

Care of the infant with setting-sun sign includes monitoring vital signs and neurologic status. Elevate the head of the crib, and monitor intake and output. Monitor ICP, restrict fluids, and insert an I.V. line to administer diuretics and corticosteroids. If ICP is severely increased, endotracheal intubation and mechanical hyperventilation may be required to reduce serum carbon dioxide and constrict cerebral vessels. Therapy to induce a barbiturate coma or hypothermia therapy may be required to lower metabolic rate.

Try to maintain a calm environment and, when the infant cries, offer comfort to help prevent stress-related ICP elevations. Encourage the parents' help, and offer them emotional support.

Skin, clammy

Clammy skin — moist, cool, and commonly pale — is a sympathetic response to stress, which triggers release of the hormones epinephrine and norepinephrine. These hormones cause cutaneous vasoconstriction and secretion of cold sweat from eccrine glands, particularly on the palms, forehead, and soles.

Clammy skin typically accompanies shock, acute hypoglycemia, anxiety reactions, arrhythmias, or heat exhaustion. As a vasovagal reaction to severe pain, it's associated with nausea, anorexia, epigastric distress, hyperpnea, tachypnea, weakness, confusion, tachycardia, or pupillary dilation. Marked bradycardia and syncope may follow.

History and physical examination

If you detect clammy skin, remember that rapid evaluation and intervention are essential. (See *Clammy skin: Know how to respond.*) Ask about a history of insulin-dependent diabetes mellitus or cardiac disorders. Is the patient currently taking any medications, especially antiarrhythmics? Is he experiencing pain, chest pressure, nausea, or epigastric distress? Does he feel weak? Does he have a dry mouth? Does he have diarrhea or increased urination?

Next, examine the pupils for dilation. Also, check for abdominal distention and increased muscle tension.

Common medical causes

♦ ***Anxiety.*** An acute anxiety attack commonly causes cold, clammy skin on the forehead, palms, or soles. Other features may include pallor, dry mouth, tachycardia or bradycardia, palpitations, or hypertension or hypotension. The patient may also develop tremors, breathlessness, headache, muscle tension, nausea, vomiting, abdominal distention, di-

EMERGENCY INTERVENTIONS

Clammy skin: Know how to respond

Clammy skin commonly accompanies emergency conditions, such as shock, acute hypoglycemia, or arrhythmias. To know what to do, review these typical clinical situations.

You detect clammy skin in a patient who appears anxious and restless.

↓

Quickly take his vital signs, noting tachycardia, hypotension, and a weak, irregular pulse, if present.

↓

Suspect *shock*.

↓

Place the patient in a supine position in bed. Elevate his legs 20 to 30 degrees to promote perfusion to vital organs.

↓

Insert an I.V. line for administration of drugs, fluids, or blood. Also, give supplemental oxygen and begin cardiac monitoring.

You detect clammy skin and possible tremors in a patient who appears irritable and anxious and reports persistent hunger.

↓

Quickly take his vital signs, noting hypotension and decreased level of consciousness. If present:

↓

Suspect *acute hypoglycemia*.

↓

Immediately draw blood for glucose studies, and test a drop with a bedside glucose monitor. Insert an I.V. line, and give a 50-ml bolus of dextrose 50%. Also, begin cardiac monitoring.

You detect clammy skin in a patient with changes in mental status, such as confusion.

↓

Quickly take his vital signs, noting hypotension and changes in pulse rate and rhythm. If present:

↓

Suspect an *arrhythmia*.

↓

Insert an I.V. line and administer antiarrhythmic drugs. Also, give supplemental oxygen and begin cardiac monitoring.

arrhea, increased urination, or sharp chest pain.

♦ ***Arrhythmias.*** Cardiac arrhythmias may cause generalized cool, clammy skin, mental status changes, dizziness, and hypotension.

♦ ***Cardiogenic shock.*** Generalized cool, moist, pale skin accompanies confusion, restlessness, hypotension, tachycardia, tachypnea, narrowing pulse pressure, cyanosis, and oliguria.

♦ ***Heat exhaustion.*** In the acute stage of heat exhaustion, generalized cold, clammy skin accompanies an ashen-gray appearance, headache, confusion, syncope, giddiness and, possibly, a subnormal temperature. The patient may exhibit a rapid and thready pulse, nausea, vomiting, tachypnea, oliguria, thirst, muscle cramps, or hypotension.

♦ ***Hypoglycemia (acute).*** Generalized cool, clammy skin or diaphoresis may accompany irritability, tremors, palpitations, hunger, headache, tachycardia, or anxiety. Central nervous system disturbances may include blurred vision, diplopia, confusion, motor weakness, hemiplegia, or coma. These symptoms typically resolve after the patient is given glucose.

♦ ***Hypovolemic shock.*** In this common form of shock, generalized pale, cold, clammy skin accompanies subnormal body temperature, hypotension with narrowing pulse pressure, tachycardia, tachypnea, and rapid, thready pulse. Other findings are flat neck veins, prolonged capillary refill time, decreased urine output, confusion, or decreased level of consciousness.

♦ ***Septic shock.*** The cold shock stage causes generalized cold, clammy skin. Associated findings include rapid and thready pulse, severe hypotension, persistent oliguria or anuria, or respiratory failure.

Special considerations

Take the patient's vital signs frequently, and monitor urine output. If clammy skin occurs with an anxiety reaction or pain, offer the patient emotional support, administer pain medication, and provide a quiet environment.

Pediatric pointers

Infants in shock don't have clammy skin because their sweat glands are immature.

Geriatric pointers

Elderly patients develop clammy skin easily because of decreased tissue perfusion. Always consider bowel ischemia in the differential diagnosis of older patients who present with cool, clammy skin — especially in the presence of abdominal pain or bloody stools.

SKIN, MOTTLED

Mottled skin is patchy discoloration indicating primary or secondary changes of the deep, middle, or superficial dermal blood vessels. It can result from hematologic, immune, or connective tissue disorders; chronic occlusive arterial disease; dysproteinemias; immobility; exposure to heat or cold; or shock. Mottled skin can be a normal reaction, such as the diffuse mottling that occurs when exposure to cold causes venous stasis in cutaneous blood vessels (cutis marmorata).

Mottling that occurs with other signs and symptoms usually affects the extremities, typically those indicating restricted blood flow. For example, livedo reticularis, a characteristic network pattern of reddish blue discoloration, occurs when vasospasm of the middermal blood vessels slows local blood flow in dilated superficial capillaries and small veins. Shock causes mottling from systemic vasoconstriction.

History and physical examination

Mottled skin may reflect an emergency condition requiring rapid evaluation and intervention. (See *Mottled skin: Know how to respond.*) However, if the patient

EMERGENCY INTERVENTIONS

Mottled skin: Know how to respond

If your patient's skin is pale, cool, clammy, and mottled at the elbows and knees or all over, he may be developing *hypovolemic shock*. Quickly take his vital signs, and be sure to note tachycardia or a weak, thready pulse. Observe for flat neck veins. Does the patient appear anxious? If you detect these signs and symptoms, place the patient in a supine position in bed with his legs elevated 20 to 30 degrees. Administer oxygen by nasal cannula or face mask, and begin cardiac monitoring. Insert a large-bore I.V. line for rapid fluid administration, and prepare to insert a central line or a pulmonary artery catheter. Also prepare to catheterize the patient to monitor urine output.

Localized mottling in a pale, cool extremity that the patient says feels painful, numb, or tingling may signal acute arterial occlusion. Immediately check the patient's distal pulses. If they're absent or diminished, you'll need to insert an I.V. line in an unaffected extremity, and prepare the patient for arteriography or immediate surgery.

isn't in distress, obtain a history. Ask if the mottling began suddenly or gradually. What precipitated it? How long has he had it? Does anything make it go away? Does the patient have other symptoms, such as pain, numbness, or tingling in an extremity? If so, do they disappear with temperature changes?

Observe the patient's skin color, and palpate his arms and legs for skin texture, swelling, and temperature differences between extremities. Also palpate for the presence (or absence) of pulses and for their quality. Note breaks in the skin, muscle appearance, and hair distribution. Also, assess motor and sensory function.

Common medical causes

◆ ***Acrocyanosis.*** In this rare disorder, anxiety or exposure to cold can cause vasospasm in small cutaneous arterioles. This results in persistent symmetrical blue and red mottling of the affected hands, feet, and nose.

◆ ***Arterial occlusion (acute).*** Initial signs include sudden temperature and color changes. Pallor may change to blotchy cyanosis and livedo reticularis. Color and temperature demarcation develop at the level of obstruction. Other effects include sudden onset of pain in the extremity and possibly paresthesia, paresis, or a sensation of cold in the affected area. Examination reveals diminished or absent pulses, cool extremities, prolonged capillary refill time, pallor, and diminished reflexes.

◆ ***Arteriosclerosis obliterans.*** Atherosclerotic buildup narrows the arterial lumen, resulting in reduced blood flow through the affected artery. Obstructed blood flow to the extremities (most commonly the lower) causes such peripheral signs and symptoms as leg pallor, cyanosis, blotchy erythema, or livedo reticularis. Related findings include intermittent claudication (most common symptom), diminished or absent pedal pulses, leg coolness, or paresthesia.

◆ ***Buerger's disease.*** This form of vasculitis causes unilateral or asymmetrical color changes and mottling, particularly livedo reticularis in the lower extremities. It also typically causes intermittent claudication and erythema along extremity blood vessels. During exposure to cold, the feet are cold, cyanotic, and numb; later they're hot, red, and tingling. Other findings include impaired peripheral pulses and peripheral neuropathy. Buerger's disease is typically exacerbated by smoking.

♦ ***Cryoglobulinemia.*** This necrotizing disorder causes patchy livedo reticularis, petechiae, and ecchymoses. Other findings include fever, chills, urticaria, melena, skin ulcers, epistaxis, Raynaud's phenomenon, eye hemorrhages, hematuria, or gangrene.

♦ ***Hypovolemic shock.*** Vasoconstriction commonly causes skin mottling, initially in the knees and elbows. As shock worsens, mottling becomes generalized. Early signs include sudden onset of pallor, cool skin, restlessness, thirst, tachypnea, and slight tachycardia. As shock progresses, associated findings include cool, clammy skin; rapid, thready pulse; hypotension; narrowed pulse pressure; decreased urine output; subnormal temperature; confusion; or decreased level of consciousness.

♦ ***Livedo reticularis (idiopathic or primary).*** Symmetrical, diffuse mottling can involve the hands, feet, arms, legs, buttocks, or trunk. Initially, networking is intermittent and most pronounced on exposure to cold or stress; eventually, mottling persists even after warming.

♦ ***Periarteritis nodosa.*** Skin findings may include asymmetrical, patchy livedo reticularis, palpable nodules along the path of medium-sized arteries, erythema, or purpura. Other manifestations include muscle wasting, ulcers, gangrene, peripheral neuropathy, fever, weight loss, or malaise.

♦ ***Polycythemia vera.*** This hematologic disorder causes livedo reticularis, hemangiomas, purpura, rubor, ulcerative nodules, and scleroderma-like lesions. Other possible symptoms include headache, a vague feeling of fullness in the head, dizziness, vertigo, visual disturbances, dyspnea, or aquagenic pruritus.

♦ ***Systemic lupus erythematosus.*** This connective tissue disorder can cause livedo reticularis, most commonly on the outer arms. Other signs and symptoms may include a butterfly rash, nondeforming joint pain and stiffness, photosensitivity, Raynaud's phenomenon, patchy alopecia, seizures, fever, anorexia, weight loss, lymphadenopathy, or emotional lability.

Other causes

♦ ***Immobility.*** Prolonged immobility may cause bluish mottling, most noticeably in dependent extremities.

♦ ***Thermal exposure.*** Prolonged thermal exposure, as from a heating pad or hot water bottle, may cause erythema ab igne—localized, reticulated, brown-to-red mottling.

Special considerations

Mottled skin typically results from chronic conditions. Teach patients to avoid tight clothing and overexposure to cold or to heating devices, such as hot water bottles and heating pads.

Pediatric pointers

A common cause of mottled skin in children is systemic vasoconstriction from shock. Other causes are the same as those for adults.

Geriatric pointers

In elderly patients, decreased tissue perfusion can cause mottled skin. In addition to arterial occlusion and polycythemia vera, conditions that commonly affect this age group, always suspect bowel ischemia in elderly patients who present with livedo reticularis, especially if they also have abdominal pain or bloody stools.

SKIN, SCALY

Scaly skin results when cells of the uppermost skin layer (stratum corneum) desiccate and shed, causing excessive accumulation of loosely adherent flakes of normal or abnormal keratin. Normally, skin cell loss is imperceptible; the appearance of scale indicates increased cell proliferation secondary to altered keratinization.

Scaly skin varies in texture from fine and delicate to coarse or stratified. Scales are typically dry, brittle, and shiny, but they can be greasy and dull. Their color ranges from whitish gray, yellow, or brown to a silvery sheen.

Usually benign, scaly skin occurs in fungal, bacterial, and viral infections (cutaneous or systemic), lymphomas, lupus erythematosus, and inflammatory skin diseases. A form of scaly skin — generalized fine desquamation — commonly follows prolonged febrile illness, sunburn, or thermal burns. Red patches of scaly skin that appear or worsen in the winter may result from dry skin (or from actinic keratosis, common in the elderly). Certain drugs also cause scaly skin. Aggravating factors include cold, heat, immobility, or frequent bathing.

History and physical examination

Begin the history by asking how long the patient has had scaly skin and whether he has had it before. Where did it appear first? Did a lesion or skin eruption, such as erythema, precede it? Has the patient used a topical skin product recently? How often does he bathe? Has he had recent joint pain, illness, or malaise? Ask the patient about work exposure to chemicals, use of prescribed drugs, and a family history of skin disorders. Find out what kinds of soap, cosmetics, skin lotion, and hair preparations he uses.

Next, examine the entire skin surface. Is it dry, oily, or moist? Observe the general pattern of skin lesions, and record their location. Note their color, shape, and size. Are they thick or fine? Do they itch? Does the patient have other lesions besides scaly skin? Examine the mucous membranes of his mouth, lips, and nose, and inspect his ears, hair, and nails.

Common medical causes

◆ ***Bowen's disease.*** This common form of intraepidermal carcinoma causes painless, erythematous plaques that are raised and indurated with a thick, hyperkeratotic scale and, possibly, ulcerated centers.

◆ ***Dermatitis.*** *Exfoliative dermatitis* begins with rapidly developing generalized erythema. Desquamation with fine scales or thick sheets of all or most of the skin surface may cause life-threatening hypothermia. Other possible complications include cardiac output failure and septicemia. Systemic signs and symptoms may include low-grade fever, chills, malaise, lymphadenopathy, or gynecomastia.

In *nummular dermatitis,* round, pustular lesions commonly ooze purulent exudate, itch severely, and rapidly become encrusted and scaly. Lesions appear on the extensor surfaces of the limbs, posterior trunk, or buttocks.

Seborrheic dermatitis begins with erythematous, pruritic scaly papules that progress to larger scaly plaques. This disorder primarily involves the center of the face, the chest and scalp or, possibly, the genitalia, axillae, or perianal region.

◆ ***Dermatophytosis.*** *Tinea capitis* causes lesions with reddened, slightly elevated borders and a central area of dense scaling; these lesions may become inflamed and pus-filled (kerions). Patchy alopecia and itching may also occur. *Tinea pedis* causes scaling and blisters between the toes. The squamous type causes diffuse, fine scales. Adherent and silvery white, they're most prominent in skin creases and may affect the entire dorsum of the foot. *Tinea corporis* causes crusty lesions. As they enlarge, their centers heal, causing the classic ringworm shape.

◆ ***Lymphoma.*** Hodgkin's disease and malignant lymphoma commonly cause scaly rashes. *Hodgkin's disease* may cause pruritic scaling dermatitis that begins in the legs and spreads to the entire body. Remissions and recurrences are common. Small nodules and diffuse pigmentation are related signs. This disease typically causes painless enlargement of the peripheral lymph nodes. Other signs and symptoms include fever, fatigue, weight loss, malaise, or hepatosplenomegaly.

In *malignant lymphoma,* initial erythematous patches with some scaling later become interspersed with nodules. Pruritus and discomfort are common; later, tumors and ulcers form. Progression causes nontender lymphadenopathy.

♦ ***Parapsoriasis (chronic).*** This disorder causes small or moderate-sized papules, with a thin, adherent scale, on the trunk, hands, or feet. Removal of the scale reveals a shiny brown surface.

♦ ***Pityriasis.*** *Pityriasis rosea* is an acute, benign, and self-limiting disorder that causes widespread scales. It begins with an erythematous, raised, oval herald patch anywhere on the body. A few days or weeks later, yellow-tan or erythematous pruritic patches with scaly edges erupt on the trunk and limbs and sometimes on the face, hands, or feet.

Pityriasis rubra pilaris, an uncommon disorder, initially causes seborrheic scaling on the scalp that progresses to the face and ears. Later, scaly red patches develop on the palms and soles, becoming diffuse, thick, fissured, hyperkeratotic, and painful. Lesions also appear on the hands, fingers, wrists, and forearms and then on wide areas of the trunk, neck, and limbs.

♦ ***Psoriasis.*** Silvery white, micaceous scales cover erythematous plaques that have sharply defined borders. Psoriasis usually appears on the scalp, chest, elbows, knees, back, buttocks, or genitalia. Associated signs and symptoms include nail pitting, pruritus, arthritis and, sometimes, pain from dry, cracked, encrusted lesions.

♦ ***Systemic lupus erythematosus.*** This disorder causes a bright-red maculopapular eruption, sometimes with scaling. Patches are sharply defined and involve the nose and malar regions of the face in a butterfly pattern — a primary sign. Similar characteristic rashes appear on other body surfaces; scaling occurs along the lower lip or anterior hair line. Other clinical features include photosensitivity, joint pain and stiffness, vasculitis (leading to infarctive lesions, necrotic leg ulcers, or digital gangrene), Raynaud's phenomenon, patchy alopecia, or mucous membrane ulcers.

♦ ***Tinea versicolor.*** This benign fungal skin infection typically causes macular hypopigmented, fawn-colored, or brown patches of various sizes and shapes. All are slightly scaly. Lesions frequently affect the upper trunk, arms, and lower abdomen, sometimes the neck and, rarely, the face.

Other causes

♦ ***Drugs.*** Many drugs — including penicillins, sulfonamides, barbiturates, quinidine, diazepam, phenytoin, and isoniazid — can cause patchy scaling.

Special considerations

If scaling results from treatment with corticosteroids, withhold the drug. Prepare the patient for such diagnostic tests as a Wood's light examination, skin scraping, or skin biopsy.

Pediatric pointers

In children, scaly skin may stem from infantile eczema, pityriasis rosea, epidermolytic hyperkeratosis, psoriasis, various forms of ichthyosis, atopic dermatitis, a viral infection (especially hepatitis B virus, which can cause Gianotti-Crosti syndrome), or an acute transient dermatitis. Desquamation may follow a febrile illness.

SKIN TURGOR, DECREASED

Skin turgor — the skin's elasticity — is determined by observing the time required for the skin to return to its normal position after being stretched or pinched. In decreased turgor, lightly pinched skin "holds" for up to 30 seconds, then slowly returns to its normal contour. Skin turgor is commonly assessed over the arm or sternum, areas normally free of wrinkles and wide variations in tissue thickness. (See *Evaluating skin turgor.*)

Decreased skin turgor results from dehydration or volume depletion. Movement of interstitial fluid into the vascular bed to maintain circulating blood volume leads to slackness in the skin's dermal layer. It's a normal finding in the elderly and in people who have lost weight rapidly.

History and physical examination

If your examination reveals decreased skin turgor, ask the patient about food and fluid intake and fluid loss. Has he recently experienced prolonged fluid loss from vomiting, diarrhea, draining wounds, or increased urination? Has he recently had a fever with sweating? Is the patient taking diuretics? If so, how often?

Next, take the patient's vital signs. Note if his systolic blood pressure while supine is abnormally low (90 mm Hg or less), if it drops 15 to 20 mm Hg or more when he stands, or if his pulse increases by 10 beats/minute when he moves from supine to sitting or from sitting to standing. If you detect these signs of orthostatic hypotension or resting tachycardia, start an I.V. line for fluid administration.

Evaluate the patient's level of consciousness (LOC) for confusion, disorientation, and signs of profound dehydration. Inspect his oral mucosa, the furrows of his tongue (especially under the tongue), and his axillae for dryness. Also, check his neck veins for flatness, and monitor his urine output.

Common medical causes

◆ ***Dehydration.*** Decreased skin turgor commonly occurs in moderate to severe dehydration. Associated findings include dry oral mucosa, decreased perspiration, resting tachycardia, orthostatic hypotension, dry and furrowed tongue, increased thirst, weight loss, oliguria, fever, or fatigue. As dehydration worsens, findings include enophthalmos, lethargy, weakness, confusion, delirium or obtundation, anuria, or shock. Hypotension persists even when the patient lies down.

EXAMINATION TIP

Evaluating skin turgor

To evaluate skin turgor in a adult, pick up a fold of skin over the sternum or the arm, as shown at top. (In an infant, roll a fold of loosely adherent skin on the abdomen between your thumb and forefinger.) Then release it. Normal skin will immediately return it its previous contour. In decreased skin turgor, the skin fold will "hold", as shown at bottom, for up to 30 seconds.

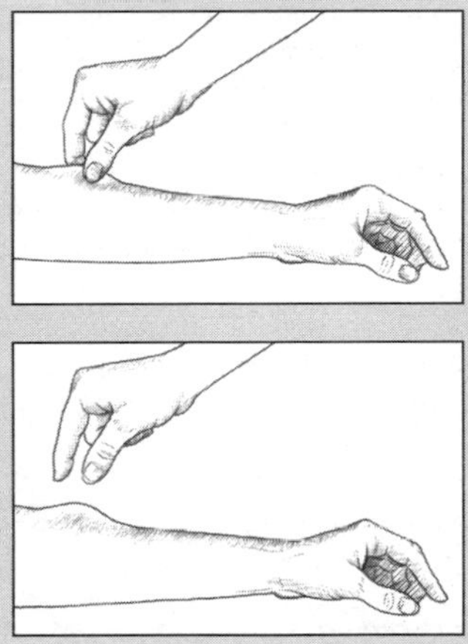

Special considerations

Even a small deficit in body fluid may be critical in patients with diminished total body fluid—young children, the elderly, the obese, and people who have rapidly lost a large amount of weight.

To prevent skin breakdown in the dehydrated patient with poor skin turgor, decreased LOC, and impaired peripheral circulation, turn the patient every 2 hours, and frequently massage his back and pressure points. Monitor his intake and output, administer I.V. fluid replacement, and offer frequent oral fluids. Weigh the patient daily at the same time on the same scale. Be alert for urine output that falls below 30 ml/hour and for continued weight loss. Also, closely monitor the patient for signs of electrolyte imbalance.

Pediatric pointers

Diarrhea secondary to gastroenteritis is the most common cause of dehydration in children, especially before age 2.

Geriatric pointers

Because it's a natural part of the aging process, decreased skin turgor may be an unreliable physical finding in elderly patients. Other signs of volume depletion, such as dry oral mucosa, dry axillae, or decreased urine output, must be carefully evaluated.

SPLENOMEGALY

Splenomegaly (an enlarged spleen) isn't a diagnostic sign by itself; it occurs in up to 5% of normal adults and is associated with many disorders. Usually, however, it points to infection, trauma, or hepatic, autoimmune, neoplastic, or hematologic disorders.

Because the spleen functions as the body's largest lymph node, splenomegaly can result from any process that triggers lymphadenopathy. For example, it may reflect reactive hyperplasia (a response to infection or inflammation), proliferation or infiltration of neoplastic cells, extramedullary hemopoiesis, phagocytic cell proliferation, increased blood cell destruction, or vascular congestion associated with portal hypertension.

Splenomegaly may be detected by light palpation under the left costal margin. (See *How to palpate for splenomegaly*.) However, because this technique isn't always advisable or effective, splenomegaly may need to be confirmed by a computed tomography or radionuclide scan.

Emergency interventions

If the patient has a history of abdominal or thoracic trauma, don't palpate the abdomen because this may aggravate internal bleeding. Instead, examine for left-upper-quadrant pain and signs of shock, such as tachycardia or tachypnea. If you detect these signs, suspect splenic rupture. Insert an I.V. line for emergency fluid and blood replacement, and administer oxygen. Also, catheterize the patient to evaluate urine output, and begin cardiac monitoring. Prepare the patient for possible surgery.

History and physical examination

If you detect splenomegaly during a routine physical examination, begin by exploring associated signs and symptoms. Ask the patient if he has been unusually tired lately. Does he frequently have colds, sore throats, or other infections? Does he bruise easily? Ask about left-upper-quadrant pain, abdominal fullness, and early satiety. Finally, examine the patient's skin for pallor and ecchymoses, and palpate his axillae, groin, and neck for lymphadenopathy.

Common medical causes

- ***Brucellosis.*** In severe cases of this rare infection, splenomegaly is a major sign. Typically, brucellosis begins insidiously with fatigue, headache, backache, anorexia, or arthralgia. Later, it may cause hepatomegaly, lymphadenopathy, weight loss, or vertebral or peripheral nerve pain on pressure.
- ***Cirrhosis.*** About one-third of patients with advanced cirrhosis develop moderate to marked splenomegaly. Among other late findings are jaundice, hepatomegaly,

EXAMINATION TIP

How to palpate for splenomegaly

Detecting splenomegaly requires skillful and gentle palpation to avoid rupturing the enlarged spleen. Follow these steps carefully.

◆ Place the patient in the supine position, and stand at her right side. Place your left hand under the left costovertebral angle, and push lightly to move the spleen forward. Then press your right hand gently under the left front costal margin.
◆ Have the patient take a deep breath and then exhale. As she exhales, move your right hand along the tissue contours under the border of the ribs, feeling for the spleen's edge. The enlarged spleen should feel like a firm mass that bumps against your fingers. Begin palpation low enough in the abdomen to catch the edge of a massive spleen.
◆ Grade the splenomegaly as slight (1 to 4 cm below the costal margin), moderate (4 to 8 cm below the costal margin), or great (8 or more cm below the costal margin).
◆ Reposition the patient on her right side with her hips and knees flexed slightly to move the spleen forward. Then repeat the palpation procedure.

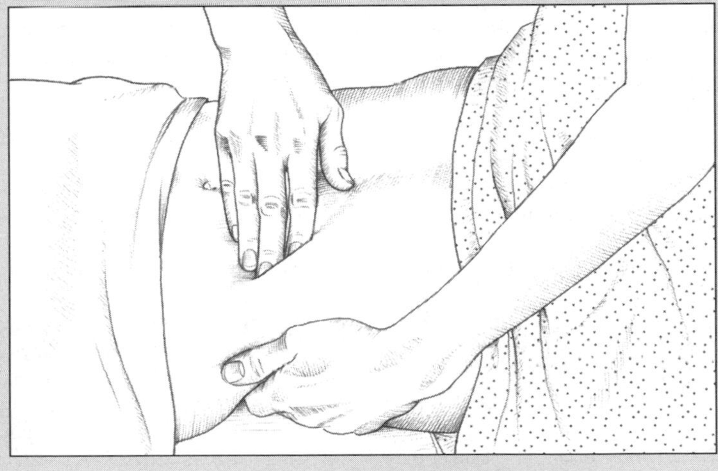

leg edema, hematemesis, and ascites. Signs of hepatic encephalopathy—such as asterixis, fetor hepaticus, slurred speech, and decreased level of consciousness that may progress to coma—are also common. Besides jaundice, skin effects may include severe pruritus, poor tissue turgor, spider angiomas, palmar erythema, pallor, or signs of bleeding tendencies. Endocrine effects may include menstrual irregularities or testicular atrophy, gynecomastia, and loss of chest and axillary hair. The patient may also develop fever and right-upper-abdominal pain that's aggravated by sitting up or leaning forward.

◆ ***Felty's syndrome.*** Splenomegaly is characteristic in this syndrome that occurs in chronic rheumatoid arthritis. Associated findings are joint pain and deformity, sensory or motor loss, rheumatoid nodules, palmar erythema, lymphadenopathy, or leg ulcers.

◆ ***Histoplasmosis.*** Acute disseminated histoplasmosis commonly causes splenomegaly and hepatomegaly. It may also cause lymphadenopathy, jaundice, fever, anorexia, emaciation, or signs of anemia, such as weakness, fatigue, pallor, or malaise. Occasionally, the patient's tongue, palate, epiglottis, and larynx become ulcerated, resulting in pain, hoarseness, and dysphagia.

◆ ***Leukemia.*** Moderate to severe splenomegaly is an early sign of acute and chronic leukemias. In chronic granulocytic leukemia, splenomegaly is sometimes painful. Accompanying it may be hepatomegaly, lymphadenopathy, fatigue, malaise, pallor, fever, gum swelling, bleeding tendencies, weight loss, anorexia, or abdominal, bone, or joint pain. At times, acute leukemia also causes dyspnea, tachycardia, and palpitations. In advanced disease, the patient may display confusion, headache, vomiting, seizures, papilledema, or nuchal rigidity.

◆ ***Mononucleosis (infectious).*** A common sign of this disorder, splenomegaly is most pronounced during the second and third weeks of illness. Typically, it's accompanied by a triad of symptoms: sore throat, cervical lymphadenopathy, and fluctuating temperature with an evening peak of 101° to 102° F (38.3° to 38.9° C). Occasionally, hepatomegaly, jaundice, or a maculopapular rash may also occur.

◆ ***Pancreatic cancer.*** This cancer may cause moderate to severe splenomegaly if tumor growth compresses the splenic vein. Other characteristic findings include abdominal or back pain, anorexia, nausea and vomiting, weight loss, GI bleeding, jaundice, pruritus, skin lesions, emotional lability, weakness, or fatigue. Palpation may reveal a tender abdominal mass and hepatomegaly; auscultation reveals a bruit in the periumbilical area and left upper quadrant.

◆ ***Polycythemia vera.*** Late in this disorder, the spleen may become markedly enlarged, resulting in easy satiety, abdominal fullness, and left-upper-quadrant or pleuritic chest pain. Clinical features accompanying splenomegaly are widespread and numerous, including deep, purplish red oral mucous membranes, headache, dyspnea, dizziness, vertigo, weakness, and fatigue. The patient may also develop finger and toe paresthesia, impaired mentation, tinnitus, blurred or double vision, scotoma, increased blood pressure, and intermittent claudication. Other signs and symptoms include pruritus, urticaria, ruddy cyanosis, epigastric distress, weight loss, hepatomegaly, and bleeding tendencies.

◆ ***Sarcoidosis.*** This granulomatous disorder may cause splenomegaly and hepatomegaly, possibly accompanied by vague abdominal discomfort. Its other signs and symptoms vary with the affected body system but may include nonproductive cough, dyspnea, malaise, fatigue, arthralgia, myalgia, weight loss, lymphadenopathy, skin lesions, irregular pulse, impaired vision, dysphagia, or seizures.

◆ ***Splenic rupture.*** Splenomegaly may result from massive hemorrhage in this disorder. The patient may also experience left-upper-quadrant pain, abdominal rigidity, and Kehr's sign.

◆ ***Thrombotic thrombocytopenic purpura.*** Splenomegaly and hepatomegaly may be accompanied by fever, generalized purpura, jaundice, pallor, vaginal bleeding, or hematuria. Other effects may include fatigue, weakness, headache, pallor, abdominal pain, and arthralgias. Eventually, the patient develops signs of neurologic deterioration and of renal failure.

Special considerations

Prepare the patient for diagnostic studies, such as a complete blood count, radionuclide and computed tomography scans of the spleen, bone marrow aspiration and biopsy, or liver function tests.

Pediatric pointers

Besides the causes of splenomegaly described above, children may develop splenomegaly in histiocytic disorders, congenital hemolytic anemia, Gaucher's disease, Niemann-Pick disease, hereditary spherocytosis, sickle cell disease, or beta-thalassemia (Cooley's anemia). Splenic abscess is the most common cause of splenomegaly in immunocompromised children.

STOOLS, CLAY-COLORED

Pale stools usually result from hepatic, gallbladder, or pancreatic disorders. Normally, bile pigments give the stool its characteristic brown color; however, hepatocellular degeneration or biliary obstruction may interfere with the formation or release of these pigments into the intestine. These stools are commonly associated with jaundice and dark urine.

History and physical examination

After documenting when the patient first noticed clay-colored stools, explore associated signs and symptoms, such as abdominal pain, nausea and vomiting, fatigue, anorexia, weight loss, and dark urine. Does the patient have trouble digesting fatty foods or heavy meals? Does he bruise easily?

Next, review the patient's medical history for gallbladder, hepatic, or pancreatic disorders. Has he ever had biliary surgery? Has he recently undergone barium studies? (Barium lightens stool color for several days.) Also, ask about antacid use because large amounts may lighten stool color. Note a history of alcoholism or exposure to other hepatotoxic substances.

After assessing the patient's general appearance, take his vital signs and check his skin and eyes for jaundice. Then examine the abdomen; inspect for distention and auscultate for hypoactive bowel sounds. Percuss and palpate for masses and rebound tenderness. Finally, obtain urine and stool specimens for laboratory analysis.

Common medical causes

◆ ***Bile duct cancer.*** Frequently a presenting sign of this cancer, clay-colored stools may be accompanied by jaundice, pruritus, anorexia and weight loss, upper abdominal pain, bleeding tendencies, and a palpable mass.

◆ ***Biliary cirrhosis.*** Clay-colored stools typically follow unexplained pruritus that worsens at bedtime, weakness, fatigue, weight loss, and vague abdominal pain; these features may be present for years. Associated findings include jaundice, hyperpigmentation, and signs of malabsorption, such as nocturnal diarrhea, steatorrhea, purpura, or bone and back pain due to osteomalacia. The patient may also develop firm, nontender hepatomegaly, hematemesis, ascites, edema, or xanthomas on his palms, soles, or elbows.

◆ ***Cholangitis (sclerosing).*** Characterized by fibrosis of the bile ducts, this chronic inflammatory disorder may cause clay-colored stools, chronic or intermittent jaundice, pruritus, right-upper-quadrant pain, or chills and fever.

◆ ***Cholelithiasis.*** Stones in the biliary tract may cause clay-colored stools when they obstruct the common bile duct (choledocholithiasis). However, if the obstruction is intermittent, the stools may alternate between normal and clay color. Associated symptoms may include dyspepsia and — in sudden, severe obstruction — biliary colic. This right-upper-quadrant pain intensifies over several hours, may radiate to the epigastrium or shoulder blades, and is unrelieved by antacids. The pain is accompanied by tachycardia, restlessness, nausea, vomiting, upper abdominal tenderness, fever, chills, or jaundice.

♦ ***Hepatic cancer.*** Before clay-colored stools develop in this disease, the patient usually experiences weight loss, weakness, and anorexia. Later, he may develop nodular, firm hepatomegaly, jaundice, right-upper-quadrant pain, ascites, dependent edema, and fever. A bruit, hum, or rubbing sound may be heard on auscultation if the cancer involves a large part of the liver.

♦ ***Hepatitis.*** In *viral hepatitis,* clay-colored stools signal the start of the icteric phase and are typically followed by jaundice within 1 to 5 days. Associated signs include mild weight loss and dark urine as well as continuation of some preicteric findings, such as anorexia or tender hepatomegaly. During the icteric phase, the patient may become irritable and develop right-upper-quadrant pain, splenomegaly, enlarged cervical lymph nodes, and severe pruritus. After jaundice disappears, the patient continues to experience fatigue, flatulence, abdominal pain or tenderness, and dyspepsia, although his appetite usually returns and hepatomegaly subsides. The posticteric phase generally lasts from 2 to 6 weeks, with full recovery in 6 months.

In cholestatic *nonviral hepatitis,* clay-colored stools occur with other signs of viral hepatitis.

♦ ***Pancreatic cancer.*** Common-bile-duct obstruction associated with this cancer may cause clay-colored stools. Classic associated features include abdominal or back pain, jaundice, pruritus, nausea and vomiting, anorexia, weight loss, fatigue, weakness, or fever. Other possible effects are diarrhea, skin lesions (especially on the legs), emotional lability, splenomegaly, or signs of GI bleeding. Auscultation may reveal a bruit in the periumbilical area or left upper quadrant.

♦ ***Pancreatitis (acute).*** This inflammatory disorder may cause clay-colored stools, dark urine, and jaundice. Typically, it also causes severe epigastric pain that radiates to the back and is aggravated by lying down. Associated findings may include nausea and vomiting, fever, abdominal rigidity and tenderness, hypoactive bowel sounds, or crackles at the lung bases. In severe pancreatitis, findings include marked restlessness, tachycardia, mottled skin, and cold, sweaty extremities.

Other causes

♦ ***Biliary surgery.*** This surgery may cause bile duct stricture, resulting in clay-colored stools.

Special considerations

Prepare the patient for diagnostic tests, such as liver enzyme and serum bilirubin levels, sonograms, computed tomography scan, or stool analysis.

Pediatric pointers

Clay-colored stools may occur in infants with biliary atresia.

Geriatric pointers

Because elderly patients with cholelithiasis have a greater risk of developing complications if the condition isn't treated, surgery should be considered early if symptoms persist.

STRIDOR

A loud, harsh, musical respiratory sound, stridor results from an obstruction in the trachea or larynx. Usually heard during inspiration, this sign may also occur during expiration in severe upper airway obstruction. It may begin as low-pitched "croaking" and progress to high-pitched "crowing" as respirations become more vigorous.

Life-threatening upper airway obstruction can stem from foreign-body aspiration, increased secretions, intraluminal tumor, localized edema or muscle spasms, or external compression by a tumor or aneurysm.

Emergency interventions

If you hear stridor, quickly check the patient's vital signs and examine him for other signs of partial airway obstruction — choking or gagging, tachypnea, dyspnea, shallow respirations, intercostal retractions, nasal flaring, tachycardia, cyanosis, or diaphoresis. Abrupt cessation of stridor signals complete obstruction, in which the patient has inspiratory chest movement but absent breath sounds. Complete lack of air movement makes the patient unable to talk and he quickly becomes lethargic and loses consciousness.

If you detect signs of airway obstruction, try to clear the airway with back blows or abdominal thrusts. Next, administer oxygen by nasal cannula or face mask, or prepare for emergency endotracheal intubation or tracheostomy and mechanical ventilation. (See *Performing emergency endotracheal intubation,* page 550.) Have equipment ready to suction aspirated vomitus or blood through the endotracheal or tracheostomy tube. Connect the patient to a cardiac monitor, and position him upright to ease his breathing.

History and physical examination

When the patient's condition permits, obtain a patient history from him or a family member. First, find out when the stridor began. Has he had it before? Does he have an upper respiratory infection? If so, how long has he had it?

Ask about a history of allergies, tumors, and respiratory and vascular disorders. Note recent exposure to smoke or noxious fumes or gases. Next, explore associated signs and symptoms. Does stridor occur with pain or a cough?

Examine the patient's mouth for excessive secretions, foreign matter, inflammation, and swelling. Assess his neck for swelling, masses, subcutaneous crepitation, and scars. Observe his chest for delayed, decreased, or asymmetrical chest expansion. Auscultate for wheezes, rhonchi, crackles, rubs, and other abnormal breath sounds. Percuss for dullness, tympany, or flatness. Finally, note burns or signs of trauma, such as ecchymoses or lacerations.

Common medical causes

◆ ***Airway trauma.*** Local trauma to the upper airway commonly causes acute obstruction, resulting in the sudden onset of stridor. Accompanying this sign are dysphonia, dysphagia, hemoptysis, cyanosis, accessory muscle use, intercostal retractions, nasal flaring, tachypnea, progressive dyspnea, and shallow respirations. Palpation may reveal subcutaneous crepitation in the neck or upper chest.

◆ ***Anaphylaxis.*** In a severe allergic reaction, upper airway edema and laryngospasm cause stridor and other signs of respiratory distress: nasal flaring, wheezing, accessory muscle use, intercostal retractions, and dyspnea. The patient may also develop nasal congestion and profuse, watery rhinorrhea. Typically, these respiratory effects are preceded by a feeling of impending doom or fear, weakness, diaphoresis, sneezing, nasal pruritus, urticaria, erythema, or angioedema. Common associated findings include chest or throat tightness, dysphagia, and possibly signs of shock, such as hypotension, tachycardia, or cool, clammy skin.

◆ ***Aspiration of a foreign body.*** Sudden stridor is characteristic in this life-threatening situation. Related findings include abrupt onset of dry, paroxysmal coughing, gagging or choking, hoarseness, tachycardia, wheezing, dyspnea, tachypnea, intercostal muscle retractions, diminished breath sounds, cyanosis, and shallow respirations. The patient typically appears anxious and distressed.

◆ ***Hypocalcemia.*** In this disorder, laryngospasm can cause stridor. Other findings include paresthesia, carpopedal spasm, or positive Chvostek's and Trousseau's signs.

EMERGENCY INTERVENTIONS

Performing emergency endotracheal intubation

If a patient has stridor, you may have to perform emergency endotracheal (ET) intubation to establish a patent airway and administer mechanical ventilation. Follow these essential steps:

- Gather the necessary equipment.
- Explain the procedure to the patient.
- Place the patient on his back with a small blanket or pillow under his head. This position aligns the axis of the oropharynx, posterior pharynx, and trachea.
- Check the cuff on the ET tube for leaks.
- After intubation, inflate the cuff, using minimal air leak technique.
- Check tube placement by auscultating for bilateral breath sounds: observe the patient for chest expansion and feel for warm exhalations at the ET tube's opening.
- Insert an oral airway or bite block.
- Secure the tube and airway with tape applied to skin treated with compound benzoin tincture.
- Suction secretions from the patient's mouth and the ET tube as needed.
- Administer oxygen or initiate mechanical ventilation (or both).

After the patient has been intubated, suction secretions as needed and check cuff pressure once every shift. Correct any air leaks with the minimal leak technique. Prepare the patient for chest X-rays to check tube placement, and restrain and reassure him as needed.

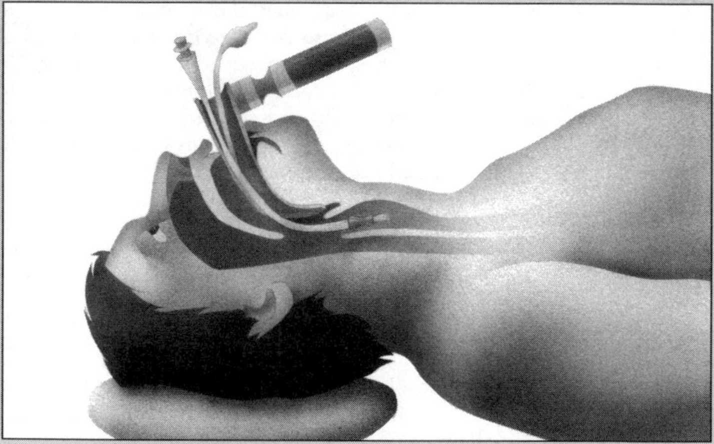

♦ ***Inhalation injury.*** Within 48 hours after inhalation of smoke or noxious fumes, the patient may develop laryngeal edema and bronchospasms, resulting in stridor. Associated signs and symptoms may include singed nasal hairs, orofacial burns, coughing, hoarseness, sooty sputum, crackles, rhonchi, wheezes, or other signs of respiratory distress, such as dyspnea, accessory muscle use, intercostal retractions, or nasal flaring.

♦ ***Mediastinal tumor.*** Commonly producing no symptoms at first, this tumor may eventually compress the trachea and bronchi, resulting in stridor. Its other effects include hoarseness, brassy cough, tracheal shift or tug, dilated neck veins, swelling of the face and neck, stertorous respirations, or suprasternal retractions on inspiration. The patient may also report dyspnea, dysphagia, or pain in the chest, shoulder, or arm.

♦ ***Retrosternal thyroid.*** This anatomic abnormality causes stridor, dysphagia, cough, hoarseness, and tracheal deviation. It can also cause signs of thyrotoxicosis.

Other causes

♦ ***Diagnostic tests.*** Bronchoscopy or laryngoscopy may precipitate laryngospasm and stridor.

♦ ***Treatments.*** After prolonged intubation, the patient may exhibit laryngeal edema and stridor when the tube is removed. Aerosol therapy with epinephrine may reduce stridor. Reintubation may be necessary. Neck surgery, such as thyroidectomy, may cause laryngeal paralysis and stridor.

Special considerations

Continue to monitor the patient's vital signs closely. Prepare him for diagnostic tests, such as arterial blood gas analysis and chest X-rays.

Pediatric pointers

Stridor is a major sign of airway obstruction in children. When you hear it, you must intervene quickly to prevent total airway obstruction. This emergency can happen more rapidly in a child because his airway is narrower than an adult's.

Causes of stridor in children include foreign-body aspiration, croup syndrome, laryngeal diphtheria, pertussis, retropharyngeal abscess, or congenital abnormalities of the larynx.

Therapy for partial airway obstruction typically involves hot or cold steam in a mist tent or hood, parenteral fluids and electrolytes, and plenty of rest.

Syncope

A common neurologic sign, syncope (or fainting) refers to transient loss of consciousness associated with impaired cerebral blood supply. It usually occurs abruptly and lasts for seconds to minutes. Typically, the patient lies motionless with skeletal muscles relaxed but sphincter muscles controlled. The depth of unconsciousness varies — some patients can hear voices or see blurred outlines; others are unaware of their surroundings.

In many ways, syncope simulates death: The patient is strikingly pale, has a slow, weak pulse, and is hypotensive; breathing is almost imperceptible. If severe hypotension lasts for 20 seconds or longer, the patient may also develop convulsive, tonic-clonic movements.

Syncope may result from cardiac and cerebrovascular disorders, hypoxemia, or postural changes in the presence of autonomic dysfunction. It may also follow vigorous coughing (tussive syncope) or emotional stress, injury, shock, or pain (vasovagal syncope, or common fainting). Hysterical syncope may follow emotional stress but isn't accompanied by other vasodepressor effects.

Emergency interventions

If you see a patient faint, ensure a patent airway and take vital signs. Then place the patient in a supine position, elevate his legs, and loosen tight clothing. Be alert for tachycardia, bradycardia, or an irregular pulse. Meanwhile, place him on a cardiac monitor to detect arrhythmias. If an arrhythmia appears, give oxygen and insert an I.V. line for drug administration. Be ready to begin cardiopulmonary resuscitation. Cardioversion, defibrillation, or insertion of a temporary pacemaker may be required.

History and physical examination

If the patient reports a fainting episode, gather information about the episode from him and his family. Did he feel weak, light-headed, nauseous, or sweaty just before he fainted? Did he get up quickly from a chair or from lying down? During the fainting episode, did he have muscle spasms or incontinence? How long was he unconscious? When he regained consciousness, was he alert or confused? Did he have a headache? Has he fainted before? If so, how often does it occur?

Next, take the patient's vital signs and examine him for injuries that may have occurred during his fall.

Common medical causes

♦ ***Aortic arch syndrome.*** The patient experiences syncope and may exhibit weak or abruptly absent carotid pulses and unequal or absent radial pulses. Early symptoms include night sweats, pallor, nausea, anorexia, weight loss, arthralgia, or Raynaud's phenomenon. He may also develop hypotension in the arms; neck, shoulder, and chest pain; paresthesia; intermittent claudication; bruits; visual disturbances; or dizziness.

♦ ***Aortic stenosis.*** A cardinal late sign, syncope is accompanied by exertional dyspnea and anginal pain. Related findings include marked fatigue, orthopnea, paroxysmal nocturnal dyspnea, palpitations, or diminished carotid pulses. Typically, auscultation reveals atrial and ventricular gallops as well as a harsh, crescendo-decrescendo systolic ejection murmur that's loudest at the right sternal border of the second intercostal space.

♦ ***Cardiac arrhythmias.*** Any arrhythmia that decreases cardiac output and impairs cerebral circulation may cause syncope. Other effects, such as palpitations, pallor, confusion, diaphoresis, dyspnea, and hypotension, usually develop first. However, in Adams-Stokes syndrome, syncope may occur without warning. During syncope, the patient develops asystole, which may precipitate spasm and myoclonic jerks if prolonged. He also displays an ashen-gray pallor that progresses to cyanosis, incontinence, bilateral Babinski's reflex, and fixed pupils.

♦ ***Hypoxemia.*** Regardless of its cause, severe hypoxemia may cause syncope. Common related effects include confusion, tachycardia, restlessness, and incoordination.

♦ ***Orthostatic hypotension.*** Syncope occurs when the patient rises quickly from a recumbent position. Look for a drop of 10 to 20 mm Hg or more in systolic or diastolic blood pressure as well as tachycardia, pallor, dizziness, blurred vision, nausea, or diaphoresis.

♦ ***Transient ischemic attacks.*** Marked by transient neurologic deficits, these attacks may cause syncope and decreased level of consciousness. Other findings vary with the affected artery; they may include vision loss, nystagmus, aphasia, dysarthria, unilateral numbness, hemiparesis or hemiplegia, tinnitus, facial weakness, dysphagia, or staggering or uncoordinated gait.

Other causes

♦ ***Drugs.*** Quinidine may cause syncope — and possibly sudden death — associated with ventricular fibrillation. Prazosin may cause severe orthostatic hypotension and syncope, usually after the first dose. Occasionally, griseofulvin, levodopa, or indomethacin can cause syncope.

Special considerations

Continue to monitor the patient's vital signs closely. Advise him to pace his activities, to rise slowly from a recumbent position, to avoid standing still for a prolonged time, and to sit or lie down as soon as he feels faint.

Pediatric pointers

Syncope is much less common in children than in adults. It may result from cardiac or neurologic disorders, allergy, or emotional stress.

T

TACHYCARDIA

Easily detected by counting the apical, carotid, or radial pulse, tachycardia is a heart rate greater than 100 beats/minute. The patient with tachycardia usually complains of palpitations or of a "racing" heart. This common sign normally occurs in response to emotional or physical stress, such as excitement, exercise, pain, or fever. It may also result from the use of stimulants, such as caffeine or tobacco. However, tachycardia may be an early sign of a life-threatening disorder, such as cardiogenic, hypovolemic, or septic shock. It may also result from cardiovascular, respiratory, or metabolic disorders or from the effects of certain drugs, tests, or treatments. (See *What happens in tachycardia*, page 554.)

Emergency interventions

After detecting tachycardia, first perform electrocardiography (ECG) to evaluate the cardiac rhythm. Then, examine the patient for reduced cardiac output, which may initiate or result from tachycardia. Take the patient's other vital signs and determine his level of consciousness (LOC). If the patient has increased or decreased blood pressure and is drowsy or confused, administer oxygen and begin cardiac monitoring. Insert an I.V. line to allow fluid and drug administration, and gather emergency resuscitation equipment.

History and physical examination

If the patient's condition permits, take a focused history. Find out if he has had palpitations before. If so, how were they treated? Explore associated symptoms. Is the patient dizzy or short of breath? Weak or fatigued? Is he experiencing chest pain? Next, ask about a history of trauma, diabetes, or cardiac, pulmonary, or thyroid disorders. Also, obtain a drug history.

Inspect the patient's skin for pallor or cyanosis. Assess pulses and look for peripheral edema. Finally, auscultate the heart and lungs for abnormal sounds or rhythms.

Common medical causes

♦ ***Adrenocortical insufficiency.*** In this disorder, tachycardia commonly occurs with a weak pulse and progressive weakness and fatigue, which may become so severe that the patient requires bed rest. Other clinical features include abdominal pain, nausea and vomiting, altered bowel habits, weight loss, orthostatic hypotension, irritability, bronze skin, decreased libido, and syncope. Some patients report an enhanced sense of taste, smell, or hearing.

♦ ***Adult respiratory distress syndrome.*** Besides tachycardia, this syndrome causes crackles, rhonchi, dyspnea, tachypnea, nasal flaring, and grunting respirations. Other findings include cyanosis, anxiety,

What happens in tachycardia

Tachycardia represents the heart's effort to deliver more oxygen to body tissues by increasing the rate at which blood passes through the vessels. This sign can reflect over-stimulation in the sinoatrial node, the atrium, the atrioventricular node, or the ventricles.

Increased heart rate can increase cardiac output (cardiac output = heart rate × stroke volume) but tachycardia can lower cardiac output by reducing ventricular filling time and stroke volume (the output of each ventricle at every contraction). If cardiac output falls, so do arterial pressure and peripheral perfusion. Tachycardia further aggravates myocardial ischemia by increasing the heart's demand for oxygen while reducing the duration of diastole — the period of greatest coronary flow.

decreased LOC, and abnormal chest X-ray findings.

♦ ***Anaphylactic shock.*** In this life-threatening condition, tachycardia and hypotension develop within minutes after exposure to an allergen, such as penicillin or an insect sting. Typically, the patient is visibly anxious and has severe pruritus, perhaps with urticaria and a pounding headache. Other findings may include flushed and clammy skin, a cough, dyspnea, nausea, abdominal cramps, seizures, stridor, change or loss of voice associated with laryngeal edema, or urinary urgency and incontinence.

♦ ***Anemia.*** Tachycardia and bounding pulse are characteristic in anemia. Associated signs and symptoms include fatigue, pallor, dyspnea and, possibly, bleeding tendencies. Auscultation may reveal an atrial gallop, a systolic bruit over the carotid arteries, and crackles.

♦ ***Aortic regurgitation.*** Accompanying tachycardia are a "water-hammer" bounding pulse and a large, diffuse apical heave. In severe regurgitation, widened pulse pressure occurs. Auscultation reveals a hallmark diastolic murmur that starts with the second heart sound; is decrescendo, high-pitched, and blowing; and is heard best at the left sternal border of the second and third intercostal spaces. An atrial or ventricular gallop, an early systolic murmur, an Austin Flint murmur (apical diastolic rumble), or Duroziez's sign (a murmur over the femoral artery during systole and diastole) also may be heard. Other findings may include anginal chest pain, dyspnea, palpitations, strong and abrupt carotid pulsations, pallor, or signs of heart failure, such as crackles and neck vein distention.

♦ ***Aortic stenosis.*** Typically, this valvular disorder causes tachycardia, a weak, thready pulse, and an atrial gallop. Its chief features, however, are exertional dyspnea, anginal chest pain, dizziness, and syncope. Aortic stenosis also causes a harsh, crescendo-decrescendo systolic ejection murmur that's loudest at the right sternal border of the second intercostal space. Other findings may include palpitations, crackles, and fatigue.

♦ ***Cardiac arrhythmias.*** Tachycardia may accompany an irregular heart rhythm. The patient may be hypotensive and report dizziness, palpitations, weakness, and fatigue. Depending on his heart rate, he may also exhibit tachypnea, decreased LOC, or pale, cool, clammy skin.

♦ ***Cardiac contusion.*** This result of blunt chest trauma may cause tachycardia, substernal pain, dyspnea, and palpitations. Assessment may detect sternal ecchymoses and a pericardial friction rub.

♦ ***Cardiac tamponade.*** In this life-threatening condition, tachycardia is commonly accompanied by pulsus paradoxus, dyspnea, and tachypnea. The patient is visibly anxious and restless and has cyanotic, clammy skin and distended neck veins. He may develop muffled

Other causes

- ***Diagnostic tests.*** Cardiac catheterization and electrophysiologic studies may induce transient tachycardia.
- ***Drugs and alcohol.*** Various drugs affect the nervous system, circulatory system, or heart muscle, resulting in tachycardia. Examples are sympathomimetics; phenothiazines; anticholinergics such as atropine; thyroid drugs; vasodilators, such as hydralazine and nifedipine; acetylcholinesterase inhibitors such as captopril; nitrates such as nitroglycerin; and alpha-adrenergic blockers such as phentolamine. Excessive caffeine intake or alcohol intoxication may also cause tachycardia.
- ***Surgery and pacemakers.*** Cardiac surgery and pacemaker malfunction or wire irritation may cause tachycardia.

Special considerations

Continue to monitor the patient closely. Explain ordered diagnostic tests, such as blood work, pulmonary function studies, and 12-lead ECG. If appropriate, prepare him for an ambulatory ECG.

Pediatric pointers

When examining a child for tachycardia, recognize that normal heart rates for children are higher than those for adults. (See *Normal pediatric vital signs.*) In children, tachycardia may result from many of the adult causes.

TACHYPNEA

A common sign of cardiopulmonary disorders, tachypnea is an abnormally fast respiratory rate — 20 or more breaths/minute. Tachypnea may reflect the need to increase minute volume — the amount of air breathed each minute. Under these circumstances, it may be accompanied by an increase in tidal volume — the volume of air inhaled or exhaled per breath — resulting in hyperventilation. Tachypnea, however, may also reflect stiff lungs or overloaded ventilatory muscles, in which case tidal volume may be reduced.

Tachypnea may result from reduced arterial oxygen tension or oxygen content, decreased perfusion, or increased oxygen demand. Fever, exertion, anxiety, or pain can heighten oxygen demand. Generally, respirations increase by 4 breaths/minute for every 1° F (0.56° C) increase in body temperature. Tachypnea may also occur as a compensatory response to metabolic acidosis or may result from pulmonary irritation, stretch receptor stimulation, or neurologic disorders that upset medullary respiratory control.

Emergency interventions

After detecting tachypnea, quickly evaluate cardiopulmonary status; check for cyanosis, chest pain, dyspnea, tachycardia, and hypotension. Administer supplemental oxygen by nasal cannula or face mask and, if possible, place the patient in semi-Fowler's position to help ease his breathing. Intubation and mechanical ventilation may be necessary if respiratory failure occurs. Also, insert an I.V. line for fluid and drug administration and begin cardiac monitoring. If the patient has paradoxical chest movement, suspect flail chest and immediately splint his chest with your hands or with sandbags.

History and physical examination

If the patient's condition permits, obtain a medical history. Find out when the tachypnea began. Did it follow activity? Has he had it before? Then have him describe associated signs and symptoms, such as diaphoresis or recent weight loss. Is he anxious about anything or does he have a history of anxiety attacks? Is he having pain? If he's taking drugs for pain relief, are the drugs effective?

Begin the physical examination by taking the patient's other vital signs, if you haven't already done so, and observing his overall behavior. Does he seem restless? Then auscultate the chest for abnormal heart and breath sounds. If the patient has a productive cough, record the color, amount, and consistency of sputum. Finally, check for jugular vein distention and examine the skin for pallor, cyanosis, edema, and warmth or coolness.

Common medical causes

♦ ***Adult respiratory distress syndrome (ARDS).*** In this life-threatening disorder, tachypnea and apprehension may be the earliest features. Tachypnea gradually worsens as fluid accumulates in the patient's lungs, causing them to stiffen. It's accompanied by accessory muscle use, grunting expirations, suprasternal and intercostal retractions, and crackles. Eventually, ARDS causes hypoxemia, resulting in tachycardia, dyspnea, cyanosis, respiratory failure, and shock.

♦ ***Anaphylactic shock.*** In this life-threatening type of shock, tachypnea develops within minutes after exposure to an allergen, such as penicillin or insect venom. Accompanying features include anxiety, pounding headache, skin flushing, intense pruritus and, possibly, diffuse urticaria. The patient may exhibit widespread edema, affecting the eyelids, lips, tongue, hands, feet, and genitalia. Other findings include cool, clammy skin; rapid, thready pulse; cough; dyspnea; stridor; and change or loss of voice associated with laryngeal edema.

♦ ***Aspiration of a foreign body.*** Upper airway obstruction by an aspirated foreign body may be life threatening. The patient with a *partial obstruction* abruptly develops a dry, paroxysmal cough with rapid, shallow respirations. Other signs and symptoms include dyspnea, gagging or choking, intercostal retractions, nasal flaring, cyanosis, decreased or absent breath sounds, hoarseness, or stridor or coarse wheezing. Typically, the patient appears frightened and distressed. A *complete obstruction* may rapidly cause asphyxia and death.

♦ ***Asthma.*** Tachypnea is common during an asthma attack. An attack usually begins with mild wheezing and a dry cough. If it continues, the patient becomes apprehensive and develops prolonged expirations, intercostal and supraclavicular retractions on inspiration, accessory muscle use, severe audible wheezing, flaring nostrils, tachycardia, diaphoresis, and flushing or cyanosis.

♦ ***Bronchitis (chronic).*** Mild tachypnea may occur in this form of chronic obstructive pulmonary disease, but it isn't typically a predominant sign. Usually, chronic bronchitis begins with a productive cough. Other characteristics include dyspnea, prolonged expirations, wheezing, scattered rhonchi, accessory muscle use, and cyanosis. Clubbing and barrel chest are late signs.

♦ ***Cardiac arrhythmias.*** Depending on the patient's heart rate, tachypnea may occur with hypotension, dizziness, palpitations, weakness, and fatigue. The patient's level of consciousness (LOC) may be decreased.

♦ ***Cardiac tamponade.*** In this life-threatening condition, tachypnea may accompany tachycardia, dyspnea, and pulsus paradoxus. Related findings include muffled heart sounds, pericardial friction rub, chest pain, hypotension, narrowed pulse pressure, and hepatomegaly. The patient is noticeably anxious and restless. His skin is clammy and cyanotic, and his neck veins are distended.

♦ ***Cardiogenic shock.*** Although many signs of cardiogenic shock appear in other types of shock, they're usually more severe in this type. Besides tachypnea, the patient commonly displays cold, pale, clammy, cyanotic skin; hypotension; tachycardia; narrowed pulse pressure; a ventricular gallop; oliguria; decreased LOC; and neck vein distention.

♦ ***Emphysema.*** This chronic pulmonary disorder commonly causes tachypnea accompanied by exertional dyspnea. Other possible findings include anorexia, malaise, pursed-lip breathing, accessory muscle use, barrel chest, and dry cough. Percussion yields a hyperresonant tone; auscultation reveals diminished breath sounds.

- ***Flail chest.*** Tachypnea usually appears early in this life-threatening disorder. Other findings include paradoxical chest wall movement, rib bruises and palpable fractures, localized chest pain, hypotension, and diminished breath sounds. The patient may also develop signs of respiratory distress, such as dyspnea and accessory muscle use.
- ***Hyperosmolar hyperglycemic nonketotic syndrome.*** Rapidly deteriorating LOC is accompanied by tachypnea, tachycardia, hypotension, seizures, oliguria, and signs of dehydration.
- ***Hypovolemic shock.*** An early sign of life-threatening hypovolemic shock, tachypnea is accompanied by cool, pale skin; restlessness; thirst; and mild tachycardia. As shock progresses, the patient's skin becomes clammy and his pulse increasingly rapid and thready. Other findings include hypotension, narrowed pulse pressure, oliguria, subnormal body temperature, or decreased LOC.
- ***Interstitial fibrosis.*** Tachypnea develops gradually and may become severe. Associated features may include dyspnea on exertion, pleuritic chest pain, a paroxysmal dry cough, crackles, fatigue, or weight loss. Clubbing is a late sign.
- ***Lung abscess.*** Tachypnea is usually paired with dyspnea and accentuated by fever. However, the chief sign is a productive cough with copious amounts of purulent, foul-smelling, commonly bloody sputum. Other findings may include chest pain, halitosis, diaphoresis, chills, fatigue, weakness, anorexia, weight loss, or clubbing.
- ***Mesothelioma (malignant).*** Commonly related to asbestos exposure, this pleural mass initially causes tachypnea and dyspnea on mild exertion. Other classic symptoms are persistent, dull chest pain and aching shoulder pain that progresses to arm weakness and paresthesia. Later signs and symptoms include a cough, insomnia associated with pain, clubbing, and dullness over the tumor.
- ***Neurogenic shock.*** Tachypnea is characteristic in this life-threatening type of shock. It's commonly accompanied by apprehension, bradycardia or tachycardia, oliguria, fluctuating body temperature, and decreased LOC, which may progress to coma. The patient's skin is warm, dry, and perhaps flushed. He may experience nausea and vomiting.
- ***Pneumonia (bacterial).*** A common sign in this infection, tachypnea is usually preceded by a painful, hacking, dry cough that rapidly becomes productive. Other signs and symptoms quickly follow, including high fever, shaking chills, headache, dyspnea, pleuritic chest pain, tachycardia, grunting respirations, nasal flaring, and cyanosis. Auscultation reveals diminished breath sounds and fine crackles; percussion yields a dull tone.
- ***Pneumothorax.*** Tachypnea, a common sign of life-threatening pneumothorax, is typically accompanied by severe, sharp, and commonly unilateral chest pain that's aggravated by chest movement. Associated signs and symptoms may include dyspnea, tachycardia, accessory muscle use, asymmetrical chest expansion, dry cough, anxiety, or restlessness. Examination of the affected lung reveals hyperresonance or tympany, subcutaneous crepitation, decreased vocal fremitus, and diminished or absent breath sounds. The patient with tension pneumothorax may also develop a deviated trachea.
- ***Pulmonary edema.*** An early sign of this life-threatening disorder, tachypnea is accompanied by exertional dyspnea, paroxysmal nocturnal dyspnea and, later, orthopnea. Other features include a dry cough, crackles, tachycardia, and a ventricular gallop. In severe pulmonary edema, respirations become increasing-

ly rapid and labored, tachycardia worsens, crackles become more diffuse, and the cough produces frothy, pink sputum. Signs of shock — such as hypotension, thready pulse, and cold, clammy skin — may also be present.

◆ ***Pulmonary embolism (acute).*** Tachypnea occurs suddenly in pulmonary embolism and is usually accompanied by dyspnea. The patient may complain of anginal or pleuritic chest pain. Other common characteristics include tachycardia, a dry cough or one producing blood-tinged sputum, low-grade fever, restlessness, and diaphoresis. Less common signs include massive hemoptysis, chest splinting, or leg edema and — with a large embolus — distended neck veins, cyanosis, and syncope. Other possible findings include pleural friction rub, crackles, diffuse wheezing, dullness on percussion, diminished breath sounds, or signs of shock, such as hypotension and a weak, rapid pulse.

◆ ***Septic shock.*** Early in septic shock, the patient usually experiences tachypnea; sudden fever; chills; flushed, warm, dry skin; and possibly nausea, vomiting, and diarrhea. He may also develop tachycardia and normal or slightly decreased blood pressure. As this life-threatening type of shock progresses, the patient may display anxiety; restlessness; decreased LOC; hypotension; cool, clammy, and cyanotic skin; rapid, thready pulse; thirst; and oliguria that may progress to anuria.

Other causes

◆ ***Salicylates.*** Tachypnea may result from an overdose of these drugs due to hyperventilation to compensate for metabolic acidosis.

Special considerations

Continue to monitor the patient's vital signs closely. Be sure to keep suction and emergency equipment nearby. Prepare to intubate the patient and to provide mechanical ventilation if necessary. Prepare the patient for diagnostic studies, such as arterial blood gas analysis, chest X-rays, or an electrocardiogram.

Pediatric pointers

When assessing a child for tachypnea, be aware that the normal respiratory rate varies with the child's age. (See *Normal pediatric vital signs,* page 556.) If you detect tachypnea, first rule out the causes listed previously. Then consider these pediatric causes: congenital heart defects, meningitis, metabolic acidosis, and cystic fibrosis. Keep in mind, however, that hunger and anxiety may also cause tachypnea.

Geriatric pointers

Tachypnea may have various causes in elderly patients, and mild increases in respiratory rate may be unnoticed.

THROAT PAIN

Throat pain — commonly known as a sore throat — refers to discomfort in any part of the pharynx: nasopharynx, oropharynx, or hypopharynx. This common symptom ranges from a sensation of scratchiness to severe pain. It's commonly accompanied by ear pain because cranial nerves IX and X innervate the pharynx as well as the middle and external ears. (See *Reviewing anatomy of the throat.*)

Throat pain may result from infection, trauma, cancer, or certain systemic disorders. It may also follow surgery or endotracheal intubation. Nonpathologic causes include dry mucous membranes associated with mouth breathing and laryngeal irritation associated with alcohol consumption, inhaling smoke or chemicals like ammonia, or vocal strain.

History and physical examination

Ask the patient when he first noticed the pain and have him describe it. Has he had throat pain before? Is it accompa-

Reviewing anatomy of the throat

The throat, or pharynx, is divided into three areas: nasopharynx (soft palate and posterior, or nasal, cavity), oropharynx (between the soft palate and the upper edge of the epiglottis), and hypopharynx (between the epiglottis and the level of the cricoid cartilage). A disorder affecting any of these areas may cause throat pain. Pinpointing the causative disorder begins with accurate assessment of the throat structures illustrated here.

FRONTAL VIEW

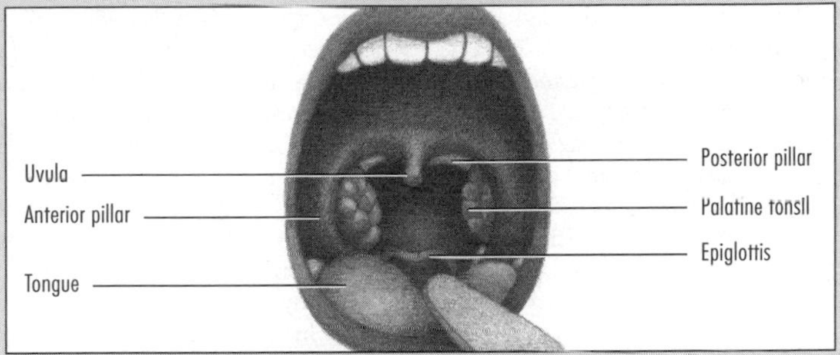

CROSS-SECTIONAL VIEW

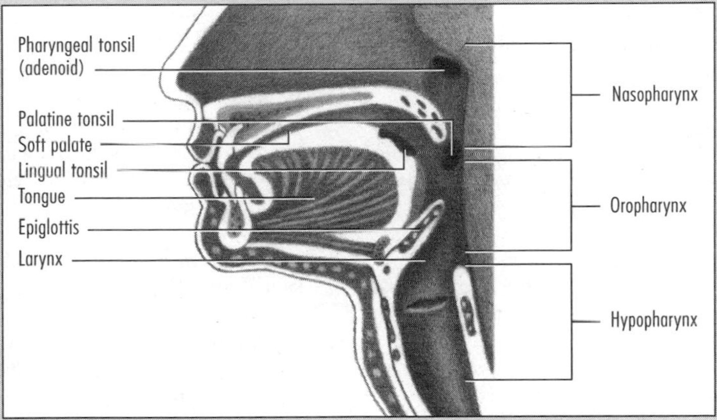

nied by fever, ear pain, or dysphagia? Review the patient's medical history for throat problems, allergies, and systemic disorders.

Next, carefully examine the pharynx, noting redness, exudate, or swelling. Examine the oropharynx, using a warmed metal spatula or a tongue blade, and the nasopharynx, using a warmed laryngeal mirror or a fiberoptic nasopharyngoscope. Laryngoscopic examination of the hypopharynx may be required. (If necessary, spray the soft palate and pharyngeal wall with a local anesthetic to prevent gagging.) Observe the tonsils for redness, swelling, asymmetry, or exudate (if present, obtain a specimen for culture). Then use a nasal speculum to examine the nose. Also check the patient's ears, especially if he reports ear pain. Finally, palpate the neck and oropharynx, tonsils and base of tongue for nodules or lymph node enlargement.

Common medical causes

- ***Agranulocytosis.*** Sore throat may accompany other signs of infection, such as fever and chills or headache. Typically, it follows progressive fatigue and weakness. Other findings may include nausea and vomiting, anorexia, and bleeding tendencies. Rough-edged ulcers with gray or black membranes may appear on the gums, palate, or perianal area.
- ***Bronchitis (acute).*** This disorder may cause lower throat pain associated with fever, chills, cough, or muscle or back pain. Auscultation reveals rhonchi, wheezing and, at times, crackles.
- ***Chronic fatigue syndrome.*** This nonspecific symptom complex is characterized by incapacitating fatigue. In addition to sore throat, associated findings include myalgia and cognitive dysfunction.
- ***Common cold.*** Sore throat may accompany cough, sneezing, nasal congestion, rhinorrhea, fatigue, headache, myalgia, or arthralgia.
- ***Contact ulcers.*** Common in men with stressful jobs, contact ulcers appear symmetrically on the posterior vocal cords, resulting in sore throat. The pain is aggravated by talking and may be accompanied by referred ear pain and, occasionally, hemoptysis. Typically, the patient also has a history of chronic throat clearing or acid reflux.
- ***Foreign body.*** A foreign body lodged in the palatine or lingual tonsil and pyriform sinus may cause localized throat pain. The pain may persist after the foreign body is dislodged until mucosal irritation resolves.
- ***Influenza.*** Patients with the flu commonly complain of sore throat, fever with chills, headache, weakness, malaise, muscle aches, cough and, occasionally, hoarseness and rhinorrhea.
- ***Laryngeal cancer.*** In *extrinsic laryngeal cancer,* the chief symptom is pain or burning in the throat when drinking citrus juice or hot liquids or a lump in the throat; in *intrinsic laryngeal cancer*, it's hoarseness that persists for longer than 3 weeks. Later clinical effects of metastasis include dysphagia, dyspnea, a cough, enlarged cervical lymph nodes, or pain that radiates to the ear.
- ***Mononucleosis (infectious).*** This disorder resembles a severe attack of acute tonsillitis with high fluctuating fever (evening peak of 101° F to 102° F [38.3° C to 38.9° C]), swollen tonsils covered with a dirty gray membrane, malaise, sore throat, significant cervical adenopathy, dysphagia, or odynophagia. Patients may have hepatomegaly, splenomegaly, skin rash, or palatal petechiae.
- ***Necrotizing ulcerative gingivitis (acute).*** Also known as trench mouth, this disorder usually begins abruptly with sore throat and tender gums that ulcerate and bleed. A gray exudate may cover the gums and pharyngeal tonsils. Related signs and symptoms include a foul taste in the mouth, halitosis, cervical lymphadenopathy, headache, malaise, or fever.
- ***Peritonsillar abscess.*** A complication of bacterial tonsillitis, this abscess typically causes severe throat pain that radiates to the ear. Accompanying the pain may be dysphagia, drooling, dysarthria, halitosis, fever with chills, malaise, and nausea. The patient usually tilts his head toward the side of the abscess. Examination may also reveal a deviated uvula, trismus, or tender cervical lymphadenopathy.
- ***Pharyngitis.*** Whether bacterial, fungal, or viral, pharyngitis may cause sore throat and localized erythema and edema. *Bacterial pharyngitis* begins abruptly with a unilateral sore throat. Associated signs and symptoms include dys-

phagia, fever, malaise, headache, abdominal pain, myalgia, and arthralgia. Inspection reveals an exudate on the tonsil or tonsillar fossae, uvular edema, soft palate erythema, or tender cervical lymph nodes.

Also known as thrush, *fungal pharyngitis* causes diffuse sore throat—commonly described as a burning sensation—accompanied by pharyngeal erythema and edema. White plaques mark the pharynx, tonsil, tonsillar pillars, base of the tongue, and oral mucosa; scraping these plaques uncovers a hemorrhagic base.

In *viral pharyngitis,* findings include diffuse sore throat, malaise, fever, and mild erythema and edema of the posterior oropharyngeal wall. The tonsils aren't inflamed, but the cervical lymph nodes may be enlarged.

♦ ***Sinusitis (acute).*** This disorder may cause sore throat with purulent nasal discharge and postnasal drip, resulting in halitosis. Other effects may include headache, malaise, cough, fever, or facial pain and swelling associated with nasal congestion.

♦ ***Tongue cancer.*** Localized throat pain may occur around a raised white lesion or ulcer. The pain may radiate to the ear and be accompanied by dysphagia.

♦ ***Tonsillar cancer.*** Sore throat is the presenting symptom of tonsillar cancer; however, the cancer is usually quite advanced before this symptom appears. The pain radiates to the ear and is accompanied by a superficial ulcer on the tonsil or one that extends to the base of the tongue from the tonsil.

♦ ***Tonsillitis.*** Mild to severe sore throat is usually the first symptom of *acute tonsillitis*. The pain may radiate to the ears and be accompanied by dysphagia and headache. Related findings include malaise, fever with chills, halitosis, myalgia, arthralgia, and tender cervical lymphadenopathy. Examination reveals edematous, reddened tonsils with a purulent exudate.

Chronic tonsillitis causes mild sore throat, malaise, and tender cervical lymph nodes. The tonsils appear smooth, pink and, possibly, enlarged; purulent debris is observed in the crypts. Halitosis and a foul taste in the mouth are other common findings.

Unilateral or bilateral throat pain just above the hyoid bone occurs in *lingual tonsillitis.* The lingual tonsils appear red and swollen and are covered with exudate. Other findings include a muffled voice, dysphagia, and tender cervical lymphadenopathy on the affected side.

♦ ***Uvulitis.*** This inflammation may cause throat pain or a sensation of "something in the throat." The uvula is usually swollen and red; it's pale, however, in allergic uvulitis.

Other causes

♦ ***Treatments.*** Endotracheal intubation and local surgery, such as tonsillectomy and adenoidectomy, commonly cause sore throat.

Special considerations

Provide analgesic sprays or lozenges to relieve throat pain. Also prepare the patient for throat culture, complete blood count, and a monospot test.

Pediatric pointers

Sore throat is a common complaint in children and may result from many of the same disorders that affect adults. Other pediatric causes of sore throat include acute epiglottiditis, herpangina, scarlet fever, acute follicular tonsillitis, and retropharyngeal abscess.

THYROID ENLARGEMENT

An enlarged thyroid can result from inflammation, physiologic changes, iodine deficiency, or thyroid tumors. Depending on the medical cause, hyperfunction or hypofunction may occur with resulting excess or deficiency, respectively, of the hormone thyroxine. If no infection is present, enlargement is usually slow and progressive. An enlarged thyroid that causes visible swelling in the front of the neck is called a *goiter*.

History and physical examination

The patient's history commonly reveals the cause of thyroid enlargement. Important data include a family history of thyroid disease, when the thyroid enlargement began, previous irradiation of the thyroid or the neck, recent infections, and the use of thyroid replacement drugs.

Begin the physical examination by inspecting the patient's trachea for midline deviation. Although you can frequently see an enlarged gland, you should always palpate it. To palpate the thyroid gland, stand in front of or behind the patient. Give the patient a cup of water, and have him extend his neck slightly. Place the fingers of both hands on the patient's neck, just below the cricoid cartilage and just lateral to the trachea. Tell the patient to take a sip of water and swallow. The thyroid gland should rise as he swallows. Use your fingers to palpate laterally and downward to feel the whole thyroid gland. Palpate over the midline to feel the isthmus of the thyroid.

During palpation, note the size, shape, and consistency of the gland, and the presence or absence of nodules. Using the bell of a stethoscope, listen over the lateral lobes for a bruit, which may be continuous.

Common medical causes

◆ ***Hypothyroidism.*** This disorder, which is most prevalent in women, usually results from a dysfunction of the thyroid gland, which may be due to surgery, irradiation therapy, chronic autoimmune thyroiditis (Hashimoto's disease), or inflammatory conditions, such as amyloidosis or sarcoidosis. Besides an enlarged thyroid, signs and symptoms may include weight gain despite anorexia; fatigue; cold intolerance; constipation; menorrhagia; slowed intellectual and motor activity; dry, pale, cool skin; dry, sparse hair; and thick, brittle nails. Eventually, periorbital edema appears, and the face assumes a dull expression.

◆ ***Iodine deficiency.*** A goiter may result from a lack of iodine in the diet. *Endemic goiter* arises from a deficiency of iodine in the food or water of a particular area. Associated signs and symptoms of an endemic goiter include dysphagia, dyspnea, and tracheal deviation.

◆ ***Thyroiditis.*** Thyroiditis, inflammation of the thyroid gland, may be classified as acute or subacute. It may be due to bacterial or viral infections, in which case associated features may include fever and thyroid tenderness. The most prevalent cause of spontaneous hypothyroidism, however, is an autoimmune reaction, as occurs in Hashimoto's thyroiditis. Autoimmune thyroiditis usually causes no symptoms other than thyroid enlargement.

◆ ***Thyrotoxicosis.*** Overproduction of thyroid hormone causes thyrotoxicosis. The most common form is Graves' disease, which may result from genetic or immunologic causes. Associated signs and symptoms include nervousness; heat intolerance; fatigue; muscle atrophy and weakness; diminished blink frequency; prominent eyes with conjunctival vein engorgement; weight loss despite increased appetite; palpitations; tremors; exophthalmos; nausea and vomiting due to increased GI motility and peristalsis; and, in females, oligomenorrhea or amenorrhea.

◆ ***Tumors.*** An enlarged thyroid may result from a malignant tumor or a nonmalignant tumor, such as an adenoma. A malignant tumor usually appears as a single nodule; a nonmalignant tumor, as multiple nodules. Associated signs and symptoms include hoarseness, loss of voice, and dysphagia.

Ovarian dermoid tumors can contain thyroid tissue that functions autonomously. Pituitary tumors that secrete thyroid stimulating hormone (TSH), a rare type, are the only cause of normal or high TSH levels associated with thyrotoxicosis. Finally, high levels of human chorionic gonadotropin, as occur in pregnancy or as secreted by trophoblastic tumors, can cause thyrotoxicosis.

Other causes

♦ ***Goitrogens.*** These drugs and substances in foods inhibit thyroxine production. Drugs include lithium, sulfonamides, phenylbutazone, and para-aminosalicylic acid. Foods containing goitrogens include peanuts, cabbage, soybeans, strawberries, spinach, rutabagas, and radishes.

Special considerations

Prepare the patient with an enlarged thyroid for scheduled tests, which may include needle aspiration, ultrasound, or radioactive thyroid scanning. Also prepare him for surgery or radiation therapy, if necessary.

The hypothyroid patient will need a warm room and moisturizing lotion for his skin. A gentle laxative and stool softener may help with constipation. Provide a high-bulk, low-calorie diet, and encourage activity to promote weight loss. Warn the patient to report infection immediately; if he develops a fever, monitor his temperature until it's stable. After thyroid hormone replacement begins, watch for signs and symptoms of hyperthyroidism, such as restlessness, sweating, and excessive weight loss. Avoid administering sedatives if possible, or reduce their dosage because hypothyroidism delays metabolism of many drugs. Check arterial blood gas levels for indications of hypoxia and respiratory acidosis to determine whether the patient needs ventilatory assistance.

For patients with thyroiditis, give antibiotics and watch for rising temperature, which suggests developing resistance to antibiotics. Check vital signs, and examine the patient's neck for unusual swelling or redness. Provide a liquid diet if the patient has difficulty swallowing. Check for signs of hyperthyroidism, such as nervousness, tremor, and weakness, which commonly occur in subacute thyroiditis. The patient with severe hyperthyroidism (thyroid storm) will need close monitoring of temperature, volume status, heart rate, and blood pressure. For patients with hyperthyroidism, encourage hydration, monitor for mental status changes as the first sign of impending hemodynamic crisis (thyroid storm). Give written instructions and explain them slowly and thoroughly. Until the thyroid levels are normal, these patients commonly have difficulty with memory and concentration.

After thyroidectomy, check vital signs every 15 to 30 minutes until the patient's condition stabilizes. Be alert for signs of tetany secondary to accidental parathyroid injury during surgery. Keep 10% calcium gluconate available for I.V. use if needed. Evaluate dressings frequently for excessive bleeding, and watch for signs of airway obstruction, such as difficulty in talking or increased swallowing. Keep tracheotomy equipment handy.

Pediatric pointers

Congenital goiter, a syndrome of infantile myxedema or cretinism, is characterized by mental retardation, growth failure, and other signs and symptoms of hypothyroidism. Early treatment can prevent mental retardation. Genetic counseling is important, as subsequent children are at risk.

Tics

A tic is an involuntary, repetitive movement of a specific group of muscles—usually those of the face, neck, shoulders, trunk, or hands. This sign typically occurs suddenly and intermittently. It may be a single isolated movement—such as lip smacking, grimacing, blinking, sniffing, tongue thrusting, throat clearing, hitching up one shoulder, or protruding the chin—or a complex set of movements. Mild tics, such as twitching of an eyelid, are especially common. Unlike minor seizures, tics aren't associated with transient loss of consciousness or amnesia.

Tics are usually psychogenic and may be aggravated by stress or anxiety. Psychogenic tics commonly begin between the ages of 5 and 10 as voluntary, coordinated, and purposeful actions that the child feels compelled to perform to decrease anxiety. Unless the tics are severe, the child may be unaware of them. The tics may subside as the child matures, or they may persist into adulthood. Tics are also associated with one rare disorder—Gilles de la Tourette's syndrome, which typically begins in childhood.

History

Begin by asking the parents how long the child has had the tic. Can they identify precipitating factors? Ask about stress in the child's life such as difficult schoolwork. Next, carefully observe the tic and describe it in detail. Is it a purposive or involuntary movement? Is it localized or generalized?

Common medical causes

◆ ***Gilles de la Tourette's syndrome.*** This syndrome, which is thought to be largely a genetic disorder, typically begins between the ages of 2 and 15 with a tic that involves the face or neck. Symptoms include both motor and vocal tics that may involve the muscles of the shoulders, arms, trunk, or legs. The tics may be associated with violent movements or outbursts of obscenities (coprolalia). The patient may snort, bark, or grunt, and he may emit explosive sounds, such as hissing, when he speaks. He may involuntarily repeat another person's words (echolalia) or movements (echopraxia). This syndrome may subside spontaneously, undergo a prolonged remission, or persist throughout life.

◆ ***Neurochemical imbalance.*** It's thought that tics may result from an abnormality of the brain's metabolism of neurotransmitters such as dopamine, serotonin, or norepinephrine.

Special considerations

Psychotherapy and administration of tranquilizers may provide relief. In many patients with Gilles de la Tourette's syndrome, haloperidol, pimozide, or other antipsychotics help to control tics.

Tinnitus

Tinnitus literally means ringing in the ears, although many other abnormal sounds fall under this term. For example, tinnitus may be described as the sound of escaping air, running water, or the inside of a seashell or as a sizzling, buzzing, or humming noise. Occasionally, it's described as a roaring or musical sound. This common symptom may be unilateral or bilateral, constant or intermittent. Although the brain can adjust to or suppress constant tinnitus, intermittent tinnitus may be so disturbing that some patients contemplate suicide as their only source of relief.

Tinnitus can be classified in several ways: for example, *subjective tinnitus,* heard only by the patient; *objective tinnitus,* also heard by the observer who places a stethoscope near the patient's affected ear, *tinnitus aurium,* noise that the

Common causes of tinnitus

Tinnitus usually results from disorders that affect the external, middle, or inner ear. Here are some of its more common causes and their locations.

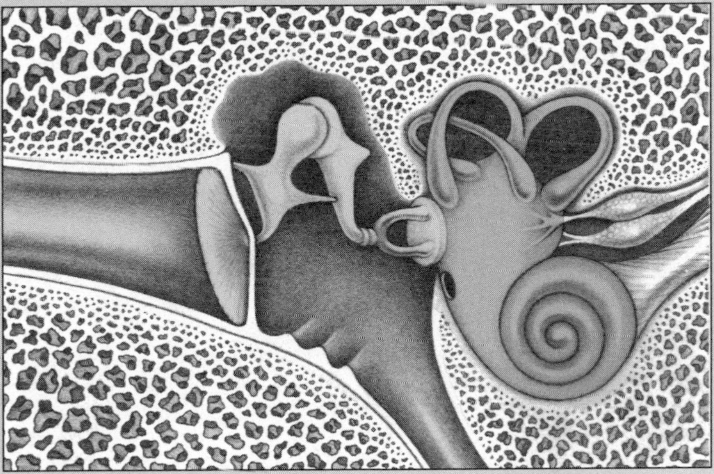

EXTERNAL EAR
- Ear canal obstruction by cerumen or a foreign body
- Otitis externa
- Tympanic membrane perforation

MIDDLE EAR
- Ossicle dislocation
- Otitis media
- Otosclerosis

INNER EAR
- Acoustic neuroma
- Atherosclerosis of the carotid artery
- Labyrinthitis
- Ménière's disease

patient hears in his ears; *tinnitus cerebri,* noise that he hears in his head.

Tinnitus is usually associated with neural injury in the auditory pathway, which causes abnormal, spontaneous firing of sensory auditory neurons. In addition to ear disorders, cardiovascular or systemic disorders or drugs can cause tinnitus. Nonpathologic causes of tinnitus include acute anxiety and presbycusis. (See *Common causes of tinnitus.*)

History and physical examination

Ask the patient to describe the sound he hears, including its onset, pattern, pitch, location, and intensity. Ask whether it's accompanied by other symptoms, such as vertigo, headache, or hearing loss. Next, take a health history, including a complete drug history.

Using an otoscope, inspect the patient's ears and examine the tympanic membrane. To check for hearing loss, perform Weber's and Rinne tests.

Also, auscultate for bruits in the neck. Then compress the jugular or carotid artery to see if this affects the tinnitus. Finally, examine the nasopharynx for masses that might cause eustachian tube dysfunction and tinnitus.

Common medical causes

♦ ***Acoustic neuroma.*** An early symptom of this cranial nerve VIII tumor, unilateral tinnitus precedes unilateral sensorineural hearing loss and vertigo. Facial paralysis, headache, nausea, vomiting, or papilledema may also occur.

♦ ***Atherosclerosis of the carotid artery.*** The patient has constant tinnitus that can be stopped by applying pressure over the carotid artery. He also feels confused, weak, and unsteady when he rises in the morning or stands up quickly. Auscultation over the upper part of the neck, on the auricle, or near the ear on the affected side may detect a bruit. Palpation may reveal a weak carotid pulse.

♦ ***Cervical spondylosis.*** In this degenerative disorder, osteophytic growths may compress the vertebral arteries, resulting in tinnitus. Typically, a stiff neck and pain aggravated by activity accompany tinnitus. Other features may include brief vertigo, nystagmus, hearing loss, paresthesia, weakness, or pain that radiates down the arms.

♦ ***Eustachian tube patency.*** Normally, the eustachian tube remains closed, except during swallowing. However, persistent patency of this tube can cause tinnitus, audible breath sounds, loud and distorted voice sounds, and a sense of fullness in the ear. Examination with a pneumatic otoscope reveals movement of the tympanic membrane with respirations. At times, breath sounds can be heard through a stethoscope placed over the auricle.

♦ ***Glomus jugulare or tympanicum tumor.*** A pulsating sound is usually the first symptom of this tumor. Other early features include a reddish-blue mass behind the tympanic membrane and progressive conductive hearing loss. Later, total unilateral deafness is accompanied by ear pain and dizziness. Otorrhagia may also occur if the tumor breaks through the tympanic membrane.

♦ ***Hypertension.*** Bilateral, high-pitched tinnitus may occur in severe hypertension. Diastolic blood pressure exceeding 120 mm Hg may also cause severe, throbbing headache, restlessness, nausea, vomiting, blurred vision, seizures, or decreased level of consciousness.

♦ ***Labyrinthitis (suppurative).*** In this disorder, tinnitus may accompany sudden, severe attacks of vertigo, unilateral or bilateral sensorineural hearing loss, nystagmus, dizziness, nausea, and vomiting.

♦ ***Ménière's disease.*** Most common in men between the ages of 55 and 65, this labyrinthine disease is characterized by attacks of low-pitched tinnitus, vertigo, and fluctuating sensorineural hearing loss. These attacks are usually unilateral and last from 10 minutes to several hours; they occur over a few days or weeks and are followed by a remission. Severe nausea, vomiting, diaphoresis, and nystagmus may also occur during attacks.

♦ ***Ossicle dislocation.*** Acoustic trauma, such as a slap on the ear, may dislocate the ossicle, resulting in tinnitus and sensorineural hearing loss. Bleeding from the middle ear also may occur.

♦ ***Otitis externa (acute).*** Although not a major complaint in this disorder, tinnitus may result if debris in the external ear canal impinges on the tympanic membrane. More typical findings include pruritus, foul-smelling purulent discharge, or severe ear pain that's aggravated by manipulation of the tragus or auricle, teeth clenching, mouth opening, and chewing. The external ear canal typically appears red and edematous and may be occluded by debris, causing partial hearing loss.

♦ ***Otitis media.*** This infection may cause tinnitus and conductive hearing loss. However, its more typical features include ear pain, a red and bulging tympanic membrane, high fever and chills, or dizziness.

♦ ***Otosclerosis.*** In this disorder, the patient may describe ringing, roaring, or whistling tinnitus or a combination of these sounds. He may also report progressive hearing loss, which may lead to bilateral deafness, and vertigo.

◆ ***Tympanic membrane perforation.*** Tinnitus is usually the chief complaint in a small perforation; hearing loss, in a larger perforation. These symptoms typically develop suddenly and may be accompanied by pain, vertigo, and a feeling of fullness in the ear.

Other causes

◆ ***Drugs or alcohol.*** An overdose of salicylates commonly causes reversible tinnitus. Quinine, alcohol, or indomethacin may also cause reversible tinnitus. Common drugs that may cause irreversible tinnitus include the aminoglycoside antibiotics (especially kanamycin, streptomycin, and gentamicin) and vancomycin.

◆ ***Noise.*** Chronic exposure to noise, especially high-pitched sounds, can damage the ear's hair cells, causing tinnitus and a bilateral hearing loss. These symptoms may be temporary or permanent.

Special considerations

Tinnitus usually can't be treated successfully. To help the patient tolerate this symptom, you may have to provide vasodilators, tranquilizers, or antiseizure drugs or encourage the use of biofeedback or tinnitus maskers. (A tinnitus masker produces a band of noise measuring about 1800 Hz, which helps block out tinnitus without interfering with hearing.)

A hearing aid may be prescribed to amplify environmental sounds, thereby obscuring tinnitus. For some patients, a device that combines features of a masker and a hearing aid may be used to block out tinnitus.

Pediatric pointers

An expectant mother's use of ototoxic drugs during the third trimester of pregnancy can cause labyrinth damage in the fetus, resulting in tinnitus. Many of the disorders described previously can also cause tinnitus in children.

TRACHEAL DEVIATION

Normally, the trachea is located at the midline of the neck — except at the bifurcation, where it shifts slightly toward the right. Visible deviation from its normal position signals an underlying condition that can compromise pulmonary function and possibly cause respiratory distress. A hallmark of life-threatening tension pneumothorax, tracheal deviation occurs when asymmetrical thoracic volume or pressure causes a mediastinal shift. A nontension pneumothorax can cause tracheal deviation to the ipsilateral side. (See *Detecting slight tracheal deviation*, page 570.)

Emergency interventions

Be alert for signs of respiratory distress: tachypnea, dyspnea, decreased or absent breath sounds, stridor, nasal flaring, accessory muscle use, asymmetrical chest expansion, restlessness, or anxiety. If possible, place the patient in semi-Fowler's position to aid respiratory excursion and improve oxygenation. Give supplemental oxygen and intubate the patient if necessary. Insert an I.V. line for fluid and drug administration. In addition, palpate the neck and chest for subcutaneous crepitation, a sign of tension pneumothorax. Chest tube insertion may be necessary to release trapped air or fluid and restore normal intrapleural and intrathoracic pressure gradients.

History

If the patient doesn't display signs of distress, ask about a history of pulmonary or cardiac disorders, trauma, or infection. If he smokes, determine how much. Ask about associated symptoms, especially breathing difficulty, pain, and cough.

EXAMINATION TIP

Detecting slight tracheal deviation

Although gross tracheal deviation is visible, detection of slight deviation requires palpation and perhaps even an X-ray. Try palpation first.

With the tip of your index finger, locate the patient's trachea by palpating between the sternocleidomastoid muscles. Then, compare the trachea's position to an imaginary line drawn vertically through the suprasternal notch. Any deviation from midline is usually considered abnormal.

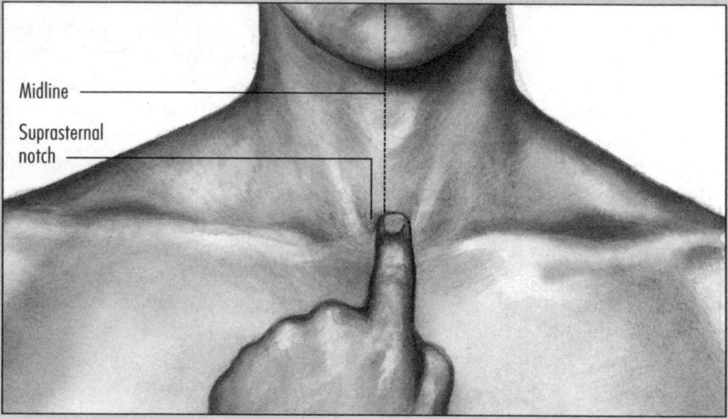

Common medical causes

◆ ***Atelectasis.*** Extensive lung collapse can cause tracheal deviation toward the affected side. Respiratory findings may include dyspnea, tachypnea, pleuritic chest pain, dry cough, dullness on percussion, decreased vocal fremitus and breath sounds, inspiratory lag, or substernal or intercostal retraction.

◆ ***Hiatal hernia.*** Intrusion of abdominal viscera into the pleural space causes tracheal deviation toward the unaffected side. The degree of attendant respiratory distress depends on the extent of herniation. Other possible effects include pyrosis, regurgitation or vomiting, or chest or abdominal pain.

◆ ***Kyphoscoliosis.*** Rib cage distortion and mediastinal shift can cause tracheal deviation toward the compressed lung. Respiratory effects include dry coughing, dyspnea, asymmetrical chest expansion and, possibly, asymmetrical breath sounds. Backache and fatigue commonly occur.

◆ ***Mediastinal tumor.*** Commonly asymptomatic in its early stages, a large tumor can press against the trachea and nearby structures, causing tracheal deviation and dysphagia. Other late findings may include stridor, dyspnea, brassy cough, hoarseness, or stertorous respirations with suprasternal retraction. The patient may experience shoulder, arm, or chest pain as well as edema of the neck, face, or arm. His neck and chest wall veins may be dilated.

◆ ***Pulmonary tuberculosis.*** A large cavitation causes tracheal deviation toward the affected side, asymmetrical chest excursion, dullness on percussion, increased tactile fremitus, amphoric breath sounds, and inspiratory crackles. Insidious early effects include fatigue, anorexia, weight loss, fever, chills, or night sweats. Productive cough, hemoptysis, pleuritic chest pain, and dyspnea develop as the disease progresses.

◆ ***Retrosternal thyroid.*** This anatomic abnormality can displace the trachea. The gland is felt as a movable neck mass above the suprasternal notch. Dysphagia, cough, hoarseness, and stridor frequently occur. Signs of thyrotoxicosis may be present.

◆ ***Tension pneumothorax.*** This acute, life-threatening condition causes tracheal deviation toward the unaffected side. It's marked by a sudden onset of respiratory distress with sharp chest pain, dry cough, severe dyspnea, tachycardia, wheezing, cyanosis, accessory muscle use, nasal flaring, air hunger, and asymmetrical chest movement. Restless and anxious, the patient may also develop subcutaneous crepitation in the neck and upper chest, decreased vocal fremitus, decreased or absent breath sounds on the affected side, distended neck veins, and hypotension. Heart sounds may shift away from the affected side.

◆ ***Thoracic aortic aneurysm.*** This disorder usually causes the trachea to deviate to the right. Highly variable associated findings may include stridor, dyspnea, wheezing, brassy cough, hoarseness, and dysphagia. Edema of the face, neck, or arm may accompany distended chest wall and neck veins. Substernal, neck, shoulder, or lower back pain may occur, possibly with paresthesia or neuralgia.

Special considerations

Because tracheal deviation usually signals a severe underlying disorder that can cause respiratory distress at any time, monitor the patient's respiratory and cardiac status constantly, and make sure that emergency equipment is readily available. Prepare the patient for diagnostic tests, such as chest X-rays, an electrocardiogram, and arterial blood gas analysis.

Pediatric pointers

Respiratory distress commonly develops more rapidly in children than in adults.

Geriatric pointers

In elderly persons, tracheal deviation to the right commonly stems from an elongated, atherosclerotic aortic arch, but this deviation isn't considered abnormal.

TRACHEAL TUGGING

[Cardarelli's sign, Castellino's sign, Oliver's sign]

A visible recession of the larynx and trachea that occurs in synchrony with cardiac systole, tracheal tugging commonly results from an aneurysm or a tumor near the aortic arch. It may signal dangerous compression or obstruction of major airways. The tugging movement, best observed with the patient's neck hyperextended, reflects abnormal transmission of aortic pulsations in the compressed and distorted heart, esophagus, great vessels, airways, and nerves.

Emergency interventions

If you observe tracheal tugging, examine the patient for signs of respiratory distress, such as tachypnea, stridor, accessory muscle use, cyanosis, or agitation. If the patient is in distress, check airway patency. Administer oxygen. Prepare to intubate the patient if necessary. Insert an I.V. line for fluid and drug access, and begin cardiac monitoring.

Tracheal tugging: Common causes and associated findings

S&S

CAUSES	Chest pain	Cough, brassy	Cough	Dyspnea	Edema of face, neck, or arm	Fever	Hemoptysis	Hoarseness	Lymphadenopathy	Murmur	Neck vein distention	Stridor
	MAJOR ASSOCIATED SIGNS AND SYMPTOMS											
Aortic arch aneurysm	◆	◆		◆	◆		◆	◆		◆	◆	◆
Hodgkin's disease				◆	◆	◆			◆		◆	◆
Thymoma	◆		◆	◆	◆			◆			◆	

History and physical examination

If the patient isn't in distress, obtain a pertinent history. Ask about associated symptoms, especially pain, and about a history of cardiovascular disease, cancer, chest surgery, or trauma.

Then examine the patient's neck and chest for abnormalities. Palpate the neck for masses, enlarged lymph nodes, abnormal arterial pulsations, and tracheal deviation. Percuss and auscultate the lung fields for abnormal sounds, and auscultate the heart for murmurs. (See *Tracheal tugging: Common causes and associated findings*.)

Common medical causes

♦ ***Aortic arch aneurysm.*** A large aneurysm can distort and compress surrounding tissues and structures, producing tracheal tugging. The cardinal sign is severe pain in the substernal area, sometimes radiating to the back or side of the chest. A sudden increase in pain may herald impending rupture—a medical emergency. Depending on the aneurysm's site and size, associated findings may include a visible pulsatile mass in the first or second intercostal space or suprasternal notch, a diastolic murmur of aortic regurgitation, or an aortic systolic murmur and thrill in the absence of peripheral signs of aortic stenosis. Dyspnea and stridor may occur with hoarseness, dysphagia, brassy cough, or hemoptysis. Distended jugular veins and edema of the face, neck, or arm may develop. Compression of the left main bronchus can cause atelectasis of the left lung.

♦ ***Hodgkin's disease.*** A tumor that develops adjacent to the aortic arch can cause tracheal tugging. Initial signs and symptoms include usually painless cervical lymphadenopathy, sustained or remittent fever, fatigue, malaise, pruritus, night sweats, and weight loss. Swollen lymph nodes may become tender and painful. Later findings include dyspnea and stridor; dry cough; dysphagia; distended neck veins; edema of the face, neck, or arm; hepatosplenomegaly; hyperpigmentation, jaundice, or pallor; or neuralgia.

♦ ***Thymoma.*** This rare tumor can cause tracheal tugging. Cough, chest pain, dysphagia, dyspnea, hoarseness, a palpable neck mass, distended neck veins, and edema of the face, neck, or upper arm are common findings.

Special considerations

Place the patient in semi-Fowler's position to ease respiration. Administer cough suppressants and prescribed pain medications, but be alert for signs of respiratory depression.

Prepare the patient for diagnostic procedures, which may include chest X-rays, computed tomography scan, lymphangiography, aortography, bone marrow biopsy, liver biopsy, echocardiography, or a complete blood count.

Pediatric pointers

In infants and children, tracheal tugging suggests a mediastinal tumor, as occurs in Hodgkin's disease and malignant lymphoma, or Marfan syndrome.

TREMORS

The most common type of involuntary muscle movement, tremors are regular rhythmic oscillations that result from alternating contraction of opposing muscle groups. They're typical signs of extrapyramidal or cerebellar disorders and can also result from certain drugs.

Tremors can be characterized by their location, amplitude, and frequency. *Resting tremors* occur when an extremity is at rest and subside with movement; they include the classic pill-rolling tremor of Parkinson's disease. *Intention tremors* occur only with movement and subside with rest. *Postural (or action) tremors* appear when an extremity or the trunk is actively held in a particular posture or position; a common type of postural tremor is called *essential tremor.*

Tremorlike movements may also occur, such as asterixis — the characteristic flapping tremor seen in hepatic failure.

Stress or emotional upset tends to aggravate a tremor. Alcohol commonly diminishes postural tremors.

History and physical examination

Begin by asking the patient about the tremor's onset (sudden or gradual) and about its duration, progression, and aggravating or alleviating factors. Does the tremor interfere with the patient's normal activities? Does he have other symptoms? Has he noticed behavioral changes or memory loss (the patient's family or friends may provide more accurate information on this)?

Explore the patient's personal and family medical history for neurologic (especially seizures), endocrine, or metabolic disorders. Obtain a complete drug history, noting especially the use of phenothiazines, and ask about alcohol use. Is the patient taking over-the-counter diet products? If so, how much is he taking?

Assess the patient's overall appearance and demeanor, noting mental status. Test range of motion and strength in all major muscle groups while observing for chorea, athetosis, dystonia, and other involuntary movements. Check deep tendon reflexes and, if possible, observe the patient's gait.

Common medical causes

- ***Alkalosis.*** Severe alkalosis may cause a severe intention tremor and twitching, carpopedal spasms, agitation, diaphoresis, and hyperventilation. The patient may complain of dizziness, tinnitus, palpitations, or peripheral and circumoral paresthesia.
- ***Benign familial essential tremor.*** This disorder of early adulthood causes a bilateral essential tremor that typically begins in the fingers and hands and may spread to the head, jaw, lips, and tongue. Laryngeal involvement may result in a quavering voice.
- ***Cerebellar tumor.*** An intention tremor is a cardinal sign of this disorder; related findings may include ataxia, nystagmus, incoordination, muscle weakness and atrophy, or hypoactive or absent deep tendon reflexes.

♦ ***Hypercapnia.*** Elevated partial pressure of carbon dioxide may result in a rapid, fine intention tremor. Other common findings include headache, fatigue, blurred vision, weakness, lethargy, and decreasing level of consciousness (LOC).

♦ ***Hypoglycemia.*** Acute hypoglycemia may cause a rapid, fine intention tremor accompanied by confusion, weakness, tachycardia, diaphoresis, and cold, clammy skin. Early patient complaints typically include mild generalized headache, profound hunger, nervousness, and blurred or double vision. The tremor may disappear as hypoglycemia worsens and hypotonia and decreased LOC become evident.

♦ ***Multiple sclerosis.*** An intention tremor that waxes and wanes may be an early sign of multiple sclerosis. Commonly, visual and sensory impairments are the earliest findings. Associated effects vary greatly and may include nystagmus, muscle weakness, paralysis, spasticity, hyperreflexia, ataxic gait, dysphagia, and dysarthria. Constipation, urinary frequency and urgency, incontinence, impotence, and emotional lability may also occur.

♦ ***Parkinson's disease.*** Tremors, a classic early sign of this degenerative disease, usually begin in the fingers and may eventually affect the foot, eyelids, jaw, lips, and tongue. The slow, regular, rhythmic resting tremor takes the form of flexion-extension or abduction-adduction of the fingers or hand, or pronation-supination of the hand. Flexion-extension of the fingers combined with abduction-adduction of the thumb yields the characteristic pill-rolling tremor.

Leg involvement causes flexion-extension foot movement. Lightly closing the eyelids causes them to flutter. The jaw may move up and down, and the lips may purse. The tongue, when protruded, may move in and out of the mouth in tempo with tremors elsewhere in the body. The rate of the tremor holds constant over time, but its amplitude varies.

Other characteristic findings include cogwheel or lead-pipe rigidity, bradykinesia, propulsive gait with forward-leaning posture, monotone voice, mask-like facies, drooling, dysphagia, dysarthria and, occasionally, oculogyric crisis (eyes fix upward, with involuntary tonic movements) or blepharospasm (eyelids close completely).

♦ ***Thalamic syndrome.*** *Central midbrain syndromes* are heralded by contralateral ataxic tremors and other abnormal movements, along with Weber's syndrome (oculomotor palsy with contralateral hemiplegia), paralysis of vertical gaze, and stupor or coma. *Anteromedial-inferior thalamic syndrome* causes varying combinations of tremor, deep sensory loss, and hemiataxia. However, the main effect of this syndrome may be an extrapyramidal dysfunction, such as hemiballismus or hemiathetosis.

♦ ***Thyrotoxicosis.*** Neuromuscular effects of this disorder include a rapid, fine intention tremor of the hands and tongue, along with clonus, hyperreflexia, and Babinski's reflex. Other common signs and symptoms include tachycardia, cardiac arrhythmias, palpitations, anxiety, dyspnea, diaphoresis, heat intolerance, weight loss despite increased appetite, diarrhea, an enlarged thyroid and, possibly, exophthalmos.

♦ ***Wernicke's encephalopathy.*** An intention tremor is an early sign of this thiamine deficiency. Other features include ocular abnormalities (such as gaze paralysis or nystagmus), ataxia, apathy, or confusion. Orthostatic hypotension or tachycardia may also develop.

♦ ***West Nile encephalitis.*** This brain infection is caused by West Nile virus, a mosquito-borne flavivirus endemic to Africa, the Middle East, and western Asia. Mild infections are common and manifest as fever, headache, and body aches, commonly accompanied by rash and swollen lymph glands. More severe infections are marked by stupor, disorientation, coma, tremors, occasional seizures, paralysis and, rarely, death.

Other causes

◆ ***Drugs.*** Phenothiazines (particularly piperazine derivatives such as fluphenazine) and other antipsychotics may cause resting and pill-rolling tremors. Infrequently, metoclopramide and metyrosine also cause these tremors. Lithium toxicity, sympathomimetics (such as terbutaline and pseudoephedrine), amphetamines, and phenytoin can all cause tremors that disappear with dose reduction.

◆ **Herb alert** Herbal products such as ephedra (ma huang) have been known to cause serious adverse effects, which may include tremors.

Special considerations

Severe intention tremors may interfere with the patient's ability to perform activities of daily living. Assist the patient with these activities as necessary, and take precautions against possible injury during such activities as walking or eating.

Pediatric pointers

A normal neonate may display coarse tremors with stiffening — an exaggerated hypocalcemic startle reflex — in response to noises and chills. Pediatric-specific causes of pathologic tremors include cerebral palsy, fetal alcohol syndrome, and maternal drug addiction.

TUNNEL VISION

[Gun barrel vision, tubular vision]

Resulting from severe constriction of the visual field that leaves only a small central area of sight, tunnel vision is typically described as the sensation of looking through a tunnel or gun barrel. It may be unilateral or bilateral and usually develops gradually. This abnormality results from chronic open-angle glaucoma and advanced retinal degeneration. Tunnel vision also can result from laser photocoagulation therapy to correct retinal detachment. Also a common complaint of malingerers, tunnel vision can be verified or discounted by visual field examination performed by an ophthalmologist.

History and physical examination

Ask the patient when he first noticed a loss of peripheral vision, and have him describe the progression of vision loss. Ask him to describe in detail exactly what and how far he can see peripherally. Explore the patient's personal and family history for ocular problems, especially progressive blindness that began at an early age.

Observe the patient as he walks; a patient with severely limited peripheral vision typically bumps into objects (and may have bruises). If your examination findings suggest tunnel vision, refer the patient to an ophthalmologist for further evaluation.

Common medical causes

◆ ***Chronic open-angle glaucoma.*** In this insidious disorder, bilateral tunnel vision occurs late and slowly progresses to complete blindness. Other late findings include mild eye pain, halo vision, and reduced visual acuity (especially at night) that's uncorrectable with glasses.

◆ ***Retinal pigmentary degeneration.*** This group of hereditary disorders, such as retinitis pigmentosa, causes an annular scotoma that progresses concentrically, causing tunnel vision and eventually resulting in complete blindness, usually by age 50. Impaired night vision, the earliest symptom, typically appears during the first or second decade of life. An ophthalmoscopic examination may reveal narrowed retinal blood vessels and a pale optic disk.

Special considerations

To protect the patient from injury, be sure to remove all potentially dangerous objects and orient him to his surroundings. Because any visual impairment is frightening, reassure the patient and clearly explain diagnostic procedures, such as tonometry, perimeter examination, and visual field testing.

Pediatric pointers

In children with retinitis pigmentosa, night blindness foreshadows tunnel vision, which usually doesn't develop until later in the disease process.

U

Urethral discharge

This excretion from the urinary meatus may be purulent, mucoid, or thin; sanguineous or clear; scant or profuse. It usually develops suddenly, most commonly in men with a prostate infection.

History and physical examination

Ask the patient when he first noticed the discharge, and have him describe its color, consistency, and quantity. Does he have pain on urination? Does he have difficulty initiating a urinary stream? Ask the patient about other associated symptoms, such as fever, chills, and perineal fullness. Explore his history for prostate problems, sexually transmitted diseases (STDs), or urinary tract infection. Ask the patient if he has had recent sexual contacts or a new sexual partner.

Inspect the patient's urethral meatus for inflammation and swelling. Using proper technique, obtain a culture specimen. Then obtain a urine specimen for urinalysis and possibly a three-glass urine specimen. (See *How to perform a three-glass urine test*, page 578.) The prostate gland may have to be palpated.

Common medical causes

♦ ***Prostatitis.*** *Acute prostatitis* is characterized by purulent urethral discharge. Initial signs and symptoms include sudden fever, chills, lower back pain, myalgia, perineal fullness, and arthralgia. Urination becomes increasingly frequent and urgent, and the urine may appear cloudy. Dysuria, nocturia, and some degree of urinary obstruction may also occur. The prostate may be tense, boggy, very tender, and warm. Prostate massage to obtain prostatic fluid is contraindicated.

Chronic prostatitis, although commonly asymptomatic, may cause a persistent urethral discharge that's thin, milky or clear, and sometimes sticky. The discharge appears at the meatus after a long interval between voidings, as in the morning. Associated effects include a dull ache in the prostate or rectum, sexual dysfunction such as ejaculatory pain, and such urinary disturbances as frequency, urgency, and dysuria.

♦ ***Reiter's syndrome.*** In this self-limiting syndrome that usually affects males, urethral discharge and other signs of acute urethritis occur 1 to 2 weeks after sexual contact. Asymmetrical arthritis, conjunctivitis of one or both eyes, and ulcerations on the oral mucosa and glans penis may also occur.

♦ ***Urethritis.*** This inflammatory disorder, which is commonly sexually transmitted (as in gonorrhea), commonly produces scant or profuse urethral discharge that's either thin and clear, mucoid, or thick and purulent. Other effects may include urinary hesitancy, urgency, and

How to perform a three-glass urine test

If your male patient complains of urinary frequency, urgency, dysuria, flank or lower back pain, or other signs of urethritis, and if his urine specimen is cloudy, perform a three-glass urine test.

First ask him to void into three conical glasses labeled with numbers 1, 2, and 3. First-voided urine goes in glass #1; midstream urine in glass #2, and the remainder in glass #3. Tell the patient to avoid interrupting the stream of urine when shifting glasses, if possible.

Next, observe each glass for pus and mucus shreds. Also, note urine color and odor. Glass #1 will contain matter from the anterior urethra, glass #2 will contain bladder contents, and glass #3 will contain sediment from the prostate and seminal vesicles.

Some common findings are shown here. However, confirming diagnosis requires microscopic examination and a bacteriology report.

	SPECIMEN 1	SPECIMEN 2	SPECIMEN 3
Acute or subacute urethritis	Cloudy	Clear	Clear
Acute posterior urethritis	Cloudy	Clear or cloudy	Cloudy
Chronic anterior urethritis	Small shreds	Clear	Clear
Chronic posterior urethritis	Large shreds	Clear	Clear
Chronic urethritis (anterior and posterior)	Small and large shreds	Clear	Clear
Prostatitis	Clear or large shreds	Clear	Cloudy or large shreds
Cystitis and pyelonephritis	Cloudy	Cloudy	Cloudy

frequency; dysuria; or itching or burning around the meatus.

Special considerations
Advise the patient with acute prostatitis to discontinue sexual activity until acute symptoms subside. However, encourage the patient with chronic prostatitis to regularly engage in sexual activity because ejaculation may relieve pain. To help this patient relieve symptoms, suggest that he take hot sitz baths several times daily, increase his fluid intake, void frequently, and avoid caffeine, tea, and alcohol. Monitor him for urine retention.

Pediatric pointers
Carefully evaluate a child with urethral discharge for evidence of sexual or physical abuse.

Geriatric pointers

Urethral discharge in elderly males isn't usually STD-related.

URINARY FREQUENCY

Urinary frequency refers to increased incidence of the urge to void. Usually resulting from decreased bladder capacity, frequency is a cardinal sign of urinary tract infection (UTI). However, it can also stem from other urologic disorders, neurologic dysfunction, or pressure on the bladder from a nearby tumor or from organ enlargement (as in pregnancy).

Urinary frequency may be reported by the patient with polyuria — an increase in total daily urine output. (See "Polyuria," page 467.)

History and physical examination

Ask the patient how many times per day he voids. How does this compare to his previous pattern of voiding? Ask about the onset and duration of the abnormal frequency and about associated urinary symptoms, such as dysuria, urgency, incontinence, hematuria, or lower abdominal pain during urination. Also ask about neurologic symptoms, such as muscle weakness, numbness, or tingling. Explore his medical history for UTI, other urologic problems or recent urologic procedures, and neurologic disorders. Ask a male patient about a history of prostatic enlargement. If the patient is a female of childbearing age, ask whether she is or could be pregnant.

Obtain a clean-catch midstream specimen for urinalysis and culture and sensitivity tests. Then palpate the patient's suprapubic area, abdomen, and flanks, noting tenderness. Examine his urethral meatus for redness, discharge, or swelling. Palpate his prostate gland.

If the patient's medical history reveals symptoms or a history of neurologic disorders, perform a neurologic examination.

Common medical causes

◆ ***Benign prostatic hyperplasia.*** Prostatic enlargement causes urinary frequency, nocturia and, possibly, incontinence or hematuria. Initial effects are those of prostatism: reduced caliber and force of the urinary stream, urinary hesitancy and tenesmus, inability to stop the urine stream, a feeling of incomplete voiding and, occasionally, urine retention. Assessment reveals bladder distention.

◆ ***Bladder calculus.*** Bladder irritation may lead to urinary frequency and urgency, dysuria, terminal hematuria, and suprapubic pain from bladder spasms. If the stone lodges in the bladder neck, greatest discomfort usually occurs at the end of micturition, overflow incontinence may occur, and pain may be referred to the lower back or heel.

◆ ***Diabetes insipidus.*** Antidiuretic hormone deficiency typically results in periodic voiding of moderate to large amounts of urine. Other possible manifestations are polydipsia, dehydration, and headache.

◆ ***Diabetes mellitus.*** In addition to urinary frequency, findings include nocturia, daytime polyuria, polydipsia, polyphagia, weight loss, fatigue, weakness and, possibly, signs of dehydration.

◆ Prostatic cancer. In advanced stages, urinary frequency may occur with hesitancy, dribbling, nocturia, dysuria, bladder distention, perineal pain, constipation, and a hard, irregularly shaped prostate.

◆ ***Prostatitis.*** *Acute prostatitis* commonly causes urinary frequency, urgency, dysuria, nocturia, and purulent urethral discharge. Other findings include fever, chills, lower back pain, myalgia, arthralgia, and perineal fullness. The prostate may be tense, boggy, very tender, and warm. Prostate massage to obtain prostatic fluid is contraindicated. Clinical features of *chronic prostatitis* are usually the same as those of the acute form, but to a lesser degree. The patient may also experience pain on ejaculation.

♦ ***Rectal tumor.*** Pressure exerted by this tumor on the bladder may cause urinary frequency. Early findings include changed bowel habits, commonly starting with an urgent need to defecate on arising or obstipation alternating with diarrhea; blood or mucus in the stool; or a sense of incomplete evacuation.

♦ ***Reiter's syndrome.*** In this self-limiting syndrome, urinary frequency occurs with symptoms of acute urethritis 1 to 2 weeks after sexual contact. Other manifestations of Reiter's syndrome include asymmetrical arthritis of knees, ankles, and metatarsophalangeal joints; unilateral or bilateral conjunctivitis; and small painless ulcers on the mouth, tongue, or glans penis.

♦ ***Reproductive tract tumor.*** A tumor in the female reproductive tract may compress the bladder, causing urinary frequency. Other findings vary but may include abdominal distention, menstrual disturbances, vaginal bleeding, weight loss, pelvic pain, and fatigue.

♦ ***Spinal cord lesion.*** Incomplete cord transection results in urinary frequency, continuous overflow, dribbling, and urgency when voluntary control of sphincter function weakens. Other urologic effects may include hesitancy or bladder distention. Effects below the level of the lesion may include weakness, paralysis, sensory disturbances, hyperreflexia, and impotence.

♦ ***Urethral stricture.*** Bladder decompensation causes urinary frequency, along with urgency and nocturia. Early signs include hesitancy, tenesmus, and reduced caliber and force of the urinary stream. Eventually, overflow incontinence may occur. Urinoma or urosepsis may develop.

♦ ***UTI.*** Affecting the urethra, the bladder, or the kidneys, this common cause of urinary frequency also may cause urgency, dysuria, hematuria, cloudy urine and, in males, urethral discharge. The patient may report bladder spasms or a feeling of warmth during urination. Women may experience suprapubic or pelvic pain. In young adult males, UTI is usually related to sexual contact.

Other causes

♦ ***Diuretics.*** These substances reduce the body's total volume of water and salt by increasing urinary excretion. Excessive intake of coffee, tea, or other caffeine-containing beverages can lead to urinary frequency.

♦ ***Treatments.*** Radiation therapy may cause bladder inflammation, leading to urinary frequency.

Special considerations

Prepare the patient for diagnostic tests, such as urinalysis, culture and sensitivity tests, imaging tests, ultrasonography, cystoscopy, cystometry, or a complete neurologic workup. If the patient's mobility is impaired, keep a bedpan, urinal, or commode near his bed.

Pediatric pointers

UTI is a common cause of urinary frequency in children, especially girls. Congenital anomalies that can cause UTI include a duplicated ureter, congenital bladder diverticulum, and an ectopic ureteral orifice.

Geriatric pointers

Men older than age 50 are prone to frequent non–sex-related UTIs. In postmenopausal women, decreased estrogen levels cause urinary frequency, urgency, and nocturia.

URINARY HESITANCY

Hesitancy — difficulty starting a urinary stream — can result from a urinary tract infection (UTI), a partial lower urinary tract obstruction, a neuromuscular disorder, or use of certain drugs. Occurring at all ages and in both sexes, it's most common in older men with prostatic enlargement. It also occurs in women with gravid uterus; tumors in the reproductive system, such as uterine fibroids; or ovarian, uterine, or vaginal carcinoma. Hesitancy usually arises gradually, commonly going unnoticed until urine retention causes bladder distention and discomfort.

History and physical examination

Ask the patient when he first noticed hesitancy and if he has had the problem before. Ask about other urinary problems, especially reduced force or interruption of the urinary stream. Ask if he has ever been treated for a prostate problem or UTI or obstruction. Obtain a drug history.

Inspect the patient's urethral meatus for inflammation, discharge, and other abnormalities. Examine the anal sphincter and test sensation in the perineum. Obtain a clean-catch specimen for urinalysis. A male patient requires prostate palpation; a female patient, gynecologic examination.

Common medical causes

♦ ***Benign prostatic hyperplasia.*** Clinical features depend on the extent of prostatic enlargement and the lobes affected. Characteristic early findings include urinary hesitancy, reduced caliber and force of urinary stream, perineal pain, a feeling of incomplete voiding, inability to stop the urinary stream and, occasionally, urine retention. As obstruction increases, urination becomes more frequent, with nocturia, urinary overflow, incontinence, bladder distention and, possibly, hematuria.

♦ ***Prostatic cancer.*** In advanced cancer, urinary hesitancy may occur, accompanied by frequency, dribbling, nocturia, dysuria, bladder distention, perineal pain, and constipation. Digital rectal examination commonly reveals a hard, nodular prostate.

♦ ***Spinal cord lesion.*** A lesion below the micturition center (controls voiding) that has destroyed the sacral nerve roots causes urinary hesitancy, tenesmus, and constant dribbling from retention and overflow incontinence. Associated findings are urinary frequency and urgency, dysuria, and nocturia.

♦ ***Urethral stricture.*** Partial obstruction of the lower urinary tract secondary to trauma or infection causes urinary hesitancy, tenesmus, and decreased force and caliber of the urinary stream. Urinary frequency and urgency, nocturia, and eventually overflow incontinence may develop. Pyuria usually reflects accompanying infection. Increased obstruction may lead to urine extravasation and formation of urinomas.

♦ ***UTI.*** Urinary hesitancy is commonly associated with frequency, possible hematuria, dysuria, nocturia, and cloudy urine. Other findings may include bladder spasms; costovertebral angle tenderness; suprapubic, lower back, pelvic, or flank pain; urethral discharge in males; or constitutional effects, such as fever, chills, malaise, nausea, and vomiting.

Other causes

♦ ***Drugs.*** Anticholinergics and drugs with anticholinergic properties (such as tricyclic antidepressants or some nasal decongestants or cold remedies) may cause urinary hesitancy. Hesitancy also may occur in patients recovering from general anesthesia.

Special considerations

Monitor the patient's voiding pattern, and frequently palpate for bladder distention. Apply local heat to the perineum or the abdomen to enhance muscle relaxation and aid urination. Also, teach how to perform a clean, intermittent self-catheterization. Prepare the patient for tests, such as cystometrography or cystourethrography.

Pediatric pointers

The most common cause of urinary obstruction in a male infant is a posterior stricture. Affected infants may have a less forceful urinary stream as well as fever due to UTI, failure to thrive, or a palpable bladder.

URINARY INCONTINENCE

Urinary incontinence, the uncontrollable passage of urine, results from bladder abnormalities or neurologic disorders. A common urologic sign, incontinence may be transient or permanent and may range from large volumes of urine to scant dribbling. It can be classified as stress, overflow, urge, or total incontinence. *Stress incontinence* is intermittent leakage resulting from a sudden physical strain, such as a cough, sneeze, or quick movement. *Overflow incontinence* is a dribble resulting from urine retention that occurs when the bladder is too full to contract with sufficient force to expel a urine stream. *Urge incontinence* is inability to suppress a sudden urge to urinate. *Total incontinence* is continuous leakage resulting from the bladder's inability to retain any urine.

History and physical examination

Ask the patient when he first noticed the incontinence and whether it began suddenly or gradually. Have him describe his typical urinary pattern: Does incontinence usually occur during the day or at night? Does he have any urinary control, or is he totally incontinent? If he sometimes urinates with control, ask him the usual times and amounts voided. Determine his normal fluid intake. Ask about other urinary problems, such as hesitancy, frequency, urgency, nocturia, and decreased force or interruption of the urinary stream. Also ask if he has sought treatment for incontinence or found a way to deal with it himself.

Obtain a medical history, especially noting urinary tract infection (UTI), prostate conditions, spinal injury or tumor, cerebrovascular accident, or surgery involving the bladder, prostate, or pelvic floor.

After completing the history, have the patient empty his bladder. Inspect the urethral meatus for obvious inflammation or anatomic defect. Have female patients bear down; note any urine leakage. Gently palpate the abdomen for bladder distention, which signals urine retention. Perform a complete neurologic assessment, noting motor and sensory function and obvious muscle atrophy.

Common medical causes

♦ ***Benign prostatic hyperplasia (BPH).*** Overflow incontinence is a common result of urethral obstruction and urine retention. BPH begins with a group of symptoms known as *prostatism:* reduced caliber and force of urinary stream, urinary hesitancy, and a feeling of incomplete voiding. As obstruction increases, urination becomes more frequent, with nocturia and, possibly, hematuria. Examination reveals bladder distention and an enlarged prostate.

♦ ***Bladder cancer.*** This disorder commonly presents with urge incontinence and hematuria; obstruction by a tumor may cause overflow incontinence. The early stages can be asymptomatic. Other urinary complaints may include frequency, dysuria, nocturia, dribbling, or suprapubic pain from bladder spasms after voiding. A mass may be palpable on bimanual examination.

♦ ***Cerebrovascular accident.*** Urinary incontinence may be transient or permanent. Associated findings reflect the site and extent of the lesion and may include impaired mentation, emotional lability, behavioral changes, altered level of consciousness, and seizures. Headache, vomiting, visual deficits, and decreased visual acuity are possible. Sensorimotor effects may include contralateral hemiplegia, dysarthria, dysphagia, ataxia, apraxia, agnosia, aphasia, or unilateral sensory loss.

♦ ***Diabetic neuropathy.*** Autonomic neuropathy may cause painless bladder distention with overflow incontinence. Related findings may include episodic constipation or diarrhea (which is commonly nocturnal), impotence and retrograde ejaculation, orthostatic hypotension, syncope, or dysphagia.

◆ ***Multiple sclerosis (MS).*** Urinary incontinence, urgency, and frequency are common urologic findings in MS. In most patients, visual problems and sensory impairment occur early. Other findings may include constipation, muscle weakness, paralysis, spasticity, hyperreflexia, intention tremor, ataxic gait, dysarthria, impotence, or emotional lability.

◆ ***Prostatic cancer.*** Urinary incontinence usually appears only in the advanced stages of this cancer. Urinary frequency and hesitancy, nocturia, dysuria, bladder distention, perineal pain, constipation, and a hard, irregularly shaped, nodular prostate are other common late findings.

◆ ***Prostatitis (chronic).*** Urinary incontinence may occur as a result of urethral obstruction by an enlarged prostate. Other findings may include urinary frequency and urgency, dysuria, hematuria, bladder distention, persistent urethral discharge, dull perineal pain that may radiate, ejaculatory pain, or decreased libido.

◆ ***Spinal cord injury.*** Complete cord transection above the sacral level causes flaccid paralysis of the bladder. Overflow incontinence follows rapid bladder distention. Other possible findings include paraplegia, sexual dysfunction, sensory loss, muscle atrophy, anhidrosis, or loss of reflexes distal to the injury.

◆ ***Urethral stricture.*** Overflow incontinence may occur and, as obstruction increases, urine extravasation may lead to formation of urinomas and urosepsis.

◆ ***UTI.*** Besides incontinence, this infection may cause urinary urgency, dysuria, hematuria, cloudy urine or, in males, urethral discharge. Bladder spasms or a feeling of warmth during urination may occur.

ALTERNATIVE THERAPY

Biofeedback to correct incontinence

Stress-related conditions such as incontinence (which involves muscle tone) have been treated successfully with biofeedback. This procedure is a type of relaxation therapy that uses electronic feedback devices to teach the patient to be aware of and to consciously control involuntary body functions, such as heart and respiratory rates, blood pressure, temperature, digestion, or muscle behavior.

Electrodes are applied to the perianal skin and lateral thigh and then attached to a sequential light display mechanism. As the patient tightens his perianal and thigh muscles in an attempt to increase muscle tone, the light illuminates, offering immediate feedback. The device can also measure the strength and duration of the muscle exercises, allowing the patient to monitor his progress.

Other causes

◆ **Surgery**. Urinary incontinence may occur after prostatectomy as a result of urethral sphincter damage.

Special considerations

Prepare the patient for diagnostic tests, such as cystoscopy, cystometry, or a complete neurologic workup. Obtain a urine specimen.

Begin management of incontinence by implementing a bladder retraining program. (See *Correcting incontinence with bladder retraining*, page 584.) To prevent stress incontinence, teach exercises to help strengthen the pelvic-floor muscles. Alternative therapies, such as biofeedback, may be beneficial. (See *Biofeedback to correct incontinence.*)

If the patient's incontinence has a neurologic basis, monitor for urine retention, which may require periodic cath-

Correcting incontinence with bladder retraining

The patient with incontinence typically feels embarrassed, frustrated and, sometimes, hopeless. Fortunately, however, his problem can usually be corrected by bladder retraining — a program that aims to establish a regular voiding pattern. Here are some guidelines for establishing such a program.

◆ Before you start the program, assess the patient's intake pattern, voiding pattern, and behavior (for example, restlessness or talkativeness) before each voiding episode.
◆ Encourage the patient to use the toilet 30 minutes before he's usually incontinent. If this isn't successful, readjust the schedule. Once he's able to stay dry for 2 hours, increase the time between voidings by 30 minutes each day until he achieves a 3- to 4-hour voiding schedule.
◆ When your patient voids, make sure the sequence of conditioning stimuli is always the same.
◆ Avoid any inhibiting stimuli; make sure that the patient has privacy while voiding.
◆ Keeping a record of continence and incontinence for 5 days may reinforce your patient's efforts to remain continent.

CLUES TO SUCCESS
Remember, both your positive attitude and your patient's are crucial to his successful bladder retraining. Here are some additional tips that may help your patient succeed.
◆ Make sure the patient is close to a bathroom or portable toilet. Leave a light on at night.
◆ If your patient needs assistance getting out of his bed or chair, promptly answer his call for help.
◆ Encourage him to wear his accustomed clothing, as an indication that you're confident he can remain continent. Acceptable alternatives to diapers include condoms for the male patient and incontinence pads or panties for the female patient.
◆ Encourage him to drink 2,000 to 2,500 ml of fluid each day. Less fluid doesn't prevent incontinence but does promote bladder infection. Limiting his intake after 5 P.M., however, will help him remain continent during the night.
◆ Reassure your patient that episodes of incontinence don't signal a failure of the program. Encourage him to maintain a persistent, tolerant attitude.

eterizations. If appropriate, teach the patient self-catheterization techniques. A patient with permanent urinary incontinence may require surgical creation of a urinary diversion.

Pediatric pointers
Causes of incontinence in children include infrequent or incomplete voiding. These may also lead to UTI. *Ectopic ureteral orifice* is an uncommon congenital anomaly associated with incontinence. A complete diagnostic evaluation usually is necessary to rule out organic disease.

Geriatric pointers
Diagnosing a UTI in an elderly patient can be problematic because many present only with urinary incontinence or changes in mental status, anorexia, or malaise. In addition, many elderly patients without UTIs present with dysuria, frequency, urgency, or incontinence.

URINARY URGENCY

A sudden compelling urge to urinate, accompanied by bladder pain, is a classic symptom of urinary tract infection

(UTI). As inflammation decreases bladder capacity, discomfort results from the accumulation of even small amounts of urine. Repeated, frequent voiding in an effort to alleviate this discomfort produces urine output of only a few milliliters at each voiding.

Urgency without bladder pain may point to an upper-motor-neuron lesion that has disrupted bladder control.

History and physical examination

Ask the patient about the onset of urinary urgency and whether he has experienced it before. Ask about other urologic symptoms, such as dysuria and cloudy urine. Also ask about neurologic symptoms, such as paresthesia. Review his medical history for recurrent or chronic UTIs or for surgery or procedures involving the urinary tract.

Obtain a clean-catch specimen for urinalysis. Note urine character, color, and odor, and use a reagent strip to test for pH, glucose, and blood. Then palpate the suprapubic area and both flanks for tenderness. If the patient's history or symptoms suggest neurologic dysfunction, perform a neurologic examination.

Common medical causes

- ***Bladder calculus.*** Bladder irritation can lead to urinary urgency and frequency, dysuria, terminal hematuria, and suprapubic pain from bladder spasms. Pain may be referred to the penis, vulva, lower back, or heel.
- ***Multiple sclerosis (MS).*** Urinary urgency can occur with or without the frequent UTIs that commonly accompany MS. Like other variable effects of MS, urinary urgency may wax and wane. Commonly, visual and sensory impairments are the earliest findings. Others include urinary frequency, incontinence, constipation, muscle weakness, paralysis, spasticity, intention tremor, hyperreflexia, ataxic gait, dysphagia, dysarthria, impotence, or emotional lability.
- ***Reiter's syndrome.*** In this self-limiting syndrome that primarily affects males, urgency occurs with other symptoms of acute urethritis 1 to 2 weeks after sexual contact. Arthritic and ocular symptoms and skin lesions usually develop within several weeks after sexual contact. These include asymmetrical arthritis of knees, ankles, or metatarsophalangeal joints; conjunctivitis; and ulcers on the penis or skin or in the mouth.
- ***Spinal cord lesion.*** Urinary urgency can result from incomplete cord transection when voluntary control of sphincter function weakens. Urinary frequency, difficulty initiating and inhibiting a urinary stream, and bladder distention and discomfort may also occur. Neuromuscular effects distal to the lesion may include weakness, paralysis, hyperreflexia, sensory disturbances, or impotence.
- ***Urethral stricture.*** Bladder decompensation causes urinary urgency, frequency, and nocturia. Early signs include hesitancy, tenesmus, and reduced caliber and force of the urinary stream. Eventually, overflow incontinence may occur.
- ***UTI.*** Urinary urgency is commonly associated with this infection. Other characteristic urinary changes include frequency, hematuria, dysuria, nocturia, and cloudy urine. Urinary hesitancy may also occur. Associated findings may include bladder spasms; costovertebral angle tenderness; suprapubic, lower back, or flank pain; urethral discharge in males; or constitutional effects, such as fever, chills, malaise, nausea, and vomiting.

Other causes

- ***Treatments.*** Radiation therapy may irritate and inflame the bladder, causing urinary urgency.

Special considerations

Prepare the patient for the diagnostic workup, including a complete urinalysis, culture and sensitivity studies and, possibly, neurologic tests. Increase the patient's fluid intake, if not contraindicated, to dilute the urine and diminish the feeling of urgency. Administer antibiotics and urinary anesthetics, such as phenazopyridine.

Pediatric pointers

In young children, urinary urgency may appear as a change in toilet habits, such as a sudden onset of bed-wetting or daytime accidents in a toilet-trained child. Urgency may also result from urethral irritation by bubble bath salts. Girls may experience vaginal discharge and vulvar soreness or pruritus.

URINE CLOUDINESS

Cloudy, murky, or turbid urine reflects the presence of bacteria, mucus, leukocytes or erythrocytes, epithelial cells, fat, or phosphates (in alkaline urine). It's characteristic of urinary tract infection (UTI) but can also result from prolonged storage of a urine specimen at room temperature.

History and physical examination

Ask about symptoms of UTI, such as dysuria; urinary urgency or frequency; or pain in the flank, lower back, or suprapubic area. Also ask about recurrent UTIs or recent surgery or treatment involving the urinary tract.

Obtain a urine specimen to check for pus or mucus. Using a reagent strip, test for blood glucose and pH. (See *How to perform a three-glass urine test,* page 578.) Palpate the suprapubic area and flanks for tenderness.

If you note cloudy urine in a patient with an indwelling urinary catheter, especially with concurrent fever, remove the catheter immediately (or change it if the patient must have one in place).

Common medical causes

◆ ***UTI.*** Cloudy urine is common here. Other urinary changes include urgency, frequency, hematuria, dysuria, nocturia and, in males, urethral discharge. Urinary hesitancy, bladder spasms, costovertebral angle tenderness, and suprapubic, lower back, or flank pain may occur. Other effects may include fever, chills, malaise, nausea, and vomiting.

Special considerations

Collect urine specimens for urinalysis and culture and sensitivity tests. Increase the patient's fluid intake and administer antibiotics and urinary anesthetics (such as phenazopyridine). Continue checking the appearance of the patient's urine to monitor the effectiveness of therapy.

Pediatric pointers

Cloudy urine in children also points to UTI.

URTICARIA

[Hives]

Urticaria is a vascular skin reaction characterized by the eruption of transient pruritic wheals — smooth, slightly elevated patches with well-defined erythematous margins and pale centers. It's caused by the local release of histamine or other vasoactive substances as part of a hypersensitivity reaction. (See *Recognizing common skin lesions*, page 444.)

Acute urticaria evolves rapidly and usually has a detectable cause — commonly hypersensitivity to certain drugs, foods, insect bites, inhalants, or contactants; emotional stress; or environmental factors. Although individual lesions usually subside within 12 to 24 hours, new groups of lesions may erupt continuously.

Urticaria lasting longer than 6 weeks is classified as chronic. The lesions may recur for months or years, and the underlying cause is usually unknown. Occasionally, a diagnosis of psychogenic urticaria is made.

Angioedema, or giant urticaria, is characterized by the acute eruption of wheals involving the mucous membranes and, occasionally, the arms, legs, or genitals.

Emergency interventions

In acute cases of urticaria, quickly evaluate respiratory status and take vital signs. Start an I.V. infusion of dextrose 5% in water if you note respiratory difficulty or signs of impending anaphylactic shock. Also, as appropriate, give local epinephrine or apply ice to the affected site to decrease absorption through vasoconstriction. Clear and maintain the airway, give oxygen as needed, and institute cardiac monitoring. Have resuscitation equipment at hand, and be prepared to begin cardiopulmonary resuscitation. Intubation or a tracheostomy may be required.

History

If the patient isn't in distress, obtain a complete history. Does the urticaria follow a seasonal pattern? Do certain foods or drugs seem to aggravate it? Is there a relationship to physical exertion? Is the patient routinely exposed to chemicals on the job or at home? Obtain a detailed drug history, including prescription and over-the-counter drugs. Note a history of chronic or parasitic infections, skin disease, or GI disorders.

Common medical causes

♦ ***Anaphylaxis.*** This acute reaction is marked by the rapid eruption of diffuse urticaria and angioedema; wheals may range from pinpoint to palm-sized or larger. Lesions are usually pruritic and stinging; paresthesia commonly precedes their eruption. Other acute findings include profound anxiety; weakness; diaphoresis; sneezing; shortness of breath; profuse rhinorrhea; nasal congestion; dysphagia; and warm, moist skin.

♦ ***Hereditary angioedema.*** In this autosomal dominant disorder, cutaneous involvement is manifested by nonpitting, nonpruritic edema of an extremity or the face. Respiratory mucosal involvement can cause life-threatening acute laryngeal edema.

♦ ***Lyme disease.*** Although not diagnostic of this tick-borne disease, urticaria may result from the characteristic skin lesion (*erythema chronicum migrans*). Later effects may include constant malaise and fatigue, intermittent headache, fever, chills, lymphadenopathy, neurologic and cardiac abnormalities, or arthritis.

Other causes

♦ ***Diagnostic tests.*** Radiographic contrast medium commonly causes urticaria, especially when administered I.V.

♦ ***Drugs.*** Among the most common are aspirin, atropine, codeine, dextrans, immune serums, insulin, morphine, penicillin, quinine, sulfonamides, and vaccines.

Special considerations

To help relieve the patient's discomfort, apply a bland skin emollient or one containing menthol and phenol. Expect to give antihistamines, systemic corticosteroids or, if stress is a suspected contributing factor, tranquilizers. Tepid baths and cool compresses may also enhance vasoconstriction and decrease pruritus. Teach the patient to avoid the causative stimulus, if identified.

Pediatric pointers

Pediatric forms of urticaria include acute papular urticaria (usually after insect bites) and urticaria pigmentosa (rare). Hereditary angioedema may be causative.

V

Vaginal Bleeding, Postmenopausal

Postmenopausal vaginal bleeding—bleeding that occurs 6 or more months after menopause—is an important indicator of gynecologic cancer. But it can also result from infection, local pelvic disorders, hormone replacement therapy, ovarian tumor, atrophy of the endometrium, or physiologic thinning and drying of the vaginal mucous membranes. It usually occurs as slight, brown or red spotting, either spontaneous or after coitus or douching, but it may also occur as oozing of fresh blood or as bright red hemorrhage. Many patients—especially those with a history of heavy menstrual flow—minimize the importance of this bleeding, delaying diagnosis.

History and physical examination

Determine the patient's current age and her age at menopause. Ask when she first noticed the abnormal bleeding. Then obtain a thorough obstetric and gynecologic history. When did she begin menstruating? Were her periods regular? If not, ask her to describe any menstrual irregularities. How old was she when she first had intercourse? How many sexual partners has she had? Has she had children? Has she had fertility problems? If possible, obtain an obstetric and gynecologic history of the patient's mother, and ask about a family history of gynecologic cancer. Determine if the patient has associated symptoms and if she's currently taking estrogen.

Observe the external genitalia, noting the character of vaginal discharge and the appearance of the labia, vaginal rugae, and clitoris. Carefully palpate the patient's breasts and lymph nodes for nodules or enlargement. The patient may require pelvic and rectal examinations.

Common medical causes

♦ ***Atrophic vaginitis.*** When bloody staining occurs, it usually follows coitus or douching. Characteristic white, watery vaginal discharge may be accompanied by pruritus, dyspareunia, and a burning sensation in the vagina and labia. Other possible findings include sparse pubic hair, a pale vagina with decreased rugae and small hemorrhagic spots, clitoral atrophy, or shrinkage of the labia minora.

♦ ***Cervical cancer.*** Early invasive cervical cancer causes vaginal spotting or heavier bleeding, usually after coitus or douching but occasionally spontaneously. Related findings include persistent, pink-tinged, and foul-smelling vaginal discharge and postcoital pain. As the cancer spreads, the patient may experience back and sciatic pain, leg swelling, anorexia, weight loss, hematuria, dysuria, or rectal bleeding.

♦ ***Cervical or endometrial polyps.*** These small, pedunculated growths may cause spotting (possibly as a mucopurulent, pink discharge) after coitus, douching, or straining at stool. Endometrial polyps are commonly asymptomatic, however.

♦ ***Endometrial hyperplasia or cancer.*** Bleeding occurs early and can be brownish and scant or bright red and profuse; it commonly follows coitus or douching. Bleeding later becomes heavier and more frequent, leading to clotting and anemia. It may be accompanied by pelvic, rectal, lower back, or leg pain. The uterus may be enlarged.

♦ ***Ovarian tumors (feminizing).*** Estrogen-producing ovarian tumors can stimulate endometrial shedding and cause heavy bleeding not associated with coitus or douching. A palpable pelvic mass, increased cervical mucus, breast enlargement, or spider angiomas may be present.

♦ ***Vaginal cancer.*** Characteristic spotting or bleeding may be preceded by a thin, watery vaginal discharge. Bleeding may be spontaneous but usually follows coitus or douching. A firm, ulcerated vaginal lesion may be present; dyspareunia, urinary frequency, bladder and pelvic pain, rectal bleeding, or vulvar lesions may develop later.

Other causes

♦ ***Drugs.*** Unopposed or cyclic estrogen replacement therapy is a common cause of abnormal vaginal bleeding, which can usually be reduced by adjusting the dose.

♦ **Herb alert** Ginseng can cause postmenopausal bleeding.

Special considerations

Prepare the patient for diagnostic tests, such as ultrasonography to outline a cervical or uterine tumor; endometrial biopsy or dilatation and fractional curettage to obtain tissue for histologic examination; testing for occult blood in the stool; and vaginal and cervical cultures to detect infection. Discontinue estrogens until a diagnosis is made.

Geriatric pointers

Eighty percent of postmenopausal vaginal bleeding is benign; endometrial atrophy is the predominant cause. Malignancy should be ruled out.

VAGINAL DISCHARGE

Common in women of childbearing age, physiologic vaginal discharge is mucoid, clear or white, nonbloody, and odorless. Produced by the cervical mucosa and, to a lesser degree, by the vulvar glands, this discharge may vary from scant to profuse with normal estrogenic stimulation and changes during the patient's menstrual cycle. However, a marked increase in discharge or a change in color, odor, or consistency should be investigated as a sign of disease. Discharge may result from infection, sexually transmitted disease, reproductive tract disease, or drug therapy. In addition, the prolonged presence of a foreign body, such as a tampon or diaphragm, can cause local irritation and an inflammatory exudate. Frequent douching, feminine hygiene products, contraceptive products, bubble baths, and colored or perfumed toilet papers can also be factors.

History and physical examination

Ask the patient to describe the onset, color, consistency, odor, and texture of her vaginal discharge. How does the discharge differ from her usual vaginal secretions? Is the onset predicable or related to her menstrual cycle? Also ask about associated symptoms, such as dysuria or perineal pruritus and burning. Does she have spotting after coitus or douching? Ask about recent changes in her sexual habits and hygiene practices. Is she or could she be pregnant? Next, ask if she has had vaginal discharge before or has been treated for a vaginal infection. What treatment did she receive? Did she complete the course of medication? Ask about her current use of medications, especially antibiotics, oral estrogens, or contraceptives.

Examine the external genitalia and note the character of the discharge. (See *Common causes of vaginal discharge*.) Observe vulvar and vaginal tissues for redness, edema, and excoriation. Palpate the inguinal lymph nodes to detect tenderness or enlargement, and palpate the abdomen for tenderness. A pelvic examination may be required. Obtain vaginal discharge specimens for testing.

Common medical causes

♦ ***Atrophic vaginitis.*** In this disorder, a thin, scant, watery white vaginal discharge may be accompanied by pruritus, burning, tenderness, and bloody spotting after coitus or douching. Sparse pubic hair, a pale vagina with decreased rugae and small hemorrhagic spots, clitoral atrophy, and shrinkage of the labia minora may also occur.

♦ ***Candidiasis.*** Infection with *Candida albicans* causes abrupt onset of a profuse, white, curdlike discharge with a yeasty, sweet odor. The infection occurs in up to 20% of nonpregnant woman and up to 40% of pregnant women. Exudate may be lightly attached to the labia and vaginal walls and is commonly accompanied by vulvar redness and edema. The inner thighs may be covered with a fine, red dermatitis and weeping erosions. The patient may report intense labial itching and burning or external dysuria.

♦ ***Chlamydia infection.*** This infection causes a yellow, mucopurulent, odorless, or acrid vaginal discharge. Other findings may include dysuria, dyspareunia, and vaginal bleeding after douching or coitus, especially following menses. Many women remain asymptomatic.

♦ ***Human papillomavirus genital warts.*** These mosaic, papular vulvar lesions can cause a profuse, mucopurulent vaginal discharge, which may be foul-smelling if the warts are infected. Patients commonly complain of burning or paresthesia in the vaginal introitus.

♦ ***Gonorrhea.*** Although 80% of women with gonorrhea are asymptomatic, others have a yellow or green, foul-smelling discharge that can be expressed from Bartholin's or Skene's ducts. Other findings include dysuria, urinary frequency and incontinence, bleeding, or vaginal redness and swelling. Severe pelvic and lower abdominal pain and fever may develop.

♦ ***Gynecologic cancer.*** Endometrial or cervical cancer produces a chronic, watery, bloody or purulent vaginal discharge that may be foul-smelling. Other findings may include abnormal vaginal bleeding and, later, weight loss; pelvic, back, and leg pain; fatigue; urinary frequency; or abdominal distention.

♦ ***Trichomoniasis.*** This infection can cause a foul-smelling discharge, which may be frothy, greenish yellow, and profuse or thin, white, and scant. Other findings may include pruritus; inflammation of the cervix and vagina with tiny petechiae; dysuria and urinary frequency; and dyspareunia, postcoital spotting, menorrhagia, or dysmenorrhea. About 50% of patients are asymptomatic.

Other causes

♦ ***Contraceptive creams and jellies.*** These products can increase vaginal secretions.

♦ ***Drugs.*** Estrogen and estrogen-inhibiting drugs can cause increased mucoid vaginal discharge. Antibiotics, such as tetracycline, may increase the risk of a monilial vaginal infection and discharge.

♦ ***Radiation therapy.*** Irradiation of the reproductive tract can cause a watery, odorless vaginal discharge.

♦ ***Tampon retention.*** A discharge may signal inadvertent retention of a tampon, especially in a patient using multiple tampons for metrorrhagia.

Common causes of vaginal discharge

The color, consistency, amount, and odor of your patient's vaginal discharge provide important clues about the underlying disorder. For quick reference, use this chart to match common characteristics of vaginal discharge and their possible causes.

CHARACTERISTICS	POSSIBLE CAUSES
Thin, scant, watery, white discharge	Atrophic vaginitis
White, curdlike, profuse discharge with yeasty, sweet odor	Candidiasis
Mucopurulent, foul-smelling discharge	Chancroid
Yellow, mucopurulent, odorless or acrid discharge	*Chlamydia* infection
Scant, serosanguineous, or purulent discharge with foul odor	Endometritis
Thin, green, or grayish white, foul-smelling discharge	*Gardnerella* vaginitis
Watery discharge	Genital herpes
Profuse, mucopurulent discharge, possibly foul-smelling	Human papillomavirus genital warts
Yellow or green, foul-smelling discharge from the cervix or occasionally from Bartholin's or Skene's ducts	Gonorrhea
Chronic, watery, bloody, or purulent discharge, possibly foul-smelling	Gynecological cancer
Frothy, greenish yellow, and profuse (or thin, white, and scant) foul-smelling discharge	Trichomoniasis

Special considerations

Teach the patient to keep her perineum clean and dry. Also tell her to avoid wearing tight-fitting clothing and nylon underwear and instead to wear cotton-crotched underwear and pantyhose. If appropriate, suggest that the patient douche with a solution of 5 tbs of white vinegar to 2 qt (1.9 L) of warm water to help relieve her discomfort.

If the patient has a vaginal infection, tell her to continue taking the prescribed medication even if her symptoms clear or she menstruates. Also advise her to avoid intercourse until her symptoms clear and then to have her partner use condoms until she completes her course of medication.

Pediatric pointers

Female newborns who have been exposed to maternal estrogens in utero may have a white mucus vaginal discharge for the first month after birth; a yellow mucus discharge indicates a pathologic condition. In the older child, a purulent, foul-smelling and, possibly, bloody vaginal discharge commonly results from a foreign object placed in the vagina. The possibility of sexual abuse should also be considered.

Geriatric pointers

The postmenopausal vaginal mucosa becomes thin due to decreased estrogen levels. Together with a rise in vaginal pH, this reduces resistance to infectious agents, increasing the incidence of vaginitis.

Vertigo

Vertigo is an illusion of movement in which the patient feels that he's revolving in space (subjective vertigo) or that his surroundings are revolving around him (objective vertigo). He may complain of feeling pulled sideways, as though drawn by a magnet.

A common symptom, vertigo usually begins abruptly and may be temporary or permanent, mild or severe. It may worsen when the patient moves and commonly subsides when he lies down. Frequently, it's confused with dizziness — a nonspecific sensation of imbalance and light-headedness. However, unlike dizziness, vertigo is commonly accompanied by nausea, vomiting, nystagmus, or tinnitus or hearing loss. Although the patient's limb coordination is unaffected, vertiginous gait may occur.

Vertigo may result from neurologic, cranial, or otologic disorders that affect the equilibratory apparatus (the vestibule, semicircular canals, eighth cranial nerve [CN VIII], vestibular nuclei in the brain stem and their temporal lobe connections, and eyes). However, this symptom may also result from alcohol intoxication, hyperventilation, postural changes (benign postural vertigo), or the effects of certain drugs, tests, or procedures.

History and physical examination

Ask your patient to describe the onset and duration of his vertigo, being careful to distinguish this symptom from dizziness. Does he feel that he's moving or that his surroundings are moving around him? How often do the attacks occur? Do they follow position changes, or are they unpredictable? Find out if the patient can walk during an attack, if he leans to one side, and if he's ever fallen. Ask if he experiences motion sickness and if he prefers one position during an attack. Obtain a recent drug history and note evidence of alcohol abuse.

Perform a neurologic assessment, focusing particularly on CN VIII function. Observe the patient's gait and posture for abnormalities. Auditory diagnostic tests may reveal sensorineural hearing loss.

Common medical causes

♦ ***Acoustic neuroma.*** This tumor of CN VIII causes mild, intermittent vertigo and unilateral sensorineural hearing loss. Other findings may include tinnitus, postauricular or suboccipital pain, or — with cranial nerve compression — facial paralysis.

♦ ***Benign positional vertigo.*** When the patient moves his head, debris in a semicircular canal causes vertigo, which lasts a few minutes. It's usually temporary and can be effectively treated with positional maneuvers.

♦ ***Brain stem ischemia.*** This condition causes sudden, severe vertigo that may become episodic and later persistent. Associated findings include ataxia, nausea, vomiting, increased blood pressure, tachycardia, nystagmus, or lateral deviation of the eyes toward the side of the lesion. Hemiparesis or paresthesia may also occur.

♦ ***Head trauma.*** Soon after injury, positional vertigo accompanies spontaneous or positional nystagmus and, if the temporal bone is fractured, hearing loss. Associated findings include headache, nausea, vomiting, and decreased level of consciousness (LOC). Behavioral changes, diplopia or visual blurring, seizures, motor or sensory deficits, or signs of increased intracranial pressure may also occur.

◆ ***Herpes zoster.*** Infection of the CN VIII causes sudden onset of vertigo accompanied by facial paralysis, hearing loss in the affected ear, and herpetic vesicular lesions in the auditory canal.

◆ ***Labyrinthitis.*** Severe vertigo begins abruptly with this inner ear infection. Vertigo may occur in a single episode or may recur over months or years. Associated findings may include nausea, vomiting, progressive sensorineural hearing loss, or nystagmus.

◆ ***Ménière's disease.*** Labyrinthine dysfunction causes abrupt onset of vertigo, lasting minutes, hours, or days. Unpredictable episodes of severe vertigo and unsteady gait may cause the patient to fall. During an attack, a sudden motion of the head or eyes can precipitate nausea and vomiting. Onset may follow middle ear infection or head trauma. Typically, this disorder is unilateral (affects only one ear). Tinnitus and hearing loss may accompany attacks.

◆ ***Multiple sclerosis (MS).*** Episodic vertigo may occur early and become persistent. Other early findings include diplopia, visual blurring, and paresthesia. MS may also cause nystagmus, constipation, muscle weakness, paralysis, spasticity, hyperreflexia, intention tremor, or ataxia.

◆ ***Seizures.*** Temporal lobe seizures may cause vertigo, usually associated with other symptoms of partial complex seizures.

Other causes

◆ ***Diagnostic tests.*** Caloric testing (irrigating the ears with warm or cold water) can induce vertigo.

◆ ***Drugs and alcohol.*** High or toxic doses of certain drugs or alcohol may cause vertigo. These drugs include salicylates, aminoglycosides, antibiotics, quinine, and oral contraceptives.

◆ ***Surgery and other procedures.*** Ear surgery may cause vertigo that lasts for several days. In addition, administration of overly warm or cold eardrops or irrigating solutions may cause vertigo.

Special considerations

Place the patient in a comfortable position, and monitor his vital signs and LOC. Keep the side rails up if he's in bed, or help him to a chair if he's standing when vertigo occurs. Darken the room and keep him calm. Administer drugs to control nausea and vomiting and meclizine or dimenhydrinate to decrease labyrinthine irritability.

Prepare the patient for diagnostic tests, such as electronystagmography, electroencephalography, and X-rays of the middle and inner ears.

Pediatric pointers

Ear infection is a common cause of vertigo in children. Vestibular neuritis may also cause this symptom.

VESICULAR RASH

A vesicular rash is a scattered or linear distribution of vesicles — sharply circumscribed lesions filled with clear, cloudy, or bloody fluid. The lesions, which are usually less than 0.5 cm in diameter, may occur singly or in groups. (See *Recognizing common skin lesions*, page 444.) They sometimes are accompanied by bullae — fluid-filled lesions larger than 0.5 cm in diameter.

A vesicular rash may be mild or severe and temporary or permanent. It can result from infection, inflammation, or allergic reactions.

History and physical examination

Ask your patient when the rash began, how it spread, and whether it has appeared before. Did other skin lesions precede eruption of the vesicles? Obtain a thorough drug history. If the patient has used a topical medication, what type did he use and when was it last applied? Also ask about associated signs and symptoms. Find out if he has a family history of skin disorders, and ask about allergies, recent infections, insect bites, and exposure to allergens.

Examine the patient's skin, noting if it's dry, oily, or moist. Observe the general distribution of the lesions and record their exact location. Note the color, shape, and size of the lesions, and check for crusts, scales, scars, macules, papules, or wheals. Palpate the vesicles or bullae to determine if they're flaccid or tense. Slide your finger across the skin to see if the outer layer of epidermis separates easily from the basal layer (Nikolsky's sign).

Common medical causes

♦ ***Burns.*** Thermal burns that affect the epidermis and part of the dermis commonly cause vesicles and bullae, erythema, swelling, and pain.

♦ ***Dermatitis.*** In *contact dermatitis,* a severe hypersensitivity reaction causes an eruption of small vesicles surrounded by redness and marked edema. The vesicles may ooze, scale, and cause severe pruritus.

Dermatitis herpetiformis, occurring most commonly in men between the ages of 20 and 50, causes a chronic inflammatory eruption marked by vesicular, papular, bullous, pustular, or erythematous lesions. Usually, the rash is symmetrically distributed on the buttocks, shoulders, extensor surfaces of the elbows and knees and, sometimes, the face, scalp, and neck. Other symptoms include severe pruritus, burning, and stinging.

In *nummular dermatitis,* groups of pinpoint vesicles and papules appear on erythematous or pustular lesions that are nummular (coinlike) or annular (ringlike). Commonly, the pustular lesions ooze a purulent exudate, itch severely, and rapidly become crusted and scaly. Two or three lesions may develop on the hands, but the lesions most commonly develop on the extensor surfaces of the limbs and on the buttocks and posterior trunk.

♦ ***Erythema multiforme.*** This acute inflammatory skin disease is heralded by a sudden eruption of erythematous macules, papules and, occasionally, vesicles and bullae. The characteristic rash appears symmetrically over the hands, arms, feet, legs, face, and neck and tends to reappear. Vesicles and bullae may also erupt on the eyes and genitalia. Most commonly, however, vesiculobullous lesions appear on the mucous membranes — especially the lips and buccal mucosa — where they rupture and ulcerate, producing a thick, yellow or white exudate. Bloody, painful crusts, a foul-smelling oral discharge, and difficulty chewing may develop. Lymphadenopathy may also occur.

♦ ***Herpes simplex.*** This common viral infection causes groups of vesicles on an inflamed base, most commonly on the lips and lower face or, in about 25% of cases, the genital region. Vesicles are heralded by itching, tingling, burning, or pain; they develop singly or in groups, are 2 to 3 mm in size, and don't coalesce. Eventually, they rupture, forming a painful ulcer followed by a yellowish crust.

♦ ***Herpes zoster.*** A vesicular rash is preceded by erythema and, occasionally, by a nodular skin eruption and unilateral, sharp, shooting chest pain that mimics a myocardial infarction. About 5 days later, the lesions erupt and commonly spread unilaterally over the thorax or vertically over the arms and legs. The pain becomes burning. Vesicles dry and scab about 10 days after eruption. Associated findings include fever, malaise, pruritus, and paresthesia or hyperesthesia of the involved area. Occasionally, herpes zoster involves the cranial nerves, producing facial palsy, hearing loss, dizziness, loss of taste, eye pain, and impaired vision.

♦ ***Insect bites.*** Vesicles appear on red hivelike papules and may become hemorrhagic.

♦ ***Pemphigoid (bullous).*** Generalized pruritus or an urticarial or eczematous eruption may precede the classic bullous rash. Bullae are large, tense, and irregular and most commonly form on an erythematous base. They usually appear on the lower abdomen, groin, inner thighs, and forearms.

◆ ***Pompholyx.*** This common, recurrent disorder causes symmetrical vesicular lesions that can become pustular. The pruritic lesions appear on the palms more frequently than on the soles and may be accompanied by minimal erythema.

◆ ***Porphyria cutanea tarda.*** Bullae — especially on areas exposed to sun, friction, trauma, or heat — result from abnormal porphyrin metabolism. Photosensitivity is also a common sign. Papulovesicular lesions evolving into erosions or ulcers and scars may appear. Chronic skin changes include hyperpigmentation or hypopigmentation, hypertrichosis, and sclerodermoid lesions. The patient's urine is pink to brown.

◆ ***Scabies.*** Small vesicles erupt on an erythematous base and may be at the end of a threadlike burrow. Burrows are a few millimeters long, and a swollen nodule or red papule contains the itch mite. Pustules and excoriations may form. In men, burrows may be on the glans, shaft, or scrotum; in women, on the nipples; in both sexes, burrows on the wrists, elbows, axilla, or waistline. Associated pruritus worsens with inactivity and warmth and at night.

◆ ***Tinea pedis.*** This fungal infection causes vesicles and scaling between the toes and, possibly, scaling over the entire sole. Severe infection causes inflammation, pruritus, and difficulty walking.

◆ ***Toxic epidermal necrolysis.*** In this immune reaction to drugs or other toxins, vesicles and large, flaccid bullae are preceded by a diffuse, erythematous rash. Prodromal signs include mucous membrane inflammation, a burning sensation in the conjunctivae, malaise, fever, and generalized skin tenderness. The bullae rupture easily, exposing extensive areas of denuded skin and leading to large-scale epidermal necrolysis and desquamation. (See *Drugs that cause toxic epidermal necrolysis.*)

Drugs that cause toxic epidermal necrolysis

Various drugs can trigger toxic epidermal necrolysis (TEN) — a rare but potentially fatal immune reaction characterized by a vesicular rash. TEN produces large, flaccid bullae that rupture easily, exposing extensive areas of denuded skin. The resulting loss of fluid and electrolytes — along with widespread systemic involvement — can lead to such life-threatening complications as pulmonary edema, shock, renal failure, sepsis, and disseminated intravascular coagulation. Here's a list of some drugs that can cause TEN:

- allopurinol
- aspirin
- barbiturates
- chloramphenicol
- chlorpropamide
- gold salts
- nitrofurantoin
- penicillin
- phenolphthalein
- phenylbutazone
- phenytoin
- primidone
- sulfonamides
- tetracycline.

Special considerations

Any skin eruption that covers a large area may cause substantial fluid loss through the vesicles, bullae, or other weeping lesions. If necessary, start an I.V. line to replace fluids and electrolytes. Keep the patient's environment warm and free from drafts, cover him with sheets or blankets as necessary, and take his rectal temperature every 4 hours because fluid loss and increased blood flow to inflamed skin may lead to hyperthermia.

Obtain cultures to determine the causative organism. Use standard precautions until infection is ruled out. Tell the patient to wash his hands often and not to touch the lesions. Be alert for signs of secondary infection. Give the patient antibiotics and apply corticosteroid or antimicrobial ointment to the lesions.

Pediatric pointers

Vesicular rashes in children are caused by staphylococcal infections (staphylococcal scalded skin syndrome is a life-threatening infection occurring in infants), varicella, hand-foot-and-mouth disease, or miliaria rubra.

VIOLENT BEHAVIOR

Marked by sudden loss of self-control, violent behavior refers to the use of physical force to violate, injure, or abuse an object or person. This behavior may also be self-directed. It may result from organic or psychiatric disorders or from the effects of drugs.

History and physical examination

Determine if the patient has a history of violent behavior. Is he intoxicated or suffering symptoms of alcohol or drug withdrawal? Does he have a history of family violence, including corporal punishment and child or spouse abuse? (See *Understanding family violence*.)

Watch for clues indicating that the patient is losing control and may become violent. Has he exhibited abrupt behavioral changes? Is he unable to sit still? Increased activity may indicate an attempt to discharge aggression. Does he suddenly cease activity (suggesting the calm before the storm)? Does he make verbal threats or angry gestures? Is he jumpy, extremely tense, or laughing? Such intensifying of emotion may herald loss of control.

If your patient's violent behavior is a new development, he may have an organic disorder. Obtain a medical history and perform a physical examination. Watch for a sudden change in his level of consciousness. Disorientation, failure to recall recent events, and display of tics, jerks, tremors, or asterixis all suggest an organic disorder.

Common medical causes

♦ ***Organic disorders.*** Many disorders may cause violent behavior resulting from metabolic and neurologic dysfunction. Common causes include epilepsy, brain tumor, encephalitis, head injury, endocrine disorders, metabolic disorders (such as uremia and calcium imbalance), or severe physical trauma.

♦ ***Psychiatric disorders.*** In psychotic disorders, such as schizophrenia, violent behavior occurs as a protective mechanism in response to a perceived threat. A similar response may occur in personality disorders, such as antisocial or borderline personality.

Other causes

♦ ***Drugs and alcohol.*** Various drugs, such as lidocaine and procaine penicillin, may cause violent behavior as an adverse effect. Alcohol abuse or withdrawal, hallucinogens, amphetamines, or barbiturate withdrawal may also cause violent behavior.

Special considerations

Violent behavior is most prevalent in emergency rooms, critical care units, and crisis and acute psychiatric units. Natural disasters and accidents also increase the potential for violent behavior, so be on guard in these situations.

If your patient becomes violent or potentially violent, your goal is to remain composed and to establish environmental control. First, protect yourself. Remain at a distance from the patient, call for assistance, and don't overreact. Remain calm, and make sure you have enough personnel for a show of force to subdue or restrain the patient if necessary. Encourage the patient to move to

Understanding family violence

Effectively managing the violent patient requires an understanding of the roots of his behavior — for example, a family history of corporal punishment or child or spouse abuse. His violent behavior may also be associated with drugs or alcohol abuse or with fixed family roles that stifle growth and individuality.

What causes family violence? Social scientists suggest that it stems from cultural attitudes fostering violence and from frustration and stress associated with overcrowded living conditions and poverty. Albert Bandura, a social learning theorist, believes that individuals learn violent behavior by observing and imitating other family members who vent their aggressive feelings through verbal abuse and physical force. (They also learn from television and the movies, especially when the violent hero gains power and recognition.) Members of families with these characteristics may have an increased potential for violent behavior, thus initiating a cycle of violence that passes from generation to generation.

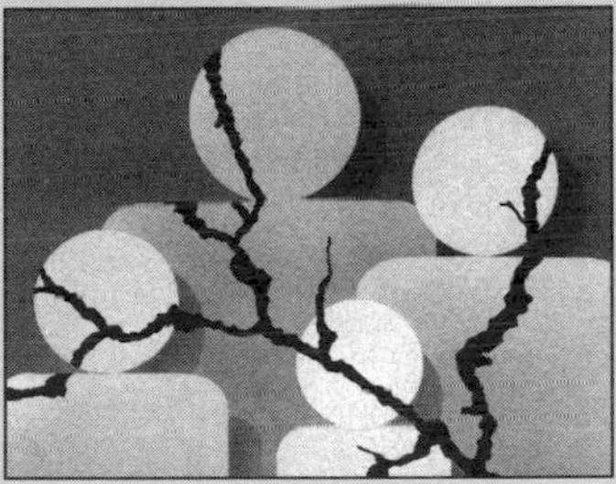

a quiet location — free of noise, activity, and people — to avoid frightening or stimulating him further. Reassure him, explain what's happening, and tell him that he's safe. Use a calm, low tone of voice. Keep verbal communication brief, using short, simple statements.

If the patient makes violent threats, take them seriously, and inform those at whom the threats are directed. Administer psychotropic medications as ordered.

Remember, your own attitudes can affect your ability to care for a violent patient. If you feel fearful or judgmental, ask another staff member for help.

Pediatric pointers

Adolescents and younger children commonly make threats resulting from violent dreams or fantasies or unmet needs. Adolescents who exhibit extreme violence can come from families with a history of physical or psychological abuse. These children may display violent behavior toward their peers, siblings, or pets.

Geriatric pointers

The elderly are particularly at risk for violent behavior caused by cognitive deficits. A patient who misinterprets his environment may feel frightened or threatened by the caregiver and may respond with violent behavior.

Vision loss

Vision loss — the inability to perceive visual stimuli — can be sudden or gradual, temporary or permanent. The deficit can range from a slight impairment of vision to total blindness. It results from ocular, neurologic, or systemic disorders as well as from trauma or reactions to certain drugs. The ultimate outcome may depend on early, accurate diagnosis and treatment.

History and physical examination

Sudden vision loss can signal an ocular emergency. (See *Managing sudden vision loss,* page 598.) Don't touch the eye if the

EMERGENCY INTERVENTIONS

Managing sudden vision loss

Sudden vision loss can signal central retinal artery occlusion or acute angle-closure glaucoma—ocular emergencies that require immediate intervention. If your patient reports sudden vision loss, immediately notify an ophthalmologist for an emergency examination and perform these interventions:

For a patient with suspected central retinal artery occlusion, perform light massage over his closed eyelid. Increase his carbon dioxide level by administering a set flow of oxygen and carbon dioxide through a Venturi mask, or have the patient rebreathe in a paper bag to retain exhaled carbon dioxide. These steps will dilate the artery and, possibly, restore blood flow to the retina.

For a patient with suspected acute angle-closure glaucoma, measure intraocular pressure (IOP) with a tonometer. (You can also estimate IOP by placing your fingers over the patient's closed eyelid. A rock-hard eyeball usually indicates increased IOP.) Expect to administer timolol drops and I.V. acetazolamide to help decrease IOP.

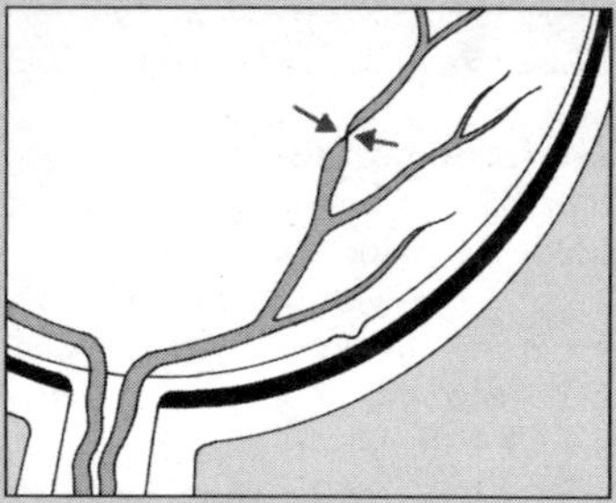

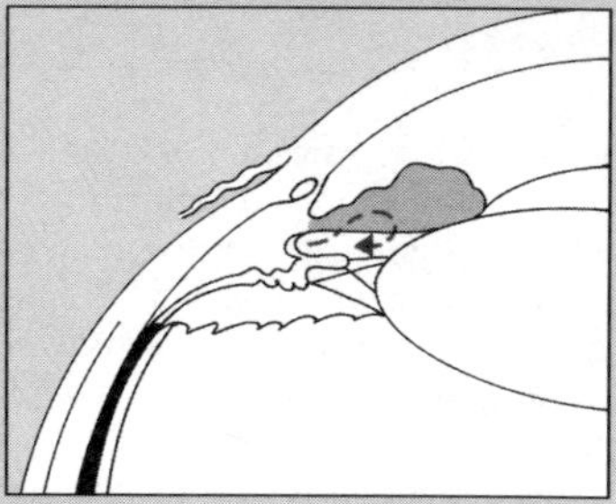

patient has perforating or penetrating ocular trauma.

If the patient's vision loss occurred gradually, ask him if it affects one eye or both and all or only part of the visual field. Is the visual loss transient or persistent? Did it occur abruptly or over hours, days, or weeks? What's the patient's age? Ask the patient if he has experienced photosensitivity, and ask him about the location, intensity, and duration of eye pain. Obtain an ocular history and a family history of eye problems or systemic diseases that may cause eye problems, such as hypertension; diabetes mellitus; thyroid, rheumatic, or vascular disease; infections; or cancer.

The first step in performing the eye examination is to assess visual acuity, with best available correction in each eye. (See *Testing visual acuity.*)

Carefully inspect both eyes, noting edema, foreign bodies, drainage, or conjunctival or scleral redness. Observe whether lid closure is complete or incomplete, and check for ptosis. Using a flashlight, examine the cornea and iris for scars, irregularities, and foreign bodies. Observe the size, shape, and color of the pupils, and test the direct and consensual light reflex (see "Pupils, nonreactive," page 498) and the effect of accommodation. Evaluate extraocular muscle function by testing the six cardinal

EXAMINATION TIP

Testing visual acuity

Use a Snellen letter chart to test visual acuity in the literate patient over age 6 years. Have the patient sit or stand 20′ (6.1 m) from the chart. Tell him to cover his left eye and read aloud the smallest line of letters that he can see. Record the fraction assigned to that line on the chart (the numerator indicates distance from the chart, the denominator indicates the distance at which the normal eye can read the chart.) Normal vision is 20/20. Repeat the test with the patient's right eye covered.

If your patient can't read the largest letter from a distance of 20 feet, have him approach the chart until he can read it. Then, record the distance between him and the chart as the numerator of the fraction. For example, if he can see the top line of the chart at a distance of 3′ (0.9 m), record the test result as 3/200.

Use a Snellen symbol chart to test children 3 to 6 years of age and illiterate patients. Follow the same procedure as for the Snellen letter chart, but ask the patient to indicate the direction of the E's fingers as you point to each symbol.

SNELLEN LETTER CHART

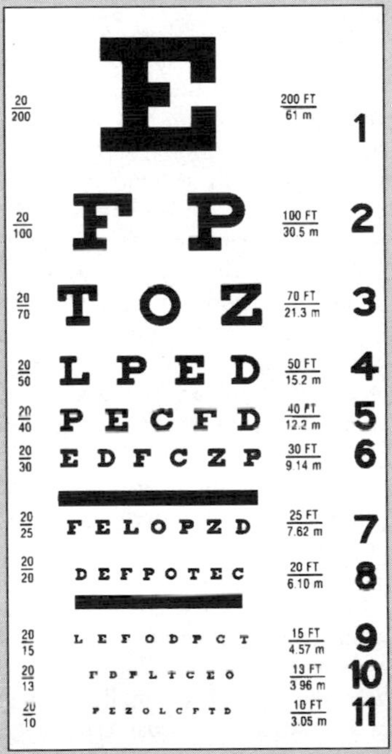

SNELLEN SYMBOL CHART

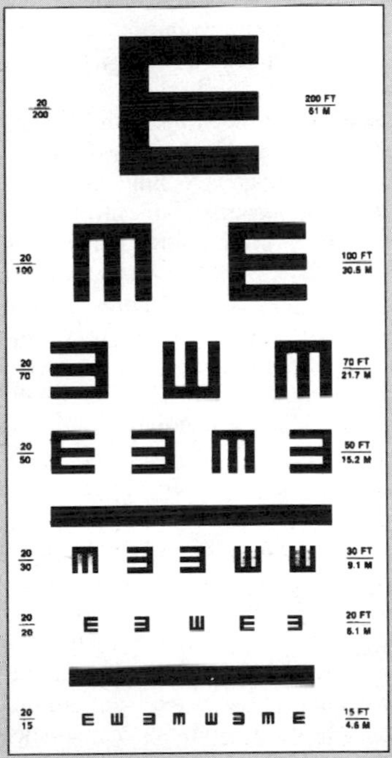

fields of gaze. (See *Testing extraocular muscles*, page 192.)

Common medical causes

♦ ***Amaurosis fugax.*** In this disorder, recurrent attacks of unilateral vision loss may last from a few seconds to a few minutes. Vision is normal at other times. Transient unilateral weakness, hypertension, and elevated intraocular pressure (IOP) in the affected eye may also occur.

♦ ***Cataract.*** Typically, painless and gradual visual blurring precedes vision loss. As the cataract progresses, the pupil turns milky white.

♦ ***Concussion.*** Immediately or shortly after blunt head trauma, vision may be blurred, double, or lost. Generally, vision loss is temporary. Other findings may include headache, anterograde or retrograde amnesia, transient loss of consciousness, nausea, vomiting, dizziness, irritability, confusion, lethargy, or aphasia.

♦ ***Diabetic retinopathy.*** Retinal edema and hemorrhage lead to visual blurring, which may progress to blindness.

♦ ***Endophthalmitis.*** Typically, this intraocular infection follows penetrating trauma, I.V. drug use, or intraocular surgery, causing possibly permanent unilateral vision loss. A sympathetic inflammation may affect the other eye.

♦ ***Glaucoma.*** This disorder causes gradual visual blurring that may progress to total blindness. *Acute angle-closure glaucoma* is an ocular emergency that may cause blindness within 3 to 5 days. Findings are rapid onset of unilateral inflammation and pain, pressure over the eye, moderate pupil dilation, nonreactive pupillary response, a cloudy cornea, reduced visual acuity, photophobia, and perception of blue or red halos around lights. Nausea and vomiting may also occur.

Chronic angle-closure glaucoma has a gradual onset and usually causes no symptoms, although blurred or halo vision may occur. If untreated, it progresses to blindness and extreme pain.

Chronic open-angle glaucoma is usually bilateral, with an insidious onset and a slowly progressive course. It causes peripheral vision loss, aching eyes, halo vision, and reduced visual acuity (especially at night).

♦ ***Ocular trauma.*** Sudden unilateral or bilateral vision loss may occur after eye injury. Vision loss may be total or partial and permanent or temporary. The eyelids may be reddened, edematous, or lacerated; intraocular contents may be extruded.

♦ ***Optic atrophy.*** Degeneration of the optic nerve can develop spontaneously or follow inflammation or edema of the nerve head, causing irreversible loss of the visual field with changes in color vision. Pupillary reactions are sluggish, and the optic disk is pale.

♦ ***Optic neuritis.*** An umbrella term for inflammation, degeneration, or demyelinization of the optic nerve, optic neuritis usually causes temporary but severe unilateral vision loss. Pain around the eye, especially with movement of the globe, may accompany visual field defects or a sluggish pupillary response to light. Ophthalmoscopic examination commonly reveals hyperemia of the optic disk, blurred disk margins, and filling of the physiologic cup.

♦ ***Pituitary tumor.*** As a pituitary adenoma grows, blurred vision progresses to hemianopsia and, possibly, unilateral blindness. Double vision, nystagmus, ptosis, limited eye movement, or headaches may also occur.

♦ ***Retinal artery occlusion (central).*** This painless ocular emergency causes sudden unilateral vision loss, which may be partial or complete. Examination reveals a sluggish direct pupillary response and a normal consensual response. Permanent blindness may occur within hours.

♦ ***Retinal detachment.*** Depending on the degree and location of detachment, painless vision loss may be gradual or sudden, total or partial. Macular involvement causes total blindness. The patient with partial vision loss may describe visual field defects or a shadow or curtain over the visual field as well as visual floaters.

◆ ***Retinal vein occlusion (central).*** Most common in geriatric patients, this painless disorder causes a unilateral decrease in visual acuity with variable vision loss. IOP may be elevated in both eyes.

◆ ***Senile macular degeneration.*** Elderly patients with this disorder experience painless blurring or loss of central vision. Vision loss may proceed slowly or rapidly, eventually affecting both eyes. Visual acuity may be worse at night.

◆ ***Stevens-Johnson syndrome.*** Corneal scarring from associated conjunctival lesions causes marked vision loss. The patient exhibits purulent conjunctivitis, eye pain, and difficulty opening the eyes. Additional findings may include widespread bullae, fever, malaise, cough, drooling, inability to eat, sore throat, chest pain, vomiting, diarrhea, myalgias, arthralgias, hematuria or, possibly, signs of renal failure.

◆ ***Temporal arteritis.*** Blurring and vision loss with a throbbing, unilateral headache characterize this disorder. Other findings include malaise, anorexia, weight loss, weakness, low-grade fever, generalized muscle aches, or confusion.

◆ ***Vitreous hemorrhage.*** Intraocular trauma, ocular tumors, or systemic disease — especially diabetes, hypertension, sickle cell anemia, or leukemia — may cause sudden onset of unilateral visual floaters and partial vision loss with a reddish haze or total vision loss in the affected eye. The vision loss may be permanent.

Other causes

◆ ***Drugs.*** Chloroquine therapy may cause patchy retinal pigmentation that typically leads to blindness. Phenylbutazone may cause vision loss and increased susceptibility to retinal detachment. Digitalis derivatives, indomethacin, ethambutol, quinine sulfate, or methanol may also cause vision loss.

Special considerations

Any degree of vision loss is extremely frightening to your patient. To ease his fears, orient him to his environment, and announce your presence each time you approach him. If the patient reports photophobia, darken the room and suggest that he wear sunglasses during the day. Obtain cultures of drainage, and instruct him not to touch the unaffected eye with anything that has come in contact with the affected eye. Instruct him to wash his hands often and to avoid rubbing his eyes. If necessary, prepare him for surgery.

Pediatric pointers

Children who complain of slowly progressive vision loss may have an optic nerve glioma (a slow-growing, usually benign tumor) or retinoblastoma (a malignant tumor of the retina). Congenital rubella or syphilis may cause vision loss in infants. Retrolental fibroplasia may cause vision loss in premature infants. Other congenital causes of vision loss include Marfan syndrome, retinitis pigmentosa, retinal detachment, optic nerve hypoplasia and atrophy, diabetic neuropathy, or amblyopia.

Geriatric pointers

In the elderly, the corneal epithelium commonly undergoes degenerative changes that slightly reduce visual acuity. The most common causes of complete vision loss are cataracts, glaucoma, macular degeneration, and diabetic neuropathy. In elderly patients, reduced visual acuity may be caused by morphologic changes in the choroid, pigment epithelium, and retina or by decreased function of the rods, cones, and other neural elements. Elderly patients commonly have difficulty turning their eyes upward or sustaining convergence. IOP pressure also increases with age.

VISUAL BLURRING

This common symptom refers to the loss of visual acuity with indistinct visual details. It may result from eye injury, neurologic and eye disorders, or disorders with vascular complications, such as diabetes mellitus. Visual blurring may also result from mucus passing over the cornea, refractive errors, improperly fitted contact lenses, or the effects of drugs.

Patients sometimes say they have double vision when they mean they have blurred vision in one eye — for example, due to a strand of mucus in the tear film.

History and physical examination

If your patient has visual blurring accompanied by sudden, severe eye pain, a history of trauma, or sudden vision loss, order an ophthalmologic examination. (See *Managing sudden vision loss*, page 598.) If the patient has a penetrating or perforating eye injury, don't touch the eye.

If the patient isn't in distress, ask him how long he has had the visual blurring. Does it occur only at certain times? Ask about associated symptoms, such as pain or discharge. If visual blurring followed injury, obtain details of the accident, and ask if vision was impaired immediately after the injury. Obtain a medical and drug history.

Inspect the patient's eye, noting lid edema, drainage, or conjunctival or scleral redness. Also note an irregularly shaped iris, which may indicate previous trauma, and excessive blinking, which may indicate corneal damage. Assess for pupillary changes, and test visual acuity in both eyes. (See *Testing visual acuity*, page 599.)

Common medical causes

♦ ***Brain tumor.*** Visual blurring may be associated with decreased level of consciousness (LOC), headache, apathy, behavioral changes, memory loss, decreased attention span, dizziness, or confusion. A tumor can also cause aphasia, seizures, ataxia, or signs of hormonal imbalance. Later effects are papilledema, vomiting, increased systolic blood pressure, widened pulse pressure, and decorticate posture.

♦ ***Cataract.*** This painless disorder causes gradual visual blurring. Other effects include halo vision (an early sign), visual glare in bright light, progressive vision loss, and a gray pupil that later turns milky white.

♦ ***Cerebrovascular accident (CVA).*** Brief attacks of bilateral visual blurring may precede or accompany a CVA. Associated findings may include a decreased LOC, contralateral hemiplegia, dysarthria, dysphagia, ataxia, unilateral sensory loss, or apraxia. CVA may also cause agnosia, aphasia, homonymous hemianopsia, diplopia, disorientation, memory loss, and poor judgment.

♦ ***Concussion.*** Immediately or shortly after blunt head trauma, vision may be blurred, double, or temporarily lost. Other findings include changes in behavior or LOC.

♦ ***Corneal abrasions.*** Visual blurring, severe eye pain, photophobia, redness, and excessive tearing may occur.

♦ ***Corneal foreign bodies.*** Visual blurring may accompany a foreign-body sensation, excessive tearing, photophobia, intense eye pain, miosis, conjunctival injection, and a dark corneal speck.

♦ ***Diabetic retinopathy.*** Retinal edema and hemorrhage cause gradual blurring, which may progress to blindness.

♦ ***Dislocated lens.*** Dislocation of the lens, especially beyond the line of vision, causes visual blurring and (with trauma) redness.

♦ ***Eye tumor.*** If the tumor involves the macula, visual blurring may be the presenting symptom. Related findings include varying visual field losses.

♦ ***Glaucoma.*** In *acute angle-closure glaucoma,* an ocular emergency, unilateral visual blurring and severe pain begin suddenly. Other findings may include halo vision; a moderately dilated, nonreactive pupil; conjunctival injection; a cloudy cornea; or decreased visual acuity. Severely elevated intraocular pressure may cause nausea and vomiting.

In *chronic angle-closure glaucoma,* transient visual blurring and halo vision may precede pain and blindness.

♦ ***Hereditary corneal dystrophies.*** Visual blurring may remain stable or may progressively worsen throughout life. Some dystrophies cause pain, vision loss, photophobia, or tearing.

♦ ***Hypertension.*** This usually asymptomatic disorder may cause visual blurring and a constant morning headache that decreases in severity during the day. If diastolic blood pressure exceeds 120 mm Hg, the patient may report a severe, throbbing headache. Associated findings may include restlessness, confusion, nausea, vomiting, seizures, or decreased LOC.

♦ ***Hyphema.*** Blunt eye trauma with hemorrhage into the anterior chamber causes visual blurring. Other effects include moderate pain, diffuse conjunctival injection, visible blood in the anterior chamber, ecchymoses, eyelid edema, or a hard eye.

♦ ***Iritis.*** Acute iritis causes sudden visual blurring, moderate to severe eye pain, photophobia, conjunctival injection, and a constricted pupil.

♦ ***Optic neuritis.*** Inflammation, degeneration, or demyelinization of the optic nerve usually causes an acute attack of visual blurring and vision loss. Related findings include scotomas and eye pain. Ophthalmoscopic examination reveals hyperemia of the optic disk, large vein distention, blurred disk margins, and filling of the physiologic cup.

♦ ***Retinal detachment.*** Sudden visual blurring may be the initial symptom of this disorder. However, sudden onset of visual floaters and recurring flashes of light is more common. Blurring worsens, and progressive detachment increases vision loss.

♦ ***Retinal vein occlusion (central).*** This disorder causes gradual unilateral visual blurring and varying degrees of vision loss.

♦ ***Senile macular degeneration.*** This retinal disorder may cause visual blurring (initially worse at night) and slowly or rapidly progressive vision loss.

♦ ***Syphilis.*** Ocular involvement in secondary syphilis may include pain, redness, photophobia, blurred vision, and floating spots. In latent syphilis, the presenting ocular complaint is blurred vision.

♦ ***Temporal arteritis.*** Most common in women older than age 60, this disorder causes sudden blurred vision accompanied by vision loss and a throbbing unilateral headache in the temporal or frontotemporal region. Prodromal symptoms include malaise, anorexia, weight loss, weakness, low-grade fever, or generalized muscle aches. Other findings include confusion; disorientation; swollen, nodular, tender temporal arteries; or erythema of overlying skin.

♦ ***Vitreous hemorrhage.*** Sudden unilateral visual blurring and varying vision loss signal this condition. The patient may report visual floaters or dark streaks.

Other causes

♦ ***Drugs.*** Visual blurring may stem from the effects of cycloplegics, guanethidine, reserpine, clomiphene, phenylbutazone, thiazide diuretics, antihistamines, anticholinergics, or phenothiazines.

Special considerations

Prepare the patient for diagnostic tests, such as tonometry, slit-lamp examination, X-rays of the skull and orbit and, if a neurologic lesion is suspected, a computed tomography scan. If necessary, teach him how to instill ophthalmic medication. If visual blurring leads to permanent vision loss, provide emotional support, orient him to his surroundings, and provide for his safety. If necessary, prepare him for surgery.

Other helpful tests include the glare test and contrast sensitivity. A potential acuity meter used in conjunction with a glare test helps to differentiate retinal from media pathology.

Pediatric pointers

Visual blurring in children may stem from congenital syphilis, congenital cataracts, refractive errors, eye injuries or infections, or increased intracranial pressure.

Test vision in school-age children as you would in adults; test children age 3 to 6 years with the Snellen symbol chart. Test toddlers with Allen cards, each illustrated with a familiar object, such as an animal. Ask the child to cover one eye and identify the objects as you flash them. Then, ask him to identify them as you gradually back away. Record the maximum distance at which he can identify at least three pictures.

VISUAL FLOATERS

Visual floaters are particles of blood or cellular debris that move about in the vitreous. As these enter the visual field, they appear as spots or dots. Chronic floaters may occur normally in elderly or myopic patients. Floaters may represent migrainous scintillations that last for several seconds or minutes. However, the sudden onset of visual floaters or particles, spiders, cobwebs, threads, worms, or dark streaks commonly signals retinal detachment, an ocular emergency.

Emergency interventions

Sudden onset of visual floaters may signal retinal detachment. Does the patient also see flashing lights or spots in the affected eye? Is he experiencing a curtainlike loss of vision? If so, notify an ophthalmologist immediately. Restrict the patient's eye movements until the diagnosis is made.

History and physical examination

If the patient's condition permits, obtain a drug and allergy history. Ask about nearsightedness (a predisposing factor), use of corrective lenses, eye trauma, or other eye disorders. Does he have a history of granulomatous disease, diabetes mellitus, or hypertension, which may have predisposed him to retinal detachment, vitreous hemorrhage, or uveitis. If appropriate, inspect his eyes for signs of injury, such as bruising or edema, and determine his visual acuity. (See *Testing visual acuity,* page 599.)

Visual floaters should never be dismissed as harmless or imaginary. A careful examination of the vitreous and retina is always indicated to identify the nature and origin of floaters and to guide management. Assume that a patient with new floaters or photopsia has retinal tears or detachment until ruled out by thorough examination of the peripheral retina with an indirect ophthalmoscope.

Common medical causes

- ***Retinal detachment.*** Floaters and light flashes appear suddenly in the portion of the visual field where the retina is detached. As the retina detaches further (a painless process), gradual vision loss occurs, likened to a cloud or curtain falling in front of the eyes. Ophthalmoscopic examination reveals a gray, opaque, detached retina with an indefinite margin. Retinal vessels appear almost black.
- ***Uveitis (posterior).*** This disorder may cause visual floaters accompanied by gradual eye pain, photophobia, blurred vision, or conjunctival injection.
- ***Vitreous hemorrhage.*** Rupture of retinal vessels causes a shower of red or black dots or a red haze across the visual field. Vision is suddenly blurred in the affected eye, and visual acuity may be greatly reduced.

Special considerations

Encourage bed rest and provide a calm environment. Depending on the cause, the patient may require eye patches, surgery, or corticosteroids or other drug therapy. If bilateral eye patches are necessary — as with retinal detachment —

ensure the patient's safety. Identify yourself when you approach the patient and orient him to time frequently. Provide sensory stimulation, such as a radio or tape player. Place pillows or towels behind the patient's head to maintain appropriate position. Be sure to warn him not to touch or rub his eyes and to avoid straining or sudden movements.

Pediatric pointers

Visual floaters in children usually follow trauma that causes retinal detachment or vitreous hemorrhage. However, they may also result from vitreous debris, a benign congenital condition with no other signs or symptoms.

VOMITING

Vomiting is the forceful expulsion of gastric contents through the mouth. Characteristically preceded by nausea, vomiting results from a coordinated sequence of abdominal muscle contractions and reverse esophageal peristalsis.

A common sign of GI disorders, vomiting also occurs with fluid and electrolyte imbalances; infections; and metabolic, endocrine, labyrinthine, central nervous system (CNS), and cardiac disorders. It can also result from drug therapy, surgery, and radiation.

Vomiting occurs normally during the first trimester of pregnancy, but its subsequent development may signal complications. It can also result from stress, anxiety, pain, alcohol intoxication, overeating, or ingestion of distasteful foods or liquids.

History and physical examination

Ask your patient to describe the onset, duration, and intensity of the vomiting. What started the vomiting? What makes it subside? If possible, collect, measure, and inspect the character of the vomitus. (See *Vomitus: Characteristics and causes*.) Explore associated complaints, particularly nausea, abdominal pain, anorexia and weight loss, changes in bowel habits or stools, excessive belching or flatus, or bloating or fullness.

EXAMINATION TIP

Vomitus: Characteristics and causes

When you collect a sample of the patient's vomitus, observe it carefully for clues to the underlying cause. Here's what this vomitus may indicate:

Bile-stained (greenish) vomitus
Obstruction below the pylorus, as from a duodenal lesion

Bloody vomitus
Upper GI bleeding, as from gastritis or peptic ulcer if bright red; if dark red, as from esophageal or gastric varices

Brown vomitus with a fecal odor
Intestinal obstruction or infarction

Burning, bitter-tasting vomitus
Excessive hydrochloric acid in gastric contents

Coffee-ground vomitus
Digested blood from slowly bleeding gastric or duodenal lesion

Undigested food
Overingestion or gastric outlet obstruction, as from gastric tumor or ulcer.

Obtain a medical history, noting GI, endocrine, and metabolic disorders; recent infections; and cancer, including chemotherapy or radiation therapy. Ask about current medication use and alcohol consumption. If the patient is a female of childbearing age, ask if she is or could be pregnant. Ask which contraceptive method she's using.

Inspect the abdomen for distention, and auscultate for bowel sounds and bruits. Palpate for rigidity and tenderness, and test for rebound tenderness. Next, palpate and percuss the liver for enlargement. Assess other body systems as appropriate.

During the examination, keep in mind that projectile vomiting not accompanied by nausea may indicate increased intracranial pressure, a life-threatening emergency. If this occurs in a patient with CNS injury, you should quickly check his vital signs. Be alert for widened pulse pressure or bradycardia.

Common medical causes

♦ ***Adrenal insufficiency.*** Common GI findings in the disorder include vomiting, nausea, anorexia, and diarrhea. Other findings include weakness, fatigue, weight loss, bronze skin, orthostatic hypotension, and weak, irregular pulse.

♦ ***Appendicitis.*** Vomiting and nausea may follow or accompany abdominal pain. Pain typically begins as vague epigastric or periumbilical discomfort and rapidly progresses to severe, stabbing pain in the right lower quadrant (McBurney's sign). Associated findings usually include abdominal rigidity and tenderness, anorexia, constipation or diarrhea, cutaneous hyperalgesia, fever, tachycardia, and malaise.

♦ ***Cholecystitis (acute).*** Nausea and mild vomiting commonly follow severe upper quadrant pain that may radiate to the back or shoulders. Associated findings include abdominal tenderness and, possibly, rigidity and distention, fever, or diaphoresis.

♦ ***Cholelithiasis.*** Nausea and vomiting accompany severe right-upper-quadrant or epigastric pain after ingestion of fatty foods. Other findings include abdominal tenderness and guarding, flatulence, belching, epigastric burning, pyrosis, tachycardia, and restlessness.

♦ ***Cirrhosis.*** Insidious early symptoms of cirrhosis typically include nausea and vomiting, anorexia, aching abdominal pain, and constipation or diarrhea. Later findings include jaundice, hepatomegaly, and abdominal distention.

♦ ***Electrolyte imbalances.*** Such disturbances as hyponatremia, hypernatremia, hypokalemia, and hypercalcemia frequently cause nausea and vomiting. Other effects may include arrhythmias, tremors, seizures, anorexia, malaise, or weakness.

♦ ***Food poisoning.*** Vomiting is a common finding of this condition, caused by preformed toxins produced by bacteria typically found in foods, such as *Bacillus cereus, Clostridium,* and *Staphylococcus.* Diarrhea and fever also usually occur in this self-limiting condition.

♦ ***Gastric cancer.*** This rare cancer may cause mild nausea, vomiting (possibly of mucus or blood), anorexia, upper abdominal discomfort, or chronic dyspepsia. Fatigue, weight loss, melena, and altered bowel habits are also common.

♦ ***Gastritis.*** Nausea and vomiting of mucus or blood are common, especially after ingestion of alcohol, aspirin, spicy foods, or caffeine. Epigastric pain, belching, or fever may occur.

♦ ***Gastroenteritis.*** This disorder causes nausea, vomiting (commonly of undigested food), diarrhea, or abdominal cramping. Fever, malaise, hyperactive bowel sounds, or abdominal pain and tenderness may also occur.

♦ ***Heart failure.*** Nausea and vomiting may occur, especially in right-sided heart failure. Associated findings include tachycardia, ventricular gallop, fatigue, dyspnea, crackles, peripheral edema, or jugular vein distention.

♦ ***Hepatitis.*** Vomiting commonly follows nausea as an early sign of viral hepatitis. Fatigue, myalgia, arthralgia, headache, photophobia, anorexia, pharyngitis, cough, or fever also occur early.

♦ ***Hyperemesis gravidarum.*** Unremitting nausea and vomiting that last beyond the first trimester characterize this disorder of pregnancy. Early in the disorder, vomitus contains undigested food, mucus, and small amounts of bile; later, it has a "coffee-ground" appearance. Associated findings include weight loss, headache, delirium, or thyroid dysfunction.

◆ ***Increased intracranial pressure (ICP).*** Projectile vomiting that isn't preceded by nausea is a sign of increased ICP. The patient may exhibit a decreased level of consciousness and Cushing's triad (bradycardia, hypertension, and respiratory pattern changes). He may also have headache, widened pulse pressure, impaired motor movement, vision disturbances, pupillary changes, or papilledema.

◆ ***Intestinal obstruction.*** Nausea and vomiting (bilious or fecal) frequently signal obstruction, especially of the upper small intestine. Abdominal pain is usually episodic and colicky but can become severe and steady. Constipation occurs early in large-intestine obstruction and late in small-intestine obstruction. Obstipation, however, may signal complete obstruction. Bowel sounds are typically high-pitched and hyperactive in partial obstruction; hypoactive or absent in complete obstruction. Abdominal distention and tenderness also occur, possibly with visible peristaltic waves or a palpable abdominal mass.

◆ ***Labyrinthitis.*** Nausea and vomiting commonly accompany this acute inner ear inflammation. Other findings include severe vertigo, progressive hearing loss, nystagmus or, possibly, otorrhea.

◆ ***Migraine headache.*** Prodromal symptoms include nausea and vomiting, fatigue, photophobia, light flashes, increased noise sensitivity or, possibly, partial vision loss or paresthesia.

◆ ***Motion sickness.*** Nausea and vomiting may be accompanied by headache, dizziness, fatigue, diaphoresis, or dyspnea.

◆ ***Pancreatitis (acute).*** Vomiting, usually preceded by nausea, is an early symptom of pancreatitis. Associated findings include steady, severe epigastric or left-upper-quadrant pain that may radiate to the back, abdominal tenderness and rigidity, hypoactive bowel sounds, or fever. Tachycardia, restlessness, hypotension, skin mottling, and cold, sweaty extremities may occur in severe cases.

◆ ***Peritonitis.*** Nausea and vomiting usually accompany acute abdominal pain in the area of inflammation. Other findings may include high fever with chills; tachycardia; hypoactive or absent bowel sounds; abdominal distention and tenderness; weakness; pale, cold skin; diaphoresis; hypotension; signs of dehydration; or shallow respirations.

◆ ***Preeclampsia.*** Nausea and vomiting are common in this disorder of pregnancy. Rapid weight gain, epigastric pain, generalized edema, elevated blood pressure, oliguria, severe frontal headache, or blurred or double vision may occur.

◆ ***Renal and urologic disorders.*** Cystitis, pyelonephritis, calculi, and other disorders of this system can cause vomiting. Accompanying findings reflect the specific disorder. Persistent nausea and vomiting are typical findings in patients with acute or worsening chronic renal failure.

Other causes

◆ ***Drugs.*** Drugs that commonly cause vomiting include antineoplastic agents, opiates, ferrous sulfate, levodopa, oral potassium, chloride replacements, estrogens, sulfasalazine, antibiotics, quinidine, or anesthetic agents, as well as overdoses of digoxin or theophylline.

◆ ***Radiation and surgery.*** Radiation therapy may cause nausea and vomiting if it disrupts the gastric mucosa. Postoperative nausea and vomiting are common, especially after abdominal surgery.

Special considerations

Draw blood to determine fluid, electrolyte, and acid-base balance. (Prolonged vomiting can cause dehydration, electrolyte imbalances, and metabolic alkalosis.) Have the patient breathe deeply to ease his nausea and help prevent further vomiting. Keep his room fresh and clean-smelling by rinsing and removing bedpans, urinals, and emesis basins promptly after use. Elevate his head or position him on his side to prevent aspiration of vomitus. Continuously monitor vital signs and intake and output (including vomitus and liquid stools). If necessary, administer I.V. fluids or have the patient sip clear liquids to maintain hydration.

Because pain can precipitate or intensify nausea and vomiting, administer pain medications promptly. If possible, give these by injection or suppository to prevent exacerbating associated nausea. If you administer antiemetics, be alert for abdominal distention and hypoactive bowel sounds, which may indicate gastric retention. If this occurs, insert a nasogastric tube.

Pediatric pointers

In a newborn, pyloric obstruction may cause projectile vomiting. Hirschsprung's disease may cause fecal vomiting. In an infant or toddler, intussusception may lead to vomiting of bile and fecal matter. Because an infant may aspirate vomitus as a result of immature cough and gag reflexes, lay him on his side or abdomen and clear vomitus immediately.

Geriatric pointers

Although elderly patients can develop several of the disorders mentioned earlier, always rule out intestinal ischemia first. It's especially common in this age group and has a high mortality rate.

VULVAR LESIONS

Vulvar cutaneous lumps, nodules, papules, vesicles, or ulcers may result from benign or malignant tumors, dystrophies, dermatoses, or infection. They can appear anywhere on the vulva and may go undetected until a gynecologic examination. Usually, however, the patient notices lesions because of associated symptoms, such as pruritus, local pain, dysuria, or dyspareunia.

History and physical examination

Ask the patient when she first noticed a vulvar lesion, and find out about associated features, such as swelling, pain, tenderness, itching, or discharge. Does she have lesions elsewhere on her body? Ask about signs of systemic illness, such as malaise, fever, or rash on other body areas. Is the patient sexually active? Could she have been exposed to a sexually transmitted disease (STD)?

In addition, examine the lesion, do a pelvic examination, and obtain cultures. (See *Recognizing common vulvar lesions.*)

Common medical causes

- ***Basal cell carcinoma.*** Occurring most commonly in postmenopausal women, this nodular tumor has a central ulcer and a raised, poorly rolled border. Typically asymptomatic, the tumor may occasionally cause pruritus, bleeding, discharge, and a burning sensation. Vulvar cancer should be suspected in patients with a history of squamous cell malignancy of the cervix or vagina.
- ***Benign cysts.*** *Epidermal inclusion cysts,* the most common vulvar cysts, appear primarily on the labia majora and are usually round and asymptomatic. Occasionally, they become erythematous and tender. *Bartholin's duct cysts* are usually unilateral, tense, nontender, and palpable. They appear on the posterior labia minora and may cause minor discomfort during intercourse or, when large, difficulty with intercourse or even walking. *Bartholin's abscess,* infection of a Bartholin's duct cyst, causes gradual pain and tenderness and possibly vulvar swelling, redness, and deformity.
- ***Benign vulvar tumors.*** Cystic or solid, tumors are usually asymptomatic.
- ***Chancroid.*** This rare STD causes painful vulvar lesions. Headache, malaise, fever to 102.2° F (39° C), and enlarged, tender inguinal lymph nodes may occur.
- ***Human papillomavirus (HPV) genital warts.*** This STD is the most common viral STD, occurring in 6% of women between ages 20 and 34. HPV

EXAMINATION TIP

Recognizing common vulvar lesions

Various disorders can cause vulvar lesions. For example, sexually transmitted diseases account for most vulvar lesions in premenopausal women; whereas vulvar tumors and cysts account for most lesions in women ages 50 to 70. The illustrations here help you recognize some of the most common lesions.

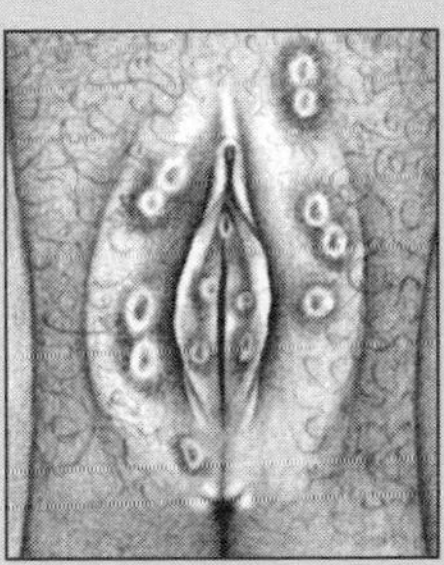

Primary genital herpes produces multiple ulcerated lesions surrounded by red halos.

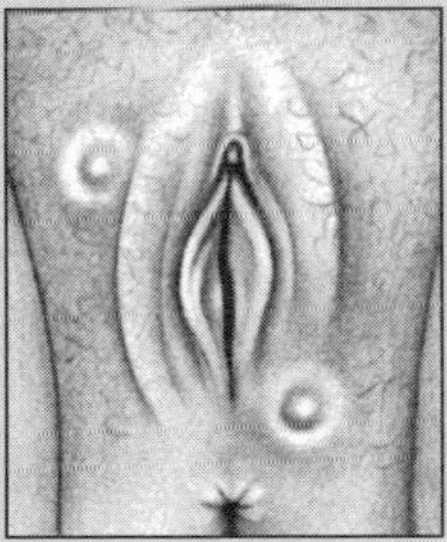

Primary syphilis produces chancres that appear as ulcerated lesions with raised borders.

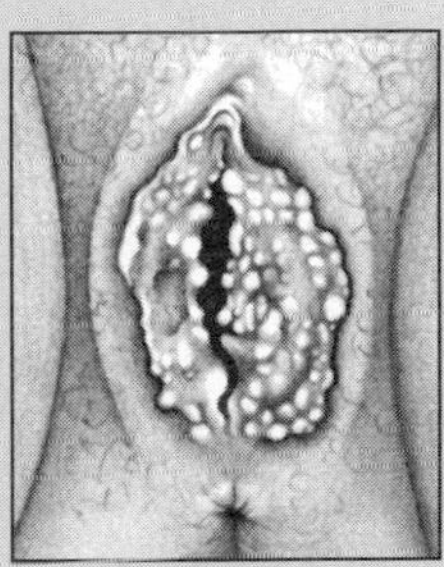

Squamous cell carcinoma can produce a large, granulomatous-appearing ulcer.

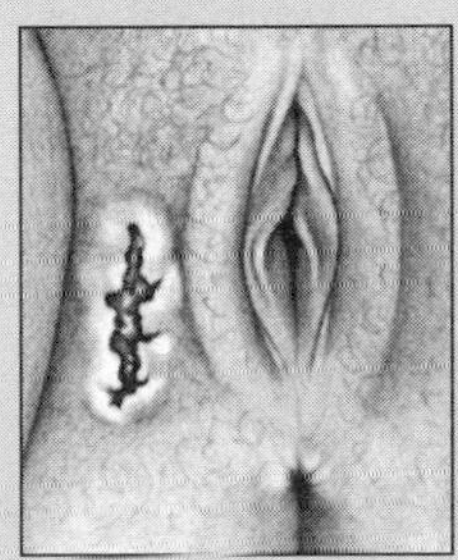

Basal cell carcinoma can produce an ulcerated lesion with raised, poorly rolled edges.

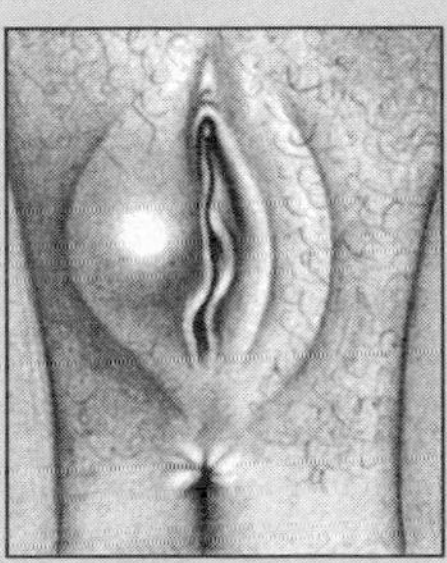

Epidermal inclusion cysts produce a round lump that usually appears on the labia majora.

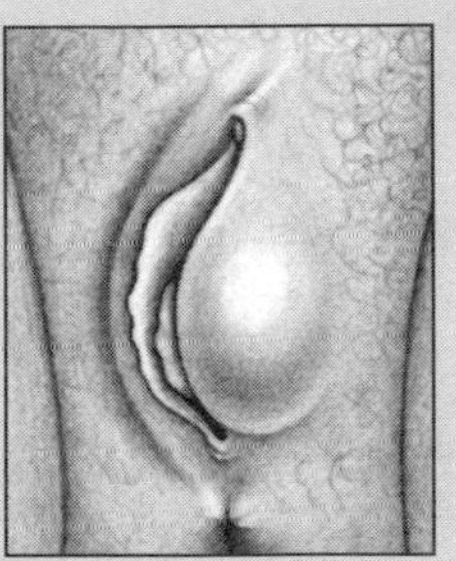

Bartholin's duct cysts produce a tense, nontender, palpable lump that usually appears on the labia majora.

causes painless warts on the vulva, vagina, and cervix. Warts start as tiny red or pink swellings that grow and become pedunculated. Multiple swellings with a cauliflower appearance are common. Other findings may include pruritus, erythema, or a profuse, mucopurulent vaginal discharge. Patients frequently complain of burning or paresthesia in the vaginal introitus.

♦ ***Gonorrhea.*** Vulvar lesions, usually confined to Bartholin's glands, may develop, along with pruritus, a burning sensation, pain, and a greenish yellow vaginal discharge, but most patients are asymptomatic. Other findings may include dysuria and urinary incontinence;

vaginal redness, swelling, bleeding, and engorgement; or severe pelvic or lower abdominal pain.

♦ ***Granuloma inguinale.*** Initially, a single painless macule or papule appears on the vulva, ulcerating into a raised, beefy red lesion with a granulated, friable border. Other painless and possibly foul-smelling lesions may occur on the labia, vagina, or cervix. These become infected and painful, and regional lymph nodes enlarge and may become tender. Fever, weight loss, or malaise may occur.

♦ ***Herpes simplex (genital).*** Fluid-filled vesicles appear on the cervix and, possibly, on the vulva, labia, perianal skin, vagina, or mouth. The vesicles, initially painless, may rupture and develop into extensive, shallow, painful ulcers, with redness and marked edema. Other findings may include tender inguinal lymph nodes, fever, malaise, or dysuria.

♦ ***Lymphogranuloma venereum.*** This bacterial infection commonly presents with a single, painless papule or ulcer on the posterior vulva that heals in a few days. Painful, swollen lymph nodes, usually unilateral, develop about 2 to 6 weeks later. Other findings may include fever, chills, headache, anorexia, myalgias, arthralgias, weight loss, or perineal edema.

♦ ***Paget's disease of the vulva.*** Eczematoid lesions are characterized by large, pale epidermal cells. In 20% of cases, it's associated with adenocarcinoma of the breast, vulva, or Bartholin's gland.

♦ ***Squamous cell carcinoma.*** Ninety percent of all vulvar cancers are of this type. *Invasive carcinoma* occurs primarily in postmenopausal women and may cause vulvar pruritus, pain, and a vulvar lump. As the tumor enlarges, it may encroach on the vagina, anus, or urethra, causing bleeding, discharge, or dysuria. *Carcinoma in situ,* most common in premenopausal women, produces a vulvar lesion that may be white or red, raised, well defined, moist, crusted, and isolated.

♦ ***Squamous cell hyperplasia.*** Formerly known as hyperplastic dystrophy, these vulvar lesions may be well delineated or poorly defined; localized or extensive; and red, brown, white, or both red and white. However, intense pruritus, possibly with vulvar pain, intense burning, and dyspareunia, is the cardinal symptom. In *lichen sclerosus,* a type of vulvar dystrophy, vulvar skin resembles parchment. Fissures may develop between clitoris and urethra or other vulvar areas.

♦ ***Syphilis.*** Chancres, the primary vulvar lesions of this STD, may appear on the vulva, vagina, or cervix 10 to 90 days after initial contact. Usually painless, they start as papules that then erode, with indurated, raised edges and clear bases. Condylomata lata, highly contagious secondary vulvar lesions, are raised, gray, flat-topped, and frequently ulcerated. Other findings may include a maculopapular, pustular, or nodular rash; headache; malaise; anorexia; weight loss; fever; nausea; vomiting; generalized lymphadenopathy; and a sore throat.

♦ ***Viral disease (systemic).*** Varicella, measles, and other systemic viral diseases may cause vulvar lesions.

Special considerations

As required, administer systemic antibiotics, antiviral agents, topical corticosteroids, topical testosterone, or an antipruritic agent.

Pediatric pointers

Vulvar lesions in children may result from congenital syphilis or gonorrhea. Evaluate for sexual abuse.

Geriatric pointers

Vulvar dystrophies and neoplasia increase in frequency with advancing age. All vulvar lesions must be considered malignant until proven otherwise. Also, many women remain sexually active well into their elder years and may come from a time when STDs weren't openly discussed. These patients should be questioned about sexual activities and educated about safer sex practices.

W XYZ

Weight gain, excessive

Weight gain occurs when ingested calories exceed body requirements for energy, causing increased adipose tissue storage. It can also occur when fluid retention causes edema. When weight gain results from overeating, emotional factors — most commonly anxiety, guilt, and depression — and social factors may be the primary causes.

Among the elderly, weight gain commonly reflects a sustained food intake in the presence of the normal, progressive fall in basal metabolic rate. In women, a progressive weight gain occurs with pregnancy, whereas periodic weight gain usually occurs with menstruation.

Weight gain, a primary symptom of many endocrine disorders, also occurs in conditions that limit activity, especially cardiovascular or pulmonary disorders. It can also result from drug therapy that increases appetite or causes fluid retention or from cardiovascular, hepatic, and renal disorders that cause edema.

History and physical examination

Determine your patient's previous patterns of weight gain and loss. Does he have a family history of obesity, thyroid disease, or diabetes mellitus? Assess his eating and activity patterns. Has his appetite increased? Does he exercise regularly or at all? Has his exercise decreased? Have his professional and personal responsibilities increased? If so, he's likely to be exercising less. Next, ask about associated symptoms. Has he experienced vision disturbances, hoarseness, paresthesia, or increased urination and thirst? Has he become impotent? If the patient is female, has she had menstrual irregularities or experienced weight gain during menstruation?

Form an impression of the patient's mental status. Is he anxious or depressed? Does he respond slowly? Is his memory poor? What medications is he currently using?

During your physical examination, measure skin-fold thickness to estimate fat reserves. (See *Evaluating nutritional status,* pages 612 and 613.) Note fat distribution and the presence of localized or generalized edema and overall nutritional status. Inspect for other abnormalities, such as abnormal body hair distribution or hair loss and dry skin. Take and record the patient's vital signs.

Common medical causes

♦ ***Acromegaly.*** This disorder causes moderate weight gain. Other findings include coarsened facial features, prognathism, enlarged hands and feet, increased sweating, oily skin, deep voice, back and joint pain, lethargy, sleepiness, and heat intolerance. Occasionally, hirsutism may occur.

♦ ***Diabetes mellitus.*** The increased appetite associated with this disorder may lead to weight gain, although weight loss sometimes occurs instead. Other findings may include fatigue, polydipsia, polyuria, nocturia, weakness, polyphagia, or somnolence.

♦ ***Hypercortisolism.*** Excessive weight gain, usually over the trunk and the back of the neck (buffalo hump), characteristically occurs in this disorder. Other cushingoid features include slender extremities, moon face, weakness, purple striae, emotional lability, and increased susceptibility to infection. Gynecomastia may occur in men; hirsutism, acne, and menstrual irregularities may occur in women.

♦ ***Hyperinsulinism.*** This disorder increases appetite, leading to weight gain. Emotional lability, indigestion, weakness, diaphoresis, tachycardia, vision disturbances, or syncope also occur.

♦ ***Hypogonadism.*** Weight gain is common in this disorder. *Prepubertal hypogonadism* causes eunuchoid body proportions with relatively sparse facial and body hair and a high-pitched voice. *Postpubertal hypogonadism* causes loss of libido, impotence, and infertility.

♦ ***Hypothalamic dysfunction.*** Such conditions as Laurence-Moon syndrome cause a voracious appetite with subsequent weight gain and altered body temperature and sleep rhythms.

♦ ***Hypothyroidism.*** Weight gain occurs despite anorexia. Related signs and symptoms include fatigue; cold intolerance; constipation; menorrhagia; slowed intellectual and motor activity; dry, pale, cool skin; dry, sparse hair; and thick, brittle nails. Myalgia, hoarseness, hypoactive deep tendon reflexes, bradycardia, and abdominal distention may occur. Eventually, periorbital edema develops, and the face assumes a dull expression.

♦ ***Menopause.*** Menopause is associated with a 10- to 20-pound weight gain as loss of endogenous estrogen causes a decline in metabolic rate.

EXAMINATION TIP

Evaluating nutritional status

If your patient has excessive weight loss or gain, you can help assess his nutritional status by measuring his skin-fold thickness and midarm circumference and by calculating his midarm muscle circumference. Skin-fold measurements reflect adipose tissue mass (subcutaneous fat accounts for about 50% of the body's adipose tissue.) Midarm measurements reflect both skeletal muscle and adipose tissue mass.

Use the steps described here to gather these measurements. Then express them as a percentage of standard by using this formula:

$$\frac{\text{Actual measurement}}{\text{Standard measurement}} \times 100 = \_\_\_\_\_$$

Standard anthropometric measurements vary according to the patient's age and sex and can be found in a chart of normal anthropometric values. The abridged chart below lists standard arm measurements for adults.

TEST	STANDARD	
Triceps skin fold	Men Women	12.5 mm 16.5 mm
Midarm circumference	Men Women	29.3 mm 28.5 mm
Midarm muscle circumference	Men Women	25.3 mm 23.2 mm

A triceps or subscapular skin-fold measurement below 60% of the standard value indicates severe depletion of fat reserves; measurement between 60% and 90%, moderate to mild depletion; above 90%, significant fat reserves.

A midarm circumference below 90% of the standard value indicates caloric deprivation; above 90%, adequate or ample muscle and fat.

A midarm muscle circumference below 90% indicates protein depletion; above 90%, adequate or ample protein reserves.

MEASURING THE TRICEPS SKIN FOLD

Locate the midpoint of the patient's upper arm, using a nonstretch tape measure. Mark the midpoint with a felt-tip pen. Then grasp the skin with your thumb and forefinger about 1 cm above the midpoint. Place the calipers at the midpoint and squeeze them for about 3 seconds. Record the measurement registered on the handle gauge to the nearest 0.5 mm. Take two more readings and average all three to compensate for any measurement error.

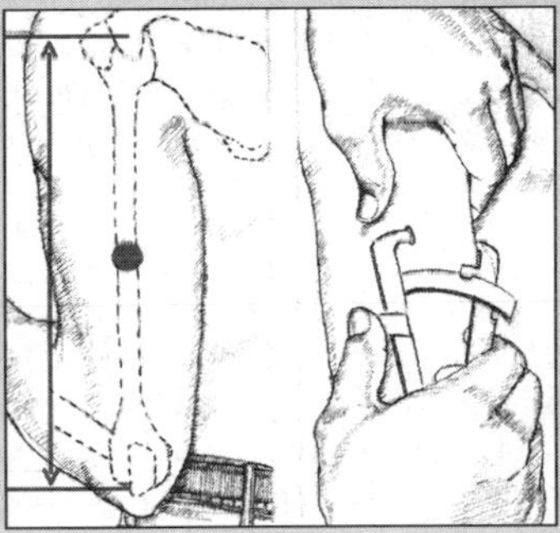

MEASURING THE SUBSCAPULAR SKIN FOLD

Use your thumb and forefinger to grasp the skin just below the angle of the scapula, in line with the natural cleavage of the skin. Apply the calipers and proceed as you would when measuring the triceps skin fold. Subscapular and triceps skin-fold measurements are reliable measurements of fat loss or gain during hospitalization.

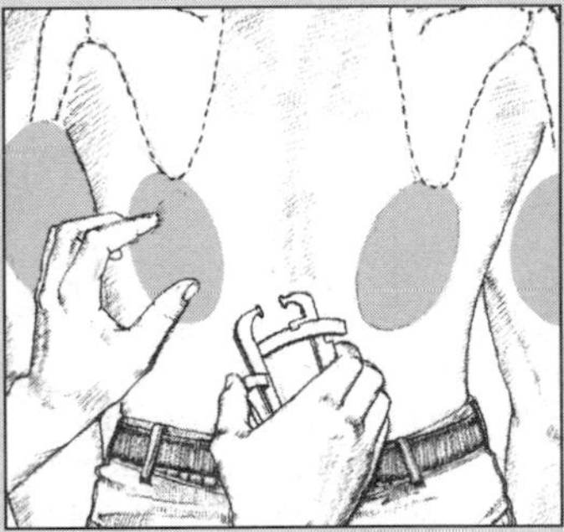

MEASURING MIDARM CIRCUMFERENCE

Return to the midpoint you marked on the patient's upper arm. Then use a tape measure to determine the arm circumference at this point. This measurement reflects skeletal muscle and adipose tissue mass and helps evaluate protein and caloric reserves. To calculate midarm muscle circumference, multiply the triceps skin-fold thickness (in centimeters) by 3.143, and subtract this figure from the midarm circumference. Midarm muscle circumference reflects muscle mass alone, providing a more sensitive index of protein reserves.

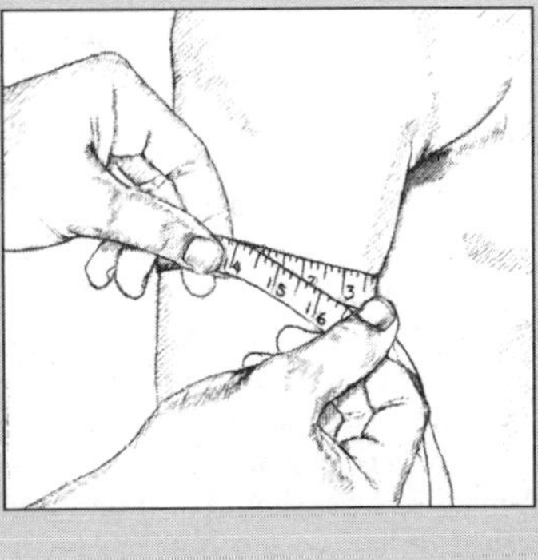

♦ ***Nephrotic syndrome.*** In this syndrome, weight gain results from edema. In severe cases, anasarca develops — increasing body weight up to 50%. Related effects include abdominal distention, orthostatic hypotension, and lethargy.

♦ ***Pancreatic islet cell tumor.*** This disorder causes excessive hunger, which leads to weight gain. Other findings include emotional lability, weakness, malaise, fatigue, restlessness, diaphoresis, palpitations, tachycardia, visual disturbances, or syncope.

♦ ***Preeclampsia.*** In this disorder, rapid weight gain (exceeding the normal weight gain of pregnancy) may accompany nausea and vomiting, epigastric pain, elevated blood pressure, or blurred or double vision.

♦ ***Sheehan's syndrome.*** Most common in women who experience severe obstetric hemorrhage, this syndrome may cause weight gain.

Other causes

♦ ***Drugs.*** Corticosteroids, phenothiazines, and tricyclic antidepressants cause weight gain from fluid retention and increased appetite. Other drugs that can lead to weight gain include oral contraceptives, which cause fluid retention; cyproheptadine, which increases appetite; and lithium, which can induce hypothyroidism.

Special considerations

Psychological counseling may be necessary for patients with weight gain, particularly when it results from emotional problems or when uneven weight distribution alters body image. If the patient is obese or has a cardiopulmonary disorder, any exercise should be monitored closely. Further study to rule out possible secondary causes should include serum thyroid-stimulating hormone determination and dexamethasone suppression testing. Laboratory tests of all patients ideally include cardiac risk factors: serum cholesterol, triglycerides, and glucose.

Pediatric pointers

Weight gain in children can result from endocrine disorders, such as hypercortisolism. Other causes include inactivity caused by Prader-Willi syndrome, Werdnig-Hoffmann disease, Down syndrome, late stages of muscular dystrophy, and severe cerebral palsy.

Nonpathologic causes include poor eating habits, sedentary recreation, and emotional problems, especially among adolescents. Regardless of the cause, discourage fad diets and provide a balanced weight loss program. The incidence of obesity is increasing among children.

Geriatric pointers

Desired weights (associated with lowest mortality rates) increase with age.

WEIGHT LOSS, EXCESSIVE

Weight loss can reflect decreased food intake, decreased food absorption, increased metabolic requirements, or a combination of the three. Its causes include endocrine, neoplastic, GI, and psychiatric disorders; nutritional deficiencies; infections; and neurologic lesions that cause paralysis and dysphagia. However, weight loss may accompany conditions that prevent sufficient food intake, such as painful oral lesions, ill-fitting dentures, or loss of teeth. It may be the metabolic sequela of poverty, fad diets, excessive exercise, or certain drugs.

Weight loss may occur as a late sign in such chronic diseases as heart failure and renal disease. In these diseases, however, it's the result of anorexia (see "Anorexia," page 36).

History and physical examination

Begin with a thorough diet history because weight loss almost always is caused by inadequate caloric intake. If the patient hasn't been eating properly, try to determine why. Ask him about previous weight and if the recent loss was intentional. Be alert to lifestyle or occupational changes that may be a source of anxiety or depression. For example, has he gotten separated or divorced? Has he recently changed jobs?

Inquire about recent or long-standing bowel habits, such as diarrhea or bulky, floating stools. Has the patient had nausea, vomiting, or abdominal pain, which may indicate a GI disorder? Has he had excessive thirst, excessive urination, or heat intolerance, which may signal an endocrine disorder? Take a careful drug history, noting especially use of diet pills or laxatives.

Carefully check the patient's height and weight, and ask about his previous weight. Take his vital signs and note his general appearance: Is he well nourished? Do his clothes fit? Is muscle wasting evident? Ask about exact weight changes (with approximate dates).

Next, examine the patient's skin for turgor and abnormal pigmentation, especially around the joints. Does he have pallor or jaundice? Examine his mouth, including the condition of his teeth or dentures. Look for signs of infection or irritation on the roof of the mouth, and note hyperpigmentation of the buccal mucosa. Also check the patient's eyes for exophthalmos and his neck for swelling; evaluate his lungs for adventitious sounds. Inspect his abdomen for signs of wasting, and palpate for masses, tenderness, and an enlarged liver.

Conventional laboratory and radiologic investigations, such as complete blood count, urinalysis, chest X-ray, and upper GI series, usually reveal the cause. Almost all physical causes are clinically evident during the initial evaluation. Cancer, GI disorders, and depression are the most common pathologic causes.

Common medical causes

♦ ***Anorexia nervosa.*** This psychogenic disorder, most common in young women, is characterized by a severe, self-imposed weight loss ranging from 10% to 50% of premorbid weight, which typically was normal or not more than 5 lb (2.3 kg) over ideal weight. Related findings include skeletal muscle atrophy, loss of fatty tissue, hypotension, constipation, dental caries, susceptibility to infection, blotchy or sallow skin, cold intolerance, hairiness on the face and body, dryness or loss of scalp hair, and amenorrhea. The patient usually demonstrates restless activity and vigor and may also have a morbid fear of becoming fat. Self-induced vomiting or self-administration of laxatives or diuretics may lead to dehydration or to metabolic alkalosis or acidosis.

♦ ***AIDS.*** Patients may present with weight loss or fever, dyspnea, diarrhea, weakness, or lassitude. Examination will reveal lymph node enlargement, wasting and malnutrition, oral thrush, or rashes. Other findings reflect the type of opportunistic infection involved.

♦ ***Cancer.*** Weight loss is frequently a sign of cancer. Other findings reflect the type, location, and stage of the tumor. They may include fatigue, pain, nausea, vomiting, anorexia, abnormal bleeding, or a palpable mass.

♦ ***Crohn's disease.*** Weight loss occurs with chronic cramping, abdominal pain, and anorexia. Other signs and symptoms may include diarrhea (possibly bloody) or constipation, nausea, fever, tachycardia, abdominal tenderness and guarding, hyperactive bowel sounds, abdominal distention, or pain. Perianal lesions or a palpable mass in the right or left lower quadrant may also be present.

♦ ***Cryptosporidiosis.*** Weight loss may signal this opportunistic protozoan infection. Other findings include profuse watery diarrhea, abdominal cramping, flatulence, anorexia, malaise, fever, nausea, vomiting, or myalgia.

♦ ***Depression.*** Weight loss may occur in the severely depressed patient, along with insomnia or hypersomnia, anorexia, apathy, fatigue, or feelings of worthlessness. Indecisiveness, incoherence, or suicidal thoughts or behavior may also occur.

♦ ***Diabetes mellitus.*** Weight loss may occur, despite increased appetite. Other findings include polydipsia, weakness, fatigue, or polyuria with nocturia.

♦ ***Esophagitis.*** Painful inflammation of the esophagus leads to temporary avoidance of eating and consequent weight loss. Intense pain in the mouth and anterior chest occurs, along with hypersalivation, dysphagia, tachypnea, or hematemesis. If a stricture develops, dysphagia and weight loss will recur.

♦ ***Gastroenteritis.*** Malabsorption and dehydration cause weight loss in this disorder. The loss may be sudden in acute viral infections or reactions or gradual in parasitic infection. Other findings include poor skin turgor, dry mucous membranes, tachycardia, hypotension, diarrhea, abdominal pain and tenderness, hyperactive bowel sounds, nausea, vomiting, fever, or malaise.

♦ ***Leukemia.*** *Acute leukemia* causes progressive weight loss accompanied by severe prostration; high fever; swollen, bleeding gums; and bleeding tendencies. Dyspnea, tachycardia, palpitations, or abdominal or bone pain may occur. As the disease progresses, neurologic symptoms may eventually develop.

Chronic leukemia, which occurs insidiously in adults, causes progressive weight loss with malaise, fatigue, pallor, enlarged spleen, bleeding tendencies, anemia, skin eruptions, anorexia, and fever.

♦ ***Lymphoma.*** *Hodgkin's disease* and *malignant lymphoma* cause gradual weight loss. Associated findings include fever, fatigue, night sweats, malaise, hepatosplenomegaly, or lymphadenopathy. Scaly rashes and pruritus may develop.

♦ ***Pulmonary tuberculosis.*** This disorder causes gradual weight loss, along with fatigue, weakness, anorexia, night sweats, and low-grade fever. Other clinical effects include a cough with bloody or mucopurulent sputum, dyspnea, and pleuritic chest pain. Examination may reveal dullness upon percussion, crackles after coughing, increased tactile fremitus, or amphoric breath sounds.

♦ ***Stomatitis.*** Inflammation of the oral mucosa (usually red, swollen, and ulcerated) causes weight loss due to decreased eating. Associated findings may include fever, increased salivation, malaise, mouth pain, anorexia, or swollen, bleeding gums.

♦ ***Thyrotoxicosis.*** Increased metabolism causes weight loss. Other characteristic signs and symptoms include nervousness, heat intolerance, diarrhea, increased appetite, palpitations, tachycardia, diaphoresis, fine tremor, or possibly an enlarged thyroid or exophthalmos. A ventricular or atrial gallop may be heard.

Other causes

♦ ***Drugs.*** Amphetamines and inappropriate dosage of thyroid preparations commonly lead to weight loss. Laxative abuse may cause a malabsorptive state that leads to weight loss. Chemotherapeutic agents cause stomatitis and vomiting, which, when severe, causes weight loss.

Special considerations

Refer your patient for psychological counseling if weight loss negatively affects his body image. If the patient has a chronic disease, administer hyperalimentation or tube feedings to maintain nutrition and to prevent edema, poor healing, and muscle wasting. Take daily calorie counts and weigh him weekly. Consult a dietitian, if necessary.

Pediatric pointers

In infants, weight loss may be caused by failure-to-thrive syndrome. In children, severe weight loss may be the first indication of diabetes mellitus. Chronic, gradual weight loss occurs in children with *marasmus,* nonedematous protein-calorie malnutrition.

Weight loss may also occur as a result of child abuse or neglect, infections causing high fevers, GI disorders causing vomiting and diarrhea, or celiac disease.

LESS COMMON SIGNS AND SYMPTOMS

SELECTED REFERENCES

INDEX

LESS COMMON SIGNS AND SYMPTOMS

This appendix supplements the main text of *Handbook of Signs & Symptoms,* Second Edition, which provides detailed coverage of about 250 signs and symptoms that are familiar, diagnostically significant, or indicative of an emergency. This appendix, in contrast, provides the definition and common causes of about 270 less familiar, accessory, or nonspecific signs and symptoms. For elicited signs, such as Chaddock's reflex, it also includes the technique for evoking the patient's response.

This appendix also covers selected pediatric signs, such as low-set ears and Allis' sign; psychiatric symptoms, such as delusions and hallucinations; and nail and tongue signs, such as nail plate hypertrophy and tongue discoloration.

A

Aaron's sign Pain in the chest or abdominal (precordial or epigastric) area that's elicited by applying gentle but steadily increasing pressure over McBurney's point. A positive sign indicates appendicitis.

Abadie's sign Spasm of the levator muscle of the upper eyelid. This sign may be slight or pronounced and may affect one eye or both eyes. It reflects an exophthalmic goiter in Graves' disease.

ALLIS' SIGN

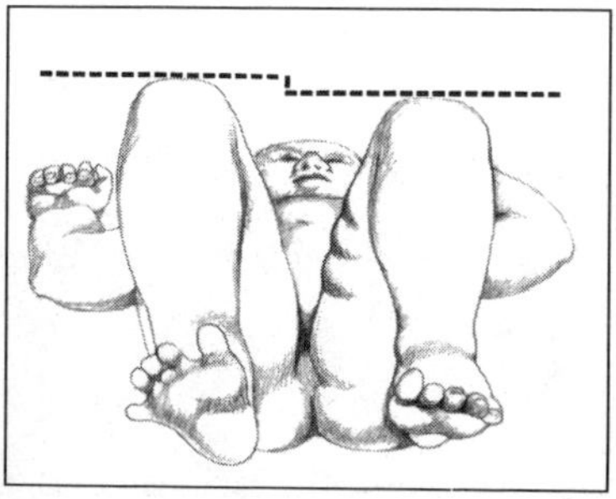

adipsia Abnormal absence of thirst. This sign commonly occurs in hypothalamic injury or tumor, head injury, bronchial tumor, or cirrhosis.

agnosia Inability to recognize and interpret sensory stimuli, even though the principal sensation of the stimulus is known. *Auditory agnosia* is the inability to recognize familiar sounds. *Astereognosis,* or *tactile agnosia,* is the inability to recognize objects by touch or feel. *Anosmia* is the inability to recognize familiar smells; *gustatory agnosia,* familiar tastes. *Visual agnosia* is the inability to recognize familiar objects by sight. *Autotopagnosia* is the inability to recognize body parts. *Anosognosia* is the denial or lack of awareness of a disease or defect (especially paralysis).

Agnosias stem from lesions that affect the association areas of the parietal sensory cortex. They're common sequelae of cerebrovascular accidents.

agraphia Inability to express thoughts in writing. *Aphasic agraphia* is associated with spelling and grammatical errors, whereas *constructional agraphia* refers to the reversal or incorrect ordering of correctly spelled words. *Apraxic agraphia* refers to the inability to form letters in the absence of significant motor impairment.

Agraphia commonly results from a cerebrovascular accident.

Allis' sign *In an adult:* relaxation of the fascia lata between the iliac crest and greater trochanter caused by a fracture of the neck of the femur. To detect this sign, place a finger over the area between the iliac crest and greater trochanter and press firmly; if your finger sinks deeply into this area, you have detected Allis' sign.

In an infant: unequal leg lengths caused by hip dislocation. To detect this sign, place the infant on his back with his pelvis flat. Then flex both legs at the knee and hip with the feet even. Next, compare the height of the knees. If they differ, suspect hip dislocation in the shorter leg.

ambivalence Simultaneous existence of conflicting feelings about a person, idea, or object (such as love and hate). It causes uncertainty or indecisiveness about which course to follow. Severe, debilitating ambivalence can occur in schizophrenia.

Amoss' sign A sparing maneuver to avoid pain on flexion of the spine. To detect this sign, ask the patient to rise from a supine to a sitting position. If he supports himself by placing his hands far behind him on the examining table, the sign is present.

anesthesia Absence of cutaneous sensations of touch, temperature, and pain. This sensory loss may be partial or total, unilateral or bilateral. To detect anesthesia, ask the patient to close his eyes. Then touch him and ask him to specify the location. If the patient's verbal skills are immature or poor, watch for movement or changes in facial expression in response to your touch.

anisocoria A difference of 0.5 to 2 mm in pupil size. Anisocoria occurs normally in about 2% of people, in whom the pupillary inequality remains constant despite changes in light. However, if anisocoria results from fixed dilation or constriction of one pupil, or slowed or impaired constriction of one pupil in response to light, it may indicate neurologic disease. Determining whether the abnormal pupil is dilated or constricted aids diagnosis.

ANISCORIA

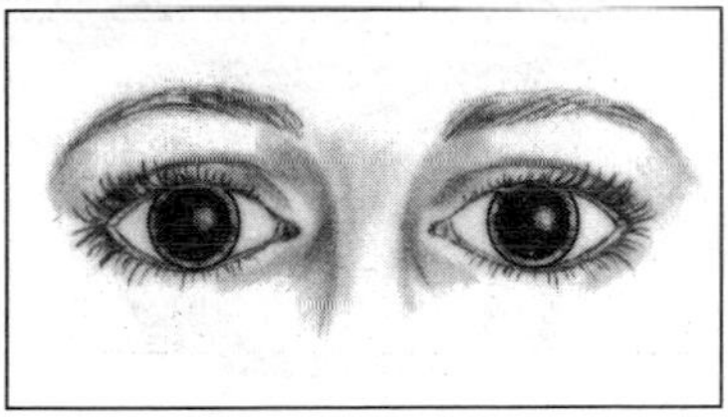

apathy Absence or suppression of emotion or interest in the external environment and personal affairs. This indifference can result from many disorders, chiefly neurologic, psychological, respiratory, or renal — as well as from alcohol or drug use or abuse. It's associated with many chronic disorders that cause personality changes and depression. Apathy may be an early indicator of a severe disorder such as a brain tumor.

aphonia Inability to produce speech sounds. This sign may result from overuse of the vocal cords, disorders of the larynx or laryngeal nerves, psychological disorders, or muscle spasm.

Argyll Robertson pupil A small, irregular pupil that constricts normally in accommodation for near vision, but poorly or not at all in response to light. Response to mydriatic drugs is poor or absent. This condition may be unilateral, bilateral, or asymmetrical. It most commonly results from chronic syphilitic meningitis or other forms of late syphilis.

arthralgia Joint pain. This symptom may have no pathologic importance or may reflect such disorders as arthritis or systemic lupus erythematosus.

asthenocoria Slow dilation or constriction of the pupils in response to light changes. Photophobia may be present if constriction occurs slowly. Asthenocoria occurs in adrenal insufficiency. It's also known as Arroyo's sign.

asynergy Impaired coordination of muscles or organs that normally function harmoniously. This extrapyramidal

BEAU'S LINES

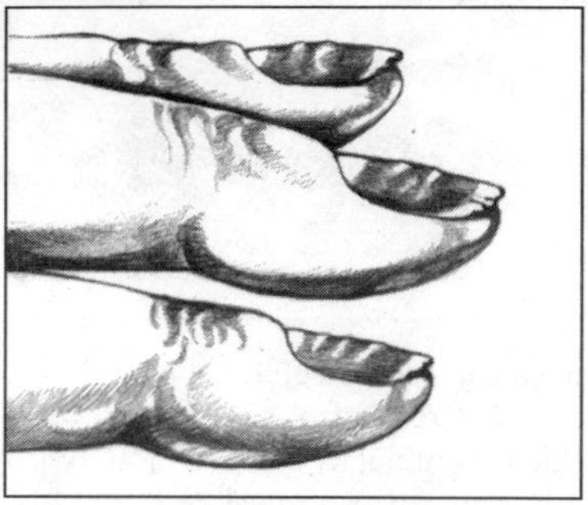

symptom stems from disorders of the basal ganglia and cerebellum.

atrophy Shrinkage or wasting away of a tissue or organ due to a reduction in the size or number of its cells. Its etiology may be physiologic—as in ovary, brain, or skin atrophy—or pathologic, as is commonly associated with neurologic disorders or spleen, liver, or thyroid abnormalities. This symptom is usually observed by means of inspection and palpation.

attention span decrease Inability to focus selectively on a task while ignoring extraneous stimuli. Anxiety, emotional upset, or dysfunction of the central nervous system may decrease the attention span.

autistic behavior Exaggerated self-centered behavior marked by a lack of responsiveness to other people. It's characterized by highly personalized speech and actions that aren't meaningful to an observer. For example, the patient may rock his body or repeatedly bang his head against the floor or wall. Autistic behavior may occur in schizophrenic children and adults.

Ballance's sign A fixed mass or area of dullness found by palpation and percussion of the left upper quadrant of the abdomen. It may indicate subcapsular or extracapsular hematoma after splenic rupture.

Ballet's sign Ophthalmoplegia, or paralysis of the external ocular muscles. The patient can't control voluntary eye movement but has normal reflexive movement and pupillary light reflexes. This sign is an indicator of thyrotoxicosis.

Bárány's symptom Warm water irrigation of the ear triggers rotary nystagmus toward the irrigated side; cold water irrigation, away from the irrigated side. Absence of this symptom indicates labyrinth dysfunction.

Barlow's sign An indicator of congenital dislocation of the hip, detected during the first 6 weeks of life. To elicit this sign, place the infant supine with the hips flexed 90 degrees and the knees fully flexed. Place your palm over the infant's knee, your thumb in the femoral triangle opposite the lesser trochanter, and your index finger over the greater trochanter. Bring the hip into midabduction while gently exerting posterior and lateral pressure with your thumb, and posterior and medial pressure with your palm. If you detect a click of the femoral head as it dislocates across the posterior lip of the acetabular socket, you have elicited this sign.

Barré's pyramidal sign Inability to hold the lower legs still with the knees flexed. To detect this sign, place the patient prone and flex his knees 90 degrees. Then ask him to hold his lower legs still. If he can't maintain this position, you have observed this sign of pyramidal tract disease.

Barré's sign Delayed contraction of the iris, seen in mental deterioration.

Beau's lines Transverse white linear depressions on the fingernails. These lines may develop after any severe illness or toxic reaction. Other common causes include malnutrition, nail bed trauma, and coronary artery occlusion.

Beevor's sign Upward movement of the umbilicus during contraction of the abdominal muscles; indicates paralysis of the lower recti abdominis muscles associated with lesions at T10. To detect this sign, position the patient supine and ask him to sit up.

Bell's sign Reflexive upward and outward deviation of the eyes that occurs when the patient with Bell's palsy attempts to close his eyes. It occurs on the affected side and indicates that the defect is supranuclear. Also known as Bell's phenomenon.

Bezold's sign Swelling and tenderness of the mastoid area. Resulting from formation of an abscess beneath the sternocleidomastoid muscle, Bezold's sign indicates mastoiditis.

Bitot's spots Triangular white or foamy gray spots, varying from a few bubbles to a frothy white coating. Appearing on the conjunctiva at the lateral margin of the cornea, they're associated with vitamin A deficiency.

blepharoclonus Excessive blinking of the eyes. This extrapyramidal sign occurs with disorders of the basal ganglia and cerebellum.

blocking A cognitive disturbance resulting in the interruption of a stream of speech or thought. It usually occurs in midsentence or before completion of a thought. Generally, the patient can't explain the interruption. Blocking may occur in normal individuals but most commonly occurs in schizophrenics.

Bonnet's sign Pain on adduction of the thigh, occurs in sciatica.

Bozzolo's sign Pulsation of arteries in the nasal mucous membrane, seen occasionally with thoracic aortic aneurysms. To detect this sign, examine both nostrils, using a speculum and light.

bradykinesia Slowness of all voluntary movement and speech, believed to be caused when reduced level of dopamine to neurons in the brain stem inhibits normal function in the central nervous system. Bradykinesia is commonly associated with parkinsonism, extrapyramidal or cerebellar disorders, or the use of certain drugs. Patients displaying bradykinesia are usually over age 50, but it may also occur in children who have suffered hypoxic accidents. Associated findings include tremor and muscle rigidity.

Braunwald sign Occurrence of a weak, rather than strong, pulse immediately after a premature ventricular contraction (PVC). To detect this sign, watch for a PVC during cardiac monitoring and check the quality of the pulse after it. Braunwald sign may reflect idiopathic hypertrophic subaortic stenosis.

breath sounds, absent or decreased Diminished loudness of breath sounds — or their absence — detected by auscultation. This may reflect reduced airflow to a lung segment caused by a tumor,

BEZOLD'S SIGN

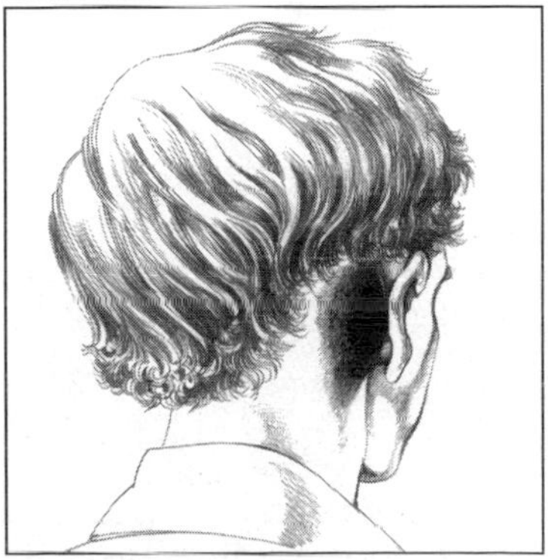

foreign body, mucous plug, or mucosal edema. It may also reflect hyperinflation of the lungs in emphysema or an asthma attack. Alternatively, it may indicate air or fluid in the pleural cavity from a pneumothorax, hemothorax, pleural effusion, atelectasis, or empyema. In an obese or extremely muscular patient, breath sounds may be diminished or inaudible because of increased thickness of the chest wall.

Broadbent's inverted sign Pulsations in the left posterolateral chest wall during ventricular systole. To detect this sign, palpate the patient's chest with your fingers and palm over areas of visible pulsation while auscultating for ventricular systole. When you feel pulsations, note their rate, rhythm, and intensity. This sign may indicate gross dilatation of the left atrium.

Broadbent's sign Visible retraction of the left posterior chest wall near the 11th and 12th ribs, occurring during systole. To detect this sign, inspect the chest wall while standing at the patient's right side. Position a strong light so that it casts rays tangential to the skin. While auscultating the heart, watch for retraction of the skin and muscles and determine its timing in the cardiac cycle. Broadbent's sign may occur in extensive adhesive pericarditis.

CHADDOCK'S TOE SIGN

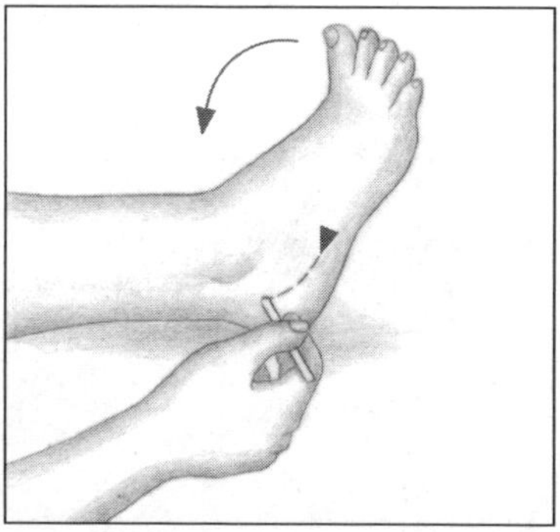

Catatonia Marked inhibition or excitation of motor behavior, occurring in psychotic disorders. *Catatonic stupor* refers to extreme inhibition of spontaneous activity or movement; *catatonic excitement,* to extreme psychomotor agitation.

Chaddock's sign *Chaddock's toe sign:* extension (dorsiflexion) of the great toe and fanning of the other toes. To elicit this sign, firmly stroke the side of the patient's foot just distal to the lateral malleolus. A positive sign indicates pyramidal tract disorders.

Chaddock's wrist sign: flexion of the wrist and extension of the fingers. To elicit this sign, stroke the ulnar surface of the patient's forearm near the wrist. A positive sign occurs on the affected side in hemiplegia. Although Chaddock's sign signals pathology in children and adults, it's a normal finding in infants up to age 7 months.

cherry red spot Appearance of the choroid as a red circular area surrounded by an abnormal gray-white retina when viewed through the fovea centralis of the eye with an ophthalmoscope. A cherry red spot suggests infantile cerebral sphingolipidosis; for example, it's detected in more than 90% of patients with Tay-Sachs disease.

circumstantiality Speech in which the main point is obscured by minute detail. Although the speaker may recognize his main point and return to it after many digressions, the listener may fail to recognize it. Circumstantiality commonly occurs in compulsive disorders, organic brain disorders, and schizophrenia.

Claude's hyperkinesis sign Increased reflex activity of paretic muscles, elicited by painful stimuli.

clavicular sign Swelling, puffiness, or edema at the medial third of the right clavicle, most common in congenital syphilis.

Cleeman's sign Slight linear depression or wrinkling of the skin superior to the patella. It usually indicates a femoral fracture with overriding bone fragments.

clenched fist sign The patient's placement of a clenched fist against his chest. This gesture may be performed by patients with angina pectoris when they're asked to indicate the location of their pain. The patient's gesture conveys the constricting, oppressive quality of substernal pain.

clicks Brief, high-frequency heart sounds auscultated during systole or diastole. *Ejection clicks* occur soon after the first heart sound. Presumably, they result from sudden distention of a dilated pulmonary artery or the aorta, or from forceful opening of the pulmonic or aortic valves. Associated with increased pulmonary resistance and hypertension, they usually occur with septal defects or patent ductus arteriosus. To best detect ejection clicks, have the patient sit upright or lie down, then auscultate the heart with the diaphragm of the stethoscope.

Systolic clicks occur most commonly in mid-to-late systole. They're characteristic of mitral valve prolapse. A click is heard most distinctly at or medial to the heart's apex, but it may also be heard at the lower left sternal border. Clicks are best heard using the diaphragm of the stethoscope.

clonus Abnormal response of a muscle to stretching. It's a sign of damage to nerve fibers that carry impulses from the motor cortex, usually to a muscle that responds to stretching by contracting once and then relaxing. In clonus, stretching sets off a series of contractions of the muscle or muscles in rapid succession. Clonuslike, or clonic, muscle contractions are also a feature of seizures in grand mal epilepsy.

Codman's sign Pain resulting from rupture of the supraspinatus tendon. To elicit this sign, have the patient relax his arm on the affected side while you abduct it. If the patient reports no pain until you remove your support and the deltoid muscle contracts, you have detected Codman's sign.

cognitive dysfunction Inability to perceive, organize, and interpret sensory stimuli, and to think and solve problems. It may arise from various causes, including central nervous system disturbances, extrapyramidal conditions, systemic illness, endocrine diseases, deficiency states, or from an unknown etiology, as in chronic fatigue syndrome.

Comolli's sign Triangular swelling over the scapula that matches its shape. This sign indicates scapular fracture.

complementary opposition sign Increased effort in lifting a paretic leg, demonstrated in the opposite leg. To elicit this sign, position the patient supine and place your hand under the heel of the unaffected leg. Then ask the patient to lift the paretic leg. If his effort produces marked downward pressure on your hand, you've detected this sign. Also known as Grasset-Gaussel-Hoover sign.

compulsion Stereotyped, repetitive behavior in which the individual recognizes the irrationality of his actions but can't stop them. An example is constant hand washing. Compulsion occurs in obsessive-compulsive disorders and occasionally in schizophrenia.

confabulation Fabrication to cover gaps in memory. Confabulation is most commonly seen in alcoholism or Korsakoff's syndrome.

conjunctival paleness Lack of color in the tissues inside the eyelid. Although the conjunctiva is a transparent mucous membrane, the portion lining the eyelids normally appears pink or red because it overlies the vasculature of the inner lid. Pale conjunctiva indicates anemia. To detect this sign, separate the eyelids widely by applying gentle pressure against the orbit of the eye. Ask the patient to look up, down, and to each side.

conversion An alteration in physical activity or function that resembles an organic disorder but lacks an organic cause. Occurring without voluntary control, conversion is generally considered symbolic of psychological conflict.

Coopernail's sign Ecchymoses on the perineum, scrotum, or labia. This sign indicates pelvic fracture.

Corrigan's pulse A jerky pulse in which a strong surge precedes an abrupt collapse. To detect this sign, hold the patient's hand above his head and palpate the carotid artery. Corrigan's pulse occurs in aortic insufficiency. It may also occur in severe anemia, patent ductus arteriosus, coarctation of the aorta, or systemic arteriosclerosis.

Cowen's sign A jerky consensual pupillary light reflex. To detect this sign, observe for constriction and dilation of one pupil while the other is stimulated by increased and decreased light. This sign occurs in Graves' disease.

crossed extensor reflex Extension of one leg in response to stimulation of the opposite leg; a normal reflex in neonates. It's mediated in the spinal cord and should disappear after age 6 months. To elicit this sign, place the neonate in a supine position with his legs extended. Tap the medial aspect of the thigh just above the patella. The neonate should respond by extending and adducting the opposite leg and fanning the toes of that foot. Persistence of this reflex beyond age 6 months indicates anoxic brain damage. Its appearance in a child signals a central nervous system lesion or injury.

crowing respirations Slow, deep inspirations accompanied by a high-pitched crowing sound — the characteristic whoop of the paroxysmal stage of pertussis.

Cruveilhier's sign Swelling in the groin associated with inguinal hernia. To detect this sign, ask the patient to flex one knee slightly while you insert your index finger in the inguinal canal on the same side. When your finger is inserted as deeply as possible, ask the patient to cough. If a hernia is present, you'll feel a mass of tissue that meets your finger and then withdraws.

Cullen's sign Irregular, bluish hemorrhagic patches on the skin around the umbilicus and occasionally around abdominal scars. Cullen's sign indicates massive hemorrhage after trauma or rupture in such disorders as duodenal ulcer, ectopic pregnancy, abdominal aneurysm, gallbladder or common bile duct obstruction, or acute hemorrhagic pancreatitis. Usually, Cullen's sign appears gradually; blood travels from a retroperitoneal organ or structure to the periumbilical area, where it diffuses through subcutaneous tissues. It may be difficult to detect in a dark-skinned patient. The extent of discoloration depends on the extent of bleeding. In time, the bluish discoloration fades to greenish yellow and then yellow before disappearing.

Dalrymple's sign Abnormally wide palpebral fissures associated with retraction of the upper eyelids. To detect this sign of thyrotoxicosis, observe the eyes while the patient focuses on a fixed point, or ask him to close his eyes. He may exhibit infrequent blinking and noticeable restriction of lid movement; he may not be able to close his eyes completely.

Darier's sign Whealing and itching of the skin after rubbing the macular lesions of urticaria pigmentosa (mastocytosis). To elicit this sign, vigorously rub the pigmented macules with the blunt end of a pen or a similar blunt object. The appearance of pruritic, red, palpable wheals around the macules follows the release of histamine when mast cells are irritated.

Dawbarn's sign Pain on palpation of the acromial process in acute subacromial bursitis. To elicit this sign, palpate the patient's shoulder while his arm hangs at his side and as he abducts it. If palpation causes pain that disappears on abduction, you have detected Dawbarn's sign.

Delbet's sign Adequate collateral circulation to the distal portion of a limb associated with aneurysmal occlusion of the main artery. Check pulses, color, and temperature in the affected limb; pulses are absent in the presence of normal color and temperature, you have detected Delbet's sign.

delirium Acute confusion characterized by restlessness, agitation, incoherence, and often hallucinations. Typically, delirium develops suddenly and lasts for a short period. It's a common effect of drug or alcohol abuse, metabolic disorders, or high fever. Delirium may also follow head trauma or seizure.

delusion A persistent false belief held despite invalidating evidence. A *delusion of grandeur,* which may occur in schizophrenia and bipolar disorders, is an exaggerated belief in one's importance, wealth, or talent. The patient may take a powerful figure, such as Napoleon, as his persona. In a *paranoid delusion,* which may occur in schizophrenia or paranoid disorders, the patient believes that he or someone close to him is the victim of an attack, harassment, or conspiracy. In a *somatic delusion,* which may occur in psychotic disorders, the patient believes that his body is diseased or distorted.

Demianoff's sign Lumbar pain caused by stretching the sacrolumbalis muscle. To elicit this sign, place the patient supine on the examining table and raise his extended leg. Lumbar pain that prevents lifting the leg high enough to form a 10-degree angle to the table — a positive Demianoff's sign — occurs in lumbago.

denial An unconscious defense mechanism used to ward off distressing feelings, thoughts, wishes, or needs. Denial occurs in normal and pathologic mental states. In terminal illness, it represents the first stage of the response to dying.

depersonalization Perception of self as strange or unreal. For example, a person may report feeling as if he's observing himself from a distance. This symptom occurs in patients with schizophrenia or depersonalization disorders, and in normal persons during periods of great stress or anxiety.

Desault's sign Alteration of the arc made by the greater trochanter during rotation of the femur; seen in fracture of the intracapsular region of the femur. In this fracture, the greater trochanter rotates only on the axis of the femur, making a small arc; normal rotation of the femur in the capsule of the hip joint normally describes the arc of a circle.

disorientation Inaccurate perception of time, place, or identity. Disorientation may occur in organic brain disorders, cerebral anoxia, drug or alcohol intoxication or, occasionally, after prolonged, severe stress.

Dorendorf's sign Fullness at the supraclavicular groove. This sign may occur in an aneurysm of the aortic arch.

Duchenne's sign Inward movement of the epigastrium during inspiration. This suggests paralysis of the diaphragm or accumulation of fluid in the pericardium.

Dugas' sign An indicator of a dislocated shoulder. To detect this sign, ask the patient to place the hand of the affected side on his opposite shoulder and to move his elbow toward his chest. Inability to perform this maneuver—a positive Dugas' sign—indicates dislocation.

Duroziez's sign A double murmur heard over a large peripheral artery, an indicator of aortic insufficiency. To detect this sign, auscultate over the femoral artery, alternately compressing the vessel proximally and then distally. If you hear a systolic murmur with proximal compression and a diastolic murmur with distal compression, you have detected this sign, also known as Duroziez's murmur.

DORENDORF'S SIGN

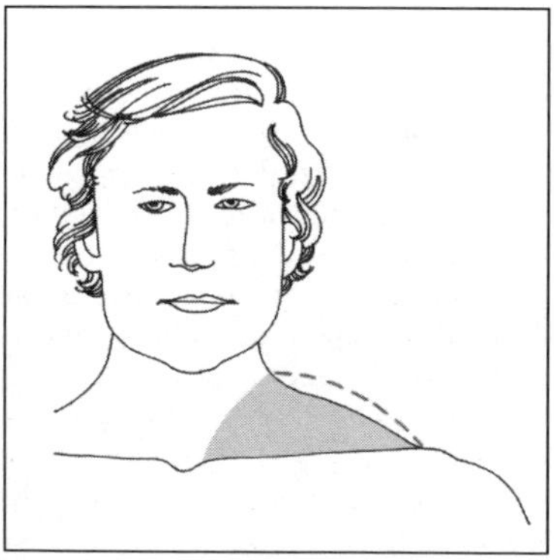

dysdiadochokinesia Difficulty in stopping one movement and starting another. This extrapyramidal sign occurs in disorders of the basal ganglia or cerebellum.

dysphonia Hoarseness or difficulty in producing voice sounds. This sign may reflect disorders of the larynx or laryngeal nerves, overuse or spasm of the vocal cords, or central nervous system disorders such as Parkinson's disease. It may also occur normally at puberty.

Echolalia In an adult: repetition of another's words or phrases with no comprehension of their meaning. This sign occurs in schizophrenia and frontal lobe disorders.

In a child: imitation of sounds or words produced by others.

echopraxia Repetition of another's movements with no comprehension of their meaning. This sign may occur in catatonic schizophrenia or certain neurologic disorders.

ectropion Eversion of the eyelid. It may affect the lower eyelid or both lids, exposing the palpebral conjunctiva. If the lacrimal puncta are everted, the eye can't drain properly, and tearing occurs. Ectropion may occur gradually as part of aging but may also reflect injury or paralysis of the facial nerve.

entropion Inversion of the eyelid. It typically affects the lower lid but may also affect the upper lid. The eyelashes may touch and irritate the cornea. Usually associated with aging, entropion may also reflect chemical burns, mechanical injuries, spasm of the orbicularis muscle, pemphigoid, Stevens-Johnson syndrome, or trachoma.

epicanthal folds Vertical skin folds that partially or fully obscure the inner canthus of the eye. These folds may make the eyes appear crossed because the pupil lies closer to the inner canthus than to the outer canthus. Epicanthal folds are a normal characteristic in many young children and Asians. They also occur as a familial trait in other ethnic groups and as an acquired trait in aging. However, the presence of epicanthal folds with oblique palpebral fissures in non-Asian children indicates Down syndrome.

ECTROPION

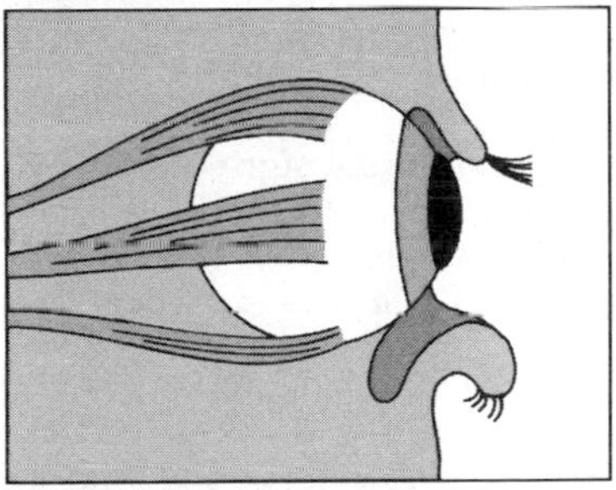

ENTROPION

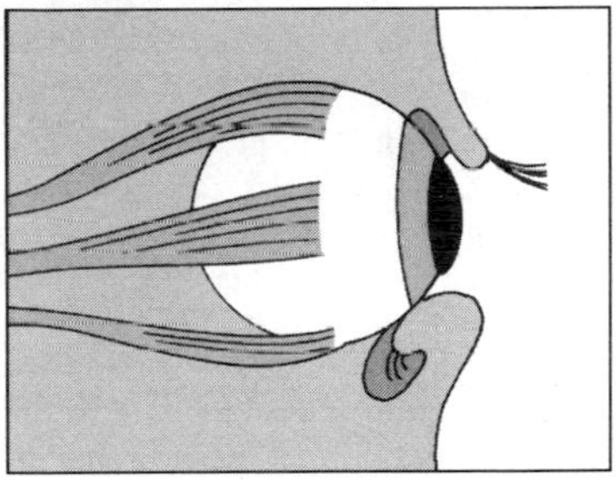

Erben's reflex Slowing of the pulse when the head and trunk are forcibly bent forward. It may indicate vagal excitability.

Erb's sign In tetany, increased irritability of motor nerves, detected by electromyography. Erb's sign also refers to dullness on percussion over the sternum's manubrium in acromegaly.

Escherich's sign Contraction of the lips, tongue, and masseters during tetany. To elicit Escherich's sign, percuss the inner surface of the lips or the tongue.

euphoria A feeling of great happiness or well-being. When euphoria doesn't accompany enlightening experiences or superb achievements, it may reflect bipolar disorder, organic brain disease, or use of such drugs as heroin, cocaine, or amphetamines.

Ewart's sign Bronchial breathing heard on auscultation of the lungs and dullness heard on percussion below the angle of the left scapula. These compression signs commonly occur in pericardial effusion. They also occur beneath the prominence of the sternal end of the first rib in some cases of pericardial effusion.

extensor thrust reflex Extension of the leg after stimulation of the sole of the foot; a normal reflex in neonates. This reflex is mediated in the spinal cord and should disappear after age 6 months. To elicit the extensor thrust reflex, place the neonate in a supine position with the leg flexed; then stimulate the sole of the foot. If the extensor thrust reflex is present, the leg will slowly extend. In premature neonates, this reflex may be weak. Its persistence beyond age 6 months indicates anoxic brain damage. Its recurrence in a child signals a central nervous system lesion or injury.

extinction *In neurology:* inability to perceive one of two stimuli presented simultaneously. To detect this sign, simultaneously stimulate two corresponding areas on opposite sides of the body. Extinction is present if the patient fails to perceive one sensation.

In neurophysiology: loss of excitability of a nerve, synapse, or nervous tissue in response to stimuli that were previously adequate.

In psychology: disappearance of a conditioned reflex resulting from lack of reinforcement.

extrapyramidal signs and symptoms Movement and posture disturbances characteristically resulting from disorders of the basal ganglia and cerebellum. These disturbances include asynergy, ataxia, athetosis, blepharoclonus, chorea, dysarthria, dysdiadochokinesia, dystonia, muscle rigidity and spasticity, myoclonus, spasmodic torticollis, and tremors.

Fabere sign Pain produced by maneuvers used in Patrick's test. It indicates an arthritic hip. The name is an acronym for maneuvers used to elicit the sign: flexion, abduction, external rotation, extension. Begin by placing the patient in a supine position and asking him to flex the thigh and knee of the leg being examined. Then have him externally rotate the leg and place the lateral malleolus on the patella of the opposite leg. Depress the knee. If he experiences pain, you have detected the fabere sign.

Fajersztajn's crossed sciatic sign In sciatica, pain on the affected side triggered by lifting the extended opposite leg. To elicit this sign, place the patient in a supine position and have him flex his unaffected hip, keeping his knee extended. Flexion at the hip will produce pain on the affected side caused by stretching of the irritated sciatic nerve.

fan sign A component of Babinski's reflex. This sign refers to the spreading apart of the patient's toes after his foot is firmly stroked.

flexor withdrawal reflex Flexion of the knee after stimulation of the sole of the foot; a normal reflex in neonates. This reflex is mediated in the spinal cord and should disappear after age 6 months. To elicit this reflex, place the neonate in a supine position, extend his legs, and pinch the sole of his foot. Normally, an neonate younger than age 6 months will respond with slow, uncontrolled flexion of the knee. This reflex may be weak in premature neonates. Its persistence beyond age 6 months may indicate anoxic brain damage. Its recurrence signals a central nervous system lesion or injury.

flight of ideas Continuous, often seemingly pressured speech with abrupt changes of topic. In contrast with loose association, a listener can discern the connection between topics based on word similarities or sounds. This sign characteristically occurs in the manic phase of a bipolar disorder.

foot malposition, congenital Anomalous positioning of the foot, present at birth in roughly 0.4% of neonates. It may reflect the fetal position of comfort, neuromuscular disease, or malformation of a joint or connective tissue. To assess this sign, observe the resting neonate's foot to determine the comfort position. Then observe the foot during spontaneous activity. Using gentle passive maneuvers, determine the full range of motion of the foot and ankle.

Fränkel's sign In tabes dorsalis, the excessive range of passive motion at the hip joint. This excessive motion stems from decreased tone in the surrounding muscles.

Galant's reflex Movement of the pelvis toward the stimulated side when the back is stroked laterally to the spinal column. Normally present at birth, this reflex disappears by age 2 months. To elicit this reflex, place the neonate in a prone position on the examining table or on your hand. Then, using a pin or

GALANT'S REFLEX

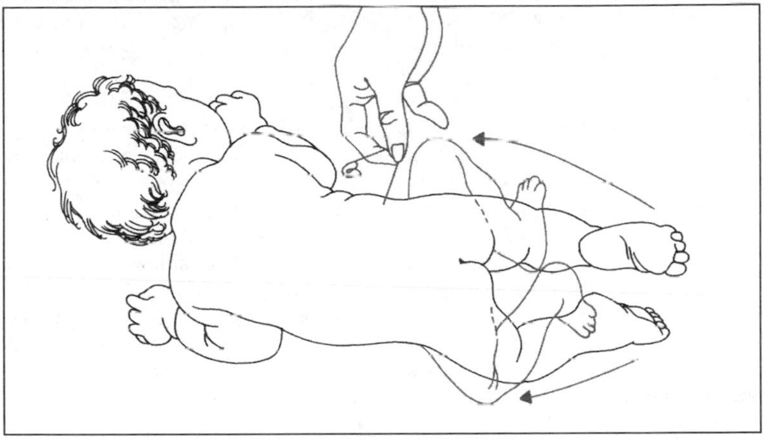

your finger, stroke the back laterally to the midline. Normally, the neonate responds by moving the pelvis toward the stimulated side, indicating integrity of the spinal cord from T1 to S1. Absence, irregularity, or asymmetry of this reflex suggests a spinal cord lesion.

Galeazzi sign Unequal leg lengths in a neonate with congenital dislocation of the hip. To detect this sign, place the neonate in a supine position on a flat, hard surface. Flex the knees and hips 90 degrees and compare the heights of the knees. With dislocation of the hip, the knee will be lower and the femur will appear shortened on the affected side.

Gifford's sign Resistance to everting the upper eyelid, seen in thyrotoxicosis. To detect this sign, attempt to raise the eyelid and evert it over a blunt object.

glabella tap reflex Persistent blinking in response to repeated light tapping on the forehead between the eyebrows. This reflex occurs in Parkinson's disease, presenile dementia, and diffuse tumors of the frontal lobes.

Goldthwait's sign Pain elicited by maneuvers of the leg, pelvis, and lower back to differentiate irritation of the sacroiliac joint from irritation of the lumbosacral or sacroiliac articulation. To elicit this sign, place the patient in a supine position and place one hand under the small of his back. With your other hand, raise the patient's leg. If the patient reports pain, suspect sacroiliac joint irritation. If he reports no pain, place your hand under his lower back and apply pressure. If the patient reports pain, suspect irritation of the lumbosacral or sacroiliac articulation.

Gowers' sign *In an adult:* irregular contraction of the iris when the eye is illuminated. This sign can be detected in certain stages of tabes dorsalis.

In a child: the characteristic maneuver used to rise from the floor or a low sitting position to compensate for proximal muscle weakness in Duchenne's or Becker's muscular dystrophy. See "Gait, waddling," page 272.

grasp reflex Flexion of the fingers when the palmar surface is touched, and of the toes when the plantar surface is touched.

In a neonate: this normal reflex develops at approximately 26 to 28 weeks gestational age but may be weak until term. Its absence, weakness, or asymmetry of this reflex during the neonatal period may indicate paralysis, central nervous system depression, or injury. To elicit this reflex, place a finger in each of the infant's palms. His reflexive grasping should be symmetrical and strong enough at term to allow him to be lifted. Elicit flexion of the toes by gently touching the ball of the foot.

In an adult: the grasp reflex is an *abnormal* finding, indicating a disorder of the premotor cortex.

Grasset's phenomenon Inability to raise both legs simultaneously, even though each can be raised separately.

In an adult: occurs in complete organic hemiplegia. To elicit it, place the patient in a supine position and lift and support the affected leg; then attempt to lift the opposite leg. In Grasset's phenomenon, the unaffected leg will drop — the result of an upper-motor-neuron lesion.

In an infant: this sign is normally present until age 5 to 7 months.

grief Deep anguish or sorrow typically felt after the loss of a loved one, a job, a goal, or an ideal. In patients with terminal illness, grief may precede acceptance of dying. Unlike depression, grief proceeds in stages and commonly resolves over time.

Griffith's sign Lagging motion of the lower eyelids during upward rotation of the eyes, seen in thyrotoxicosis. Ask the patient to focus on a steadily rising point such as your moving finger. If the lower lid doesn't follow eye motion smoothly, you have observed this sign.

Guilland's sign Quick, energetic flexion of the hip and knee in response to pinching of the contralateral quadriceps muscle. This sign indicates meningeal irritation.

H

Hallucination A sensory perception without corresponding external stimuli. Hallucinations may occur in depression, schizophrenia, bipolar disorder, organic brain disorders, or drug- or toxin-induced conditions.

An *auditory hallucination* is perception of nonexistent sounds — typically voices but occasionally music or other sounds. Occurring in schizophrenia, this is the most common type of hallucination.

An *olfactory hallucination* — a perception of nonexistent odors from the patient's own body or from some other person or object — is typically associated with somatic delusions. It occurs most commonly in temporal lobe lesions and may also occur in schizophrenia.

A *tactile hallucination* is the perception of nonexistent tactile stimuli, generally described as something crawling on or under the skin. It occurs mainly in toxic conditions or addiction to certain drugs. Formication — the sensation of insects crawling on the skin—most commonly occurs in alcohol withdrawal syndrome or cocaine abuse.

A *visual hallucination* is a perception of images of nonexistent people, flashes of light, or other scenes. It occurs most commonly in acute, reversible organic brain disorders but may also occur in drug or alcohol intoxication, schizophrenia, febrile illness, or encephalopathy.

A *gustatory hallucination* is the perception of nonexistent, usually unpleasant tastes.

Hamman's sign A loud, crushing, crunching sound synchronous with the heartbeat. Auscultated over the precordium, it reflects mediastinal emphysema, which occurs in such life-threatening conditions as pneumothorax or rupture of the trachea or bronchi. To detect this sign, place the patient in a left lateral recumbent position and gently auscultate over the precordium.

harlequin sign A benign, erythematous color change occurring especially in low-birth-weight neonates. This reddening of one longitudinal half of the body appears when the neonte is placed on either side for a few minutes. When he's placed on his back, the sign usually disappears immediately but may persist up to 20 minutes.

hemorrhage, subungual Bleeding under the nail plate. Hemorrhagic lines, called splinter hemorrhages, that run proximally from the distal edge reflect subacute bacterial endocarditis or trichinosis. Large hemorrhagic areas generally reflect nail bed injury.

Hill's sign A femoral systolic pulse pressure 60 to 100 mm Hg higher in the right leg than in the right arm. Hill's sign suggests severe aortic insufficiency. To detect it, place the patient in a supine position and take blood pressure readings, first in the right arm and then in the right leg, noting the difference.

Hoehne's sign Absence of uterine contractions during delivery, despite repeated doses of oxytocic drugs. This sign indicates a ruptured uterus.

Hoffmann's sign Flexion of the terminal phalanx of the thumb and the second and third phalanges of another finger when the nail of the index, middle, or ring finger is snapped. A bilateral or strongly unilateral response suggests a pyramidal tract disorder such as spastic hemiparesis. To elicit this sign, dorsiflex the patient's wrist, have him flex his fingers, and then snap the nail of his index, middle, or ring finger.

SUBUNGUAL HEMORRHAGE

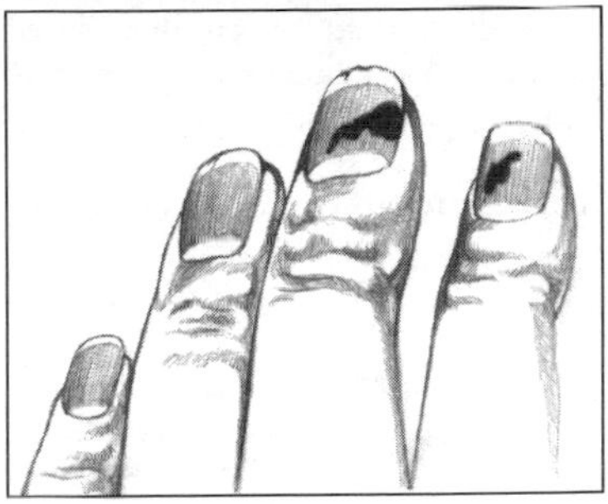

Hoffmann's sign also refers to increased sensitivity of sensory nerves to electrical stimulation, as in tetany.

Hoover's sign Inward movement of one or both costal margins during inspiration. Bilateral movement occurs in emphysema with acute respiratory distress. Unilateral movement occurs in intrathoracic disorders that cause flattening of one half of the diaphragm. A contralateral leg-lifting movement occurs when a patient is directed to press his leg against the examination table. This movement is absent in hysteria and malingering.

hyperacusis Abnormally acute hearing caused by increased irritability of the auditory neural mechanism. It results in an unusually low hearing threshold.

hyperesthesia Increased or altered cutaneous sensitivity to touch, temperature, or pain.

hypernasality A voice quality reflecting excessive expiration of air through the nose during speech. It's commonly associated with symptoms of dysarthria and possibly with swallowing defects. The sudden onset of hypernasality may indicate a neuromuscular disorder. This sign may also accompany cleft palate, or a short soft and hard palate, abnormal nasopharyngeal size, or partial or complete velar paralysis. To detect this sign, ask the patient to extend vowel sounds first with the nostrils open, then closed (pinched). A significant shift in tone may indicate hypernasality.

hypoesthesia Decreased cutaneous sensitivity to touch, temperature, or pain.

Idea of reference A delusion that other people, statements, actions, or events have a meaning specific to oneself. This delusion occurs in schizophrenia and paranoid states. Also known as delusion of reference.

illusion A misperception of external stimuli — usually visual or auditory — such as the sound of the wind being perceived as a voice. Illusions occur normally as well as in schizophrenia and toxic states.

Jellinek's sign Also known as Rasin's sign. Brownish pigmentation on the eyelids, usually more prominent on the upper lid than on the lower one. This sign appears in Graves' disease.

Joffroy's sign Immobility of the facial muscles with upward rotation of the eyes, associated with exophthalmos in Graves' disease. To detect this sign, observe the patient's forehead as he quickly rotates his eyes upward.

Joffroy's sign also refers to the inability to perform simple mathematics — a possible early sign of organic brain disorder.

KOPLIK'S SPOTS

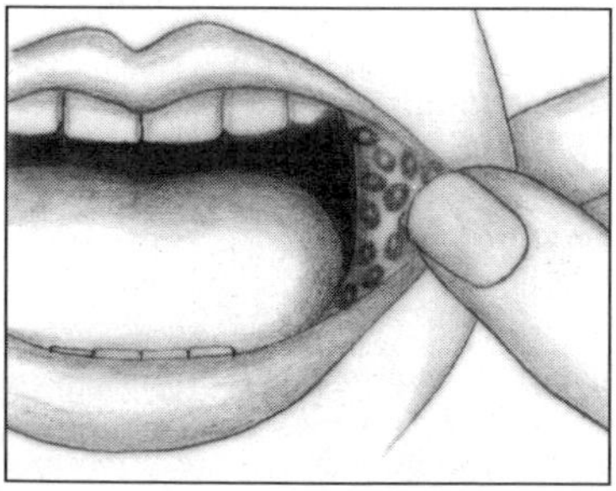

Kanavel's sign An area of tenderness in the palm, caused by inflammation of the tendon sheath of the little finger. To detect this sign, apply pressure to the palm proximal to the metacarpophalangeal joint of the little finger.

Keen's sign Increased ankle circumference in Pott's fracture of the fibula. To detect this sign, measure the ankles at the malleoli and compare their circumferences.

Kleist's sign Flexion, or hooking, of the fingers when passively raised, associated with frontal lobe and thalamic lesions. To elicit this sign, have the patient turn his palms down, then gently raise his fingers. If his fingers hook onto yours, you have detected this sign.

Koplik's spots Also known as Koplik's sign. Small red spots with bluish white centers on the lingual and buccal mucosa characteristic of measles. After this sign appears, the measles rash usually erupts in 1 to 2 days.

Kussmaul's respirations An abnormal breathing pattern characterized by deep, rapid sighing respirations, generally associated with metabolic acidosis.

Kussmaul's sign Distention of the jugular veins on inspiration, occurring in constrictive pericarditis and mediastinal tumor. Kussmaul's sign also refers to a paradoxical pulse and to seizures and coma that result from absorption of toxins.

L

Langoria's sign Relaxation of the extensor muscles of the thigh and hip joint, resulting from intracapsular fracture of the femur. To elicit this sign, place the patient in a prone position, then press firmly on the gluteus maximus and hamstring muscles on both sides, noting greater muscle relaxation on the affected side. (The muscles are soft and spongy.)

large for gestational age Neonatal weight that exceeds the 90th percentile for the neonate's gestational age. The high-birth-weight neonate is at increased risk for birth trauma, respiratory distress, hypocalcemia, hypoglycemia, and polycythemia.

Lasègue's sign Pain on passive movement of the leg that distinguishes hip joint disease from sciatica. To elicit this sign, place the patient in a supine position, raise one of his legs, and bend the knee to flex the hip joint. Pain with this movement indicates hip joint disease. With the hip still flexed, slowly extend the knee. Pain with this movement results from stretching an irritated sciatic nerve, indicating sciatica.

Laugier's sign An abnormal spatial relationship of the radial and ulnar styloid processes, resulting from fracture of the distal radius. Normally more distal than the ulnar process, the radial process may migrate proximally in the fracture of the distal radius, so that it's level with the ulnar process. To detect this sign, compare the patient's wrists.

lead-pipe rigidity Diffuse muscle stiffness occurring, for example, in Parkinson's disease.

Leichtenstern's sign Pain elicited by gentle tapping of the bones of an extremity; occurs in cerebrospinal meningitis. The patient may wince, draw back suddenly, or cry out loudly.

Lhermitte's sign Sensations of sudden, transient, electric-like shocks spreading down the back and into the extremities, precipitated by forward flexion of the head. This sign occurs in multiple sclerosis, spinal cord degeneration, and cervical spinal cord injury.

Lichtheim's sign Inability to speak associated with subcortical aphasia. However, the patient can indicate with his fingers the number of syllables in the word he wants to say.

Linder's sign Pain upon neck flexion, indicating sciatica. To elicit this sign, place the patient in a supine or sitting position with his legs fully extended. Then passively flex his neck, noting if he experiences pain in the lower back or the affected leg, resulting from stretching of the irritated sciatic nerve.

Lloyd's sign Referred loin pain elicited by deep percussion over the kidney. This sign is associated with renal calculi.

loose association A cognitive disturbance marked by absence of a logical link between spoken statements. It occurs in schizophrenia, bipolar disorders, and other psychotic disorders.

low-set ears A position of the ears in which the superior helix lies lower than the eyes. This sign appears in several genetic syndromes, including Down, Apert's, Turner's, Noonan's, and Potter's, and may appear in other congenital abnormalities.

Ludloff's sign Inability to raise the thigh while sitting, with edema and ecchymosis at the base of Scarpa's triangle (the depressed area just below the fold of the groin). Occurring in children, this

LUMBOSACRAL HAIR TUFT

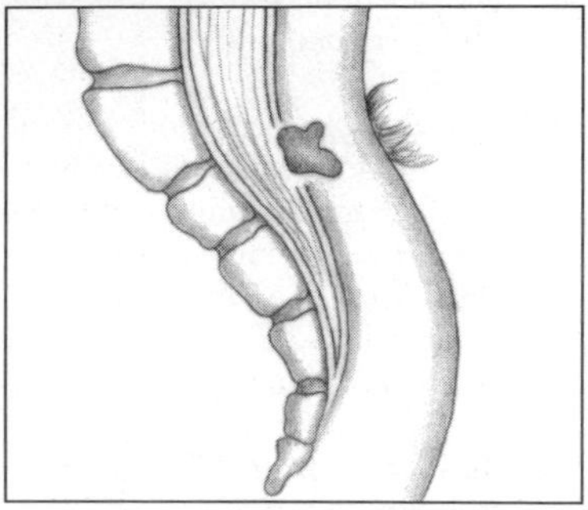

sign indicates traumatic separation of the epiphyseal growth plate of the greater trochanter.

lumbosacral hair tuft Abnormal growth of hair over the lower spine, possibly accompanied by skin depression or discoloration. This may mark the site of spina bifida occulta or spina bifida cystica.

Macewen's sign A "cracked pot" sound elicited by light percussion with one finger over an infant's or young child's anterior fontanel. An early indicator of hydrocephalus, this sign may also reflect cerebral abscess.

Maisonneuve's sign Hyperextension of the wrist in Colles' fracture. Hyperextension results when a fracture of the lower radius causes posterior displacement of the distal fragment.

malaise Listlessness, weariness, or absence of the sense of well-being. This nonspecific symptom may begin suddenly or gradually and may precede characteristic signs of an illness by several days or weeks. Malaise may reflect the metabolic alterations that precede or accompany infectious, endocrine, or neurologic disorders.

malingering Exaggeration or simulation of symptoms to avoid an unpleasant situation or to gain attention or some other goal.

mania An alteration in mood characterized by increased psychomotor activity, euphoria, flight of ideas, and pressured speech. It occurs most commonly in the manic phase of a bipolar disorder.

Mannkopf's sign Elevated pulse rate elicited by application of pressure over a painful area. It can help distinguish real pain from simulated pain — the sign doesn't occur in the latter.

Marcus Gunn's phenomenon Unilateral reflexive elevation of an upper ptotic eyelid, associated with movement of the lower jaw. This occurs in misdirectional syndrome, involving the oculomotor and trigeminal nerves (cranial nerves III and V). To elicit this sign, ask the patient to open his mouth and move his lower jaw from side to side.

Marcus Gunn's pupillary sign Paradoxical dilation of a pupil in response to afferent visual stimuli. However, vision loss in the affected eye is minimal. This sign results from an optic nerve lesion or severe retinal dysfunction. To detect this sign, darken the room and instruct the patient to focus on a distant object. Shine a bright beam of light into the unaffected eye, and observe for bilateral pupillary constriction. Then shine the light into the affected eye; you'll observe brief bilateral dilatation. When you return the light beam to the unaffected eye; you'll observe prompt and persistent bilateral pupillary constriction.

masklike facies A total loss of facial expression, resulting from bradykinesia — usually caused by extrapyramidal damage. The rate of eye blinking drops to 1 to 4 blinks per minute, producing a characteristic "reptilian" stare. Although a neurologic disorder is the most common cause, masklike facies can result from certain systemic diseases or from the effects of certain drugs or toxins.

Mayo's sign In deep anesthesia, relaxation of the lower jaw.

Mean's sign Lagging eye motion when the patient looks upward. In this sign of Graves' disease, the globe of the eye moves more slowly than the upper lid.

meconium staining of amniotic fluid The presence of greenish brown or yellow meconium in the amniotic fluid during labor. Although not necessarily indicative of distress, this sign signals the need for close fetal monitoring to detect decreased variability, or deceleration, of heart rate. It may also signal the need for neonate intubation and resuscitation at delivery to prevent meconium aspiration into the lungs.

menorrhagia Abnormally heavy menstrual flow occurring at the normal time but abnormally prolonged, saturating a pad or tampon in less than 1 hour.

metrorrhagia Vaginal bleeding or spotting between menses.

Möbius' sign Inability to maintain convergence of the eyes. To detect this sign of Graves' disease, observe the patient's attempt to focus on any small object, such as a pencil, as you move it toward him in line with his nose.

Moro's reflex A infant's generalized response to a loud noise or sudden movement. Usually, this reflex disappears by about age 3 months. Its persistence after age 6 months may indicate brain damage. To elicit this reflex, make a sudden loud noise near the infant, or carefully hold his body with one hand, while allowing his head to drop a few centimeters with the other hand. In a complete response, the infant's arms extend and abduct, and his fingers open; then his arms adduct and flex over his chest in a grasping motion. The infant may also extend his hips and legs and cry briefly. A bilaterally equal response is normal; an asymmetrical response suggests a fractured clavicle or brachial nerve damage. The absence of a response may indicate hearing loss or severe central nervous system depression.

Murphy's sign The arrest of inspiratory effort when gentle finger pressure beneath the right subcostal arch and below the margin of the liver causes pain during deep inspiration. This classic (but not always present) sign of acute cholecystitis may also occur in hepatitis.

muscle rigidity Muscle tension, stiffness, and resistance to passive movement. This extrapyramidal symptom occurs in disorders affecting the basal ganglia and cerebellum, such as Parkinson's disease, Wilson's disease, Hallervorden-Spatz disease in adults, or kernicterus in infants.

myalgia Diffuse muscle pain, usually accompanied by malaise, occurring in many infectious diseases, including brucellosis, dengue, influenza, leptospirosis, measles, and poliomyelitis. Myalgia also occurs in arteriosclerosis obliterans, fibrositis, fibromyositis, Guillain-Barré syndrome, hyperparathyroidism, hypoglycemia, hypothyroidism, muscle tumor, myoglobinuria, myositis, and renal tubular acidosis. In addition, various drugs may cause myalgia, including amphotericin B, chloroquine, clofibrate, and corticosteroids.

Nail dystrophy Changes in the nail plate, such as pitting, furrowing, splitting, or fraying. It usually results from injury, chronic nail infection, neurovascular disorders affecting the extremities, or collagen disorders. It also occurs secondary to repeated wetting and drying of the nails associated with frequent immersion in water.

nail plate discoloration A change in the color of the nail plate, resulting from infection or drugs. Blue-green discoloration may occur in *Pseudomonas* infection; brown or black, fungal infection or fluorosis; bluish gray, excessive use of silver salts.

nail plate hypertrophy Thickening of the nail plate resulting from the accumulation of irregular keratin layers. This condition is commonly associated with fungal infection of the nails, although it can be hereditary.

nail separation Separation of the nail plate from the nail bed. This occurs primarily in injury or infection of the nail, and in thyrotoxicosis.

nasal obstruction This symptom may result from inflammatory, neoplastic, endocrine, or metabolic disorders, structural abnormalities, or traumatic injuries. It may cause discomfort, alter the sense of smell and taste, and cause voice changes. Although commonly benign, nasal obstruction may herald basilar skull fracture or malignant tumor.

neologism A new word or condensation of several words with special meaning for the patient but not readily understood by others. This coining occurs in schizophrenia and organic brain disorders.

NODULE

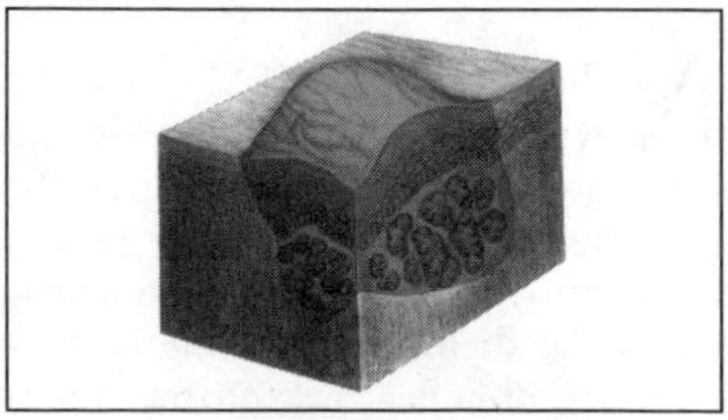

neuralgia Severe, paroxysmal pain over an area innervated by specific nerve fibers. The cause is commonly unknown, but it may be precipitated by pressure, cold, movement, or stimulation of a trigger zone. Usually brief, neuralgia may be accompanied by vasomotor symptoms, such as sweating or tearing.

Nicoladoni's sign Bradycardia resulting from finger pressure on an artery proximal to an arteriovenous fistula, also known as Branham's sign.

nightblindness Impaired vision in the dark, especially after entering a darkened room or while driving at night. This symptom of choroidal and retinal degeneration occurs in various ocular disorders. It may be an early indicator of vitamin A deficiency.

nodules Small, solid, circumscribed masses of differentiated tissue, detected by palpation.

Obsession A persistent, usually disturbing thought or image that can't be eliminated by reason or logic. It's associated with an obsessive-compulsive disorder or, occasionally, schizophrenia.

obturator sign Pain in the right hypogastric region after flexion of the right leg at the hip with the knee bent and internally rotated.

In adults, it indicates irritation of the obturator muscle.

In children, this sign may signal acute appendicitis because the appendix lies rectocecally over the obturator muscle.

oculocardiac reflex Refers to bradycardia in response to vagal stimulation, caused by application of pressure to the eyeball or carotid sinus. This reflex can help diagnose angina or relieve anginal pain. *Caution:* Repeated application of pressure to the eye to elicit this response may precipitate retinal detachment. Also known as Aschner's phenomenon.

orbicularis sign Inability to close one eye at a time, occurring in hemiplegia.

orgasmic disorders Transient or persistent inhibition of the orgasmic phase of sexual excitement.

In females: delayed or absent orgasm following a phase of sexual excitement. This usually results from psychological or interpersonal problems. Other causes include chronic disorders, congenital anomalies, and chronic vaginal or pelvic infections.

In males: delayed or absent ejaculation following a phase of sexual excitement. Its causes include psychological problems, neurologic disorders, and the effects of antihypertensive drugs. See "Impotence," page 329.

orthotonos A form of tetanic spasm producing a rigid, straight line of the neck, limbs, and body.

Osler's nodes Tender, raised, pea-sized, red or purple lesions that erupt on the palms, soles or, especially, the pads of the fingers and toes. They're rare but reliable signs of infective endocarditis and are pathognomonic of the subacute form. However, these nodes usually develop after other telling signs and symptoms disappear spontaneously within several days. How and why they develop is uncertain; they may develop from emboli caught in peripheral capillaries or may reflect an immunologic reaction to the causative organism. Osler's nodes must be distinguished from the even less common Janeway's lesions — small, painless, erythematous lesions that erupt on the palms and soles.

ostealgia Bone pain associated with such disorders as osteomyelitis.

otorrhagia Bleeding from the ear occurring with a tumor, severe infection, or injury affecting the auricle, external canal, tympanic membrane, or temporal bone.

Palmar crease abnormalities An abnormal line pattern on the palms, resulting from faulty embryonic development during the second to fourth months of gestation. This pattern may occur normally but usually accompanies Down syndrome as a single transverse crease formed by fusion of the proximal and distal palmar creases (called the simian crease). It also occur in Turner's syndrome and congenital rubella syndrome.

paradoxical respirations An abnormal breathing pattern marked by paradoxical movement of an injured portion of the chest wall — it contracts on inspiration and bulges on expiration. This ominous sign is characteristic of flail chest — a thoracic injury involving multiple free-floating, fractured ribs.

paranoia Extreme suspiciousness related to delusions of persecution by another person, group, or institution. This may occur in schizophrenia, drug-induced or toxic states, or paranoid disorders.

Pastia's sign Petechiae or hemorrhagic lines appearing along skin creases in such areas as the antecubital fossa, groin, and wrists. They accompany the rash of scarlet fever as a response to the erythrogenic toxin produced by scarlatinal strains of group A streptococci.

Pel-Ebstein fever A recurrent pattern characterized by several days of high fever alternating with afebrile periods that last for days or weeks. Typically, the fever becomes progressively higher and continuous. Pel-Ebstein fever occasionally occurs in Hodgkin's disease. Also known as Pel-Ebstein symptom or Pel-Ebstein pyrexia.

Perez's sign Crackles or friction sounds auscultated over the lungs when a seated patient raises and lowers his arms. This sign commonly occurs in fibrous mediastinitis and may occur in aortic arch aneurysm.

peroneal sign Dorsiflexion and abduction of the foot elicited by tapping over the common peroneal nerve. To elicit this sign of latent tetany, tap over the lateral neck of the fibula with the patient's knee relaxed and slightly flexed.

phobia An irrational and persistent fear of an object, situation, or activity. Occurring in phobic disorders, it may interfere with normal functioning. Typical manifestations include faintness, fatigue, palpitations, diaphoresis, nausea, tremor, or panic.

pica Craving and ingesting of normally inedible substances, such as plaster, charcoal, clay, wool, ashes, paint, or dirt.

In children, the most commonly affected group, it results from nutritional deficiencies.

In adults, it may reflect a psychological disturbance. Depending on the substance eaten, pica can lead to poisoning and GI disorders.

Piotrowski's sign Dorsiflexion and supination of the foot elicited by percussion of the anterior tibial muscle. Excessive flexion may indicate a central nervous system disorder.

Pitres' sign In tabes dorsalis, hyperesthesia of the scrotum and testes. This sign also refers to the anterior deviation of the sternum in pleural effusion.

Plummer's sign Inability to ascend stairs or step up onto a chair. This sign can be demonstrated in Graves' disease.

pneumaturia The passage of gas in the urine while voiding. Causes include a fistula between the bowel and bladder, sigmoid diverticulitis, rectosigmoid cancer or, rarely, gas-forming urinary tract infections.

postnasal drip A sinus or nasal discharge that flows behind the nose and into the throat. It typically results from infection, allergies, or environmental irritants.

Pool-Schlesinger sign In tetany, muscle spasm of the forearm, hand, and fingers or of the leg and foot. To detect this sign, forcefully abduct and elevate the patient's arm with his forearm extended. Alternatively, forcefully flex the patient's extended leg at the hip. Spasm results from tension on the brachial plexus or the sciatic nerve. Also known as Pool's phenomenon or Schlesinger's sign.

Potain's sign Dullness on percussion over the aortic arch, extending from the manubrium to the third costal cartilage on the right. This occurs in aortic dilatation.

Prehn's sign Relief of pain with elevation and support of the scrotum, occurring in epididymitis. This sign differentiates epididymitis from testicular torsion. Both disorders produce severe pain, tenderness, and scrotal swelling.

pressured speech Verbal expression that's accelerated, difficult to interrupt, and at times unintelligible. This may accompany flight of ideas in the manic phase of a bipolar disorder.

Prévost's sign Conjugate deviation of the head and eyes in hemiplegia. Typically, the eyes gaze toward the affected hemisphere.

prognathism An enlarged, protuberant jaw associated with normal mandible condyles and temporomandibular joints. This sign usually appears in acromegaly.

pulsus biferiens A hyperdynamic, double-beating pulse characterized by two systolic peaks separated by a midsystolic dip. Both peaks may be equal or one may be larger; usually, the first peak is taller or more forceful than the second. The first peak (percussion wave), is believed to be the pulse pressure and the second peak (tidal wave), reverberation from the periphery. This sign occurs in conditions in which a large volume of blood is rapidly ejected from the left ventricle such as aortic insufficiency. The pulse can be palpated in peripheral arteries or observed on an arterial pressure wave recording.

To detect pulses biferiens, lightly palpate the carotid, brachial, radial, or femoral artery while listening to the heart sounds to determine if the two palpable peaks occur during systole. If they do, you'll feel the double pulse between the first and second heart sounds.

purple striae Thin, purple streaks on the skin that characteristically occur in hypercortisolism with other cushingoid signs, such as buffalo hump and moonface. Striae usually result from excessive use of glucocorticoid drugs.

pyrosis A substernal burning sensation that rises in the chest and may radiate to the neck or throat; commonly known as heartburn. Caused by reflex of gastric contents into the esophagus, pyrosis is commonly accompanied by regurgitation. It usually develops after meals or when the patient lies down, bends over, lifts heavy objects, or exercises vigorously. It may worsen with swallowing and improves when the patient sits upright or takes antacids.

Quinquaud's sign Trembling of the fingers in alcoholism. To detect this sign, have the patient spread his hand, flex his fingers at the metacarpophalangeal joints, and touch your palm with his fingers at a 90-degree angle to your hand.

Rectal pain Discomfort that arises in the anorectal area. This pain may result from or be aggravated by diarrhea, constipation, or passage of hardened stools. It may also be aggravated by intense pruritus and continued scratching associated with drainage of mucus, blood, or fecal matter that irritates the skin and nerve endings.

rectal tenesmus Spasmodic contraction of the anal sphincter with a persistent urge to defecate and involuntary, ineffective straining. This occurs in inflammatory bowel disorders, such as ulcerative colitis and Crohn's disease, and in rectal tumors. Typically painful, rectal tenesmus usually accompanies passage of small amounts of blood, pus, or mucus.

regression Return to a behavioral level appropriate to an earlier developmental age. This defense mechanism may occur in various psychiatric and organic disorders. It may also result from worsening of symptoms or a disease process.

repression Unconscious retreat or thrusting back from awareness of unacceptable ideas or impulses. This defense mechanism may occur normally or may accompany psychiatric disorders.

Romberg's sign An inability to maintain balance when standing erect with the feet together and eyes closed. This sign indicates a disorder of the spinal tracts that carry proprioceptive information. Insufficient vestibular or proprioceptive information causes an in-

RUMPEL-LEEDE SIGN

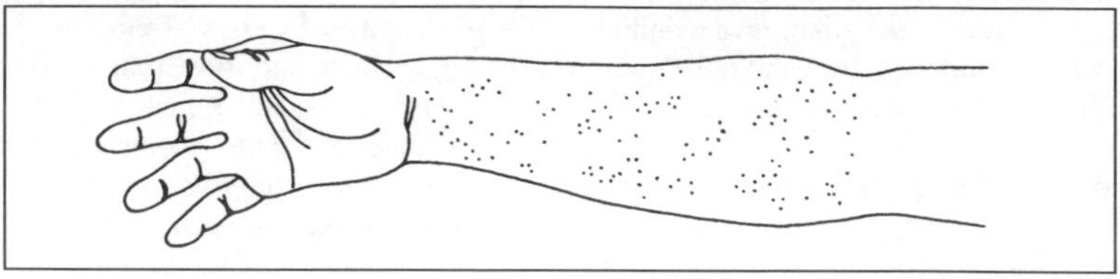

ability to execute precise movements and maintain balance without visual cues.

Rosenbach's sign Absence of the abdominal skin reflex, associated with intestinal inflammation and hemiplegia. This sign also refers to the fine, rapid tremor of gently closed eyelids in Graves' disease; and to the inability to close the eyes immediately on command, as in neurasthenia.

Rotch's sign Dullness on percussion over the right lung at the fifth intercostal space. This sign occurs in pericardial effusion.

Rovsing's sign Pain in the right lower quadrant elicited by palpation and quick withdrawal of the fingers in the left lower quadrant. This referred rebound tenderness suggests appendicitis.

Rumpel-Leede sign Extensive petechiae distal to a tourniquet placed around the upper arm and left for 5 to 10 minutes; indicates capillary fragility in scarlet fever or severe thrombocytopenia. Also known as Rumpel-Leede phenomenon.

SIEGERT'S SIGN

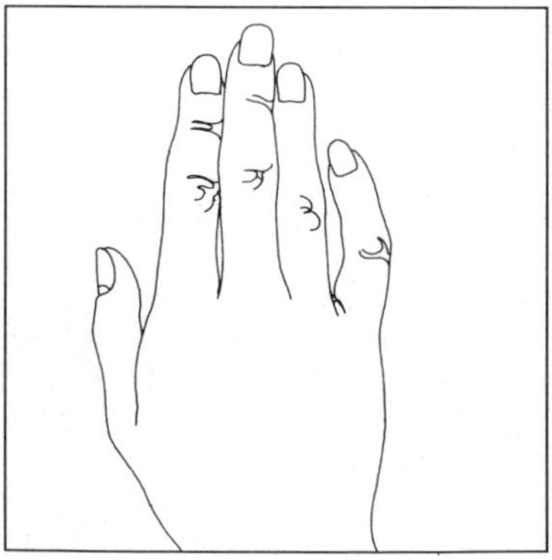

Salivation, decreased Diminished production or excretion of saliva (also known as dry mouth or xerostomia). This sign usually results from mouth breathing but other possible causes are Sjögren's syndrome, the use of anticholinergics and other drugs, radiation effects, or even vigorous exercise or autonomic stimulation — for example, by fear.

salivation, increased This uncommon condition may result from GI disorders, especially of the esophagus. It also accompanies certain systemic disorders and may result from difficulty swallowing. See "Dysphagia," page 206.

Seeligmüller's sign Pupillary dilation on the affected side, in facial neuralgia.

Siegert's sign Short, inwardly curved little fingers, typically appearing in Down syndrome.

Signorelli's sign Extreme tenderness on palpation of the retromandibular point; associated with meningitis.

Simon's sign Incoordination of the movements of the diaphragm and thorax, occurring early in meningitis. Also refers to retraction or fixation of the umbilicus during inspiration.

Soto-Hall sign Pain in the area of a lesion, occurring after passive flexion of the spine. To elicit this sign, place the patient in a supine position and progressively flex his spine from the neck downward. The patient will complain of pain at the area of the lesion.

spasmodic torticollis Intermittent or continuous spasms of the shoulder and neck muscles that turn the head to one side. Commonly transient and idiopathic, this sign can occur in extrapyramidal disorders. It can also occur in patients with shortened neck muscles. See "Dystonia," page 215.

spider angioma A fiery red vascular lesion with an elevated central body, branching spiderlike legs, and a surrounding flush. Ranging from a few millimeters to several centimeters in diameter, spider angiomas usually appear on the face and neck and may occur singly or in multiples. On palpation, they may be slightly warmer than the surrounding skin and may have a pulsating central body. This sign is usually associated with cirrhosis but may also occur in the second to third month of pregnancy and in elderly patients.

spoon nails Malformation of the nails characterized by a concave instead of the normal convex outer surface. This commonly occurs in severe hypochromic anemia but occasionally may be hereditary.

Stellwag's sign Incomplete and infrequent blinking, usually related to exophthalmos in Graves' disease.

stepping reflex In the neonate, spontaneous stepping movements that simulate walking. This reciprocal flexion and extension of the legs disappears after about age 4 weeks. However, scissoring movements with persistent extension and crossing of the legs or asymmetrical stepping is abnormal, possibly indicating central nervous system damage. To elicit this sign, hold the infant erect with the soles of his feet touching a hard surface.

STEPPING REFLEX

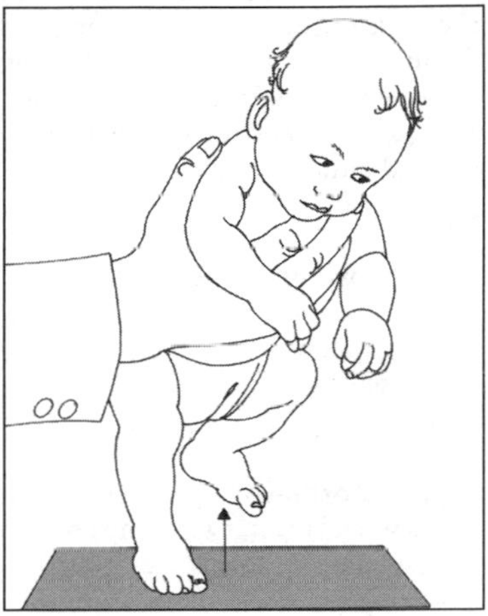

Strunsky's sign Pain on plantar flexion of the toes and forefoot, caused by inflammatory disorders of the anterior arch. To detect this sign, have the patient assume a relaxed position with his foot exposed, then grasp his toes and quickly plantarflex his toes and forefoot.

succussion splash A splashing sound heard over a hollow organ or body cavity, such as the stomach or thorax, after rocking or shaking the patient's body. Indicating the presence of fluid or air and gas, this sound may be auscultated in pyloric or intestinal obstruction, a large hiatal hernia, or hydropneumothorax. However, it may also be auscultated over a normal, empty stomach.

sucking reflex Involuntary circumoral sucking movements in response to stimulation. Present at about 26 weeks gestational age, this reflex is initially weak and isn't synchronized with swallowing. It persists through infancy, becoming more discriminating during the first few months and disappearing by age 1. To elicit this response, place your finger in the infant's mouth. Rhythmic sucking movements are normal. Weakness or absence of these movements may indicate elevated intracranial pressure.

T

tangentiality Speech characterized by tedious detail that prevents ever reaching the point of the statement. This occurs in schizophrenia and organic brain disorders.

taste abnormality This sign encompasses several types of taste impairment: *ageusia* (complete loss or taste), *hypogeusia* (partial loss of taste), *dysgeusia* (distorted sense of taste), and *cacogeusia* (unpleasant or even revolting sense of taste). Any factor that interrupts transmission of taste stimuli to the brain, such as trauma, infection, vitamin or mineral deficiency, neurologic or oral disorders, and the effects of drugs, may cause taste abnormalities. Aging and heavy smoking may also play a role.

tearing increase Excessive production of tears (also known as lacrimation) caused by stimulation of the lacrimal glands. *Psychic lacrimation* is usually a response to emotional or physical stress such as pain. *Neurogenic lacrimation* is triggered by a reflex stimulation associated with ocular trauma, inflammation, or exposure to environmental irritants (such as strong light, wind, or airborne allergens); it may also accompany eyestrain, yawning, vomiting, and laughing.

Terry's nails A white, opaque surface over more than 80% of the nail and a normal pink distal edge. This sign is commonly associated with cirrhosis.

testicular pain Unilateral or bilateral pain localized in or around the testicle and possibly radiating along the spermatic cord and into the lower abdomen. It usually results from trauma, infection, or torsion. Typically, its onset is sudden and severe; however, its intensity can vary from sharp pain accompanied by nausea and vomiting to a chronic, dull ache. In a child, sudden onset of severe testicular pain is a urologic emergency. Assume torsion is the cause until disproven. If a young male complains of abdominal pain, always carefully examine the scrotum because abdominal pain commonly precedes testicular pain in testicular torsion.

Thornton's sign Severe flank pain resulting from nephrolithiasis.

thrill A palpable sensation resulting from the vibration of a loud murmur or from turbulent blood flow in an aneurysm. Thrills are associated with heart murmurs of grades IV to VI and may be palpable over major arteries. See "Bruits," page 109, and "Murmurs," page 380.

tibialis sign Involuntary dorsiflexion and inversion of the foot elicited by brisk, voluntary flexion of the patient's knee and hip, occurring in spastic paralysis of the lower limb. Also known as Strümpell's sign.

To detect this sign, place the patient in a supine position and have him flex his leg at the hip and knee so that the thigh touches the abdomen. Alternatively, you can place the patient in a prone position, and have him flex his leg at the knee so that the calf touches the thigh. If this sign is present, you may observe dorsiflexion of the great toe, or of all toes, as the foot dorsiflexes and inverts. Normally, this action elicits plantar flexion of the foot.

Tommasi's sign Absence of hair on the posteroexternal aspect of the leg, occurring in males with gout.

Tinel's sign Distal paresthesia on percussion over an injured nerve in an extremity, as in carpal tunnel syndrome.

This sign indicates a partial lesion or the early regeneration of the nerve. To elicit this sign in the patient's wrist, tap over the median nerve on the wrist's flexor surface.

tongue, hairy Hypertrophy and elongation of the tongue's filiform papillae. Normally white, the papillae may turn yellow, brown, or black from bacteria, food, tobacco, coffee, or dyes in drugs and food. Hairy tongue may result from antibiotic therapy, irradiation of the head and neck, chronic debilitating disorders, or habitual use of mouthwashes containing oxidizing or astringent agents.

tongue, magenta, cobblestone Swelling and hyperemia of the tongue, forming rows of elevated fungiform and filiform papillae that give the tongue a magenta-colored or cobblestone appearance. It's most commonly a sign of vitamin B_2 (riboflavin) deficiency.

tongue, red Patchy or uniform redness (ranging from pink to magenta) of the tongue, which may be swollen and smooth, rough, or fissured. It usually indicates glossitis, resulting from emotional stress or nutritional disorders, such as pernicious anemia, Plummer-Vinson syndrome, pellagra, sprue, or folic acid or vitamin B deficiency.

tongue, smooth Absence or atrophy of the filiform papillae, causing a smooth (patchy or uniform), glossy, red tongue. This primary sign of undernutrition results from anemia and vitamin B deficiency.

tongue, white A uniform white coating or plaques on the tongue. Lesions associated with a white tongue may be premalignant or malignant and may require a biopsy. *Necrotic white lesions*—collections of cells, bacteria, and debris—are painful and can be scraped from the tongue. They commonly appear in children, usually resulting from candidiasis or thermal burns. *Keratotic white lesions*—thickened, keratinized patches—are usually asymptomatic and can't be scraped away. These lesions commonly result from alcohol use and local irritation from tobacco smoke or other substances.

HAIRY TONGUE

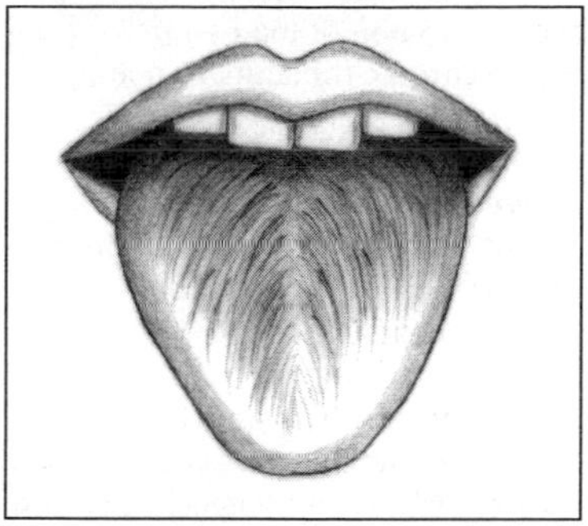

TONGUE FISSURES

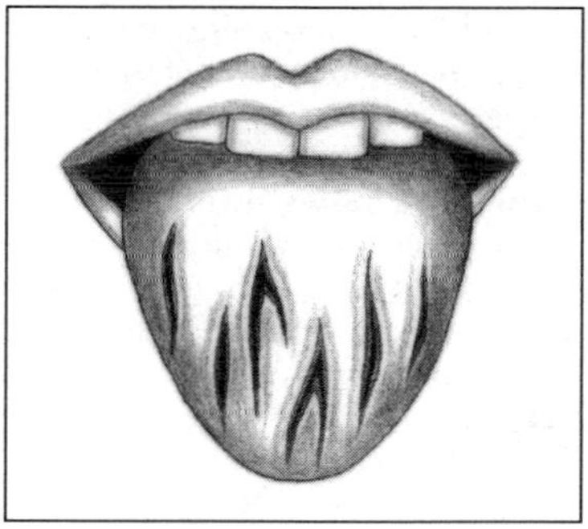

tongue enlargement An increase in the tongue's size, causing it to protrude from the mouth. Causes include Down syndrome, acromegaly, lymphangioma, Beckwith's syndrome, and congenital micrognathia. Other possible causes are cancer of the tongue, amyloidosis, or neurofibromatosis.

tongue fissures Shallow or deep grooving of the dorsum of the tongue. Usually a congenital defect, tongue fissures occur normally in about 10% of the population. Deep fissures may promote collection of food particles, leading to chronic inflammation and tenderness.

tongue swelling Edema of the tongue. Common causes include pernicious anemia, pellagra, hypothyroidism, or allergic angioneurotic edema.

tongue ulcers Circumscribed necrotic lesions of the dorsum, margin, tip, and inferior surface of the tongue. Ulcers usually result from biting, chewing, or burning of the tongue. They may also reflect Type 1 herpes simplex virus, tuberculosis, histoplasmosis, or cancer of the tongue.

tonic neck reflex Extension of the limbs on the side to which the head is turned and flexion of the opposite limbs. In the neonate, this normal reflex appears between 28 and 32 weeks gestational age, diminishes as voluntary muscle control increases, and disappears by age 3 or 4 months. The absence or persistence of this reflex may indicate central nervous system damage. To elicit this response, place the infant in a supine position, then turn his head to one side.

tooth discoloration Bluish yellow or gray teeth may result from hypoplasia of the dentin and pulp, nerve damage, or caries. Yellow teeth may indicate caries. Mottling and staining suggest fluorine excess or may be associated with the effects of certain drugs such as tetracycline. Tooth discoloration (and small tooth size) may occur in osteogenesis imperfecta.

tophi Deposits of sodium urate crystals in cartilage, soft tissue, synovial membranes, and tendon sheaths, producing painless nodular swellings, a classic symptom of gout. Tophi commonly appear on the ears, hands, and feet. They may erode the skin, producing open lesions, and cause gross deformity, limiting joint mobility. Inflammatory flare-ups may occur.

transference Unconscious process of transferring feelings and attitudes originally associated with important figures, such as parents, to another. Used therapeutically in psychoanalysis, transference can also occur in other settings and relationships.

Trendelenburg's test A demonstration of valvular incompetence of the saphenous vein and inefficiency of the communicating veins at different levels. To perform this test, raise the patient's legs above the heart level until the veins empty; then rapidly lower his legs. If the valves are incompetent, the veins immediately distend.

trismus Prolonged and painful spasms of the lower jaw muscles, commonly known as lockjaw. Trismus is a characteristic early sign of tetanus, but it can also result from drug therapy. A milder form may occur in neuromuscular involvement in other disorders or in infection or disease of the jaw, teeth, parotid glands, or tonsils.

Troisier's sign Enlargement of a single lymph node, usually in the left supraclavicular group. It indicates metastasis from a primary carcinoma in the upper abdomen, commonly the stomach. To detect this sign, have the patient sit erect facing you. Palpate the region behind the sternocleidomastoid muscle as the patient performs Valsalva's maneuver. Although the enlarged node typically lies so deep that it escapes detection, it may rise and become palpable with this maneuver.

Trousseau's sign In tetany, carpopedal spasm in response to ischemic compression of the upper arm. To elicit this sign, apply a blood pressure cuff to the patient's arm; then inflate the cuff to a pressure between the patient's diastolic and systolic readings and maintain it for 4 minutes. The patient's hand and fingers assume the "obstetrical hand" position, with wrist and metacarpophalangeal joints flexed, interphalangeal joints extended, and fingers and thumb adducted. Also known as Trousseau's phenomenon. See "Carpopedal spasm," page 115.

Turner's sign A bruiselike discoloration of the skin of the flanks. This sign appears 6 to 24 hours after onset of retroperitoneal hemorrhage in acute pancreatitis.

twitching Nonspecific intermittent contraction of muscles or muscle bundles. See "Fasciculations," page 247, and "Tics," page 566.

Urinary tenesmus Persistent, ineffective, painful straining to empty the bladder. This results when infection or an indwelling catheter irritates nerve endings in the bladder mucosa.

Vaginal bleeding abnormalities Passage of blood from the vagina at times other than menses. It may indicate abnormalities of the uterus, cervix, ovaries, fallopian tubes, or vagina. It may also indicate an abnormal pregnancy. See "Menorrhagia," page 373, "Metrorrhagia," page 374, and "Vaginal bleeding, postmenopausal," page 588.

vein sign A palpable, bluish, cordlike swelling along the line formed in the axilla by the junction of the thoracic and superficial epigastric veins. This sign appears in tuberculosis and obstruction of the superior vena cava.

Weill's sign In infantile pneumonia, absence of expansion in the subclavicular area of the affected side on inspiration.

Westphal's sign Absence of the knee jerk reflex, occurring in tabes dorsalis.

Wilder's sign Subtle twitching of the eyeball on medial or lateral gaze. This early sign of Graves' disease is discernible as a slight jerk of the eyeball when the patient changes his direction of gaze.

Yawning, excessive Persistent involuntary opening of the mouth, accompanied by attempted deep inspiration. In the absence of sleepiness, excessive yawning may indicate cerebral hypoxia.

SELECTED REFERENCES

American Heart Association. *Handbook of Emergency Cardiac Care for Healthcare Providers,* 2000.

Armstrong, D., and Cohen, J., eds. *Infectious Diseases.* St. Louis: Mosby–Year Book, Inc., 1999.

Baigent, C., et al. "Premature Cardiovascular Disease in Chronic Renal Failure," *Lancet* 356(9224):147-52, July 2000.

Ball, P., and Gray, J.A. *Infectious Diseases,* 2nd ed. Philadelphia: W.B. Saunders Co., 1999.

Boudoulas, H., and Wooley, C.F., eds. *Mitral Valve: Floppy Mitral Valve, Mitral Valve Prolapse, Mitral Valve Regurgitation,* 2nd rev. ed. Armonk, N.Y.: Futura Pub. Co., 2000.

Centers for Disease Control and Prevention. Web site: *www.cdc.gov.*

De Sepulveda, L.B., and Clawson, L.L. "Amylotrophic Lateral Sclerosis: Managing the Disease," *Nurseweek* 12 (10):16-18, May 1999.

Diseases, 3rd ed. Springhouse, Pa.: Springhouse Corp., 2001.

Doenges, M.E., et al. *Nursing Care Plans: Guidelines for Individualizing Patient Care,* 5th ed. Philadelphia: F.A. Davis Co., 2000.

Emergency Nurses Association. *Emergency Nurses Pediatric Course,* 2000.

Eto, T. "Arterial Stenting and Balloon Angioplasty in Renal Artery Stenosis," *Internal Medicine* 39(6):483-89, June 2000.

Fahey, V.A. *Vascular Nursing,* 3rd ed., Philadelphia: W.B. Saunders Co., 1999.

Fauci, A.S., et al. *Harrison's Principles of Internal Medicine,* 15th ed. New York: McGraw-Hill Book Co., 2001.

Guell, R., et al. "Long-Term Effects of Outpatient Rehabilitation of COPD: A Randomized Trial," *Chest* 117(4): 976-83, April 2000.

Handbook of Diagnostic Tests, 2nd ed. Springhouse, Pa.: Springhouse Corp., 1999.

Handbook of Diseases, 2nd ed. Springhouse, Pa.: Springhouse Corp., 2000.

Ignatavicius, D.D., et al. *Medical-Surgical Nursing Across the Health Care Continuum,* 3rd ed. Philadelphia: W.B. Saunders Co., 1999.

Jones, A., and Rowe, B.H. "Bronchopulmonary Hygiene Physical Therapy in Bronchiectasis and Chronic Obstructive Pulmonary Disease: A Systematic Review," *Heart & Lung* 29(2):125-35, March-April 2000.

Kozier, B., et al. *Fundamentals of Nursing: Concepts, Process, and Practice,* 6th ed. Upper Saddle River, N.J.: Prentice Hall, 2000.

Labson, L.H. "Current Approaches to the Lymphomas," *Patient Care* 33(8): 65-66 passim, April 1999.

Lankisch, P.G. "Progression from Acute to Chronic Pancreatitis: A Physician's View," *Surgical Clinics of North America* 79(4):815-27, August 1999.

Lee, G.R., et al., eds. *Wintrobe's Clinical Hematology*, 10th ed. Philadelphia: Lippincott Williams & Wilkins, 1999.

Lemone, P., and Burke, K.M. *Medical Surgical Nursing: Critical Thinking in Client Care,* 2nd ed. Upper Saddle River, N.J.: Prentice Hall, 2000.

Lewis, S.M., et al. *Medical-Surgical Nursing, Assessment and Management of Clinical Problems,* 5th ed. St. Louis: Mosby–Year Book, Inc., 2000.

Lippincott Williams & Wilkins. Web sites: *www.springnet.com* and *www.nursingcenter.com.*

Luukinen, H., et al. "Head Injuries and Cognitive Decline Among Older Adults: A Population-based Study," *Neurology* 52(3):557-62, February 1999.

McDonald, E.S., and Windebank, A.J. "Mechanisms of Neurotoxic Injury and Cell Death," *Neurologic Clinics* 18(3):525-40, August 2000.

Ministry of Health and Welfare, Japan. "Asthma Prevention and Management Guidelines," *International Archives of Allergy and Immunology* 121(suppl 1): I-VIII, 1-77, 2000.

National Center for Health Statistics. *Health, United States, 2000 with Adolescent Health Chartbook*. Hyattsville, Md.: U.S. Department of Health and Human Services, Centers for Disease Control and Prevention, 2000.

National Institutes of Health. Web site: *www.nih.gov* and *www.clinicaltrials.gov.*

Nursing Diagnoses: Definitions and Classification 2001-2002. Philadelphia: North American Nursing Diagnosis Association, 2001.

Phipps, W.J., et al. *Medical-Surgical Nursing: Concepts and Clinical Practice*, 6th ed. St. Louis: Mosby–Year Book, Inc., 1999.

Potter, P.A., and Perry, A.J. *Fundamentals of Nursing*, 5th ed. St. Louis: Mosby–Year Book, Inc., 2001.

Professional Guide to Diseases, 7th ed. Springhouse, Pa., Springhouse Corp., 2001.

Schlant, R.C., "Timing of Surgery for Patients with Nonischemic Severe Mitral Regurgitation," *Circulation* 99(3): 338-39, January 1999.

Smeltzer, S.C., and Bare, B.G. *Brunner and Suddarth's Textbook of Medical-Surgical Nursing,* 9th ed. Philadelphia: Lippincott Williams & Wilkins, 2000.

Sparks, S.M., and Taylor, C.M. *Nursing Diagnosis Reference Manual*, 5th ed. Springhouse, Pa.: Springhouse Corp., 2001.

Tierney, Jr., L.M., et al. *Current Medical Diagnosis and Treatment,* 40th ed. New York: Lange Medical Books/McGraw-Hill Book Co., 2001.

Turnbull, G.K. "Lactose Intolerance and Irritable Bowel Syndrome," *Nutrition* 16(7-8):665-66, July-August 2000.

Wong, D.L., et al. *Whaley & Wong's Nursing Care of Infants and Children*, 6th ed. St. Louis: Mosby–Year Book, Inc., 1999.

Voegtle, T.A. "A Different Kind of Chest Pain," *AJN* 100(7):65, July 2000.

INDEX

A

i refers to an illustration; t refers to a table.

i refers to an illustration; t refers to a table.

i refers to an illustration; t refers to a table.

i refers to an illustration; t refers to a table.

i refers to an illustration; t refers to a table.

i refers to an illustration; t refers to a table.

D

i refers to an illustration; t refers to a table.

i refers to an illustration; t refers to a table.

i refers to an illustration; t refers to a table.

i refers to an illustration; t refers to a table.

G

i refers to an illustration; t refers to a table.

i refers to an illustration; t refers to a table.

i refers to an illustration; t refers to a table.

i refers to an illustration; t refers to a table.

i refers to an illustration; t refers to a table.

i refers to an illustration; t refers to a table.

i refers to an illustration; t refers to a table.

P

i refers to an illustration; t refers to a table.

i refers to an illustration; t refers to a table.

i refers to an illustration; t refers to a table.

i refers to an illustration; t refers to a table.

S

i refers to an illustration; t refers to a table.

i refers to an illustration; t refers to a table.

i refers to an illustration; t refers to a table.

i refers to an illustration; t refers to a table.

U

i refers to an illustration; t refers to a table.

i refers to an illustration; t refers to a table.